# SALMONELLA – A DANGEROUS FOODBORNE PATHOGEN

Edited by **Barakat S. M. Mahmoud**

**Salmonella – A Dangerous Foodborne Pathogen**
Edited by Barakat S. M. Mahmoud

**Published by InTech**
Janeza Trdine 9, 51000 Rijeka, Croatia



**Notice**
Statements and opinions expressed in the chapters are these of the individual contributors and not necessarily those of the editors or publisher. No responsibility is accepted for the accuracy of information contained in the published chapters. The publisher assumes no responsibility for any damage or injury to persons or property arising out of the use of any materials, instructions, methods or ideas contained in the book.

**Publishing Process Manager** Adriana Pecar

**Technical Editor** Teodora Smiljanic

**Cover Designer** InTech Design Team

**Image Copyright** wacpan, 2011. DepositPhotos

Additional hard copies can be obtained from orders@intechopen.com

Salmonella – A Dangerous Foodborne Pathogen, Edited by Barakat S. M. Mahmoud
p. cm.
978-953-307-782-6

For EU product safety concerns:
IN TECH d.o.o., Prolaz Marije Krucifikse Kozulić 3, 51000 Rijeka, Croatia,
info@intechopen.com or visit our website at intechopen.com.

# Meet the editor

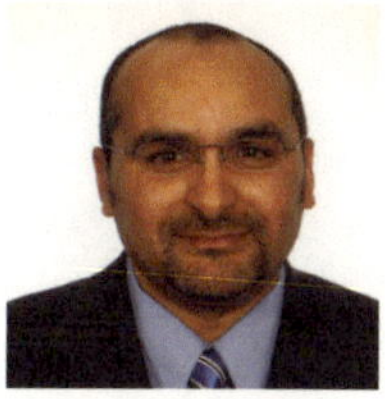

Dr. Mahmoud is an Assistant Professor of Food Safety/ Microbiology and Extension Specialist at Mississippi State University. His research addresses a broad spectrum of problematic issues in food safety, microbiology, quality, and shelf life. His work focuses on using novel non-thermal technologies to reduce the risk of foodborne illnesses, with an interest in both modern molecular (RT–PCR) and traditional methods for the detection of pathogens in food. Dr. Mahmoud is well recognized as an International Scientist, and has received many awards. He has worked in many countries, including USA, UAE, Canada, Japan, Oman, Portugal, Thailand, Korea, and Egypt. He published more than 50 publications, and two book chapters. He is serving as an editor-in-chief for three international journals, a professional member and spokesman for the Institute of Food Technologists, and has conducted a number of interviews with popular domestic and international newspaper and magazines.

# Contents

# Preface

Salmonella is a gram-negative microorganism, widely dispersed in nature and often found in the intestinal tract of animals and humans. More than 2,500 serotypes of Salmonella exist, but only some of these serotypes have been frequently associated with food-borne illnesses. The pathogenic *Salmonella* is a life-threatening bacterium, and it is a leading cause of food-borne bacterial illnesses in humans. After Campylobacter, Salmonella is the second most predominant bacterial cause of food-borne gastroenteritis worldwide. Salmonella pathogens may primarily spread through the feces of wildlife and domestic animals, contaminated water, poor fertilization methods, and other agricultural practices. Salmonella serotypes can grow and survive in many different foods. The behavior of Salmonella in foods is governed by a variety of environmental and ecological factors. These include water activity, pH, chemical composition, the presence of natural or added antimicrobial agents, and storage temperature and processing factors, such as the application of heat and physical manipulation.

Food-borne infections from Salmonella are obtained through ingesting contaminated food or water. Poultry, eggs, beef, and milk products are the main vehicles in the salmonellosis outbreak, and secondary sources are foods, such as fruits, vegetables, and seafood. Since 1962, registered cases of human salmonellosis caused by contaminated food have been steadily increasing. Salmonellosis, or Salmonella infection, caused by nontyphoid strains is the most common food-borne disease reported from population-based, active laboratory surveillance in the United States. However, since the 1980s, food-borne salmonellosis from Salmonella serotypes Typhimurium and Enteritidis has increased. The Centers for Disease Control and Prevention (CDC) revealed that the incidence of Salmonella infections in 2010 was significantly higher than during the period 2006–2008.

Often, most people who suffer from Salmonella infections may have temporary gastroenteritis, which usually does not require treatment. However, when infection becomes invasive, antimicrobial treatment is mandatory. Symptoms generally occur 8 to 72 hours after ingestion of the pathogen and can last 3 to 5 days. Children, the elderly, and immunocompromised individuals are the most susceptible to salmonellosis infections. The annual economic cost due to food-borne Salmonella infections in the United States alone is estimated at $2.4 billion, with an estimated 1.4

million cases of salmonellosis and more than 500 deaths annually. Many milder cases are not reported, making the estimated number of salmonellosis cases in the United States thirty times the number of reported cases.

The chapters contained in this book describe a range of different topics, such as the role of foods in Salmonella infections, food-borne outbreaks caused by Salmonella, biofilm formation by Salmonella (Salmonella grows predominantly as biofilm in most of its natural habitats). Additional topics include antimicrobial drug resistance of Salmonella isolates (the multidrug resistance of Salmonella, which reduces the therapeutic options in cases of invasive infections and could potentially be associated with an increased burden of illness), methods for controlling Salmonella in food, and Salmonella isolation and identification methods to ensure the safety of food. Contributing to this book are internationally renowned scientists who have provided a diverse and global perspective of the issues of concern with the Salmonella pathogen. This book serves as an excellent resource for those interested in Salmonella. In fact, this book is intended to be primarily a reference book. However, it also summarizes the current state of knowledge regarding Salmonella, and it contains ideas for future research. The editor is indebted to the participating authors for their state-of-the-art contributions in providing authoritative views resulting from their research on this dangerous Salmonella pathogen.

**Barakat S. M. Mahmoud, PhD**
A. Professor of Food Safety and Microbiology
Mississippi State University
USA

1

# The Burden of Salmonellosis in the United States

Patricia L. Cummings[1,2], Frank Sorvillo[1,2] and Tony Kuo[2,3]
[1]*University of California, Los Angeles (UCLA) School of Public Health*
[2]*Los Angeles County Department of Public Health*
[3]*David Geffen School of Medicine at UCLA*
*USA*

## 1. Introduction

Salmonellosis or *Salmonella* infection caused by nontyphoid strains is the most common foodborne disease reported from population-based, active laboratory surveillance in the United States (U.S.) (Figure 1). The overall incidence of laboratory confirmed *Salmonella*

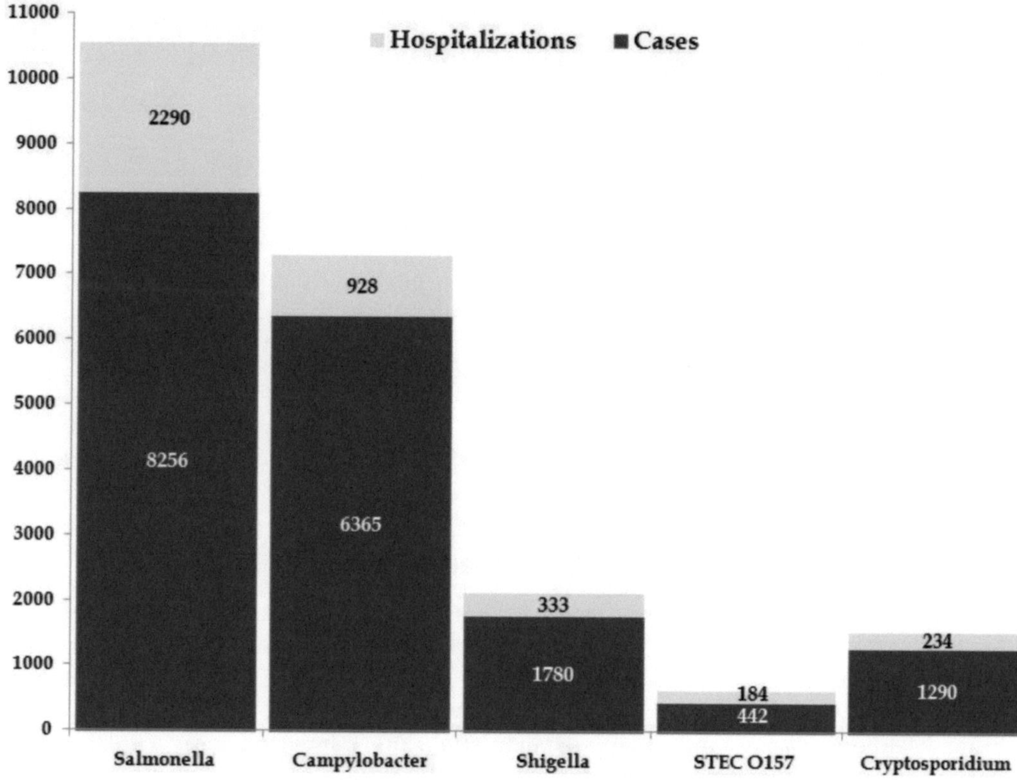


Fig. 1. Total number of laboratory-confirmed bacterial and parasitic infection cases and hospitalizations by pathogen in the United States (CDC, 2011).

infection was 17.6 cases per 100,000 persons in 2010. This was more than twice the U.S. Healthy People 2010 objective of 6.8 cases per 100,000 persons (Figure 2) (Matyas et al.,2010). Moreover, a recent report released by the Centers for Disease Control and Prevention (CDC) revealed that the incidence of *Salmonella* infections in 2010 was significantly higher than during 2006-2008 representing an increase of about 10% (95% Confidence Interval (CI), 4-17%). However, other foodborne infections, such as *Campylobacter, Listeria, Shigella,* STEC O157, *Vibrio,* and *Yersinia,* have all actually decreased during this same period (CDC, 2011). The disease burden of salmonellosis has remained substantial in the United States in spite of ongoing public health and regulatory efforts to prevent and control this infectious disease.

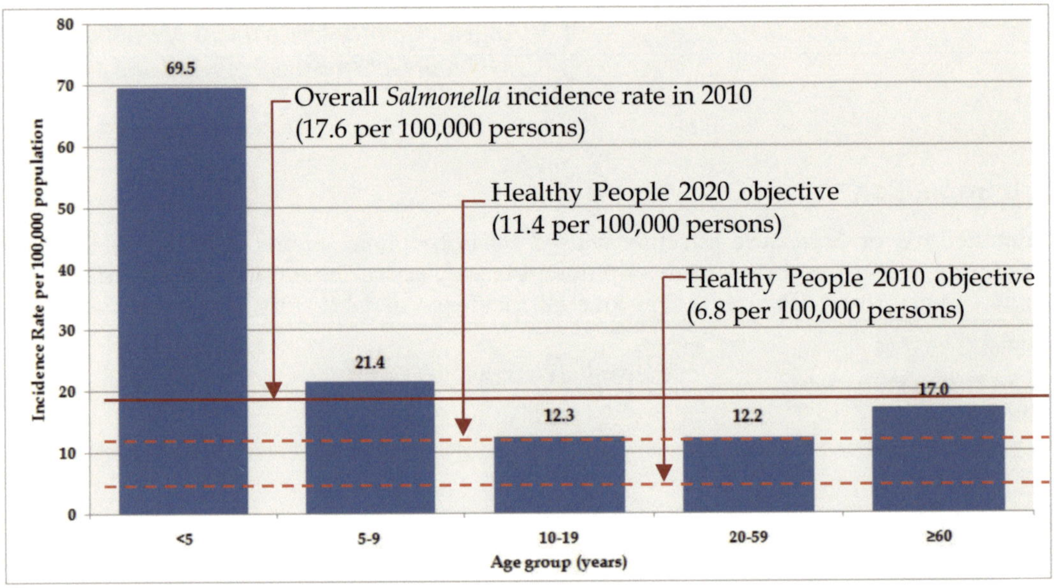


Fig. 2. Laboratory-confirmed *Salmonella* incidence rate per 100,000 population, by age group, as compared to the overall incidence rate and the national health objectives (Healthy People) for 2010 and 2020, United States, 2010 (CDC, 2011).

The present chapter discusses the trends in morbidity, mortality, and years of potential life lost attributed to human salmonellosis in the United States. In addition, this chapter provides a snapshot of U.S. public health measures and control policies that are currently in place to protect the public against *Salmonella* infection.

## 2. The burden of salmonellosis in the United States

Salmonellosis causes more disease burden than any other foodborne pathogen. An estimated 93.8 million cases (90% CI, 61.8-131.6 million) of gastroenteritis caused by *Salmonella* species occur globally each year and of these, nearly 80.3 million cases are foodborne (Majowicz et al., 2010). In the United States, an estimated 1 million incident cases of human salmonellosis occur annually (Scallan et al., 2011); however, only a small portion of these cases are recognized clinically (*see section 2.2*). In industrialized countries as few as 1% of clinical cases are actually reported (Heymann, 2008). Collectively, *Salmonella* infections in the United States account for roughly 19,336 hospitalizations, 17,000 quality adjusted life years lost (QALYs), and $3.3 billion in total medical expenditures and lost productivity each year (Batz et al., 2011).

### 2.1 Clinical manifestations, serotypes, and outbreaks

*Salmonella* gastroenteritis is usually a self-limited disease in which the symptom of fever typically resolves within 48 to 72 hours and diarrhea within three to seven days. Complications from the infection may include severe dehydration, shock, collapse, and/or septicemia. Symptoms are usually more severe among infants, young children, elderly, and those who are immune-compromised (Scallan et al., 2011).

Although there are many serotypes of *Salmonella* that are pathogenic to both humans and animals (i.e., approximately 2,500 serotypes have been identified), the vast majority of human *Salmonella* isolates are serotype *S. enterica* subsp. *enterica* (Heymann, 2008). Serovars Typhi and Paratyphi of this serotype, *S. enterica* subsp. *enterica,* are the etiologic agents that cause typhoid and paratyphoid fevers. These types are also common, but are generally found in developing countries, such as those in South America, Africa, and parts of Asia (Heymann, 2008). In developed countries where there is active, coordinated foodborne disease surveillance, other serovars such as Typhimurium and Enteritidis are frequently reported.

Sixty to eighty percent of all human salmonellosis cases in the United States occur intermittently and sporadically throughout the population. Clusters of large outbreaks in restaurants, institutions for children, hospitals, and nursing homes have occurred recently and remain major public health threats. These outbreaks are usually the product of contamination from a production source, such as chicken farms, feed blending mills, and slaughterhouses. One of the more well-known *Salmonella* outbreaks in the United States occurred in 2010. This outbreak resulted from contamination in the food production chain, leading to a massive egg recall of over half a billion eggs and more than 2,000 reported cases of *Salmonella*-related illness (Hutchison, 2010). Although less common, outbreaks from food handling by an ill person or carrier have been reported in recent years (Cruickshank et al., 1987; Khuri-Bulos et al., 1994). For instance, in 2000 an ill food handler in a bakery that supplied hamburger buns to restaurants was found responsible for an outbreak among several burger restaurants across Southern California and Arizona. This outbreak was atypical in that it resulted from consumption of commercially distributed bread, which is a highly unusual vehicle for most foodborne infectious agents (Kimura et al., 2005).

Outbreaks from person-to-person transmission can also be of particular concern, especially among hospital workers who have the potential to spread the bacterium with their hands or through contaminated instruments. Outbreaks of *Salmonella* infection have occurred in places like maternity wards where staff members with contaminated hands and/or the use of contaminated medical instruments result in the transmission of *Salmonella* to babies and mothers (Rowe et al., 1969). In 2008, an outbreak strain of *Salmonella* serotype Tennessee occurred in a neonatal intensive care unit in the United States, where limited access to sinks for hand washing likely facilitated the transmission to infants (Boehmer, 2009).

### 2.2 Salmonellosis incidence – FoodNet data

Based on FoodNet surveillance data (*see section 4.1*) for nine selected foodborne pathogens from 10 states and three federal agencies (CDC, U.S. Food and Drug Administration, and U.S. Department of Agriculture), a total of 19,089 laboratory-confirmed cases of foodborne infections, 4,247 hospitalizations, and 68 deaths were identified for the year 2010 in the U.S.

(CDC, 2011). Of the nine pathogens monitored, including *Campylobacter, Listeria, Salmonella, Shigella,* STEC O157, *Vibrio, Yersinia, Cryptosporidium,* and *Cyclospora,* salmonellosis was the most common infection reported and had the highest number of associated hospitalizations and deaths. A total of 8,256 infections (17.6 illnesses per 100,000 persons); 2,290 hospitalizations; and 29 deaths were attributed to this pathogen in 2010. Ninety-two percent (7,564 out of 8,256) of these isolates were subsequently serotyped through PulseNet (*see section 4.1*), with Enteritidis (22%), Newport (14%), and Typhimurium (13%) representing the most common serotypes. The FoodNet data indicate that the rate of infection from *Salmonella* remains substantially high and has not declined for over a decade, as compared to the other eight foodborne pathogens tracked through FoodNet. These data support ongoing control efforts in the United States that target *Salmonella,* particularly in response to the costs associated with treatment of this infection - approximately $365 million in direct medical costs each year (CDC, 2011).

### 2.3 Salmonellosis-related mortality

Current estimates indicate that there are about 155,000 salmonellosis-related deaths each year worldwide (Majowicz et al., 2010); between 400-600 of them are in the United States (Mead et al., 1999; CDC, 2008). While risk of death and actual deaths from salmonellosis are not typically common in the general population, the infection can be particularly virulent in vulnerable groups, especially among young children, older adults, and those who are immune-compromised (*see section 3*).

Table 1 presents the most updated analysis of multiple cause-of-death (MCD) data based on death certificates in the United States. From 1990 to 2007, there were 1,372 nontyphoidal *Salmonella*-related deaths. Among these reported deaths, *Salmonella* was listed as an underlying cause of death on 785 (57.2%) death certificates and as an associated cause of death on 587 (42.8%) death certificates. Fifty-six deaths occurred in 2007 alone, resulting in an age-adjusted mortality rate of 0.018 per 100,000 population (95% CI, 0.013-0.022). The average age-adjusted mortality rate over the entire study period, from 1990 to 2007, was 0.028 per 100,000 population (95% CI, 0.027-0.030; n=1,372). This represents a total of 21,417 years of potential life lost (Table 1).

Between 1990 and 2006 the age-adjusted mortality rate for human salmonellosis declined from 0.06 per 100,000 population (95%CI, 0.05-0.07; n=136 deaths) to 0.01 per 100,000 population (95%CI, 0.01-0.02; n=45 deaths). The variance between deaths and incidence, in terms of trends over the past decade show that deaths have decreased (Cummings PL et al., 2010), but incidence has increased (CDC, 2011). This difference could potentially be the result of better medical treatment or other contributing factors accounting for the decline in deaths. In 2007, however, a slight increase (albeit not significant) in the frequency and rate of *Salmonella*-related deaths was observed (Figure 3). The mean age of decedents with *Salmonella* infection listed on their death certificate for the period 1990-2007 was 63.1 years. Overall, males were more likely than females to have *Salmonella* listed as a cause of death (either underlying or associated) on their death certificate and have more years of potential life lost - 13,447 years for males versus 7,970 years for females (Table 1). Infants (< 1 year of age) and older adults (> 65 years of age) had the highest frequency of *Salmonella*-related deaths over the 18-year period (Table 1). The highest age-specific mortality rates during this period were observed among infants (0.086 per 100,000 population), those aged 75-84 (0.160 per 100,000 population), and those 85 years and older (0.314 per 100,000 population). Asian, black, and Hispanic race/ethnicity had higher rates of mortality from Salmonella infection as compared to whites.

| | Frequency (N%) | Age-Adjusted Mortality Rate (95% CI) | Age-Adjusted Rate Ratio (95% CI) | Age-adjusted Rates of Potential Life Years Lost |
|---|---|---|---|---|
| **Sex** | | | | |
| Female | 583 (42.5%) | 0.021 (0.019-0.022) | Referent | 7,970 |
| Male | 789 (57.5%) | 0.038 (0.035-0.041) | 1.84 (1.68-2.02) | 13,447 |
| **Race/Ethnicity**† | | | | |
| White | 893 (65.1%) | 0.023 (0.021-0.024) | Referent | 9,768 |
| Asian/Pacific Islander | 76 (5.5%) | 0.059 (0.045-0.073) | 2.63 (2.45-2.82) | 1,256 |
| Black | 279 (20.3%) | 0.057 (0.050-0.064) | 2.53 (2.36-2.72) | 7,095 |
| Hispanic | 116 (8.5%) | 0.031 (0.025-0.038) | 1.39 (1.28-1.50) | 3,050 |
| Native American | 7 (0.5%) | 0.025 (0.005-0.045) | 1.11 (1.02-1.21) | 173 |
| **Age group (years)***† | | **Age-Specific Mortality Rate** | | |
| <1 | 61 (4.4%) | 0.086 (0.064-0.107) | -- | 4,575 |
| 1-4 | 18 (1.3%) | 0.006 (0.003-0.009) | -- | 1,315 |
| 5-14 | 12 (0.9%) | 0.002 (0.007-0.003) | -- | 797 |
| 15-24 | 22 (1.6%) | 0.003 (0.002-0.005) | -- | 1,204 |
| 25-34 | 85 (6.2%) | 0.012 (0.009-0.014) | -- | 3,797 |
| 35-44 | 91 (6.6%) | 0.012 (0.009-0.014) | -- | 3,236 |
| 45-54 | 128 (9.3%) | 0.020 (0.017-0.024) | -- | 3,262 |
| 55-64 | 134 (9.8%) | 0.030 (0.025-0.035) | -- | 2,004 |
| 65-74 | 243 (17.7%) | 0.073 (0.064-0.082) | -- | 1,227 |
| 75-84 | 342 (24.9%) | 0.160 (0.143-0.177) | -- | 0 |
| >85 | 235 (17.1%) | 0.314 (0.274-0.354) | -- | 0 |
| Total | 1,372 | 0.028 (0.027-0.030) | N/A | 21,417 |

Note: 95% CI = confidence interval; Years of Potential Life Lost were calculated by subtracting the age in years at the time of death from 75 years. *Mortality rates are age-specific rates, not age-adjusted rates. †Numbers may not add up to total, due to missing data.

Table 1. Age-adjusted nontyphoidal *Salmonella*-related mortality rates per 100,000 population and mortality rate ratios by sex, race/ethnicity and age group, United States, 1990-2007.

Asians had the highest age-adjusted rate ratio of 2.63 (95% CI, 2.45-2.82; n=76 deaths) relative to whites, the referent group (Table 1). While whites had the highest absolute number of deaths (n = 893), they had the lowest age-adjusted mortality rate (0.023 per 100,000 population; 95% CI, 0.021-0.024). Reasons for disparities in *Salmonella* mortality based on gender and race/ethnicity have been discussed in a previously published paper (Cummings PL et al., 2010). California and New York had the highest number of deaths (n=219 and n=105, respectively), but relatively low age-adjusted mortality rates (0.04 per 100,000 population, 95% CI, 0.04-0.05 and 0.03 per 100,000 population, 95% CI, 0.02-0.04, respectively). Although Hawaii and District of Columbia had smaller numbers, they had the highest age-adjusted mortality rates during 1990-2007 (0.08 per 100,000 population, 95% CI, 0.04-0.12; n=18 and 0.08 per 100,000 population, 95% CI, 0.02-0.13; n=8, respectively).

Methods used in this updated analysis are similar to those previously described in Cummings PL et al., 2010. Briefly, years of potential life lost (YPLL) were calculated by subtracting the age in years at the time of death from 75 years (Gardner, 1990). Deaths were defined as any observation listed as either the underlying cause or the associated cause of death with the following International Classification of Diseases, 9th revision (ICD-9) and 10th revision (ICD-10) codes: 003.0-003.9 and A02.0-A02.9, respectively. These ICD codes included infection or foodborne intoxication due to any *Salmonella* species, other than serovars Typhi and Paratyphi, which are the microbial agents that cause typhoid and paratyphoid fevers. Since these latter conditions are rare in the United States and predominately occur in developing countries (e.g., countries in Southeast Asia, Africa, and South America), serovars Typhi and Paratyphi were excluded from the analysis.

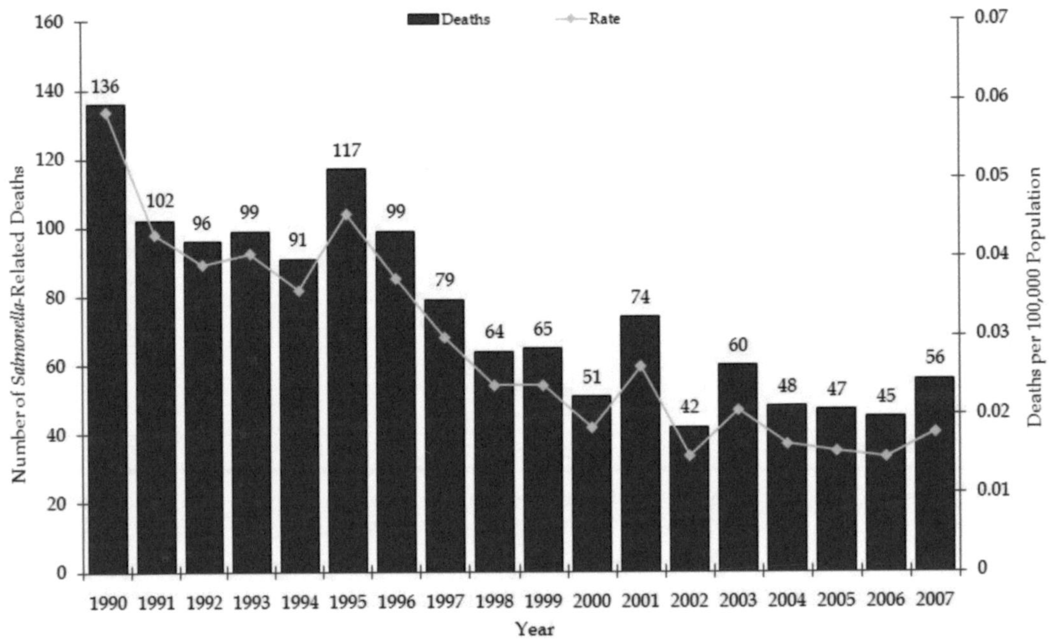


Fig. 3. Number of nontyphoidal *Salmonella*-related deaths and age-adjusted mortality rates per 100,000 population by year, United States, 1990-2007.

### 2.4 Changing trends in factors that may contribute to human salmonellosis

Although mortality rates are important indicators of health status, they often do not tell the entire story. Factors such as the aging population; increased burden of chronic diseases that can suppress immunity; and an increasingly global market in meats, poultry, vegetables, fruits, farm animals, and pets (e.g., chicks and reptiles) are all emerging influences that can potentially amplify the risk and burden of human salmonellosis in the United States.

### 2.4.1 An aging population and increased burden of chronic disease

As the present generation of baby boomers (those born between 1946 and 1964) reach age 65 and older, the trend in *Salmonella*-related deaths is expected to change, suggesting that more deaths could ensue, given that older adults frequently experience more severe infections and require hospitalization more often from this foodborne illness than younger adults (Kennedy et al., 2004). Trends showing increased chronic disease prevalence in the population for such conditions as cancer, autoimmune disorders, and other diseases requiring treatment with immune-suppressive therapies parallel the aging of the population and foreshadow the continual burden of human salmonellosis in the United States (Altekruse et al., 1997).

### 2.4.2 An increasingly global market

Today's global market in meats, poultry, vegetables, fruits, farm animals, and pets, represents potential sources of *Salmonella* contamination that are complex and sometimes difficult to control. For example, in 2008 there was a multi-state outbreak of *Salmonella* Typhimurium associated with frozen vacuum-packed rodents that are used to feed snakes (Fuller et al., 2008). This occurrence represents a rare, but wide-spread outbreak associated with commercially distributed rodents. Likewise, the illicit selling and importation of many animals from abroad have caused several unanticipated salmonellosis outbreaks, as well as agricultural problems for the region. In Los Angeles County, the illegal selling of red-eared slider turtles (< 4 inches in diameter) has become an important public health problem. Because caring for these animals is exceedingly difficult, they are often abandoned or dumped by their owners into wildlife preserves and adquaducts. A local animal control agency in Los Angeles County found that an increasing number of turtles have been dumped over the years; they impounded over 6,000 illegally sold, undersized red-eared slider turtles from 2000-2007 (unpublished data). The upward trend in the abandonment of turtles and the turtles' high fecundity rates may also increase the risk of transmission to native species (Perez-Santigosa et al., 2008). Nearly 10% of all reported cases of human salmonellosis in Los Angeles County have been attributed to direct or indirect contact with reptiles, namely the red-eared slider turtle, the most common reptile source found in more than 50% of these cases (LACDPH, 2008). Continual monitoring and targeted improvements to regulate the illegal selling of these animals remain key control measures for protecting the public against acquiring *Salmonella* infections from reptiles.

## 3. Salmonellosis in vulnerable groups with comorbid conditions

Clinical evidence suggests that infection with nontyphoid *Salmonella* often results in more severe manifestations of clinical disease than from any other foodborne pathogen (Helms et al., 2006). Comorbid health conditions and their related immuno-suppressive treatments may be particularly problematic, especially among vulnerable groups at high risk of progressing to severe forms of salmonellosis (Trevejo et al., 2003; Cummings PL et al., 2010). For example, those with HIV/AIDS, certain types of cancers (e.g., leukemia, bone marrow), or autoimmune disorders are at significantly greater risk for death, as compared to persons without these conditions. In the updated analysis of *Salmonella*-related mortality as described in *section 2.3*, a matched case-control study showed that HIV (matched odds ratio (MOR) =7.42; 95% CI, 5.26-10.47), leukemia (MOR=2.95; 95% CI, 1.48-5.88), connective tissue disorders (MOR=2.36, 95%CI, 1.42-3.93), lupus (MOR=3.83; 95% CI, 1.72-8.55), and rheumatoid arthritis (MOR=2.24; 95% CI, 1.10-4.55) were more likely to be reported on death certificates with *Salmonella* infection listed as an underlying or associated cause of death than controls when matched on age, sex, and race/ethnicity (Table 2). Other conditions found to be listed with *Salmonella* infection on death certificates included: septicemia; various types of renal failure and disorders of fluid, electrolyte, and acid-base balance; and sickle-cell disorders (Table 2). The matched analysis examined comorbid conditions most often listed on death certificates of those who died from *Salmonella* infection, as either an underlying cause or associated cause of death. Table 2 lists these diseases within a broader category (e.g., all types of cancer, all types of renal failure) and their corresponding ICD codes. For example, Leukemia is one type of cancer that affects the bone marrow.

| Comorbid condition | ICD-9 and ICD-10 codes (respectively) | Salmonella-related deaths (N=1,371),[a] N(%)[b] | Matched control deaths (N=5,484), N(%)[b] | Matched odds ratios (95%CI) |
|---|---|---|---|---|
| Alcohol and drug abuse | 303-305, K70, F10-F19 | 40 (2.92) | 237 (4.32) | 0.65 (0.46-0.92) |
| Cancer (all types) | 140-239, C00-D48 | 192 (14.00) | 1,373 (25.04) | 0.47 (0.40-0.56) |
| - Malignant neoplasm (bone, connective tissue, skin, breast) | 170-175, C40-C49 | 13 (0.95) | 102 (1.86) | 0.50 (0.28-0.90) |
| - Malignant neoplasm (digestive organs, peritoneum) | 150-159, C15-C26 | 33 (2.41) | 336 (6.13) | 0.37 (0.26-0.54) |
| Cancers affecting bone marrow (all types) | 200, 203-205, C85, C88, C90-C92 | 46 (3.36) | 92 (1.68) | 2.01 (1.41-2.87) |
| - Leukemia | 204, C91 | 14 (1.02) | 19 (0.35) | 2.95 (1.48-5.88) |
| Connective tissue disorders (all types) | 710, 714, M05-M06, M08, M32-M35 | 24 (1.75) | 43 (0.78) | 2.36 (1.42-3.93) |
| - Lupus* | 695.4, 710, L93, M32 | 12 (0.88) | 14 (0.26) | 3.83 (1.72-8.55) |
| - Rhumatoid arthritis | 714, M05-M06, M08 | 12 (0.88) | 22 (0.40) | 2.24 (1.10-4.55) |
| Diabetes | 250, E10-E11, E14 | 109 (7.95) | 422 (7.70) | 1.04 (0.83-1.30) |
| Diseases of the circulatory system | 390-459, I00-I99 | 674 (49.16) | 2,938 (53.57) | 0.82 (0.73-0.93) |
| Endocrine, nutritional, metabolic diseases, and immunity disorders (all types) | 240-279, E00-E90 | 242 (17.65) | 669 (12.20) | 1.56 (1.32-1.83) |
| - Disorders of fluid, electrolyte, acid-base balance | 276, E87 | 57 (4.16) | 78(1.42) | 3.03 (2.12-4.31) |

| Comorbid condition | ICD-9 and ICD-10 codes (respectively) | Salmonella-related deaths (N=1,371),[a] N(%)[b] | Matched control deaths (N=5,484), N(%)[b] | Matched odds ratios (95%CI) |
|---|---|---|---|---|
| Flu/Pneumonia (organism unspecified) | 480-488, J10-J18, P23 | 107 (7.80) | 445 (8.11) | 0.95 (0.76-1.18) |
| Diseases of the digestive system (all types) | 520-579, K00-K93 | 246 (17.94) | 447 (8.15) | 2.46 (2.08-2.92) |
| - Liver diseases | 570-573, K70-K77 | 72 (5.25) | 201 (3.67) | 1.51 (1.14-2.00) |
| HIV | 042, B20-B24 | 133 (9.70) | 121 (2.21) | 7.42 (5.26-10.47) |
| Renal Failure (all types) | 580-589, N17-N19 | 197 (14.37) | 374 (6.82) | 2.38 (1.96-2.87) |
| - Acute renal failure | 584, N17 | 74 (5.40) | 71 (1.29) | 4.31 (3.09-6.01) |
| - Chronic renal failure | 585, N18 | 26 (1.90) | 106 (1.93) | 0.98 (0.63-1.52) |
| - Unspecified renal failure | 586, N19 | 96 (7.00) | 203 (3.70) | 2.00 (1.55-2.58) |
| Septicemia (including other septicemia) | 038, A40.9, A41 | 193 (14.08) | 304 (5.54) | 2.73 (2.25-3.32) |
| Sickle-cell disorders | 282, D57 | 13 (0.95) | 6 (0.11) | 10.2 (3.16-32.91) |

[a] One case was excluded due to missing variables. [b] Numbers may not add up to total due to missing data.

Table 2. Comorbid conditions associated with nontyphoidal *Salmonella* mortality in the United States, 1990-2007.

## 4. Current surveillance efforts, prevention, and next steps

### 4.1 Current surveillance efforts in the United States

In the United States, surveillance for *Salmonella* infections has been an ongoing effort since 1996. Managed by the CDC, the Foodborne Diseases Active Surveillance Network (FoodNet) collects active, population-based surveillance data on laboratory-confirmed infections for nine different pathogens that are commonly transmitted through food (as listed in *section 2.2*). These pathogens include *Campylobacter, Listeria, Salmonella, Shigella,* STEC O157, *Vibrio, Yersinia, Cryptosporidium,* and *Cyclospora* (the latter two are parasites). This surveillance effort includes 10 state health departments (i.e., California, Colorado, Connecticut, Georgia, Maryland, Minnesota, New Mexico, New York, Oregon, Tennessee), the U.S. Department of Agriculture's Food Safety and Inspection Service (USDA-FSIS), the Food and Drug Administration (FDA), and the CDC. The total surveillance area accounts for approximately 15% of the United States population, representing about 46 million people.

The national *Salmonella* database in PulseNet, which is the national molecular subtyping network for foodborne disease surveillance, was established by the CDC to subtype bacterial foodborne pathogens. PulseNet routinely subtypes *E. coli* O157:H7, nontyphoid *Salmonella* serotypes, *Listeria* monocytogenes, and *Shigella*. The database encompasses 46 states, two local public health laboratories, and the food safety laboratories of the Food and Drug Administration and the U.S. Department of Agriculture. The national database of pulsed-field gel electrophoresis (PFGE) for foodborne bacterial pathogens helps track potentially unrelated cases in isolated geographic areas and identifies outbreak strains.

### 4.2 Salmonellosis transmission, prevention, and next steps

The most common mode of *Salmonella* transmission is through the ingestion of the bacterium in food derived from an infected animal or contaminated by feces of an infected animal or person (Mead et al., 1999). This includes raw and undercooked eggs or egg products, raw milk or milk products, poultry, meat, contaminated water, and any other food item that uses potentially contaminated ingredients. Farm animals used to produce these ingredients can become infected by eating feed and fertilizers prepared from contaminated meat scraps and bones. The infection can then spread by bacterial multiplication during rearing and slaughter. This chain of transmission can eventually lead to person-to-person fecal-oral transmission when a person comes in contact with contaminated feces and transmits it to others through a vehicle (e.g., food) or by direct transmission.

Other sources of transmission may occur from handling *Salmonella*-contaminated pet turtles, iguanas, chicks, and unsterilized pharmaceuticals of animal origin. Contact with pet turtles and other reptiles can be a very serious health risk to infants, small children, and adults with weakened immune systems (LACDPH, 2008). Hand-to-mouth and object-to-mouth behaviors are common among young children and can increase their risk for contracting salmonellosis. This resulted in a nationwide ban on the sale of turtles less than four inches in diameter in 1975 (US-CFR, 2010).

More recently, there have been several outbreaks of salmonellosis traced to consumption of raw fruits and vegetables, generally contaminated from manure on the outer surface of the fruit or vegetable. Manure contamination can be from the farm or during packing (Harris et al., 2003). In 1999, a multi-state outbreak of *Salmonella enterica* serotype Baildon (a rare serotype) was associated with raw, domestic tomatoes in the United States (Cummings K et al., 2001). This large outbreak resulted in 86 confirmed cases of salmonellosis.

Since there are several species of domestic and wild animals that can harbor *Salmonella* (e.g., poultry, swine, cattle, rodents and pets such as iguanas, tortoises, turtles, terrapins, chicks, dogs and cats), control policies and measures for preventing *Salmonella* infection are often more complex than for other foodborne pathogens. The fact that humans can also carry this bacterium either as mild, unrecognized cases or as convalescent carriers (i.e., those who have recovered from symptomatic illness, but are still capable of transmitting the pathogen to others) also contributes to this complexity. As carriers, humans can be particularly effective in spreading the disease in the population. Fortunately, chronic carrier states are rare in humans; they are, however, prevalent in animals.

Given that the most common mode of transmission is from handling and consuming infected food, the risk of exposure to salmonellosis can occur at multiple points in the food distribution chain, including retail food establishments and homes. Since the food distribution chain directly and indirectly affects all individuals, vigilant monitoring and regulation at multiple points in the chain are vital.

#### 4.2.1 Food distribution chain

*Salmonella* prevention can be implemented in a number of ways, one of which is through environmental or system policies that improve regulation of potential sources of contamination. For example, the U.S. Department of Agriculture's Food Safety and Inspection Service currently recommends establishing facilities for irradiation of meats and eggs (USDA-FSIS, 2005). In addition, the need for improved sanitation inspection and supervision of abattoirs, food-processing plants, feed-blending mills, and egg grading stations is growing, as these are top sources of contamination for common foodborne pathogens in the United States (Batz *et al.*, 2011). Multiple regulatory outlets are currently responsible for monitoring different aspects of the U.S. food distribution chain. The Food and Drug Administration is responsible for the safety of approximately 80% of the nation's food supply, while other government entities, including the U.S. Department of Agriculture oversee the remainder. In covering such a broad enforcement responsibility, these agencies are continuously striving to reduce gaps in coordination and frequently collaborate on multiple efforts to ensure food safety. The World Health Organization (WHO) recommends strong communication, infrastructure, and coordination efforts among private, local, and federal regulatory sectors. The WHO also recommends the establishment of enhanced food safety standards in feed control regulation; cleaning and disinfection; vector control; and adequate cooking or heat-treating (including pasteurization or irradiation) of animal-derived foods prepared for animal consumption (e.g., meat or bone or fishmeal and pet foods). U.S. agencies follow these standards.

The regulatory policies currently in place have been developed over many years in the United States. Starting in the early 1990s, farm-to-table egg safety efforts were developed by the Food and Drug Administration and the USDA Food Safety and Inspection Service (FSIS). Over the years, FSIS gained more regulatory authority in enforcing laws, including the Federal Meat Inspection Act (FMIA), the Poultry Products Inspection Act (PPIA), and the Egg Products Inspection Act. These particular laws or regulations required federal inspection and regulation of meat, poultry, and processed egg products prepared for distribution. In conjunction with these laws, the Food and Drug Administration and the FSIS conducted a joint *Salmonella Enteritidis* risk assessment in 1998. This assessment found that a broad-based policy encompassing multiple interventions from farm-to-table is more likely to be effective in eliminating egg-associated salmonellosis cases than a single policy directed solely at one stage of the production-to-consumption continuum.

The lessons learned from the Food and Drug Administration (FDA) and the FSIS joint evaluation efforts contributed to the development and implementation of the FDA's new food safety strategy - coined as the "new egg rule" (Figure 4). This rule is considered very comprehensive and is aimed at preventing *Salmonella Enteritidis* in shelled eggs during production, storage, and transportation. Ironically, (as mentioned in section 2.1) one of the largest Salmonella outbreaks in U.S. history that led to a massive recall of about half a billion eggs and more than 2,000 reported illnesses occurred just prior to implementation of these new regulations during the summer of 2010 (Hutchison, 2010). The new egg rule requires production plants to implement intense rodent control, limits on contamination from people and equipment, regular egg tests, egg storage temperatures that retard *Salmonella* growth, and a requirement that egg producers maintain records documenting their compliance with these regulations. Modeled after several existing state programs (e.g., Pennsylvania Egg Quality Assurance Program), the new egg rule will, according to some farms, increase costs of production to about a penny per dozen (Hutchison, 2010). However, the Food and Drug

Administration projected an average annual cost of about $24,100 per farm site, which translates into about $0.30 cents per *layer* (i.e., a layer is a chicken that produces eggs) (USDA-APHIS, 1999). One of the benefits of this new egg rule, if properly regulated, is that it can potentially outweigh the healthcare-associated costs of treating salmonellosis. The Food and Drug Administration expects that the rule will decrease *Salmonella* in plants by 60%, save more than 30 lives each year, and avert more than 79,000 cases of salmonellosis annually (USDHHS, 2009). The preventive measures that were included in this new rule have been demonstrated to be relatively effective for preventing the spread of *Salmonella Enteritidis* (USDHHS, 2009). Moreover, shelled eggs were targeted by these measures because they are the predominant source of foodborne *Salmonella Enteritidis*-related outbreaks in the United States (USDHHS, 2009).

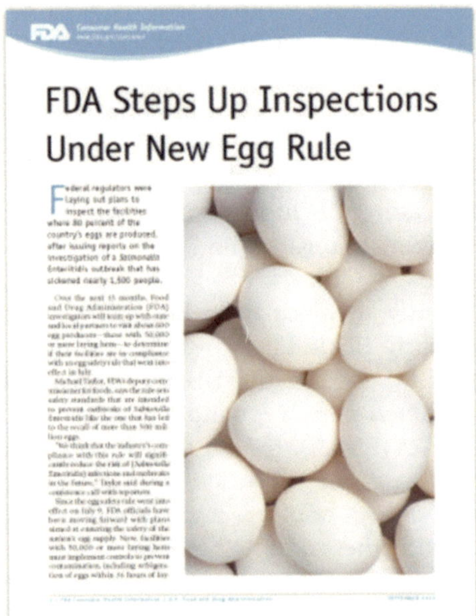
FDA Steps Up Inspections Under New Egg Rule

Federal regulators were laying out plans to inspect the facilities where 80 percent of the country's eggs are produced, after issuing reports on the investigation of a Salmonella Enteritidis outbreak that has sickened nearly 1,500 people.

Fig. 4. Consumer health information guide released by the Food and Drug Administration and the U.S. Department of Agriculture on September 2010 outlining the new egg rule.

One of the anticipated hurdles of the new egg rule may be implementation barriers, such as the limited capacity of smaller facilities to comply with the required preventive measures. Smaller farms may not be as prepared as larger farms to meet the rule's requirements during the initial stages of implementation. More specifically, they may be less likely to have adequate refrigeration capacity, effective rodent control, an efficient biosecurity program, and the necessary measures in place to limit laying hens' exposure to manure on building floors. The Food and Drug Administration (FDA) has anticipated this need to assist smaller farms. Currently, there is an FDA exemption in place for producers with small flocks (i.e., less than 3,000 laying hens). The agency's strategic decision to target the largest producers is based on its goal of having the greatest impact in terms of farm-to-table distribution of eggs. This is a reasonable approach, at least in the initial years of implementation. Eventually, consideration for expanding this rule to apply to smaller farms may be beneficial.

### 4.2.2 Restaurant and retail food environments

**United States, California**

On July 1, 2011, in the state of California (U.S.A.), a food handler card law was implemented. This law requires that all employees of retail food establishments who prepare, store or serve food, must have a California Food Handler Card. This regulation applies to servers, chefs/head chefs/cooks/head cooks, bartenders, bussers (i.e., those who help assist the server by cleaning tables and other duties), and hosts and hostesses who handle food. Supervisors, including the general manager, may also need to carry the card if they do not already have a Food Protection Manager Certification. To receive a card or become certified, a person must take a basic food safety training course and pass a test with a score of 70% or better; the card is only valid for up to three years. Thus, food service employees must take the course every three years. Currently, the U.S. National Restaurant Association (ServSafe® California Food Handler Program), ProMetric, and the U.S. National Registry for Food Safety Professionals are the only three providers that can issue cards within California.

Implementation of this program demonstrates the importance of preventive measures at the restaurant and/or retail level. For instance, not all food handlers at the different stages of food preparation in a given establishment may be entirely aware of raw products that are contained in certain foods, dishes, or recipes handed down to them by restaurant management or by other food handlers. A few examples include raw or partially cooked eggs (e.g., 'over easy' or 'sunny side up,' eggnogs, and homemade ice cream), the use of dirty or cracked eggs, pooled eggs (i.e., combining multiple eggs together), and dishes containing eggs that are not immediately cooked. Generally, all of these practices should be avoided or at least substituted with the use of pasteurized egg products (or irradiated egg products) if use of raw eggs is necessary for a recipe.

Other preventive measures should include prohibiting individuals with diarrhea from food preparation. Known *Salmonella* carriers may require isolation or long-term monitoring and should definitely be discouraged from preparing food for others as long as they shed the organism.

**Los Angeles County, California (U.S.A.)**

In December 1997, in response to increased media attention of foodborne illness stemming from unsafe and unhygienic food handling practices in restaurants, the County of Los Angeles government passed an ordinance that focused on increasing transparency and consumer awareness of hygiene and sanitation practices at restaurants and other retail food establishments through restaurant inspections (Fielding, 2008; Zhe Jin and Leslie, 2003). Prior to its passage, the Department of Health Services routinely conducted hygiene inspections among restaurants in Los Angeles County. However, the results of these inspections were not made public. Thus, under the new mandate, inspection results were required to be posted as a letter grade corresponding to an aggregated inspection score (i.e., 90-100 = A, 80-89 = B, 70-79 = C, etc.) (Figure 5). Specifically, it required that restaurants and other retail food facilities publicly post their assigned letter grade (using a standardized-format grade card, see Figure 5), typically near the entrance, within five feet of the point of entry so the score would be visible to patrons (Simon, et al. 2005; Zhe Jin and Leslie, 2003).

A month prior to the adoption of the ordinance, as a direct response to the need for transparency and consumer awareness, the County of Los Angeles Board of Supervisors requested that the Department of Health Services, which at the time included the Department of Public Health, draft a 17-point action plan to enhance the existing restaurant inspection process (Fielding, 2008). The recommendations outlined by this plan laid the groundwork for the ordinance. The plan called for establishing inspection scoring criteria, adopting letter grading, and increasing transparency of inspection results (Fielding, 2008). It also specified several enhancements to the existing program, such as requiring Environmental Health (EH) staff to undergo rigorous training to learn the new inspection procedures; restaurant managers and workers receive food safety training; a 24-hour restaurant hotline be established so that the public could report complaints about food establishments; and development of a new inspection schedule (Fielding, 2008). The drafting of the action plan and the subsequent passage of the ordinance led to the 1998 establishment of an improved inspection program, now known as the Restaurant Hygiene Inspection Program (RHIP). The program is currently under the supervision of the Los Angeles County Department of Public Health.

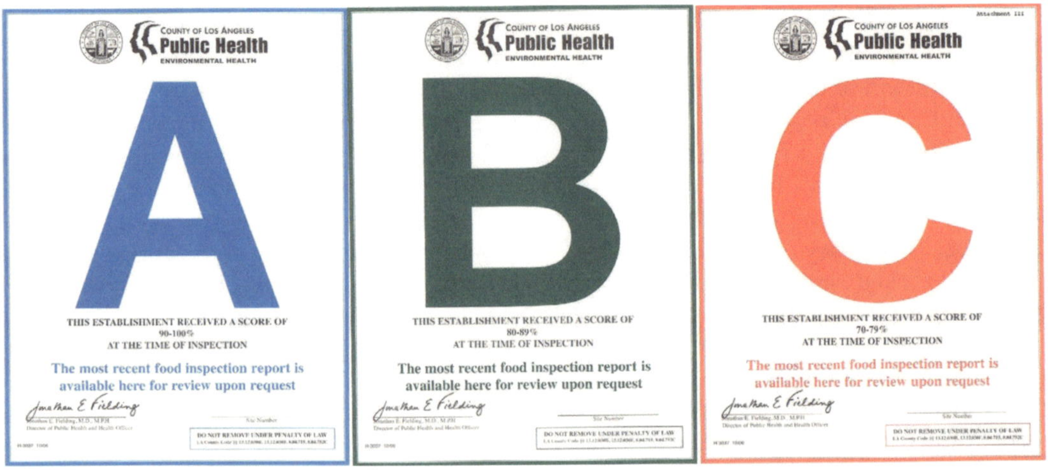


Fig. 5. Standardized-format grade cards given to restaurants and other retail food establishments upon receiving an inspection score. Los Angeles County, California, USA, 2011.

On July 1, 2011, an addendum to the RHIP's policy and procedures manual was added to the program. This addendum provided guidance on inspection frequency requirements, outlining inspection frequencies for food facilities based on risk assessment results for the facility. Risk assessment designation or category is defined as "the categorization of a food facility based on the public health risk associated with the food products served, the methods of food preparation, and the operational history of the food facility" (Environmental Health Policy and Operations Manual, 2011). Currently, there are four risk assessment categories used to evaluate restaurants (Table 3).

Since implementation, the Restaurant Hygiene Inspection Program in Los Angeles County has been considered a relatively effective strategy for reducing the burden of foodborne disease in the region. Credited for improving hygiene standards among food facilities in the county, the program has been theorized by some to have helped reduce foodborne illness hospitalizations (Figure 6). In the year following implementation of the RHIP (1998), the grading program was associated with a 13.1 percent decrease ($p<0.01$) in the number of foodborne disease hospitalizations in Los Angeles County (Simon et al., 2005), albeit other factors may have also been attributed to this decrease, including random chance. Figure 6 shows the number of hospitalizations in the county, as compared to the rest of California (Simon et al., 2005).

| Risk Category | Applies to, but not limited to: | Number of Inspections per year |
|---|---|---|
| High-Risk Category (Risk Assessment I) | -Meat Markets<br>-Full service restaurants | 3 inspections per year |
| Moderate-Risk Category (Risk Assessment II) | -Retail food stores with unpackaged foods<br>-Fast food chains that sell chicken and beef<br>-Quick service operations | 2 inspections per year |
| Low-Risk Category (Risk Assessment III) | -Liquor stores<br>-Food warehouses (retail & prepackaged)<br>-Ice cream operations in drug stores<br>-Operations that sell candy<br>-Kitchen-less bars<br>-Snack bars located in theatres | 1 inspection per year*<br><br>** If inspection score falls below 90, facility may be subject to additional inspections throughout the year.* |
| Temporary-Risk Category (Risk Assessment IV) | -Applies to facilities that have existing suspensions, violations, or investigations. | Establishments in this category will increase number of inspections by one (i.e., a restaurant in the low-risk category assigned to risk assessment IV will go from the typical 1 inspection per year to 2 inspections per year). |

Table 3. The four risk assessment categories used to evaluate restaurants and other retail food establishments in Los Angeles County, California, USA.

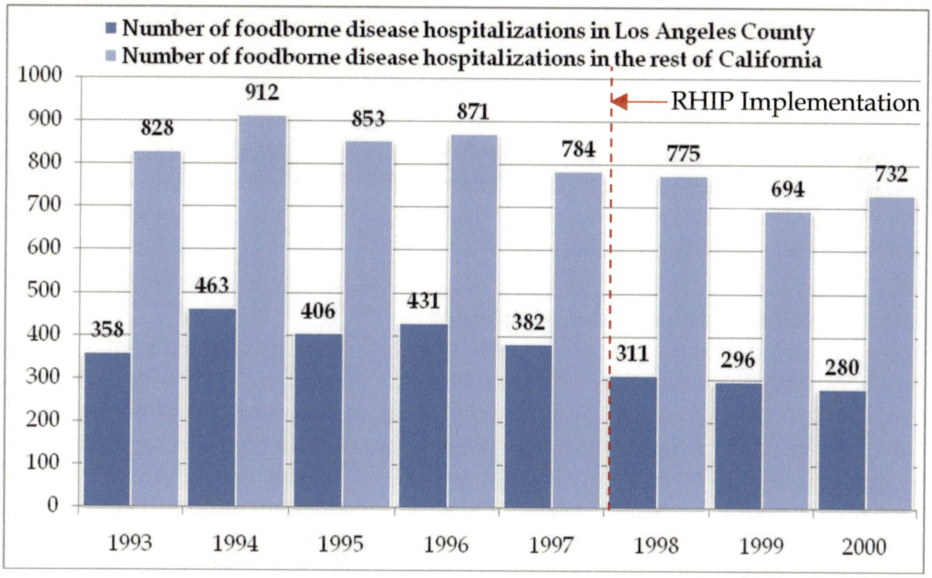


Fig. 6. Number of Foodborne-Disease Hospitalizations by Year, Los Angeles County and the Rest of California, 1993-2000, USA.

### 4.2.3 Home kitchens

Although restaurant inspections by local health departments routinely assess food-safety practices among food handlers in the retail food environment, similar scrutiny of home kitchens are rarely applied in most jurisdictions across the United States. In response to this potential risk in the home setting, the Los Angeles County Department of Public Health launched its Home Kitchen Self-Inspection Program in the spring of 2006 to promote safer food handling and preparation practices among the county's residents, using a voluntary self-inspection and education program. The program included the use of a web-based, self-assessment questionnaire, called the Food Safety Quiz (FSQ) that was based on emerging evidence indicating that online, interactive learning strategies are conducive to problem-based learning, improving self-efficacy and increasing self-mastery of selected skills (Kuo et al., 2010). The educational program stressed the importance of such preventive measures as hand washing before, during and after food preparation; refrigerating prepared foods in small containers; thoroughly cooking all foodstuffs derived from animal sources, particularly poultry, pork, egg products and meat dishes; avoiding recontamination within the kitchen after cooking is completed; and maintaining a sanitary kitchen and protecting prepared foods against rodent and insect contamination (Heymann, 2008; Scott, 2003).

During its initial program period from 2006-2008, more than 13,000 individuals participated in the program and completed the FSQ. Recent evaluation of program progress revealed that if home kitchens were graded similarly to restaurants in Los Angeles County, 61% would have received an **A** or **B** rating, as compared to 98% for the full-service restaurants based on rating criteria derived from the California Food Safety Code (Kuo et al., 2010). Among the program participants, approximately 27% reported not storing partially cooked food that was not used immediately in the refrigerator before final cooking; 26% reported that their kitchen shelves and cabinets were not clean and free from dust; and 36% said they did not have a properly working thermometer inside their refrigerators (Kuo et al., 2010).

The program evaluators concluded that even among interested and motivated persons who took the time to participate in the Home Kitchen Self-Inspection Program, food handling and preparation deficiencies were common in the home kitchen setting. This innovative, ongoing educational program in Los Angeles County underscores the importance of educating the public about home kitchen safety. Such programs, which emphasize feedback and interactive teaching about food safety, can complement the efforts of established restaurant hygiene rating programs to reduce foodborne illnesses in jurisdictions across the United States.

## 4.3 Exploring new strategies and technologies

New research on control measures is underway to investigate additional strategies for reducing foodborne illnesses, especially for *Salmonella* prevention. Advances in non-thermal technologies for microbial inactivation of *Salmonella*, such as the use of cold plasma, high pressure, and carbon dioxide are currently being evaluated (Bermúdez-Aguirre et al., 2011). Another approach that is currently being considered is the use of antimicrobial bottle coatings (i.e., packaging for liquid foods) to inactivate *Salmonella* in liquid egg albumen (Jin and Gurtler, 2011). Scientists are also actively exploring an experimental chlorate product that can be introduced into drinking water and feed for hens (McReynolds et al., 2005). Although promising, these innovations are not standalone interventions and are expected to augment existing control measures at various levels of the food distribution chain.

## 5. Conclusion

Salmonellosis caused by nontyphoid strains remains the most common foodborne illness reported in the United States. In spite of effective public health and regulatory efforts to control and prevent this infectious disease, the morbidity, mortality, and years of potential life lost due to this foodborne pathogen continue to be substantial. The overall incidence of laboratory confirmed *Salmonella* infection was 17.6 cases per 100,000 persons in 2010, which remains higher than the Healthy People 2020 objective of 11.4 cases per 100,000 persons (Figure 2). Active surveillance and continual efforts in developing and implementing control policies have helped federal and local health agencies in the United States make significant strides in combating this disease. Lessons learned from these efforts, including ways to work collaboratively across agencies at different levels of the food distribution chain have been invaluable for informing present and future *Salmonella* control policies and preventive measures in the United States. These lessons may have global implications for other jurisdictions abroad.

## 6. Acknowledgement

The authors would like to thank Brenda Robles, Mirna Ponce, Lana Sklyar, Gloria Kim, and Phyllis Thai for their technical assistance and contributions to this chapter.

## 7. References

Altekruse SF, Cohen ML, Swerdlow DL. (1997). Emerging foodborne diseases. *Emerging infectious diseases*, Vol. 3, No. 3, (July-September, 1997), pp. 285-293.

Batz MB, Hoffmann S, Morris JG, Jr. (2011). *Ranking the risks: The 10 Pathogen-Food Combinations with the Greatest Burden on Public Health.* Gainesville, FL: Emerging Pathogens Institute, University of Florida.

Bermúdez-Aguirre D and Corradini MG. Inactivation kinetics of *Salmonella* spp. Under thermal and emerging treatments: A review. *Food Research International,* article in press – Epub, available online June 24, 2011.

Boehmer TK, Bamberg WM, Ghosh TS, et al. (2009). Health care-associated outbreak of Salmonella Tennessee in a neonatal intensive care unit. *American Journal of Infection Control,* Vol. 37, No. 1, (February 2009), pp. 49-55.

(CDC) Centers for Disease Control and Prevention. (2008). *Salmonellosis*. Retrieved May 8, 2011, Available from: www.cdc.gov/salmonella

(CDC) Centers for Disease Control and Prevention. (2011). Vital signs: incidence and trends of infection with pathogens transmitted commonly through food --- foodborne diseases active surveillance network, 10 U.S. Sites, 1996--2010. *MMWR Morbidity and Mortality Weekly Report*, Vol. 60, No. 22, (June, 2011), pp. 749-55.

Cruickshank JG and Humphrey TJ. (1987). The carrier food-handler and non-typhoid salmonellosis. *Epidmeiology and Infection*, Vol. 98, No. 3, (June, 1987), pp. 223-230.

Cummings K, Barrett E, Mohle-Boetani JC, et al. (2001). A multi-state outbreak of *Salmonella enterica* serotype Baildon associated with domestic raw tomatoes. *Emerging Infectious Diseases,* Vol. 7, No. 6, (November-December 2001), pp. 1046-1048.

Cummings PL, Sorvillo F, Kuo T. (2010). Salmonellosis-related mortality in the United States, 1990-2006. *Foodborne Pathogens and Disease*, Vol. 7, No. 11, (November, 2010) pp. 1393-1399.

Environmental Health - Policy and Operations Manual. (2011). County of Los Angeles Public Health, Environmental Health. Risk Assessment, Policy No. 205.08, effective July 1, 2011. (Internal document).

Fielding, JE. (2008). Board memo. *Los Angeles County - Department of Public Health: 10-year review of restaurant and food facility grading program.* (January, 2008). Los Angeles, CA: Los Angeles County Department of Public Health.

Fuller CC, Jawahir SL, Leano FT, et al. (2008). A multi-state *Salmonella* Typhimurium outbreak associated with frozen vacuum-packed rodents used to feed snakes. *Zoonoses and Public Health,* Vol. 55, pp. 481-487.

Gardner JW and Sanborn JS. (1990). Years of potential life lost (YPLL) - What does it measure? *Epidemiology,* Vol. 1, pp. 322-329.

Harris LJ, Farber JN, Beuchat LR, et al. (2003). Outbreaks associated with fresh produce: incidence, growth, and survival of pathogens in fresh and fresh-cut produce. *Comprehensive Reviews in Food Science and Food Safety* , Vol. 2, No. supplement, pp. 78-141.

Helms M, Simonsen J, Molbak K. (2006). Foodborne bacterial infection and hospitalization: a registry-based study. *Clinical Infectious Disease,* Vol. 42, No. 4, (February, 2006) pp. 498-506.

Heymann, DL. (Ed.) (2008). *Control of Communicable Diseases Manual (19th Edition).* American Public Health Association, 978-0-87553-189-2, Washington, D.C.

Hutchison, C. (2010, August 23). *ABC News*. Retrieved July 26, 2011, from ABC News Medical Unit, Available at: http://abcnews.go.com/Health/Wellness/salmonella-outbreak-egg-recall-shows-fda-flaws/story?id=11445664&sms_ss=email&at_xt=4dc5bfad22557dc5%2C0

Jin T and Gurtler JB. (2011). Inactivation of *Salmonella* in liquid egg albumen by antimicrobial bottle coatings infused with allyl isothiocyanate, nisin and zinc oxide nanoparticles. *Journal of Applied Microbiology,* Vol. 110, No. 3, (January 2011), pp.704-712.

Kennedy M, Villar R, Vugia DJ, et al. (2004). Hospitalizations and deaths due to Salmonella infections, FoodNet, 1996-1999. *Clinical Infectious Diseases*, Vol. 38, Supplement 3, pp. S142-S148.

Khuri-Bulos NA, Khalaf MA, Shehabi A, Shami K. (1994). Foodhandler-associated Salmonella outbreak in a university hospital despite routine surveillance cultures of kitchen employees. *Infection Control and Hospital Epidemiology,* Vol. 15, No. 5, (May 1994), pp. 311-314.

Kimura AC, Palumbo MS, Meyers H, et al. (2005). A multi-state outbreak of *Salmonella* serotype Thompson infection from commercially distributed bread contaminated by an ill food handler. *Epidemiology and Infection,* Vol. 133, pp. 823-828.

Kuo T, Dela Cruz H, Redelings M, et al. (2010). Use of a self-assessment questionnaire for food safety education in the home kitchen - Los Angeles County, California, 2006-2008. MMWR *Morbidity and Mortality Weekly Report,* Vol. 59, No. 34, (September 2010), pp. 1098-1101.

(LACDPH) Los Angeles County Department of Public Health. (2008, January 31). *Veterinary Public Health.* Retrieved July 27, 2011, from Los Angeles County Department of Public Health, Available at: http://publichealth.lacounty.gov/vet/docs/TurtleBeforeYouBuySalmonellaColor.pdf

Majowicz SE, Musto J, Scallan E, et al. (2010). The global burden of nontyphoidal Salmonella gastroenteritis. *Clinical Infectious Disease,* Vol. 50, No. 6, pp. 882-889.

Matyas B, Cronquist A, Cartter M, et al. (2010). Preliminary FoodNet data on the incidence of infection with pathogens transmitted commonly through food - 10 states, 2009. *MMWR Morbidity and Mortality Weekly Report,* Vol. 59, No. 14, pp. 418-422.

McReynolds J, Kubena L, Byrd J, et al. (2005). Evaluation of *Salmonella enteritidis* in molting hens after administration of an experimental chlorate product (for nine days) in the drinking water and feeding an alfalfa molt diet. *Poultry Science,* Vol. 84, pp. 1186-1190.

Mead P, Slutsker L, Dietz V, et al. (1999). Food-related illness and death in the United States. *Emerging Infectious Disease,* Vol. 5, No. 5, pp. 607-625.

Newell DG, Koopmans M, Verhoef L, et al. (2010). Foodborne diseases - the challenges of 20 years still persist while new ones continue to emerge. *International Journal of Food Microbiology* , Vol. 139, Supplement 1, (May 2010), pp. S3-15.

Perez-Santigosa N, Diaz-Paniagua C, Hidalgo-Vila J. (2008). The reporductive ecology of exotic Trachemys scripta elegans in an invaded area of southern Europe. *Aquatic Conservation: Marine and Freshwater Ecosystems,* Vol. 18, (June, 2008), pp. 1302-1310.

Redelings MD, Wise M. (2007). Using multiple cause-of-death data to investigate associations and causality between conditions listed on the death certificate. *American Journal of Epidemiology* , Vol. 166, pp.104-108.

Rowe B, Giles C, Brown GL. (1969). Outbreak of gastroenteritis due to *Salmonella* virchow in a maternity hospital. *British Medical Journal,* Vol. 3, (September 6, 1969), pp. 561-564.

Scallan E, Hoekstra RM, Angulo FJ, et al. (2011). Foodborne illness acquired in the United States - major pathogens. *Emerging Infectious Disesae,* Vol. 17, No. 1, pp. 7-15.

Scott E. (2003). Food safety and foodborne disease in 21$^{st}$ century homes. *Canadian Journal of Infectious Disease,* Vol. 14, No. 5, (September-October, 2003), pp. 227-280.

Simon P, Leslie P, Run G, et al. (2005). Impact of restaurant hygiene grad cards on foodborne-disease hospitalizations in Los Angeles County. *Journal of Environmental Health,* Vol. 67, No. 7, (March, 2005), pp. 32-36.

Trevejo RT, Courtney JG, Starr M, and Vugia DJ. (2003). Epidemiology of salmonellosis in California, 1990-1999: morbidity, mortality, and hospitalization costs. *American Journal of Epidemiology,* Vol. 157, No. 1, (July, 2002), pp. 48-57.

(USDHHS) United States Department of Health & Human Services and the U.S. Food and Drug Administration. (2009). Federal Register Final Rule (July 9, 2009, 74 FR 33030): Prevention of Salmonella Enteritidis in shell eggs during production, storage, and transportation. *Federal Register (FR)* , FR: Vol. 74, No. 130.

(USDA) United States Department of Agriculture, Animal and Plant Health Inspecttion Service (APHIS). (October 1999). *Part I: Reference of 1999 table egg layer management in the U.S.* Fort Collins, CO : Centers for Epidemiology and Animal Health.

(USDA) United States Department of Agriculture, Food Safety and Inspection Service (FSIS). (2005). Production & Inspection: Irradiation and Food Safety (Fact Sheet). Retrieved on September 2, 2011 from: http://www.fsis.usda.gov/Fact_Sheets/Irradiation_and_Food_Safety/index.asp

(US-CFR) United States Government. (2010). *U.S. Code of Federal Regulations. 21 CFR 1240.* Washington, DC: Government Printing Office.

Zhe JG and Leslie P. (2003). The effect of information on product quality: evidence from restaurant hygiene grade cards. *The Quarterly Journal of Economics*, Vol. 118, No. 2, (May, 2003), pp. 409-451.

# 2

# The Role of Foods in *Salmonella* Infections

Carlos Alberto Gómez-Aldapa[1], Ma. del Refugio Torres-Vitela[2],
Angélica Villarruel-López[2] and Javier Castro-Rosas[1*]
*[1]Center of Chemical Research, Institute of Basic Sciences and Engineering
Autonomous University of Hidalgo State, City of Knowledge
Carretera Pachuca-Tulancingo, Mineral de la Reforma, Hidalgo
[2]Laboratory of Food Safety, University Center of Exact Sciences and Engineering
University of Guadalajara, Marcelino García Barragán, Guadalajara, Jalisco
México*

## 1. Introduction

*Salmonella* is one of the most common causes of foodborne disease worldwide. It also generates negative economic impacts due to surveillance investigation, and illness treatment and prevention. Salmonellosis is a zoonotic infection caused by *Salmonella*; for example, *S.* Enterica causes gastroenteritis, typhoid fever and bacteremia. Transmission is by the fecal–oral route whereby the intestinal contents of an infected animal are ingested with food or water. Human carriers are generally less important than animals in transmission of *Salmonella* strains. A period of temperature abuse which allows the *Salmonella* spp. to grow in food and/or inadequate or absent final heat treatment are common factors contributing to outbreaks. Meat, poultry, egg, dairy products, and fruits and vegetables are primary transmission vehicles; they may be undercooked, allowing the *Salmonella* strains to survive, or they may cross-contaminate other foods consumed without further cooking. Cross-contamination can occur through direct contact or indirectly via contaminated kitchen equipment and utensils. This chapter is a review of the role foods play in *Salmonella* infections and provides an overview of the main food chain- associated *Salmonella* risks.

## 2. *Salmonella* contamination sources in foods

*Salmonella* is found in the environment and the gastrointestinal tract of wild and farmed animals. Animals may become infected with *Salmonella* through environmental contamination, other animals or contaminated feed. Both animals and humans can function as *Salmonella* reservoirs. In addition to sheep, goats, cattle, chickens and pigs, other animals which can become infected with *Salmonella* include geese and other birds, lizards and other reptiles, shellfish, and amphibians such as turtles. Indeed, most *Salmonella* contamination is of animal origin.

Among livestock production systems, *Salmonella* is more frequently isolated from poultry (chicken, turkey, duck, and pheasants) than from other animals (Freitas et al., 2010).

---

* Corresponding Author

*Salmonella*-infected animals shed the microorganism in the feces from where it can spread into soil, water, crops and/or other animals. All *Salmonella* serotypes can be harbored in the gastrointestinal tract of livestock. The most common chain of events leading to this foodborne illness involves healthy carrier animals which subsequently transfer the pathogen to humans during production, handling and/or consumption.

*Salmonella* transmission to food processing plants and food production equipment is a serious public health issue. *Salmonella* can enter the food chain at any point: crop, farm, livestock feed, food manufacturing, processing and retailing (Wong et al., 2002). A number of workers handle animals during slaughter and processing, and contamination is possible when *Salmonella* or any other pathogen is present on the equipment or the workers' hands or clothing. Contamination most often occurs during specific slaughter stages: bleeding, skinning (or defeathering in poultry), evisceration (removal of chest and abdomen contents, also known as gutting) and pre-processing carcass handling. Cattle may be asymptomatically infected with *Salmonella* and beef can be contaminated during slaughter and processing via gastrointestinal content, and by milk during milking. *Salmonella* Dublin which is highly pathogenic to humans, is strongly associated with cattle (host-adapted). This makes cattle an important target for *Salmonella* control efforts.

*Salmonella* can frequently be isolated from most species of live poultry, such as broilers, turkeys, ducks and geese. Levels in poultry can vary depending on country, production system and the specific control measures in place. Contamination in poultry products can occur at several stages in the slaughter process, be it feces during evisceration or cross-contamination from contaminated products or surfaces on the production line. Particular contamination 'hot spots' in the poultry slaughter process include defeathering, evisceration and cutting; chilling in a water bath reduces the *Salmonella* load but may in turn facilitate cross-contamination (Corry *et al.*, 2002; Fluckey *et al.*, 2003; Northcutt *et al.*, 2003).

Pork and pork products are increasingly recognized as important sources of human salmonellosis (Nielsen and Wegener, 1997). *Salmonella* colonizes pigs on the farm, and pork is then contaminated during slaughter or subsequent processing. Control of *Salmonella* in pork can be implemented on the farm, at slaughter and during processing. Pre-harvest control consists of monitoring *Salmonella* at the herd level, and implementing *Salmonella* reduction measures in infected herds through hygiene, animal separation, feeding strategy and strict control of *Salmonella* in the breeder and growing-finishing pig supply chain.

Until recently, most human *Salmonellosis* cases have been caused by contaminated food animals, but in recent years an array of new food vehicles in foodborne disease transmission has been identified. Foods previously thought to be safe are now considered to be hazardous. These new food vehicles share several features. Contamination typically occurs early in the production process, rather than just before consumption. Consumer preferences and the globalized food market result in ingredients from many countries being combined in a single product, making it difficult to trace the specific contamination source. Many foods also have fewer barriers to microbial growth, such as added salt, sugar or preservatives. Their consequent short shelf life means they are often eaten or discarded by the time an outbreak is recognized. Under these circumstances, efforts to prevent contamination at the source are very important. Fresh produce such as fruits and vegetables have gained attention as transmission vehicles since contamination can occur at any one of the multiple steps in the processing chain (Bouchrif et al., 2009). Factors influencing the rise in salmonellosis outbreaks linked to vegetables include changes in agricultural practices and eating habits, as well as greater worldwide commerce in fresh produce (Collins, 1997).

Contamination with *Salmonella* strains from fresh produce apparently stems mainly from horticultural products. The principal contamination routes are probably use of animal-source organic fertilizers, irrigation with wastewater, humans and other animals (Islam et al., 2004; Natvig et al., 2002). Presence of *Salmonella* in the environment may also lead to contamination in fruits and vegetables because *Salmonella* can survive for long periods in the environment. Multiple pathogenic microorganism sources occur during food packaging, distribution and marketing.

Studies of environmental sources of *Salmonella* contamination indicate that water is an important source, particularly irrigation water containing manure, wildlife feces or sewage effluents (Islam et al., 2004; Reilly et al., 1981). Insects or birds may also transmit *Salmonella* to different foods. Flies are a known *Salmonella* carrier (Greenberg & Klowden, 1972), and can transmit various pathogenic microorganisms, as well as viruses such as polioviruses, coxsackie viruses, infectious hepatitis and anthrax (Ugbogu et al., 2006). Moore *et al.* (2003) mentioned the possibility that *Chironomus* genus insects were direct or indirect vectors of enteric bacteria contamination in water and food.

In general, non-typhoid *Salmonella* is a persistent contamination hazard in all raw foods, including animals, poultry, wild birds, eggs, fruit, vegetables, dairy products, fish and shellfish and cereals.

## 3. *Salmonella* in foods

*Salmonella* spp. are the most common pathogenic bacteria associated with a variety of foods. Although myriad foods can serve as *Salmonella* sources, meat and meat products, poultry and poultry products, and dairy products are significant sources of foodborne pathogen infections in humans. Presence of *Salmonella* spp. in fresh raw products can vary widely (Harris et al., 2003). Frequency usually ranges from 1 to 10 %, depending on a range of factors including organism, farming and/or food production practices, and geographical factors (Harris et al., 2003). Research on *Salmonella* frequency in different countries is extensive, and *Salmonella* serotypes have been isolated in a variety of foods (Table 1). Poultry and egg products have long been recognized as an important *Salmonella* source (Skov et al., 1999); in fact, contaminated poultry, eggs and dairy products are probably the most common cause of human Salmonellosis worldwide (Herikstad et al., 2002). *Salmonella* can contaminate eggs on the shell or internally, and egg shells are much more frequently contaminated than the white/yolk. Furthermore, egg surface contamination is associated with many different serotypes, while infection of the white/yolk is primarily associated with *S.* Enteritidis (Table 1).

Poultry and poultry products are a common foodborne illness vector. Poultry can carry some *Salmonella* serovars without any outwards signs or symptoms of disease. *Salmonella* can be introduced to a flock via multiple environmental sources, such as feed, water, rodents or contact with other poultry. The gastrointestinal tract of one or more birds may harbor *Salmonella*-and, if damaged during slaughter, may contaminate other carcasses. Cross-contamination can also occur from a *Salmonella*-positive flock or contaminated slaughter equipment to the carcasses of a *Salmonella*-free flock, as well as via handling of raw poultry during food preparation. Sufficient heating will eliminate *Salmonella* from contaminated poultry and poultry products.

Pasteurization effectively kills *Salmonella* in milk, but consumption of unpasteurized milk and milk products is a well documented risk factor for salmonellosis in humans.

Inadequately pasteurized milk as well as post-pasteurization contamination of milk and milk products are recognized sources of human disease.

| Country | Food | Serotypes | Reference |
|---|---|---|---|
| United States | Papaya | Agona | CDC, 2011 |
| United States | Cantaloupe | Panama | CDC, 2011 |
| United States | Raw milk | Anatum, Cerro, Dublin, Infantis, Kentucky, Mbdanka, Montevideo, Muenster | Van Kessel et al., 2011 |
| United States | Oysters served raw in restaurants | Newport, Mbandaka, Braenderup, Cerro, Muenchen, I:4,12:i:- | Brillhart & Joens, 2011 |
| Mexico | Chili peppers | ND | Castro-Rosas et al., 2011 |
| Mexico | Cheese | Amsterdam, Anatum, Montevideo, Brandenburg, Give, Kiambu, Nyborg, Bredeney, Typhimurium, Meleagridis, Kentucky | Torres-Vitela et al., 2011 |
| China | Beef | Enteritidis, Typhimurium | Yang et al., 2010 |
| Iran | Chicken | Thompson | Dallal et al., 2010 |
| Brazil | Poultry carcass | Enteritidis | Freitas et al., 2010 |
| Turkey | Retail Meat Products | Typhimurium, *S. bongori*, *S. enterica* subsp. *diarizonae* | Arslan & Eyi, 2010 |
| Uruguay | Poultry and Eggs | Enteritidis, Derby, Gallinarum, Panama | Betancor et al., 2010 |
| Mexico | Zucchini squash | ND | Castro-Rosas et al., 2010 |
| Bangladesh | Chick egg | Typhimurium | Hasan et al., 2009 |
| Senegal | Chicken Carcasses and Street-Vended Restaurants | Brancaster, Goelzau, Kentucky, Hadar, Agona, Poona, Bandia, Bessi, Brunei, Hull, Istanbul, Javiana, Magherafelt, Molade, Oxford, Rubislaw, Tamale, and Zanzibar | Dione et al., 2009 |
| United States | Chicken carcasses from retail stores | Kentucky, Hadar, Enteritidis, Braenderup, Montevideo, Thompson, Mbandaka, Agona | Lestari et al., 2009 |

| Country | Food | Serotypes | Reference |
|---|---|---|---|
| United States | Broiler carcasses | Kentucky, Heidelberg, Typhimurium, Typhimurium var. 5-; 4,5,12:I: -; Schwarzengrund, Montevideo, Ohio, Kiambu, Betha, Thompson; 4,12:I: -; Senftenberg, Enteritidis, Worthington, Hadar; 8,(20): -:z6; Mbandaka; 8,(20):I: -; Infantis | Berrang et al., 2009 |
| Republic of Ireland | Retail pork | Typhimurium | Prendergast et al., 2009 |
| Mexico | Parsley, coriander, cauliflower, lettuce, spinach | Typhimurium, Choleraesuis, Gallinarum, Anatum , Agona, Edinburg, Enteritidis, Typhi, Pullorum, Bongor | Quiroz-Santiago et al, 2009 |
| Japan | Imported Seafood | Weltevreden | Asai et al., 2008 |
| Iran | Raw poultry | Enteritidis, Baibouknown | Jalali et al., 2008 |
| Mexico | Hydroponic Tomatoes | Typhimurium, Agona, Thompson, Montevideo, C1 monophasic | Orozco et al., 2008 |
| Australia | Retail Raw Meats | Typhimuriuam, Infantis | Phillips et al., 2008 |
| Turkey | Chicken | Infantis | Cetinkaya et al., 2008 |
| Germany | Sushi from sushi bars and retailers | ND | Atanassova et al., 2008 |
| Vietnam | Pork, beef, chicken, Shellfish | London, Havana, Anatum, Hadar, Albany, Typhimurium | Van et al., 2007 |
| Brazil | Poultry meat | ND | Reiter et al., 2007 |
| New Zealand | Uncooked retail meats | Infantis, Typhimurium, Enteritidis, Brandenberg, 4,5,12:-:-, 4,12:-:-, 4:-:2, 6,7:k:- | Wong et al., 2007 |
| Canada | Chicken nuggets and strips | Heidelberg, Orion, Kentucky, Hadar, Indiana, Infantis, Enteritidis, Mbandaka, | Bucher et al., 2007 |

| Country | Food | Serotypes | Reference |
|---|---|---|---|
| Malaysia | Street food, fried chicken, kerabu jantung pisang, sambal fish, mix vegetables | Biafra, Braenderup, Weltevreden | Tunung et al., 2007 |
| United States | Almonds | 35 different serotypes | Danyluk et al., 2007 |

ND: not determined

Table 1. *Salmonella* serotypes identified in different foods and countries.

*Salmonella* spp. have been isolated from filter feeder seafood species such as oysters, clams and mussels (Table 1). These species acquire their food from the water flowing through their bodies, but also ingest anything else that happens to be in the water. If oceans, lakes and bays are contaminated with fecal matter, the shellfish living in them intake any waterborne pathogens and harbor them in their intestines. The highest potential infection risk is from oysters, since they are most often eaten raw on the half shell. A single raw oyster can contain enough bacteria to cause an infection in the human gut. Mussels and clams pose less of a risk because they are usually steamed, killing *Salmonella* and most other bacteria. The above constitute only a sampling of the principal ways in which animals and animal products cause lead to *Salmonella* infection.

Fresh produce as a possible disease vehicle has become the focus of increasing concern since contamination can occur at multiple steps along the food chain. *Salmonella* is among the most worrisome of the pathogenic microorganisms found in minimally-processed fresh produce (CDC, 2009; Heaton et al., 2008). Bacterial contamination of whole or minimally-processed fresh vegetables can occur at different processing stages (i.e. harvest, trimming, washing, slicing, soaking, dehydrating, blending and/or packaging) (Harris el al., 2003). Produce can also be contaminated with human or animal source pathogens (Beuchat, 2006; Natvig, 2002). *Salmonella* spp. are the most common etiological agent associated with fresh produce related infection in the United States (US). A range of fresh fruit and vegetable products have been implicated in *Salmonella* infection, most frequently lettuce, sprouted seeds, melons and tomatoes (Table 2). *Salmonella* spp. are often isolated during routine surveys of produce such as lettuce, cauliflower, sprouts, mustard cress, endive and spinach (Thunberg et al., 2002); mushrooms (Doran et al., 2005); bean sprouts, alfalfa sprouts, unpasteurized juices and fresh salad fruits and vegetables (CDC, 2009).

In Mexico, *Salmonella* has been isolated from raw vegetables such as alfalfa sprouts (Castro-Rosas and Escartín, 1999), parsley, cilantro, cauliflower, lettuce and spinach (Quiroz-Santiago et al., 2009). It has also been identified from zucchini squash (*Cucurbita pepo*) (Castro-Rosas et al., 2010), and jalapeño and serrano chili peppers (Castro-Rosas et al., 2011). In 2008, 600,000 tons of zucchini were produced in Mexico: 419,768 tons for the domestic market (SAGARPA, 2010) and approximately 200,000 tons for the US market (USDA, 2010). This squash is most commonly consumed cooked in Mexico and other countries, but can be eaten raw (e.g. green salads). In 2009, over 1,981,500 tons of chili peppers were produced in Mexico; of these 613,308 tons were jalapeño peppers and 216,617 tons were serrano peppers (SAGARPA, 2010). These peppers are most commonly consumed raw [e.g. green salads or Mexican sauce (salsa)], both in Mexico and other countries.

We studied the frequencies of coliform bacteria (CB), thermotolerant coliforms (TC), *Escherichia coli* and *Salmonella* in zucchini squash (Castro-Rosas et al., 2010) and jalapeño and serrano peppers (Castro-Rosas et al., 2011). In zucchini squash, infection was detected in 100% of cases for CB, 70% for TC, 62% for *E. coli* and 10% for *Salmonella* spp. Concentration range was 3.8 to 7.4 log CFU/fruit for CB, and <3 to 1000 MPN/fruit for TC and *E. coli*. In serrano chili peppers infection was detected in 100% of cases for CB, 90% for TC, 50% for *E. coli* and 10% for *Salmonella* spp., while in jalapeño peppers frequencies were 100% for CB, 86% for TC, 32% for *E. coli* and 12% for *Salmonella* spp. All *Salmonella*-positive samples were also *E. coli*-positive. For CB, concentration range was 3.8 to 7.9 log CFU/serrano sample and 5.3 to 8.2 log CFU/jalapeño sample, whereas TC and *E. coli* concentrations ranged from <3 to 1100 MPN/serrano and jalapeño samples (Castro-Rosas, et al., 2010; 2011). As is the case with other vegetables consumed raw, zucchini squash, and jalapeño and serrano peppers are potential pathogen vehicles. Sources of pathogenic microorganisms in the field include soil, water, wild and domestic animals, drift and runoff from adjacent farms and manure (Beuchat, 2006; Natvig, 2002). Once harvested and used in food preparation, zucchini squash, jalapeño and serrano peppers are all potential sources of cross contamination with pathogenic microorganisms.

Salmonellosis infection is an increasing problem and recent salmonellosis outbreaks have been associated with a wider variety of vegetables, even those that were not previously considered to imply a risk (e.g. jalapeño peppers; CDC, 2008a). Data on frequency of incidence for pathogenic bacteria such as *Salmonella* are clearly needed for a wide variety of vegetables which are consumed raw. Preventing contamination is vital to avoiding salmonellosis outbreaks, but it is also important to understand the potential survival and growth rates of *Salmonella* on specific substrates such as zucchini, jalapeño and serrano peppers. Our results suggest that both chili peppers and zucchini squash may be significant factors contributing to the endemicity of *Salmonella* in Mexico.

*Salmonella* has been isolated from fruits and vegetables such as cantaloupes, melons, tomatoes, lettuce, and especially alfalfa sprouts (Table 1). These products can become contaminated by several routes, therefore, consumers need to thoroughly wash all fresh foods before consumption to reduce risk of illness from fruits and vegetables. With alfalfa sprouts and lettuce, washing can merely drive bacteria deeper into the lower layers of lettuce leaves or sprouts, so the outside three layers of lettuce leaves need to be removed and sprouts need to separated before careful washing.

Finally, consumer awareness needs to be promoted that many other foods may carry *Salmonella*, even those not normally thought to be contamination sources. Most users know to handle raw chicken properly and to cook chicken and eggs thoroughly to avoid *Salmonella* contamination. But foods such as almonds, pecans and chocolate can also harbor *Salmonella*. In addition, as the food chain becomes completely global and highly complex, and international trade continues to develop, new foods will surely be linked to salmonellosis outbreaks.

## 4. *Salmonella* outbreaks

Disease surveillance reports frequently identify poultry, meat and milk products as the main vehicles in salmonellosis outbreaks. However, in recent years foodborne illness outbreaks have been increasingly associated with greater consumption of fresh fruits and vegetables (CDC, 2009). *Salmonella* is responsible for frequent foodborne illness outbreaks in the developed world, and *Salmonella* outbreaks have been associated with different *Salmonella* serovars (Table 2). Over 2000 *Salmonella* serotypes are known, but only a small fraction of these are commonly associated with foodborne illness. Which serotypes cause illness is influenced by serotype geographical distribution and serovar or strain pathogenicity. In the US, *Salmonella* Typhimurium has been considered the principal causative agent of foodborne salmonellosis, but both *S.* Typhimurium and Enteritidis have been increasingly identified in foodborne salmonellosis since the 1980s (Table 2); the exact cause of the predominance of these *Salmonella* serotypes is not yet clearly understood.

Most developed countries have laboratory-based *Salmonella* infection surveillance programs, and many countries have systems for recording outbreaks and notification systems where clinicians submit data on patients with *Salmonella* infections to national public health institutions. Official *Salmonella* infection numbers are usually derived from laboratory-based surveillance in which clinical microbiology laboratories report positive findings and, in some countries, submit *Salmonella* isolates to national reference laboratories for serotyping and other characterization. These data are necessary for measuring trends over time and detecting outbreaks. However, official figures do not quantify the burden of illness, and degree of surveillance differs between countries. Moreover, reported incidence is a composite measure of several factors, including true *Salmonella* infection incidence, the health-care seeking behavior of patients with gastroenteritis, and the likelihood that the physician requests a stool culture. Furthermore, access to laboratories and microbiological methods varies widely, as does the precision of findings reported to public health authorities. Finally, comparisons between different geographical areas can be difficult because public health jurisdictions with a tradition of active case-searching as part of outbreak investigations or extensive testing of contacts of known patients or food-handlers are likely to report higher numbers of infections than jurisdictions with only passive surveillance. As a result, the precise incidence of *Salmonella* food poisoning in all countries is not known, since small outbreaks often remain unreported.

*Salmonella* spp. and *S.* Typhi infections are endemic in many developing countries. In Mexico, there were 709,278 salmonellosis cases and 228,206 typhoid fever cases reported from 2004-2009 (Secretaría de Salud, 2011). In addition, *S.* Gaminara and *S.* Montevideo have been associated with several cases of human illness in Mexico (Gutiérrez-Cogco et al., 2000). A certain proportion of salmonellosis and typhoid fever cases in Mexico may be associated with consumption of raw vegetables exposed to fecal contamination, probably due to the continued but limited practice of irrigating vegetable crops with untreated wastewater.

Centers for Disease Control and Prevention (CDC) data for the US indicate that over 40,000 salmonellosis cases occur annually, with about 500 resulting deaths. As is the case for staphylococcal gastroenteritis, the largest salmonellosis outbreaks typically occur at banquets or similar functions. However, the two largest recorded salmonellosis outbreaks occurred under rather unusual circumstances. The largest occurred in 1994 and involved over 224,000 cases in 41 states. The serovar was *S.* Enteritidis and the vehicle food was ice cream produced from milk transported in tanker trucks which had previously hauled liquid eggs. The second largest occurred in 1985 and involved nearly 200,000 cases. *S.* Typhimurium was the etiological agent and the vehicle was 2% milk produced by a single dairy plant in Illinois. The third largest outbreak occurred in 1974 on the Navajo Indian Reservation, when 3,400 persons became ill with the *S.* Newport serovar. Human carriers are generally less important than animals in transmission of salmonellosis. Human transmission can occur if hands contaminated with infected fecal matter come in contact with food which is then consumed without adequate cooking, often after an intervening period in which microbial growth occurs. Exactly this chain of events led to a major outbreak affecting an international airline in 1984. A total of 631 passengers were infected after eating food containing an aspic glaze prepared by a food service worker who returned to work after a bout of salmonellosis but was still excreting *Salmonella* Enteritidis PT4. The serotype Typhimurium has participated in most recent outbreaks, although it is likely that this serotype's involvement in salmonellosis cases worldwide is far greater than reported. *Salmonella* surveillance sensitivity may vary widely between countries but it is still crucial to identifying trends and detecting outbreaks. Surveillance which includes serotyping is particularly useful for this purpose. Available data suggest that the incidence of *Salmonella* infections has increased over the last twenty years, that new *Salmonella* serotypes often emerge in several countries at near the same time, and that multi-state or international outbreaks call for a coordinated response. In response, several national and international networks currently address the problem of emerging *Salmonella* infections. An important objective in preventing *Salmonella* outbreaks is improvement and enhancement of surveillance, including serotyping.

| Country | Food vehicle | Serotypes | Number of cases | Reference |
|---|---|---|---|---|
| United States | Papaya | Agona | 99 | CDC, 2011a |
| United States | Alfalfa sprouts and spicy sprouts | Enteritidis | 25 | CDC, 2011b |
| United States | Turkey Burgers | Hadar | 12 | CDC, 2011c |
| United States | Cantaloupe | Panama | 20 | CDC, 2011d |
| United States | Alfalfa sprouts | I 4,[5],12:i:- | 140 | CDC, 2011e |
| Denmark | Salami | Typhimurium | 20 | Kuhn et al, 2011 |
| England | Sandwiches and prepared salads | Typhimurium | 179 | Boxall et al., 2011 |
| Australia | Raw egg mayonnaise | Typhimurium | 87 | Jardine et al, 2011 |
| Ireland, United Kingdom (England, Wales, Northern Ireland, Scotland), France, Luxembourg, Sweden, Finland, Austria | Pre-cooked meat products | Agona | 163 | Nicolay et al., 2011 |
| South Africa | Food served in a school | Enteritidis | 18 | Niehaus et al., 2011 |

| Country | Food vehicle | Serotypes | Number of cases | Reference |
|---|---|---|---|---|
| Japan | Boxed lunches | Braenderup | 176 | Mizoguchi et al., 2011 |
| England | Multiples foods | Enteritidis | 63 | Janmohamed et al., 2011 |
| United States | Shell Eggs | Enteritidis | 1,939 | CDC, 2010a |
| United States | Cheesy chicken rice frozen entrée | Chester | 44 | CDC, 2010b |
| United States | Frozen mamey fruit pulp | Typhi | 9 | CDC, 2010c |
| United States | Alfalfa Sprout | Newport | 44 | CDC, 2010d |
| United States | Red and Black Pepper/Italian-Style Meats | Montevideo | 272 | CDC, 2010e |
| United States | Potato salad | Schwarzengrund, Typhimurium | 9 | CDC, 2010f |
| United States | Cilantro and chicken meat | Montevideo | 58 | Patel et al, 2010 |
| Netherlands | Fresh fruit juice | Panama | 33 | Noël et al., 2010 |
| France | Dried pork sausage | 4,12:i:- | 90 | Bone et al., 2010 |
| China | Water | *S.* Paratyphi A | 267 | Yang et al., 2010 |
| United Kingdom | Raw bean sprouts | Bareilly | 231 | Cleary et al., 2010 |
| Netherlands | Raw or undercooked beef products | Typhimurium | 23 | Whelan et al., 2010 |
| Australia | Dessert containing raw egg | Typhimurium | 20 | Reynolds et al., 2010 |
| New Zealand | Watermelon | Typhimurium | 15 | McCallum et al., 2010 |
| Spain | Infant formula | Kedougou | 42 | Rodriguez-Urrego et al., 2010 |
| United States | Alfalfa Sprouts | Saintpaul | 228 | CDC, 2009a |
| United States | Peanut butter | Typhimurium | 529 | CDC, 2009b |
| United States | Unpasteurized orange juice | Typhimurium and Saintpaul | 152 | Jain et al., 2009 |
| United States | Vegetable-coated ready-to-eat snack food | Wandsworth, Typhimurium | 69 | Sotir et al., 2009 |
| Australia | Eggs | Typhimurium | 22 | Dyda et al., 2009 |
| Australia | Bread dumpling loaf prepared with eggs | Enteritidis | 8 | Much et al., 2009 |
| Australia | Papaya | Litchfield | 26 | Gibbs et al., 2009 |

| Country | Food vehicle | Serotypes | Number of cases | Reference |
|---|---|---|---|---|
| Denmark, Norway and Sweden | Pork meat and pork products | Typhimurium | 41 | Bruun et al., 2009 |
| Australia | Eggs | Typhimurium | 19 | Slinko et al., 2009 |
| Mauritius | Marlin mousse | Typhimurium | 53 | Issack et al., 2009 |
| Pakistan | Drinking water | *S. typhi* | 300 | Farooqui et al., 2009 |
| France | Cheese made from raw milk | Montevideo | 23 | Dominguez et al., 2009 |
| France | Goat's cheese | Muenster | 25 | Van Cauteren et al., 2009 |
| Denmark | Pasta salad with pesto | Anatum | At least 4 | Pakalniskiene et al., 2009 |
| Netherlands | Hard cheese made from raw milk | Typhimurium | 224 | Van Duynhoven et al., 2009 |
| Australia | Chocolate mousse | Typhimurium | 8 | Roberts-Witteveen et al., 2009 |
| United States | Jalapeño peppers | Saintpaul | at least 1,442 | CDC, 2008a |
| United States | Frozen Pot Pies | I 4,5,12:i:-* | 401 | CDC, 2008b |
| United States | Fruit salad | Litchfield | 30 | CDC, 2008c |
| United States | Unpasteurized Mexican-style aged cheese | Newport | 85 | CDC, 2008d |
| England and Wales | Fresh basil | Senftenberg | 32 | Pezzoli et al., 2008 |
| Norway | Rucola lettuce | Thompson | 21 | Nygård et al., 2008 |
| Bulgaria | Minced meat | Typhimurium | 22 | Pekova et al., 2008 |
| Switzerland | Soft cheese | Stanley | 82 | Pastore et al., 2008 |
| Denmark | Pork products | Typhimurium | 1,054 | Ethelberg et al., 2008 |
| Japan | Snapping turtle | Typhimurium | 4 | Fukushima et al., 2008 |
| Ireland | Meat products | Agona | 119 | O'Flanagan et al., 2008 |

Table 2. Recent reported *Salmonella* outbreaks, including country (ies) affected, food vehicle and serovar.

## 5. Interaction of *Salmonella* with foods

*Salmonella* serotypes can grow and survive on a large number of foods (Harris et al., 2003). Their behavior in foods is controlled by a variety of environmental and ecological factors, including water activity, pH, Eh, chemical composition, the presence of natural or added antimicrobial compounds and storage temperature; as well as processing factors such as heat application and physical handling. For example, optimum pH for growth in *Salmonella* is approximately neutral, with values > 9.0 and < 4.0 being bactericidal. Minimum growth in some serotypes can occur at pH 4.05 (with HCl and citric acids), although this minimum can occur at pH as high as 5.5, depending on the acid used to lower pH (Harris, et al., 2003). Growth in *Salmonella* can continue at temperatures as low as 5.3 °C (*S.* Heidelberg) and 6.2 °C (*S.* Typhimurium), and temperatures near 45 °C (temperatures ≥ 45 °C are bactericidal). In addition, available moisture (aw) inhibits growth at values below 0.94 in neutral pH media, although higher aw values are required as pH declines to near the minimum growth values (Harris, et al., 2003).

Extensive data is available on the effects of individual environmental factors on *Salmonella* strains, but the effects of their interactions are not as well understood. Parish et al. (1997) determined survival for several *Salmonella* serotypes in orange juice. To achieve a 6 log reduction in *Salmonella* serotypes, orange juice (pH 3.5) had to be stored at 4 °C for 15-24 days. A similar reduction took 43-57 days when the orange juice was at pH 4.1 and 4 °C. Using apple juice, Uljas & Ingham (1999) demonstrated that *S.* Typhimurium DT104 could be reduced by at least 5 log units at pH 3.3 after storage at 25 °C for 12 hours or at 35 °C for 2 hours. These treatments did not achieve a 5 log reduction in *E.* coli O157. At pH 4.1, a 5 log reduction in *S.* Typhimurium DT104 was produced by storage at 35 °C for 6 hours in the presence of 0.1% sorbic acid or by a combination of storage at elevated temperature (25 °C for 6 hours or 35 °C for 4 hours) followed by a freeze/thaw cycle without sorbic acid (Uljas & Ingham, 1999). In the field, the physical environment of vegetables surfaces is considered to be inhospitable for growth and survival of *Salmonella* (for example, temperature and humidity fluctuations, and ultraviolet light) (Dickinson, 1986). Environmental conditions, however, can greatly influence bacterial populations; the presence of free moisture on vegetable surfaces from precipitation, dew or irrigation can promote survival and growth of bacterial populations (Shaper et al., 2006). Certain conditions such as sunlight, particularly shorter ultraviolet wavelengths, can damage bacterial cells (Shaper et al., 2006); selection therefore occurs for bacteria with adaptations to stressful conditions. Microorganisms' ability to survive on plants depends on the environmental, physicochemical and genetic features of the plant and specific properties (Shaper et al., 2006). Many microorganisms have developed mechanisms to attach to, survive and/or grow in microniches on different vegetables (Shaper et al., 2006). For instance, surface moisture on vegetables may provide a protective environment for *Salmonella* strains. On vegetable surfaces, microorganisms interact in aggregates and may compete for the limited nutrients available in microniches at the junction of epidermal cells, where water accumulates, cuticular waxes are less dense and nutrients are more available than in other sites (Shaper et al., 2006). Free water in the surface apertures of vegetables (e.g. stomata) constitutes a water channel connecting a plant's apoplast with its external environment. Microorganisms can enter vegetables through these water channels in various ways. Once internalized, the microorganisms are protected from environmental stress (Shaper et al., 2006). Survival of pathogenic microorganisms on or in raw produce is also dictated by its metabolic capabilities. However, the manifestations of these capabilities can be greatly influenced by intrinsic (e.g. vegetable moisture surface) and extrinsic ecological factors naturally present in the raw produce or imposed at one or more points during production, processing and distribution (Harris et al., 2003). *Salmonella* strains may be able to enter a viable but nonculturable state (VBNC) on the surface of fruit and vegetables, resulting in underestimation of viable population size by direct plating on culture medium. Brandl and Mandrell (2002), suggested that *S.* Thompson may enter into a VBNC state on *Cilantro phyllosphere* due to exposure to dry pre-harvest conditions on the plant surface. Improved understanding of microbial ecosystems on the surface of foods such as raw fruits and vegetables would be extremely useful in developing strategies to minimize contamination, prevent pathogen growth, and kill or remove pathogens at different stages in production, processing, marketing and preparation for consumption. Food ecosystems are extremely diverse and complex. *Salmonella* survival and/or growth on foods are influenced by the organism, produce item and environmental conditions in the field and post-harvest, including storage conditions.

For many years, the interaction of *Salmonella* with animal hosts and animal-origin foods has received intense attention. In contrast, little research has been done on the interaction between *Salmonella* spp. and fruits and vegetables, and more specifically on its frequency and behavior in fruits and vegetables which may pose a special risk to humans [e.g. radish root (*Raphanus sativus*), beetroot (*Beta vulgaris* var. *conditiva*), jicama (*Pachyrhizus erosus*), loroco (*Fernaldia pandurata*), prickly pear (*Opuntia* spp.), zucchini squash (*Cucurbita pepo*), chili peppers (Jalapeño and Serrano peppers) and others]. It is particularly urgent to study fruits and vegetables not previously considered health hazards and those with the potential to function as pathogen microorganism vehicles but are as yet unidentified.

In a recent *Salmonella* outbreak in the US, jalapeño and serrano peppers were the food vehicle and the isolated serovar was Saintpaul (CDC, 2008). It affected at least 1,442 persons in 43 states, the District of Columbia and Canada, and was traced back to distributors in the United States which had received produce grown and packed in Mexico. The outbreak strain was isolated from samples of jalapeño peppers collected from a US warehouse and a patient's home, as well as from samples of serrano peppers and water collected from a farm in Mexico. We have studied the behavior of *Salmonella* serotypes in zucchini squash and chili peppers. In zucchini, we tested the behavior of four *Salmonella* serotypes (Typhimurium, Typhi, Gaminara and Montevideo) and a cocktail of three *Escherichia coli* strains on whole and sliced zucchini squash at 25±2 and 3-5 °C. No growth was observed for any of the tested microorganisms or the cocktail on whole fruit stored at 25±2 or 3-5 °C. After 15 days at 25±2 °C, the tested *Salmonella* serotypes had decreased from an initial inoculum level of 7 log CFU to <1 log and at 3-5 °C they decreased to approximately 2 log (Figure 1). Among the *E. coli* strains, survival was significantly higher than for the *Salmonella* strains at the same times and temperatures: after 15 days at 25±2 °C, *E. coli* cocktail strains had decreased to 3.4 log CFU/fruit and at 3-5 °C they decreased to 3.6 log CFU/fruit (Figure 1).

The observed differences in survival between the *Salmonella* and *E. coli* strains on zucchini squash fruit could be due to factors such as the area inoculated, fruit ripeness and physical and chemical characteristics of the studied fruit and strains. Different strains of *E. coli* O157:H7, *Pseudomonas*, *Salmonella*, and *Listeria monocytogenes* attach to different regions of cut lettuce leaves, indicating different and specific attachment mechanisms among different species or strains (Takeuchi et al., 2000).

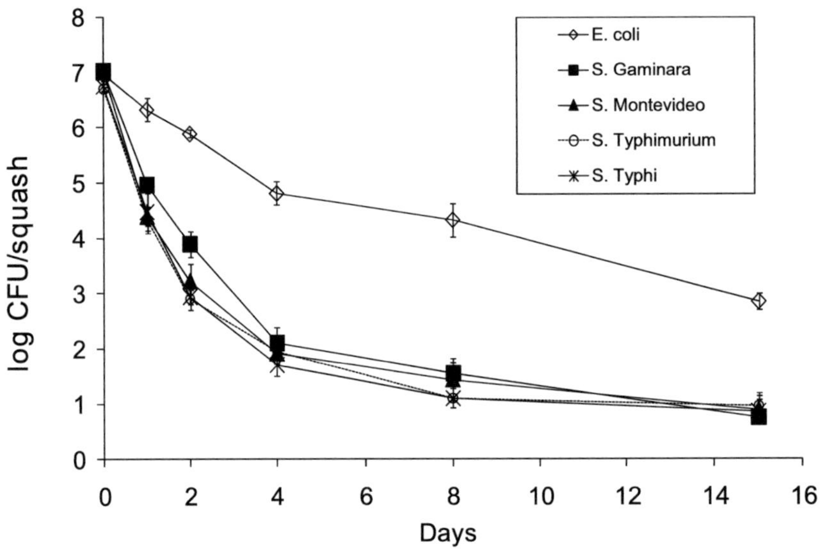


Fig. 1. Behavior of 4 *Salmonella* serotypes and *E. coli* on zucchini squash at 25±2 °C (Castro-Rosas et al., 2010).

When inoculated onto zucchini squash slices and incubated at 25±2 °C, the studied *Salmonella* and *E. coli* strains grew (Figure 2). After a short lag period (approx. 4 h), the *Salmonella* and *E. coli* populations increased from 2 log to 6 log CFU/slice at 24 h, and the *E. coli* strains increased a further 1 log CFU by 72 h. Initial *Salmonella* and *E. coli* inocula levels were close to that of Aerobic Plate Count bacteria (APC) in the studied zucchini squash fruit (approx. 2.5 log CFU/slice), and the APC growth rate (7.6 log CFU/slice by 24 h; 8.9 log CFU/slice by 72 h) was comparable to the studied strains (Figure 2). The behavior of *Salmonella* under these conditions does not differ greatly from that of *Salmonella* strains in other foods. For instance, *S.* Typhimurium inoculated in shredded cooked beef and stored at 20 °C/8 h, increased from 2.3 to 3.4 log CFU/g *(16)*, while after 22 h incubation on sliced tomatoes *S.* Montevideo increased by ca. 1.5 log CFU/g at 20 °C and 2.5 log CFU/g at 30 °C (Zhuang et al. 1995).

Under refrigeration (3-5 °C), growth in the *Salmonella* serotypes and *E. coli* strains was inhibited (Figure 4): bacterial concentration at 5 days was essentially similar to initial inocula levels. Nonetheless, survival of even a small concentration of *E. coli* and/or *Salmonella* under refrigeration poses a serious health hazard to consumers since salmonellosis outbreaks have been reported as originating in different foods at low pathogen concentrations (Greenwood and Hopper, 1983).

In a separate study, we tested the growth behavior of the same four *Salmonella* serotypes and three *E. coli* strains at the same temperatures (25±2 and 3-5 °C) on whole and sliced jalapeño and serrano peppers, as well as in a blended chili pepper sauce (Castro-Rosas et al., 2011). The sauce was an aqueous suspension containing mixed peppers, tomatoes, coriander, onion and salt (NaCl) in specific proportions. Both types of microorganisms exhibited similar behavior on/in the serrano and jalapeño peppers. No growth was observed in rifampicin-resistant *Salmonella* and *E. coli* strains on the surface of whole serrano and jalapeño peppers stored at 25±2 or 3-5 °C. After 6 days at 25±2 °C, the tested *Salmonella* serotypes and *E. coli* had decreased from an initial inoculum level of 5 log CFU to 1 log on the serrano peppers and to 2.5 log on the jalapeño peppers (Figure 3). At 3-5 °C they decreased to approximately 1.8 log in the serrano peppers and to 1.2 log on the jalapeño peppers. In contrast, when inoculated onto slices of both peppers and into the blended sauce, the *Salmonella* serotypes and *E. coli* grew: after 24 h at 25±2 °C, both bacteria types had grown to approximately 4 log CFU on the slices and 5 log CFU in the sauce (Figures 4-5). Bacterial growth was inhibited at 3-5 °C. In summary, the four tested *Salmonella* serotypes can survive on whole or sliced zucchini squash, serrano and jalapeño peppers and in sauce made of raw chili peppers, indicating them to be effective transmission vehicles and potential public health threats.

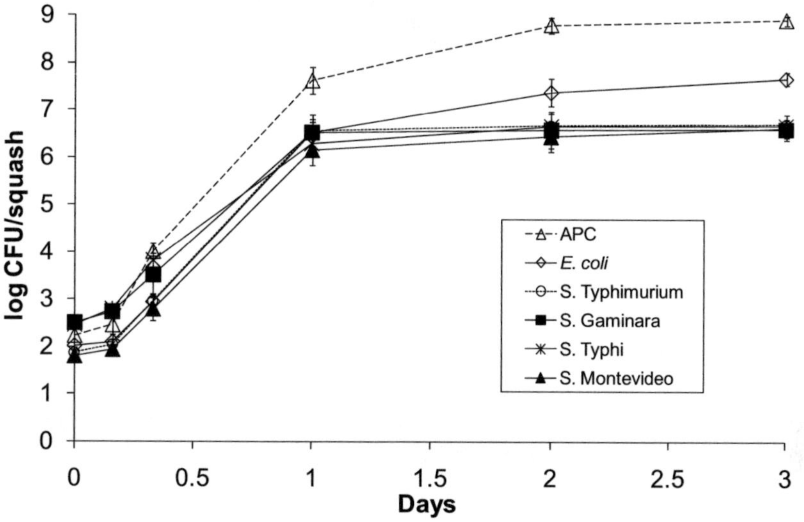


Fig. 2. Behavior of 4 *Salmonella* serotypes, *E. coli* and Aerobic Plate Count on zucchini slices at 25±2 °C (Castro-Rosas et al., 2010).

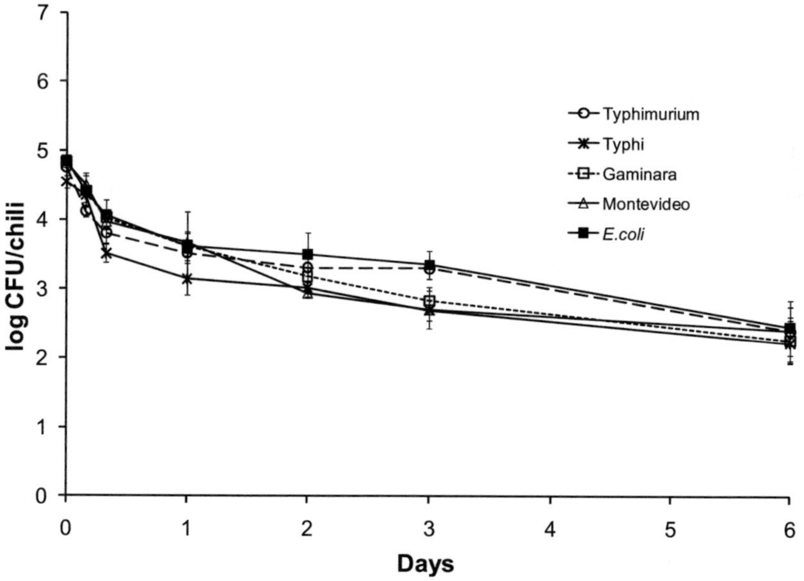


Fig. 3. Behavior of 4 *Salmonella* serotypes and a cocktail of three *E. coli* strains on whole jalapeño peppers at 25±2 ° C (Castro-Rosas, 2011).

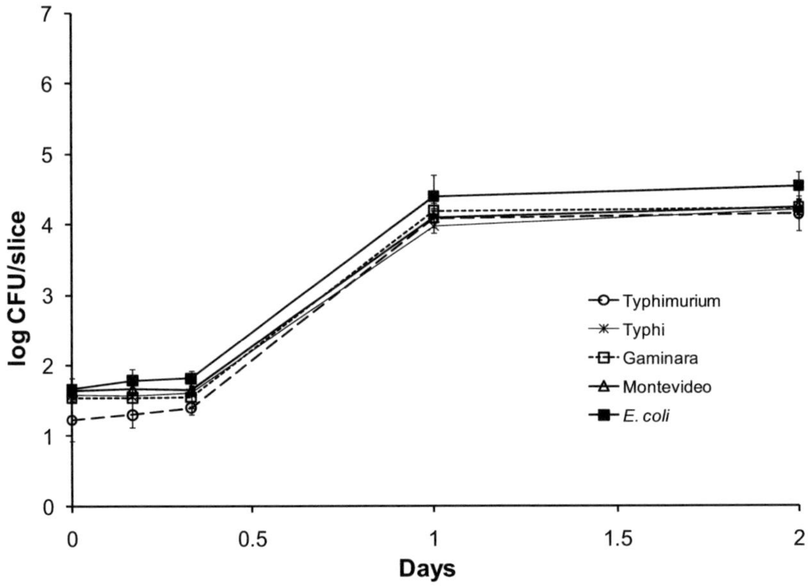


Fig. 4. Behavior of 4 *Salmonella* serotypes and a cocktail of three *E. coli* strains in jalapeño peppers slices at 25±2° C (Castro-Rosas, 2011).

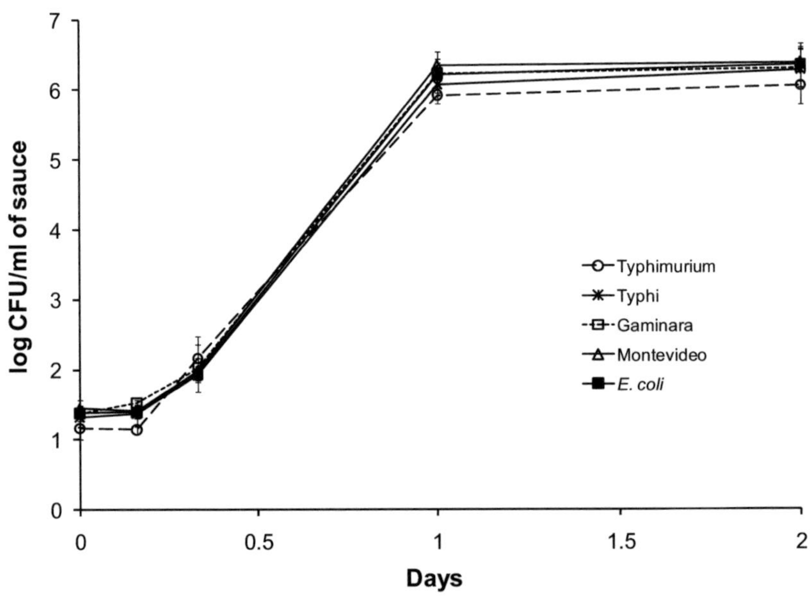


Fig. 5. Behavior of 4 *Salmonella* serotypes and a cocktail of three *E. coli* strains in a chili pepper sauce at 25±2 °C (Castro-Rosas, 2011).

## 6. Conclusion

Food is clearly a major *Salmonella* infection vehicle. This vital role in salmonellosis outbreaks calls for strict measures to minimize transmission, such as appropriate animal husbandry and agriculture practices, protection of feeds and water from contamination, adequate waste disposal methods and an overall effort to maintain a clean environment around food from farm to fork. Additionally, much of the risk posed by *Salmonella* can be mitigated through proper handling and correct food safety practices, including thorough washing and disinfection, prevention of pre-consumption, human-borne contamination during preparation and storage, leftovers disposal, cooking before consumption and refrigerated storage (3-5 °C). Continuous monitoring and generation of data on *Salmonella* and salmonellosis outbreaks, and improved surveillance measures are also vital to controlling this public health hazard. A deeper understanding of *Salmonella* and its behavior in foods is still needed to ensure food safety and quality.

## 7. References

Arslan, S. & Eyi, A. (2010). Occurrence and antimicrobial resistance profiles of *Salmonella* species in retail meat products. *Journal of Food Protection*, Vol.73, No.9, (September 2010), pp. 1613-1617, ISSN 0362-028X

Asai, Y., Kaneko, M., Ohtsuka. K., Morita, Y., Kaneko, S., Noda, H., Furukawa, I., Takatori, K. & Hara-Kudo, Y. (2008). *Salmonella* prevalence in seafood imported into Japan, *Journal of Food Protection*, Vol.71, No.7, (July 2008), pp. 1460-1464, ISSN 0362-028X

Atanassova, V., Reich, F. & Klein, G. (2008). Microbiological quality of sushi from sushi bars and retailers, *Journal of Food Prot*ection, Vol.71, No.4, (April 2008), pp. 860-864, ISSN 0362-028X

Berrang, M.E., Bailey, J.S., Altekruse, S.F., Shaw, W.K. Jr., Patel, B.L., Meinersmann, R.J. & Fedorka-Cray, P.J. (2009). Prevalence, serotype, and antimicrobial resistance of *Salmonella* on broiler carcasses postpick and postchill in 20 U.S. processing plants, *Journal of Food Protection,* Vol.72, No.8, (August 2009), pp. 1610-1615, ISSN 0362-028X

Betancor, L., Pereira, M., Martinez, A., Giossa, G., Fookes, M., Flores, K., Barrios, P., Repiso, V., Vignoli, R., Cordeiro, N., Algorta, G., Thomson, N., Maskell, D., Schelotto, F. & Chabalgoity, J.A. (2010). Prevalence of *Salmonella* enterica in poultry and eggs in Uruguay during an epidemic due to *Salmonella* enterica serovar Enteritidis, *Journal of Clinical Microbiology*, Vol.48, No.7, (July 2010), pp. 2413-2423, ISSN: 0095-1137

Beuchat, L. R. (1996). Pathogenic microorganisms associated with fresh produce, *Journal of Food Protection*, Vol.59, No.2, (February 1996), pp. 204-216, ISSN 0362-028X

Bone, A., Noel, H., Le-Hello, S., Pihier, N., Danan, C., Raguenaud, M.E., Salah, S., Bellali, H., Vaillant, V. Weill, F.X. & Jourdan-da Silva N. (2010). Nationwide outbreak of *Salmonella enterica* serotype 4,12:i:- infections in France, linked to dried pork sausage, March-May 2010, *Eurosurveillance*, Vol.15, No.24, (June 2010) pp. 2-4, ISSN 1560-7917

Bouchrif, B., Paglietti, B., Murgia, M., Piana, A., Cohen, N., Ennaji, M., Rubino, S. & Timinouni, M. (2009). Prevalence and antibiotic-resistance of *Salmonella* isolated from food in Morocco. *Journal of Infection in Developing Countries*, Vol.28, No.3, (February, 2009), pp. 35-40, ISSN 19722680

Boxall, N.S., Adak, G.K., D.E., Pinna. E. & Gillespie, I.A. (2011). A *Salmonella* Typhimurium phage type (PT) U320 outbreak in England, 2008: continuation of a trend involving ready-to-eat products. *Epidemiology and Infection,* (January 2011) Available on CJO 2011 doi:10.1017/S0950268810003080, ISSN 1469-4409

Brandl, M.T., & Mandrell, R.E. (2002). Fitness of *Salmonella enterica* serovar Thompson in the Cilantro Phyllosphere, *Applied and Environmental Microbiolog,* Vol.68, No.7, (July 2002), pp. 3614-2621, ISSN 0099-2240

Brillhart, C.D. & Joens, L.A. (2011). Prevalence and characterization of *Salmonella* serovars isolated from oysters served raw in restaurants, *Journal of Food Protection,* Vol.74, No.6, (June 2011), pp. 1025-1029, ISSN 0362-028X

Bruun, T., Sørensen, G., Forshell, L.P., Jensen, T., Nygard, K., Kapperud, G., Lindstedt, B.A., Berglund, T., Wingstrand,.A., Petersen, R.F., Müller, L., Kjelsø, C., Ivarsson, S., Hjertqvist, M., Löfdahl, S. & Ethelberg, S. (2009). An outbreak of *Salmonella* Typhimurium infections in Denmark, Norway and Sweden, *Eurosurveillance,* Vol.14, No.10, (March 2009) pp. 91-96, ISSN 1560-7917.

Bucher, O., Holley, R.A., Ahmed. R., Tabor, H., Nadon, C., Ng, L.K. & D'Aoust, J.Y. (2007). Occurrence and characterization of *Salmonella* from chicken nuggets, strips, and pelleted broiler feed, *Journal of Food Protection,* Vol.70, No.10, (October 2007), pp. 2251-2258, ISSN 0362-028X

Castro-Rosas J, Santos López EM, Gómez-Aldapa CA, González Ramírez CA, Villagomez-Ibarra JR, Gordillo-Martínez AJ, López AV, del Refugio Torres-Vitela M. (2010). Incidence and behavior of *Salmonella* and *Escherichia coli* on whole and sliced zucchini squash (Cucurbitapepo) fruit, *Journal of Food Protection,* Vol.73, No.8, (August 2010), pp. 1423-1429, ISSN 0362-028X

Castro-Rosas, J., and E.F. Escartín. (1999). Incidence and germicide sensitivity of *Salmonella typhi* and *Vibrio cholerae* O1 in alfalfa sprouts, *Journal of Food Safety,* Vol.19, No.2, (August 1999), pp. 137-146, ISSN 0149-6085

Castro-Rosas, J., Gómez-Aldapa, C,A., Acevedo-Sandoval, O.A., González Ramírez, C.A., Villagomez-Ibarra, J.R., Hernández, N.C., Villarruel-López, A. & Torres-Vitela, M. del R. (2011). Frequency and Behavior of *Salmonella* and *Escherichia coli* on Whole and Sliced Jalapeño and Serrano Peppers, *Journal of Food Protection,* Vol.74, No.6, (June 2011), pp. 874-881, ISSN 0362-028X

CDC (center for disease control and prevention). (2008)a. Outbreak of *Salmonella* Serotype Saintpaul Infections Associated with Multiple Raw Produce Items --- United States, *MMWR,* Vol.57, No.34, (August 2008), pp.929-934, ISSN 0149-2195

CDC. (2008)b. Multistate outbreak of *Salmonella* infections associated with frozen pot pies--United States, 2007, *Morbidity and Mortality Weekly Report* (*MMWR*), Vol.57, No.47, (November 2008), pp.1277-1280, ISSN 0149-2195

CDC. (2008)c. *Salmonella* Litchfield outbreak associated with a hotel restaurant--Atlantic City, New Jersey, 2007, *MMWR,* Vol.57, No.28, (July 2008), pp.775-779, ISSN 0149-2195

CDC. (2008)d. Outbreak of multidrug-resistant *Salmonella* enterica serotype Newport infections associated with consumption of unpasteurized Mexican-style aged cheese--Illinois, March 2006-April 2007, *MMWR,* Vol.57, No.16, (April 2008), pp.432-435, ISSN 0149-2195

CDC. (2009)a. Outbreak of *Salmonella* Serotype Saintpaul Infections Associated with Eating Alfalfa Sprouts — United States, 2009, *MMWR*, Vol.58, No.18, (May 2009), pp.500-503, ISSN 0149-2195

CDC. (2009)b. Surveillance for Foodborne Disease Outbreaks - United States, 2006. *MMWR*, Vol.58, No.22, (June 2009), pp.609-636, ISSN 0149-2195

CDC. (2009)c. Multistate outbreak of *Salmonella* infections associated with peanut butter and peanut butter-containing products--United States, 2008-2009, *MMWR*, Vol.58, No.4, (February 2009), pp.85-90, ISSN 0149-2195

CDC. (2010)a. Investigation Update: Multistate Outbreak of Human *Salmonella* Enteritidis Infections Associated with Shell Eggs. In: *Salmonella Outbreaks*, 20.7.2011, Available from: http://www.cdc.gov/salmonella/enteritidis/index.html

CDC. (2010)b. Investigation Update: Multistate Outbreak of Human *Salmonella* Chester Infections. In: *Salmonella Outbreaks*, 20.7.2011, Available from: http://www.cdc.gov/salmonella/enteritidis/index.html

CDC. (2010)c. Investigation Update: Multistate Outbreak of Human Typhoid Fever Infections Associated with Frozen Mamey Fruit Pulp. In: *Salmonella Outbreaks*, 20.7.2011, Available from: http://www.cdc.gov/salmonella/typhoidfever/index.html

CDC. (2010)d. Investigation Update: Multistate Outbreak of Human *Salmonella* Newport Infections Linked to raw alfalfa sprouts. In: *Salmonella Outbreaks*, 20.7.2011, Available from: http://www.cdc.gov/salmonella/newport/index.html

CDC. (2010)e. Investigation Update: Multistate Outbreak of Human *Salmonella* Montevideo Infections. In: *Salmonella Outbreaks*, 20.7.2011, Available from: http://www.cdc.gov/salmonella/montevideo/index.html

CDC. (2010)f. Multiple-serotype *Salmonella* gastroenteritis outbreak after a reception --- Connecticut, 2009, *MMWR*, Vol.59, No.34, (September 2010), pp.1093-1097, ISSN 0149-2195

CDC. (2011)a. Investigation Update: Ongoing Multistate Outbreak of Human *Salmonella* Agona Infections Linked to Whole, Fresh Imported Papayas. In: *Salmonella Outbreaks*, 20.7.2011, Available from: http://www.cdc.gov/salmonella/agona-papayas/index.html

CDC. (2011)b. Investigation Update: Multistate Outbreak of Human *Salmonella* Enteritidis Infections Linked to Alfalfa Sprouts and Spicy Sprouts. In: *Salmonella Outbreaks*, 20.7.2011, Available from: http://www.cdc.gov/salmonella/sprouts-enteritidis0611/070611/index.html

CDC. (2011)c. Investigation Announcement: Multistate Outbreak of *Salmonella* Hadar Infections Associated with Turkey Burgers. In: *Salmonella Outbreaks*, 20.7.2011, Available from: http://www.cdc.gov/salmonella/hadar0411/040411/index.html

CDC. (2011)d. Investigation Update: Multistate Outbreak of *Salmonella* Panama Infections Linked to Cantaloupe. In: *Salmonella Outbreaks*, 20.7.2011, Available from: http://www.cdc.gov/salmonella/panama0311/062311/index.html

CDC. (2011)e. Investigation Update: Multistate Outbreak of Human *Salmonella* I 4,[5],12:i:- Infections Linked to Alfalfa Sprouts. In: *Salmonella Outbreaks*, 20.7.2011, Available from: http://www.cdc.gov/salmonella/i4512i-/021011/index.html

Cetinkaya, F., Cibik, R., Soyutemiz, G.E., Ozakin, C., Kayali, R. & Levent, B. (2008). *Shigella* and *Salmonella* contamination in various foodstuffs in Turkey, *Food Control*, Vol.19, No.11, (November 2008), pp. 1059-1063, ISSN 0956-7135

Cleary, P., Browning, L., Coia, J., Cowden, J., Fox, A., Kearney, J., Lane, C., Mather, H., Quigley, C., Syed, Q. & Tubin-Delic, D. (2010). A foodborne outbreak of *Salmonella* Bareilly in the United Kingdom, *Eurosurveillance*, Vol.15, No.48, (December 2010) pp. 8-10, ISSN 1560-7917.

Collins, J.E. (1997). Impact of changing consumer lifestyles on the emergence/reemergence of foodborne pathogens. *Emerging Infectious Diseases*. Vol.3, No.4, (October-December 1997) pp. 471-479, ISSN 1080-6059.

Corry, J.E., Allen, V.M., Hudson, W.R., Breslin, M.F. & Davies, R.H. (2002). Sources of *Salmonella* on broiler carcasses during transportation and processing, modes of contamination and methods of control, *Journal of Applied Microbiology*, Vol.92, No.3, (March 2002), pp. 424-432, ISSN 1364-5072

Dallal, M.M.S., Doyle, M.P., Rezadehbashi, M., Dabiri, H., Sanaei, M., Modarresi, S., Bakhtiari, R., Sharifiy, K., Taremi, M., Zali, M.R. & Sharifi-Yazdi, M.K. (2010). Prevalence and antimicrobial resistance profiles of *Salmonella* serotypes, *Campylobacter* and *Yersinia* spp. isolated from retail chicken and beef, Tehran, Iran, *Food Control*, Vol.21, No.4, (April 2010), pp. 388-392, ISSN 0956-7135

Danyluk, M.D., Jones, T.M., Abd, S.J., Schlitt-Dittrich, F., Jacobs, M., Harris, L.J. (2007). Prevalence and amounts of *Salmonella* found on raw California almonds, *Journal of Food Protection*, Vol.70, No.4, (April 2007), pp. 820-827, ISSN 0362-028X

Dickinson, C.H. (1986). *Adaptations of micro-organisms to climatic conditions affecting aerial plant surfaces*. In: Fokkema NJ, van den Heuvel J, editors. Microbiology of the phyllosphere. ISBN 0521323444, New York: Cambridge Univ. p 77-100.

Dione, M.M., Ieven, M., Garin, B., Marcotty, T. & Geerts, S. (2009). Prevalence and antimicrobial resistance of *Salmonella* isolated from broiler farms, chicken carcasses, and street-vended restaurants in Casamance, Senegal, *Journal of Food Protection*, Vol.72, No.11, (November 2009), pp. 2423-2427, ISSN 0362-028X

Dominguez, M., Jourdan-Da Silva, N., Vaillant, V., Pihier, N., Kermin, C., Weill, F.X., Delmas, G., Kerouanton, A., Brisabois, A. & De Valk, H. (2009). Outbreak of *Salmonella* enterica serotype Montevideo infections in France linked to consumption of cheese made from raw milk, *Foodborne Pathogens and Disease*, Vol.6, No.1, (January-February 2009), pp. 121-128, ISSN 1535-3141

Doran, G., Sheridan, F., DeLappe, N., O'Hare, C., Anderson, W., Corbett-Feeney, G. & Cormican, M. (2005). *Salmonella enterica* serovar Kedougou contamination of commercially grown mushrooms, *Diagnostic Microbiology and Infectious Disease*, Vol.51, No.1, (January 2005), pp. 73-76, ISSN 0732-8893

Dyda, A., Hundy, R., Moffatt, C.R. & Cameron, S. (2009). Outbreak of *Salmonella* Typhimurium 44 related to egg consumption, *Communicable Diseases Intelligence*, Vol.33, No.4, (December 2009), pp. 414-418, ISSN 0725-3141

Ethelberg, S., Wingstrand, A., Jensen, T., Sorensen, G., Muller, L., Lisby, M., Nielsen, E. & Molbak, K. (2008). Large outbreaks of *Salmonella* Typhimurium infection in Denmark in 2008, *Eurosurveillance*, Vol.13, No.44, (October 2008) pp. 11-13, ISSN 1560-7917

Farooqui, A., Khan, A. & Kazmi, S.U. (2009). Investigation of a community outbreak of typhoid fever associated with drinking water. *BMC Public Health*, Vol.9, (December 2009), pp. 476, doi:10.1186/1471-2458-9-476, ISSN 1471-2458

Fluckey, W.M., Sanchez, M.X., McKee, S.R., Smith, D., Pendleton, E. & Brashears, M.M. (2003). Establishment of a microbiological profile for an air-chilling poultry operation in the United States, *Journal of Food Protection*, Vol.66, No.2, (February 2003), pp. 272-279, ISSN 0362-028X

Freitas, C.G.d., Santana, A.P., Silva, P.H.C.d., Goncalves, V.S.P., Barros, M.d.A.F., Torres, F.A.G., Murata, L.S. & Perecmanis, S. (2010). PCR multiplex for detection of *Salmonella* Enteritidis, Typhi and Typhimurium and occurrence in poultry meat, *International Journal of Food Microbiology*, Vol.139, No. 1-2, (April 2010), pp. 15-22, ISSN 0168-1605

Fukushima, H., Okuno, J., Fujiwara, Y., Hosoda, T., Kurazono, T., Ohtsuka, K., Yanagawa, K. & Yamaguchi M. (2008). An outbreak of *Salmonella* food poisoning at a snapping turtle restaurant, *Japanese Journal of Infectious Diseases*, Vol.61, No.4, (July 2008), pp. 328, ISSN 1344-6304

Gibbs, R., Pingault, N., Mazzucchelli, T., O'Reilly, L., MacKenzie, B., Green, J., Mogyorosy, R., Stafford, R., Bell, R., Hiley, L., Fullerton, K. & Van Buynder, P. (2009). An outbreak of *Salmonella enterica* serotype Litchfield infection in Australia linked to consumption of contaminated papaya, *Journal of Food Protection*, Vol.72, No.5, (May 2009), pp. 1094-1098, ISSN 0362-028X

Greenberg, B & Klowden M. (1972). Enteric bacterial interections in insects. *The American Journal of Clinical Nutrition*. Vol.25 (December 1972), pp 1459-1466, ISSN 0002-9165

Greenwood, M.H., & Hopper, W.L. (1983). Chocolate bars contaminated with *Salmonella napoli:* An infectivity study, *British Medical Journal,*Vol.286, No.6375 (April, 1983), pp. 1394, ISSN 0959 8138

Gutiérrez-Cogco, L., Montiel-Vázquez, E., Aguilera-Pérez, P. & González-Andrade, M. C. (2000). Serotipos de *Salmonella* identificados en los servicios de salud de México. *Salud Pública Méx*. Vol.42, No. 6, (November-December 2000) pp. 490–495. ISSN 0036-3634

Harris, L. J., J. N. Farber, L. R. Beuchat, M. E. Parish, T. V. Suslow, E. H. Garrett, & F. F. Busta. (2003). Outbreaks Associated with Fresh Produce: Incidence, Growth, and Survival of Pathogens in Fresh and Fresh Cut Produce. *Comprehensive Reviews in Food Science and Food Safety*, Vol.2, (May 2003), pp. 78-141, ISSN 1541-4337

Hasan, M.N., Ara, N., Mamun, S.A., Rahman, M.M. & Rahman, M. H. (2009). Prevalence of *Salmonella* spp. in chicken egg from Khulna city, *Journal of Innovation and Development Strategy*, Vol.3, No.3, (May 2009), pp. 1-6, ISSN 2075-1648

Heaton, J.C. & Jones, K. (2008). Microbial contamination of fruit and vegetables and the behaviour of enteropathogens in the phyllosphere: a review, *Journal of Applied Microbiology*, Vol.104, No.3, (March 2008), pp. 613-626, ISSN 1364-5072

Herikstad, H., Motarjemi, Y. & Tauxe, R.V. (2002). *Salmonella* surveillance, a global survey of public health serotyping, *Epidemiology and Infection*, Vol.129, No.1, (August 2002), pp. 1-8, ISSN 1469-4409

Islam, M., Morgan, J. Doyle, M.P., Phatak, S.C., Millner, P. & Jiang, X. (2004), Fate of *Salmonella enterica* Serovar Typhimurium on carrots and radishes grown in fields treated with contaminated manure composts or irrigation water, *Applied and Environmental Microbiolog,* Vol.70, No.4, (April 2004), pp. 2497–2502, ISSN 0099-2240

Islam, M., Morgan, J., Doyle, M.P., Phatak, S.C., Millner, P. & Jiang, X. (2004). Persistence of *Salmonella enterica* serovar Typhimurium on lettuce and parsley and in soils on which they were grown in fields treated with contaminated manure composts or irrigation water, *Foodborne Pathogens and Disease,* Vol.1, No.1, (July 2004), pp. 27-35, ISSN 1535-3141

Issack, M.I., Hendriksen, R.S., Lun, P.L., Lutchun, R.K. & Aarestrup, F.M. (2009). *Salmonella* enterica serovar Typhimurium in Mauritius linked to consumption of marlin mousse, *Foodborne Pathogens and Disease,* Vol.6, No.6, (July-August 2009), pp.739-741, ISSN 1535-3141

Jain, S., Bidol, S.A., Austin, J.L., Berl, E., Elson, F., Lemaile-Williams, M., Deasy, M.3rd, Moll, M.E., Rea, V., Vojdani, J.D., Yu, P.A., Hoekstra, R.M., Braden, C.R. & Lynch, M.F. (2009). Multistate outbreak of *Salmonella* Typhimurium and Saintpaul infections associated with unpasteurized orange juice--United States, 2005. *Clinical Infectious Disease,* Vol.48, No.8, (April 2009) pp. 1065-1071, ISSN 1058-4838

Jalali, M., Abedi, D., Pourbakhsh, S.A. & Ghoukasin, K. (2008). Prevalence of *Salmonella* spp. in raw and cooked foods in Isfahan-Iran, *Journal of Food Safety,* Vol.28, No.3, (August 208), pp. 442-452, ISSN 0149-6085

Janmohamed, K., Zenner, D., Little, C., Lane, C., Wain, J., Charlett, A., Adak, B. & Morgan, D. (2011). National outbreak of *Salmonella* Enteritidis phage type 14b in England, September to December 2009: case-control study, *Eurosurveillance,* Vol.16, No.15, (April 2011) pp. 5-10, ISSN 1560-7917

Jardine, A., Ressler, K.A., Botham, S., Irwin, M.J., Shadbolt, C., Vally, H. & Ferson, M.J. (2011). An Outbreak of *Salmonella* Typhimurium 108/170 at a Privately Catered Barbeque at a Sydney Sports Club, *Foodborne Pathogens and Disease, In Press,* doi:10.1089/fpd.2011.0918, ISSN 1535-3141

Kuhn, K., Torpdahl, M., Frank, C., Sigsgaard, K. & Ethelberg, S. 2011. An outbreak of *Salmonella* Typhimurium traced back to salami, Denmark, April to June 2010. *Eurosurveillance,* Vol.16, No.19, (May 2011), pp. 13-16, ISSN 1560-7917

Lestari, S.I., Han, F., Wang, F. & Ge, B. 2009. Prevalence and antimicrobial resistance of *Salmonella* serovars in conventional and organic chickens from Louisiana retail stores, *Journal of Food Protection,* Vol.72, No.6, (June 2007), pp. 1165-1172, ISSN 0362-028X

McCallum, L., Torok, M., Dufour, M.T., Hall, A. & Cramp, G. 2010. An outbreak of *Salmonella typhimurium* phage type 1 associated with watermelon in Gisborne, January 2009, *The New Zealand Medical Journal,* Vol.123, No.1322, (September 2010), pp. 39-45, ISSN 0028-8446

Mizoguchi, Y., Suzuki, E., Tsuchida, H., Tsuda, T., Yamamoto, E., Nakase, K., Doi, H. (2011). Outbreak of *Salmonella* Braenderup infection originating in boxed lunches in Japan in 2008, *Acta Medica Okayama,* Vol.65, No.2, (April 2011), pp. 63-69. ISSN 0386300X

Moore, B.C., Martinez, E., Gay, J.M. & Rice, D.H. (2003). Survival of *Salmonella enterica* in freshwater and sediments and transmission by the aquatic midge *Chironomus tentans* (Chironomidae: Diptera), *Applied and Environmental Microbiolog,* Vol.69, No.8, (August 2003), pp. 4556–4560, ISSN 0099-2240

Much, P., Pichler, J., Kasper, S., Lassnig, H., Kornschober, C., Buchner, A., König, C. & Allerberger, F. (2009). A foodborne outbreak of *Salmonella* Enteritidis phage type 6 in Austria, 2008, *Wiener Klinische Wochenschrift*, Vol.121, No.3-4, pp. 132-136. ISSN. 0043-5325

Natvig, E.E., Ingham, S. C., Ingham, B. H., Cooperband, L. R. & Roper, T. R. (2002). *Salmonella* enterica serovar Typhimurium and *Escherichia coli* contamination of root and leaf vegetables grown in soils with incorporated bovine manure, *Applied and Environmental Microbiolog*, Vol.68, No.6 (June 2002), pp. 2737-2744, ISSN 0099-2240

Nicolay, N., Thornton, L., Cotter, S., Garvey, P., Bannon, O., McKeown, P., Cormican, M., Fisher, I., Little, C., Boxall, N., DE Pinna E, Peters, T.M., Cowden, J., Salmon, R., Mason, B., Irvine, N., Rooney, P. & O'Flanagan, D. 2011. *Salmonella* enterica serovar Agona European outbreak associated with a food company, *Epidemiology and Infection*, Vol.139, No.8, (August 2011), pp. 1272-1280, ISSN 1469-4409

Niehaus, A.J., Apalata, T., Coovadia, Y.M., Smith, A.M. & Moodley, P. (2011). An outbreak of foodborne salmonellosis in rural KwaZulu-Natal, South Africa, *Foodborne Pathogens and Disease*, Vol.8, No.6, (June 2011), pp. 693-697, ISSN 1535-3141

Nielsen, B. & Wegener, H.C. (1997). Public health and pork and pork products, regional perspectives of Denmark, *Rev. Sci. Tech.* Vol.16, No.2, (August 1997), pp. 513–524,

Noël, H., Hofhuis, A., De Jonge, R., Heuvelink, A.E., De Jong, A., Heck, M.E., De Jager, C. & Van Pelt, W. 2010. Consumption of fresh fruit juice: how a healthy food practice caused a national outbreak of *Salmonella* Panama gastroenteritis, *Foodborne Pathogens and Disease*, Vol.7, No.4, (April 2010), pp. 375-381, ISSN 1535-3141

Northcutt, J.K., Berrang, M.E., Dickens, J.A., Fletcher, D.L. & Cox, N.A. (2003). Effect of broiler age, feed withdrawal, and transportation on levels of coliforms, *Campylobacter, Escherichia coli* and *Salmonella* on carcasses before and after immersion chilling. *Poultry Science*, Vol.82, No.1, (January 2003), pp. 169–173. ISSN: 0032-5791

Nygård, K., Lassen, J., Vold, L., Andersson, Y., Fisher, I., Löfdahl, S., Threlfall, J., Luzzi, I., Peters, T., Hampton, M., Torpdahl, M., Kapperud, G. & Aavitsland, P. (2008). Outbreak of *Salmonella* Thompson infections linked to imported rucola lettuce, *Foodborne Pathogens and Disease*, Vol.5, No.2, (April 2008), pp. 165-173, ISSN 1535-3141

O'Flanagan, D., Cormican, M., McKeown, P., Nicolay, N., Cowden, J., Mason, B., Morgan, D., Lane, C., Irvine, N., Browning, L. 2008. A multi-country outbreak of *Salmonella* Agona, February - August 2008, *Eurosurveillance*, Vol.13, No.27-39, (July-september 2008), pp. 453-454, ISSN 1560-7917

Orozco, L., Rico-Romero, L. & Escartín, E.F. (2008). Microbiological profile of greenhouses in a farm producing hydroponic tomatoes, *Journal of Food Protection*, Vol.71, No.1, (January 2008), pp. 60-65, ISSN 0362-028X

Pakalniskiene, J., Falkenhorst, G., Lisby, M., Madsen, S.B., Olsen, K.E., Nielsen, E.M., Mygh, A., Boel, J. & Mølbak, K. (2009). A foodborne outbreak of enterotoxigenic *Escherichia coli* and *Salmonella* Anatum infection after a high-school dinner in Denmark, November 2006, *Epidemiology and Infection*, Vol.137, No.3, (March 2009), pp. 396-401, ISSN 1469-4409

Parish, M.E., Narciso, J.A. & Friedrich, L.M. (1997). Survival of *Salmonellae* in orange juice, *Journal of Food Safety*, Vol.17, No.4, (December 1997), pp. 273-281, ISSN 0149-6085

Pastore, R., Schmid, H., Altpeter, E., Baumgartner, A., Hächler, H., Imhof, R., Sudre, P. & Boubaker, K. (2008). Outbreak of *Salmonella* serovar Stanley infections in Switzerland linked to locally produced soft cheese, September 2006 - February 2007, *Eurosurveillance*, Vol.13, No.27-39, (July-september 2008), pp. 403-407, ISSN 1560-7917

Patel, M.K., Chen, S., Pringle, J., Russo, E., Viñaras, J., Weiss, J., Anderson, S., Sunenshine, R., Komatsu, K., Schumacher, M., Flood, D., Theobald, L., Bopp, C., Wannemuehler, K., White, P., Angulo, F.J., Behravesh, C.B. (2010). A prolonged outbreak of *Salmonella* Montevideo infections associated with multiple locations of a restaurant chain in Phoenix, Arizona, 2008, *Journal of Food Protection*, Vol.73, No.10, (October 2010), pp. 1858-1063, ISSN 0362-028X

Pekova, L. (2008). An epidemic outbreak of *Salmonella* typhimurium in a Romany ethnic community--a clinical-epidemiological survey, *Acta Clinica Croatica*, Vol.47, No.1, (March 2008), pp. 9-12, ISSN:0353-9466

Pezzoli, L., Elson, R., Little, C.L., Yip, H., Fisher, I., Yishai, R., Anis, E., Valinsky, L., Biggerstaff, M., Patel, N., Mather, H., Brown, D.J., Coia, J.E., Van Pelt, W., Nielsen, E.M., Ethelberg, S., de Pinna, E., Hampton, M.D., Peters, T. & Threlfall, J. (2008). Packed with *Salmonella*--investigation of an international outbreak of *Salmonella* Senftenberg infection linked to contamination of prepacked basil in 2007, *Foodborne Pathogens and Disease*, Vol.5, No.5, (October 2008), pp. 661-668, ISSN 1535-3141

Phillips, D., Jordan, D., Morris, S., Jenson, I. & Sumner, J. (2008). A national Survey of the Microbiological Quality of Retail Raw Meats in Australia, *Journal of Food Protection*, Vol.71, No.6, (June 2008), pp. 1232-1236, ISSN 0362-028X

Prendergast, D.M., Duggan, S.J., Gonzales-Barron, U., Fanning, S., Butler, F., Cormican, M. & Duffy, G. (2009). Prevalence, numbers and characterizations of *Salmonella* spp. on Irish retail pork, *International Journal of Food Microbiology*, Vol.131, No. 2-3, (May 2009), pp. 233-239, ISSN 0168-1605

Quiroz-Santiago, C., Rodas-Suárez, O.R., Vázquez, C.R., Fernández, F.J., Quiñones-Ramírez, E.I. & Vázquez-Salinas, C. (2009). Prevalence of *Salmonella* in Vegetables from Mexico, *Journal of Food Protection*, Vol.72, No.6, (June 2009), pp. 1279-1282, ISSN 0362-028X

Reilly, W.J., Forbes, G.I., Paterson, G.M. & Sharp, J.C. (1981). Human and animal salmonellosis in Scotland associated with environmental contamination, 1973–79. *Veterinary Record*, Vol.108, No.26, (June 1981), pp 553–555, ISSN 0042-4900

Reiter, M.G., Fiorese, M.L., Moretto, G., López, M.C., Jordano, R. (2007). Prevalence of *Salmonella* in a poultry slaughterhouse, *Journal of Food Protection*, Vol.70, No.7, (July 2007), pp. 1723-1725, ISSN 0362-028X

Reynolds, A., Moffatt, C.R., Dyda, A., Hundy, R.L., Kaye, A.L., Krsteski, R., Rockliff, S., Kampen, R., Kelly, P.M. & O'Brien, E.D. (2010). An outbreak of gastroenteritis due to *Salmonella* Typhimurium phage type 170 associated with consumption of a dessert containing raw egg, *Communicable Diseases Intelligence*, Vol.34, No.3, (September 2010), pp. 329-333, ISSN 0725-3141

Roberts-Witteveen, A.R., Campbell, B.A., Merritt, T.D., Massey, P.D., Shadbolt, C.T. & Durrheim, D.N. (2009). Egg-associated *Salmonella* outbreak in an aged care facility, New South Wales, 2008, *Communicable Diseases Intelligence*, Vol.33, No.1, (March 2009), pp. 49-52, ISSN 0725-3141

Rodriguez-Urrego, J., Herrera-Leon, S., Echeita-Sarriondia, A., Soler, P., Simon, F. & Mateo, S. (2010). Nationwide outbreak of *Salmonella* serotype Kedougou associated with infant formula, Spain, 2008. *Eurosurveillance*, Vol.15, No.22, (June 2010), pp. 19-23, ISSN 1560-7917

SAGARPA (Secretaria de Agricultura, Ganadería, Recursos naturales, Pesca y Alimentación, México). 2010. Cierre de la producción agrícola por cultivo, México, In: Servicio de Información Agroalimentaria y Pesquera, 20.7.2011, Available from: http://www.siap.gob.mx/index.php?option=com_wrapper&view=wrapper&Itemid=350

Sapers, G.M., Gorny, J.R. & Yousef, A.E. (ed.). 2006. *Microbiology of Fruits and Vegetables*. ISBN 0849322618, CRC Press,. Boca Raton, FL.

Secretaria de Salud. (2011). Enfermedades Infecciosas y Parasitarias del Aparato Digestivo, In *Boletín Epidemiología. México.* 20.7.2011, Available from: http://www.dgepi.salud.gob.mx/boletin/boletin.htm

Slinko, V.G., McCall, B.J., Stafford, R.J., Bell, R.J., Hiley, L.A., Sandberg, S.M., White, S.A. & Bell, K.M. (2009). Outbreaks of *Salmonella* Typhimurium phage type 197 of multiple genotypes linked to an egg producer. *Communicable Diseases Intelligence,* Vol.33, No.4, (December 2009), pp. 419-425, ISSN 0725-3141

Sotir, M.J., Ewald, G., Kimura, A.C., Higa, J.I., Sheth, A., Troppy, S., Meyer, S., Hoekstra, R.M., Austin, J., Archer, J., Spayne, M., Daly, E.R. & Griffin, P.M. (2009). Outbreak of *Salmonella* Wandsworth and Typhimurium infections in infants and toddlers traced to a commercial vegetable-coated snack food, *The Pediatric Infectious Disease Journal,* Vol.28, No.12, (December 2009) pp. 1041-1046, ISSN 0891-3668

Takeuchi, K., Matute, C.M. Hassan, A. N. & Frank, J.F. (2000). Comparison of the Attachment of *Escherichia coli* O157:H7, *Listeria monocytogenes, Salmonella* Typhimurium, and *Pseudomonas fluorescens* to Lettuce Leaves, *Journal of Food Protection,* Vol.63, No.10, (October 2000), pp. 1433-1437, ISSN 0362-028X

Thunberg, R.L., Tran, T.T., Bennett, R.W. & Matthews, R.N. (2002). Microbial evaluation of selected fresh produce obtained at retail markets, *Journal of Food Protection,* Vol.65, No.4, (April 2002), pp. 677-682, ISSN 0362-028X

Torres-Vitela, M.R., Mendoza-Bernardo, M., Castro-Rosas, J., Gomez-Aldapa, C.A, Garay-Martinez, L.E., Navarro-Hidalgo, V., Villarruel-López A. (2011). Frequency of *Salmonella, Listeria monocytogenes, Escherichia coli* O157:H7 and staphylococcal toxin in two types of fresh cheese, *Journal of Food Protection, In press,* ISSN 0362-028X

Tunung, R., Chai, L.C., Usha, M.R., Lee, H.Y., Fatimah, A.B., Farinazleen, M.G. & Son, R. (2007). Characterization of *Salmonella enterica* isolated from street food and clinical samples in Malaysia, *ASEAN Food Journal,* Vol.14, No.3, pp. 161-173, ISSN: 01277324.

Ugbogu, O. C., Nwachukwu, N. C. & Ogbuagu, U. N. (2006). Isolation of *Salmonella* and *Shigella* species from house flies (*Musca domestica* l.) in Uturu, Nigeria, *African Journal of Biotechnology,* Vol.5, No.11, (June 2006), pp. 1090-1091, ISSN 1684–5315

Uljas, H.E. & Ingham, S.C. (1999). Combinations of intervention treatments resulting in 5-$\log_{10}$ unit reductions in numbers of *Escherichia coli* O157:H7 and *Salmonella* typhimurium DT104 organisms in apple cider, *Applied and Environmental Microbiology,* Vol.65, No.5 (May 1999), pp. 1924-1929, ISSN 0099-2240

USDA (United States Department of Agriculture). (2010). Agricultural Marketing Service, Fruit and Vegetable Programs, Market News Branch. Daily Movement Report - All F & V. 20.7.2011, Available from: http://search.ams.usda.gov/mndms/2010/01/FV20100108DDAILY_MOVE.PDF#xml=http://search.ams.usda.gov/mnsearch/hiliteinfo.aspx?i=1&docid=FV20100108DDAILY_MOVE.PDF.

Van Cauteren, D., Jourdan-da Silva, N., Weill, F.X., King, L., Brisabois, A., Delmas, G., Vaillant, V. & de Valk, H. (2009). Outbreak of *Salmonella* enterica serotype Muenster infections associated with goat's cheese, France, March 2008. *Eurosurveillance*, Vol.14, No.26-38, (July-September 2009), pp. 380-382, ISSN 1560-7917

Van Duynhoven, Y.T., Isken, L.D., Borgen, K., Besselse, M., Soethoudt, K., Haitsma, O., Mulder, B., Notermans, D.W., De Jonge, R., Kock, P., Van Pelt, W., Stenvers, O. & Van Steenbergen, J. (2009). A prolonged outbreak of *Salmonella* Typhimurium infection related to an uncommon vehicle: hard cheese made from raw milk, *Epidemiology and Infection*, Vol.137, No.11, (November 2009), pp. 1548-1557, ISSN 1469-4409

Van Kessel, J.A, Karns J.S., Lombard, J.E. & Kopral, C.A. (2011). Prevalence of *Salmonella enterica, Listeria monocytogenes*, and *Escherichia coli* Virulence Factors in Bulk Tank Milk and In-Line Filters from U.S. Dairies, *Journal of Food Protection*, Vol.74, No.5, (May 2011), pp. 759-768, ISSN 0362-028X

Van, T.T.H., Moutafis, G., Istivan, T., Tran, L.T. & Coloe, P. J. (2007). Detection of *Salmonella* spp. in retail raw food samples from Vietnam and characterization of their antibiotic resistance, *Applied and Environmental Microbiolog*, Vol.73, No.21, (November 2007), pp. 6885-6890, ISSN 0099-2240

Whelan, J., Noel, H., Friesema, I., Hofhuis, A., de Jager, C.M., Heck, M., Heuvelinkm A. & Van Pelt, W. (2010). National outbreak of *Salmonella* Typhimurium (Dutch) phage-type 132 in the Netherlands, October to December 2009, *Eurosurveillance*, Vol.15, No.44, (November 2010), pp. 6-10, ISSN 1560-7917

Wong, D. M. A.L. F., Hald, T., Wolf, P.J.v.d. & Swanenburg, M. (2002). Epidemiology and control measures for *Salmonella* in pigs and pork, *Livestock Production Science*, Vol.76, No.3, (September 2002), pp. 215-222, ISSN 0301-6226

Wong, T.L., Nicol, C., Cook, R. & MacDiarmid, S. (2007). *Salmonella* in uncooked retail meats in New Zealand, *Journal of Food Protection*, Vol.70, No.6, (June 2007), pp. 1360-1365, ISSN 0362-028X

Yang, B., Qu, D., Zhang, X., Shen, J., Cui, S., Shi, Y., Xi, M., Sheng, M., Zhi, S. & Meng, J. (2010). Prevalence and characterization of *Salmonella* serovars in retail meats of marketplace in Shaanxi, China, *International Journal of Food Microbiology*, Vol.141, No. 1-2, (June 2010), pp. 63-72, ISSN 0168-1605

Yang, H.H., Gong, J., Zhang, J., Wang, M.L., Yang, J., Wu, G.Z., Quan, W.L., Gong, H.M., Szu, S.C. (2010). An outbreak of *Salmonella* Paratyphi A in a boarding school: a community-acquired enteric fever and carriage investigation, *Epidemiology and Infection*, Vol.138, No.12, (December 2010), pp. 1765-1774, ISSN 1469-4409

Zhuang, R.Y., Beuchat, L.R., & Angulo, F.J. (1995). Fate of *Salmonella montevideo* on and in raw tomatoes as affected by temperature and treatment with chlorine, *Applied and Environmental Microbiology*, Vol.61, No.6 (June 1995), pp. 2127-2131, ISSN 0099-2240

# 3

# Food as Cause of Human Salmonellosis

Valerio Giaccone, Paolo Catellani and Leonardo Alberghini
*Faculty of Veterinary Medicine, University of Padua*
*Italy*

## 1. Introduction

Foodborne salmonellosis is still today a serious public health issue: very common in poor developing countries, due to the bad general hygiene conditions, it is also largely widespread in developed countries. In the latter, 95% of recorded clinical cases are foodborne (Liu *et al.*, 2011). According to EFSA epidemiological data (2011), in the European Union (EU) *Salmonella* is the second cause of foodborne disease after *Campylobacter* and it is still first in many EU States, such as Italy. Unlike *Campylobacter*, *Salmonella* often cause very large *multistate outbreaks* of food infection; this proves the greater resistance of this pathogen in the external environment and in food. In developed countries the main source of salmonellosis is still today food of animal origin, particularly meat (fresh and processed) and shell eggs. Also fresh fruits and vegetables can convey the bacteria to humans, as well as undrinkable water. *Salmonella* is quite resistant to adverse conditions and this allows them to persist in the environment and spread along the food chain, from the animals to the food of animal origin, or to plants that are fertilized with animal manure. Two species are currently registered into the genus *Salmonella*: *S. enterica* and *S. bongori*. The former is better adapted than the latter to live in the intestine of man and warm-blooded animals, whereas *S. bongori* travels in the external environment and is detectable in the intestinal contents of warm-blooded animals, so it is rare for it to be found in food for human consumption. The dangers for human health mainly arise from food contaminated with *Salmonella enterica*, which is often present in the intestines of livestock and pets, without causing any infection to the animals ("healthy carrier" condition). Humans can be healthy carriers of *S. enterica* in the intestine too. This may be a potential hazard to food hygiene, if the healthy carriers are the people involved in producing and handling the food. Usually a healthy carrier eliminates *Salmonella* in their faeces for several months after the episode of gastroenteritis through which they became carrier. In the case of *Salmonella* ser. Typhi, however, it has been demonstrated that humans can be asymptomatic carriers of the bacterium for decades (Weill, 2009). The genus *Salmonella* has more than 2,500 serotypes, and over 1,600 of these are within the *enterica* species, but not all serotypes have the same affinity for human and/or animals and they are not all found in the food that humans consume. Some serotypes (Typhy, Paratyphi A and C, some clones of Paratyphi B and Sendai) travel almost exclusively among men, and express their pathogenicity only when they infect a human being. Few serotypes travel exclusively among animals and do not infect humans, if not seldom (e.g. Abortusovis in sheep and Gallinarum-Pullorum in poultry). On the contrary, approximately 150 serotypes travel more or less constantly between the animal reservoir, the environment, food and man, starting from *Salmonella* ser. Typhimurium. Some serotypes, however, have a particular preference for some animal species: Enteritidis, Hadar, Heidelberg, Saintpaul,

Virchow, Senftenberg, Infantis and Kottbus find their main distribution channel in chickens, turkeys and ducks; Dublin and Bovismorbificans mainly infect cattle, while the Derby, Brandenburg and Panama serotypes frequently circulate among pigs (Weill, 2009). From the intestinal contents of livestock, the salmonellae can contaminate fresh meat, raw milk and egg shells. If the necessary hygienic precautions are not taken in the early stages of the production line (slaughter, milking, egg collecting), there is a risk that the salmonellae may then spread along each of their production chain, even polluting products such as cured meats, dairy products and egg-based dishes if they were made using raw milk or unpasteurized eggs. Moreover, through the faeces of animals and man, salmonellae can contaminate farmland, surface water flow and vegetables if they are fertilized with animal manure or dung that is not properly fermented. Vegetables, therefore, can be a source of disease to humans just like fresh meat, milk, shell eggs and by-products. Besides in animals, *Salmonella* can adhere well to the work surfaces, and from there spread to other foodstuffs by cross-contamination (Møretrø *et al.*, 2011). The examples are numerous and blatant: in the U.S. a major *Salmonella* ser. Enteritidis outbreak occurred and was associated with the consumption of industrial ice cream premix which was transported in tanks that had been used for carrying unpasteurized liquid eggs and were not properly sanitized (Hennessy *et al.*, 1996). An outbreak of salmonellosis due to *S.* Ealing caused by dehydrated powdered milk was traced back to the inadequate sanitization of production equipment (Rowe *et al.*, 1987). The thorough cleaning of work surfaces, both in food manufacturing facilities and in domestic kitchens, is therefore one of the main strategies for the prevention of foodborne salmonellosis (Møretrø et al., 2011). Generally, forms of gastroenteritis caused by non-typhoid *Salmonella* are moderately serious diseases with a quick recovery and without the need to resort to specific therapies. Although in some cases – when young children, elderly, or immunocompromised subjects are affected – salmonellosis may also lead to the patient's death (Pathan *et al.*, 2010). The severity of *Salmonella* infections can also be aggravated by the fact that in recent years more and more *Salmonella* strains have been spreading and they are resistant to one or more of the antibiotics which are widely used in human medicine, such as fluoroquinolones and third generation cephalosporins. In addition to the Typhimurium serotype, *Salmonella* strains which are multiresistant to many antibiotics have also been detected in the Agona, Anatum, Choleraesuis, Derby, Dublin, Heidelberg, Kentucky, Newport, Pullorum, Schwarzengrund, Senftenberg, and Uganda serotypes (Yan *et al.*, 2010). In most cases, human infection manifests itself through diarrhoea, persistent fever and abdominal cramps which appear 12 to 72 hours after the infection. The disease is self-limiting and clears up by itself within 4-7 days, but it has rather significant side effects: it takes months for the patient to regain proper bowel function and they can remain healthy carriers for months. In addition, chronic complications may occur such as widespread polyarthritis (Reiter's syndrome), ocular and urinary disorders, and even occasional cases of endocarditis and appendicitis. All these diseases are hard to treat even with antibiotics (Castillo *et al.*, 2011).

### 1.2 The infective dose "issue"

According to the regulations currently in force in the European Union, it is the manufacturer's responsibility to ensure the hygiene of their production processes on a daily basis, seeing to prevent any possible *hazard* that may contaminate food and be harmful to human health. The system used by food manufacturers to control processing hygiene in their facilities is the well-known HACCP system. In view of the fundamental principles of HACCP, if *Salmonella* contaminates a food, this is a *Hazard* because its presence could potentially cause harm to human health. It is, however, a hypothetical danger, as, for it to become real, the food has to present some specific conditions. One of these is certainly the "minimal infective dose", i.e. the lowest charge that *Salmonella* must reach in the food for it to become dangerous to human health. Generally, it is accepted that *Salmonella* becomes truly dangerous for humans when it reaches in a food a charge of at least $10^4$ cfu/g. However, it should be reminded that the bibliography reports some foodborne salmonellosis outbreaks caused by foods that contained less than 100 and sometimes less than 10 cfu of bacteria per gram of product. Fatty foods, such as cheeses, butter and chocolate, better protect the bacteria from the digestive enzymes in the stomach. In addition, the low water activity of these foods keeps the salmonellae in a latent phase, and this means that they do not proliferate in the food substrate, but can survive for very long time (Jansson *et al.*, 2011; Finstad *et al.*, 2011). The infective charge in one episode of salmonellosis which occurred in Canada and was caused by chocolate was estimated as low as 0,005 cfu/g (Komitopoulou & Penaloza, 2009). It is important to underline that the foods contaminated with Salmonella do not usually show any modification in their sensory characteristics even though the pathogens within have reached very high levels, concretely harmful to human health (Lindhardt *et al.*, 2009).

### 1.3 Epidemiology of foodborne human salmonellosis in the EU

According to the latest "European Union Summary Report on Trends and Sources of Zoonoses, Zoonotic Agents and Food-borne Outbreaks" (EFSA, 2011), in 2009 in the 27 EU Member States, the health authorities in charge have reported a total of 108,614 confirmed cases of human salmonellosis, with a prevalence of 23.7 cases/100,000 population. If we compare these levels with their equivalents reported from 2005 onwards, we discover that in the 2005/2009 period the cases of human salmonellosis have considerably dropped, estimated at -13%. In comparison, cases of campylobacteriosis have increased by +12%. In particular, between 2008 and 2009 there was a sharp decline in clinical cases of human salmonellosis caused by *Salmonella* ser. Enteritidis. All this indicates that the efforts made by health authorities and policies of individual EU states are obtaining positive and effective results. Furthermore, if we analyze the data regarding the spread of *Salmonella* among farm animals, we can find out that the importance of *Salmonella* as a cause of human foodborne disease is decreasing, also thanks to the decline in the spread of bacteria among livestock, starting with fowl. The decline in cases of foodborne salmonellosis among human beings does not tend to be consistent or regular in all 27 EU Members. The variations in the epidemiological pattern can be noticeable from one State to another. 10 states recorded a significant decline in cases; for 14 other states (including Italy) the epidemiological situation of human salmonellosis in food has remained essentially stable over the past five years, while Malta reported a sharp rise in cases (+24% compared to 2008), in contrast with the rest of the EU countries. Scandinavian and Central European countries are among the member states with the highest prevalence of human cases of foodborne salmonellosis while prevalence of salmonellosis among the population reported by the states bordering the Mediterranean are well below the previous. Epidemiologists interpret this as a sign of the single EU members' health authorities' increased awareness about the health of the populations under their responsibility. This increased attention to identify and report cases of foodborne salmonellosis explains the higher prevalence of human cases of salmonellosis in some northern European countries compared with the levels observed in Southern European countries. In most EU states food salmonellosis is a disease that patients contract "in their own country". Only Sweden, Finland, Denmark and the UK count a number of cases imported from abroad because they were contracted by people when they were out of the country. It should, however, be pointed out that some of the EU countries were not able to ascertain and report to the EFSA the proportion of "national" cases of salmonellosis and those "acquired" from abroad. We would like to recall that in 2005 the EU issued the 2073/2005 (EC) Regulation which identified the *food safety criteria* for some of the major food groups most at risk of transmitting diseases to man. *Salmonella* was adopted as a parameter for the safety of fresh meat and products derived from it, raw milk and dairy products made with it, edible bivalve molluscs, as well as for pre-cut fruits and vegetables. In accordance with the EU provisions, *Salmonella* must be absent from 25 or 10 grams of examined sample of these foods in order for them to be destined for human consumption. In the EU which foodstuffs did not comply with this criterion and exceeded it? In 2009, as in 2008, the highest percentage of non-compliance was found in food derived from fresh meat, and particularly from minced meat and meat preparations containing chicken or turkey (8.7% of the total non-complying foods). Secondly, in order of prevalence, are bivalve molluscs and echinoderms, which are often traditionally consumed raw or hardly cooked (3.4% of all samples). Much less at risk are currently liquid eggs which go through a pasteurization process before entering the food manufacturing industry. Some concern arises from the fact that there are rather large percentages of non-compliance even among meat preparations for raw human consumption (the samples tested positive for *Salmonella* during official tests ranged from 1,2% to 1,7 % of the total tested samples).

## 2. Animals as *Salmonella* reservoir

The transmission cycle of *Salmonella* to humans through food presents many complexities because it involves animal reservoirs, vector food and the environment (Graziani *et al.*, 2005). Mammals, birds, rodents, reptiles, amphibians and insects act as environmental reservoirs of *Salmonella* and can transfer the pathogen to man (D'Aoust, 2007). On intensive farming facilities the role of the "healthy carriers" is important: even if they do not show any symptoms of the disease, they contaminate the environment and contribute to spreading salmonellae on the farm, sometimes creating endemic situations. The absence of symptoms in most of the infected animals and the technical difficulties in detecting the carriers during the inspection of the meat cause a continuous contamination of foods of animal origin.

Graziani *et al.* (2005) argue that various *Salmonella* serotypes may prefer various animal species: some are considered specific to one animal species (S. Gallinarum in chickens), others are defined as "host-adapted" because they prefer one host over another (S. Dublin for cattle, S. Enteritidis in egg-laying hens, S. Hadar in birds); on the other hand, other serotypes, such as S. Typhimurium, are ubiquitous. The role as reservoir is played by many animal species, but poultry and pigs are the predominant reservoirs for *Salmonella* (Cantoni & Bersani, 2010). In birds, species-specific serotypes are present, such as S. Pullorum and S. Gallinarum (Cantoni & Ripamonti, 1998), as well as host-adapted serotypes, such as S. Hadar and S. Enteritidis in chickens in Italy, while S. Blockley is found more predominantly in turkeys (Graziani *et al.*, 2005). The importance of broilers and other farm birds as *Salmonella* reservoirs should not be underestimated (D'Aoust, 2007). Although *S.* Pullorum and *S.* Gallinarum have been eradicated from industrial production thanks to *in loco* monitoring and eradication programs in reproducers, it is known that infections by S. Enteritidis and S. Typhimurium have been quite common in farm birds recently, therefore strict hygiene rules must be followed to prevent the contamination of finished products.

For pigs, the pathogenic salmonellae are *S.* Choleraesuis and S. Typhi suis (Cantoni & Ripamonti, 1998). Over the past ten years a marked increase in the prevalence of *S. enterica* serovar 4, [5], 12:i- has been observed in many European countries (Hopkins *et al.*, 2010). It is resistant to ampicillin, streptomycin, sulphonamides and tetracycline in food-borne infections, in pigs and pork. The results indicate that genetically related strains of serovar 4, [5], 12:i:- of the DT193 and DT120 phage types with resistance to ampicillin, streptomycin, sulphonamides and tetracycline have emerged in many European countries and that pigs are the likely reservoir of the infection. A survey by the European Food Safety Authority has established the prevalence of *Salmonella* in pigs for slaughter in the EU-25 plus Norway (EFSA, 2008). This survey, as well as discovering that one pig every ten is affected, also identified the prevalent serotypes in infected pigs (*S.* Typhimurium and *S.* Derby), the same ones as in the cases of human infection.

Cattle are often colonized by S. Dublin and S. Typhimurium, with infections that vary in duration and clinical manifestation (Graziani *et al.*, 2005). Cattle are particularly susceptible to infection by *Salmonella* in the first weeks of life (Cantoni & Ripamonti, 1998). S. Dublin can stay in the host for a long time, in some cases all its life and often causes serious bouts of illness (Graziani *et al.*, 2005). As healthy carriers, they can pass S. Dublin and S. Typhimurium in their faeces, and those can remain viable in the outside for at least six months (Cantoni & Ripamonti, 1998).

In the meat-processing industry, eggs and poultry meat are the main groups of raw materials which usually carry *Salmonella* (D'Aoust & Maurer, 2007) and in many States they overshadow other sources such as pork, beef and mutton as a means of infection (WHO, 1988). To conclude, we can say that the biological cycle of *Salmonella* spp. is complex (see Table 1) and involves animals, environment and food (D'Aoust & Maurer, 2007), and that animals act as the most important reservoirs for its conservation (Graziani et al., 2005).

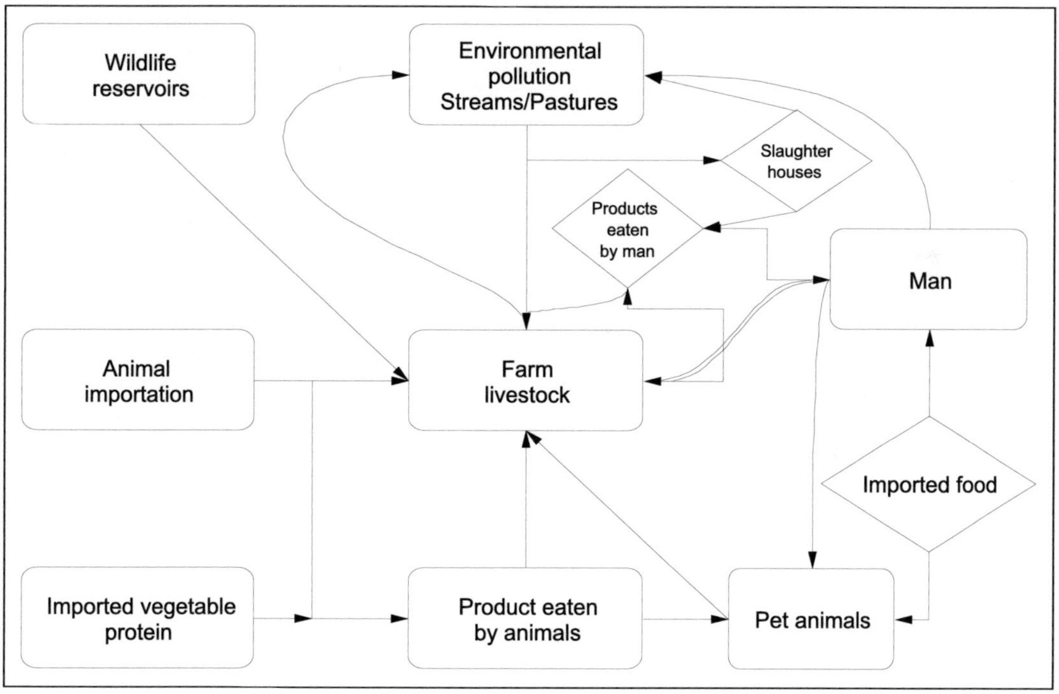


Table 1. *Salmonella* life cycle and transmission to humans (adapted from WHO, 1988).

## 3. Dynamics of the *Salmonella* population: Ecological factors

Foods are generally considered ecosystems made up of a habitat and a community of living organisms (biocenosis) that can influence each other and, in turn, be influenced by the habitat itself. Given the minute size of the microorganisms, the environment that affects them, at least in a solid matrix, is very small - of the order of a few millimeters or centimeters - so very heterogeneous physical and chemical conditions can exist in food (different conditions between the surface and the inside). In addition, a succession of microbial communities can be observed in food. The original microbial load, largely depending on the initial sources of contamination, is then replaced by new microbial communities that depend on the set of factors that appear during production and conservation processes. The factors that influence the development and survival of contaminating microorganisms are: (i) intrinsic factors, i.e. the characteristics of the food, arising from its composition or structure, pH levels, water activity ($A_w$) and redox potential (OR-value); (ii) environmental, extrinsic factors which come into action during the processing or storage of the food (storage or treatment temperature; relative humidity, light, storage environment); they may affect the intrinsic factors; (iii) implicit factors derive from the interaction between populations during manufacturing or storage. They can either be positive, such as mutualism and commensalism, or negative, such as competition, antagonism and parasitism.

Although it is possible to control the growth or survival of an individual or a group of microorganisms acting on only one of these factors, this is not always desirable, because it could have excessive consequences on the sensorial and nutritional qualities of food. As modern consumers are increasingly in demand of foods that look "natural" or "fresh", that are safe and have a relatively long shelf life, it is often necessary to act using a combination of factors, each of which is present at sublethal levels, but that, together, ensure the desired level of control. Therefore, instead of using a single barrier, combinations of barriers are used (the so called "hurdle effect") which cause, if the exposure to these conditions is prolonged, such damage that the microorganisms irreparably lose the ability to multiply, reaching their inactivation. *Vice versa*, if the microorganisms are subjected to lower levels of stress (sublethal conditions), they can adapt by activating a number of protection mechanisms, synthesizing proteins and other substances that improve their resistance to the stress in question or different stress. In recent decades, specific mathematical models have been implemented to describe the phenomena such as the growth, the production of metabolites and the death of the microorganisms found in various conditions, useful both for the conservation and for the hygienic safety of food. Predictive models, in particular, see to formulate mathematical models using adequate experimental designs which should provide information about the danger or conservation of food and about the possibility of growth, death or production of a toxin from pathogenic microorganisms. So, in view of the previous observations, we can predict microbial behaviour in similar environmental conditions (Ross & McMeekin, 1994). These approaches, however, are not disadvantage free, such as the variation of strains and the biomolecular knowledge for understanding which factors are responsible for pathogenicity. As regards *Salmonella* the ranges of the factors that favour their growth, death or survival are shown in **Table 2**.

| Conditions | Minimum | Optimum | Maximum |
|---|---|---|---|
| T °C | 7.0 (5.2 *) | 35-43 | 46.2 (49.3 *) |
| pH | 4.00 (3.80 *) | 7.00-7.50 | 9.50 |
| $A_w$ | 0.940 (0.900 *) | -- | -- |
| Tolerance to salt (%) | -- | -- | 4 |

Table 2. Limits and optimum growth in relation to intrinsic and extrinsic factors for Salmonella spp. Notes. *: Some serotypes. (Source: ICMSF, 1996; amended).

**Temperature**

In particular, we can say that the minimum temperature for the growth of *Salmonella* is 7 °C (at 8 °C generation time is 22-35 hours); under 15 °C its development is still low. The storage of food at temperatures below 5 °C therefore prevents the multiplication of all serotypes; the only one able to develop up to 5.3 °C is *S.* Heidelberg (Matches & Liston, 1968). The highest mortality occurs during the slow freezing phase (0 to -10 °C), while in the deep-freezing one, for reaching temperatures below -17 °C rapidly, its survival is more likely, as damage to the cell membrane is minor. However, freezing does not guarantee the destruction of *Salmonella*: they have been found in frozen foods stored for years (ICMSF, 1996; Farkas, 1997), due to the changes and the production of cold shock and cold acclimation proteins (Scherer & Neuhaus, 2002). Maximum development temperature is 49.3 °C, beyond which *Salmonella* begin to die due to the denaturation of cell wall components and to the inactivation of heat-sensible enzymes. Although a temperature of 55 °C is sufficient to kill them, the legal limit for the storage of cooked foods meant to be eaten hot is normally 63 °C. *Salmonella* is not particularly resistant, so a pasteurization process is more than enough to destroy it. Several authors agree that the most heat-resistant serotype is *S.* Senftenberg 775W which registers $D_{65}$= 0.29-2.0 and $D_{60}$=1.0-9.0 when the substrate is in normal conditions, but the D value decreases if you move away from the optimal range for growth. Finally, its z value is 5,6-6,4 (°C). Resistance to heat is influenced by other factors, such as:

1. water activity: the lower it is, the greater the pathogen's heat resistance, since the presence of water favours the thermal break of the peptide bonds and in their absence more energy is needed for achieving the same result;
2. the composition of the food, and its fat content, which enhance its resistance, as well as the glycerol or sucrose contents;
3. pH levels, which, if maintained at around neutrality, allow for greater heat resistance of the pathogen, whereas sensitivity increases if it is lowered or raised;
4. the age of the microbial cells, since the young ones are more sensitive to heat in logarithmic growth phase;
5. adaptation to high incubation temperatures, for a genetic selection that favours the development of strains which are more resistant to heat (Jay, 1996).

**Water activity ($A_w$)**

Minimum water activity is 0,940, below which multiplication does not cease, but the bacterial charge decreases, without disappearing though. *Salmonella* can survive for long periods in conditions of dehydration. This was detected several times in sweets, including chocolate, which led to outbreaks of food infection (Werber *et al.*, 2005). In fact, the high fat and sugar content of sweet, may lead to a protective effect against it. Of course, in chocolate, there cannot be any growth, but rather a sublethal stress which leads to an adaptation of the pathogen (Jasson *et al.*, 2011). In the presence of NaCl concentrations between 3 and 4%, the development of *Salmonella* is usually inhibited. However, it appears that the inhibitory action of salt increases with increasing storage temperature. Variations depending on the serotype can be noticed (ICSFM, 1996).

**pH value**

The minimum pH is 3.80, but it all depends on the type of acid used, among which acetic acid seems to be more effective. Over the past twenty years, the survival of *Salmonella* under varying conditions of acid stress (Acid Tolerance Response ATR) has been extensively studied, especially regarding sublethal exposure with organic acids, which make the pathogen adapt to the acid used. The complex molecular mechanisms and environmental factors involved in ATR have been studied. An interesting discussion on this topic can be found in the article by Álvarez-Ordóñez *et al.* (2011). The increase in resistance to acids is very consistent, not only for the chances of survival of *Salmonella* in food, but also because it can lead the pathogen to resist to gastric pH (<1.5) and thus pass through the intestine unharmed. Generally speaking, we can say that *Salmonella* is very sensitive to acetic acid and lactic acid, while it is much more resistant to citric acid, used to acidify foods. In turn, these acids are more active if storage or treatment temperatures are close to the pathogen's minimum or maximum values of growth. Finally, we also have to underline that the acidification and/or heat treatment should not be applied to food in sublethal conditions, in order to avoid adaptation phenomena of pathogenic strains to the same treatment or even to different treatments (salt, water activity, etc.). Leyer & Johnson (1993) tested a strain of adapted to acid *S.* Typhimurium by constantly lowering the pH, finding out that the adaptation was not only due to the rebalance of intracellular pH, but also to a change in membrane proteins and not in the lipopolysaccharidic component.

**Disinfectants**

An incorrect method of disinfection and sanitization can make *Salmonella* persist on tools and utensils used in the food industry and kitchens, with the ability to form *biofilm* and, therefore, enable the spread of the pathogen.

Møretrø *et al.* (2009), using a treatment with a concentration of 100 ppm chlorine or 50 ppm of iodine for 15 minutes, noticed a biofilm can be completely removed, while with sodium hypochlorite (approximately 400 ppm) or cationic surfactants (benzalkonium chloride) for 5 minutes, *Salmonella* biofilm can resist on stainless steel surfaces. 70% ethanol for 5 min. is unable to remove the biofilm (Ramesh *et al.*, 2002).

## 4. *Salmonella* in vegetables

Compared to foods of animal origin, which are usually consumed once cooked, fruit and vegetables are mostly eaten raw and therefore a significant part of foodborne outbreaks due to the consumption of raw vegetables has been attributed to *Salmonella* (Cantoni & Bersani, 2010). Animal faeces and irrigation water are the main ways for *Salmonella* to spread to crops (Islam *et al.*, 2004). The water can contaminate the food if it is used for irrigation, for washing or for handling it (Rondanelli *et al.*, 2005). The salmonellae present in not perfectly ripened manure or in irrigation water invade the plants by gripping to the roots or contaminating the leaves (Cantoni & Bersani, 2010). Studies headed by Professor

Gadi Frankel (2008) of the Imperial College, London, UK, have revealed how salmonellae use their flagella to stick to salad and basil leaves. The results were presented at the 21st ICFMH International Symposium "Food Micro 2008" held in Aberdeen. This ability to attach itself to vegetables is described for a certain strain, *S. enterica* ser. Senftenberg, but not for *S.* Typhimurium (Frankel, 2009). Increased understanding of the mechanism that pathogens such as *Salmonella* use to adhere to vegetables is important if scientists are to develop new methods to prevent this type of contamination and the disease it causes (Berger *et al.*, 2010). Schikora *et al.* (2008) have shown that *S.* Typhimurium, until now considered dangerous only for animals, can be a real danger for the vegetable kingdom too. Like any other plant pathogen, *S.* Typhimurium triggers the plant's immune defences and does not just cover the root surface, but enters physically into the plant's cells. The researchers attached a fluorescent probe to the bacterium and injected it, following its route: in just 17 hours the root cells were infected. Moreover, the infection later occurred simply by placing the plant (*Arabidopsis*) and the bacterium in the same liquid. *Salmonella* strains were detected in: aubergines, green salads, fennel, lettuce, onions, mustard, orange juice, pepper, parsley, spinach, strawberries, tomatoes, watermelons, coconuts, cereals, barley, chocolate and soy sauce (Cantoni & Bersani, 2010; Cantoni & Ripamonti, 1998). Today more and more ready-to-eat (RTE) vegetables are available in supermarket fridges because they are offered to the consumer as a convenience food, every part can be used, and, being already washed, peeled and chopped, they are quick and easy to prepare (Catellani *et al.*, 2005). For their packing, various techniques are used, such as modified atmosphere packaging (MAP) – the gaseous composition of which varies according to the vegetable –, vacuum packaging, and ordinary atmosphere packaging. For the first two methods, the product should be packaged at refrigeration temperature, while with ordinary atmosphere it just needs to be kept cool. $CO_2$ has the function to slow the breathing and the appearance of rotting, to inhibit pectinolytic enzymes and the development of *Pseudomonas* and other Gram-negative bacteria (Galli & Franzetti, 1998). Manvell & Ackland (1986) show that RTE vegetables can host various saprophytic microbial forms: 80-90% are Gram negative spoiling bacteria (including *Pseudomonas* spp, *Enterobacter* spp, *Erwinia* spp) and the rest are yeasts and moulds. If Good Manufacture Practices are respected, pathogens (*Salmonella* spp., *L. monocytogenes*, *E. coli* O157, enterovirus) or protozoa (*Giardia*, *Entamoeba*, *Cryptosporidium*) are detected only occasionally (Catellani *et al.*, 2005). The study of *Salmonella* has dramatically contributed to the knowledge of the epidemiology of these infections. Large-scale distribution, particularly of fruit and vegetables, sets the conditions for events that touch a very wide area, involve the exposure of a big number of individuals, and that are difficult to recognize for lack of sophisticated surveillance systems that should involve international collaboration networks.

## 5. *Salmonella* in eggs and egg products

Eggs laid by healthy animals are generally safe to eat because if they kept in sound hygiene conditions they can be considered almost sterile inside, especially as regards bacterial agents of food diseases (Bozzo, 2008; Galli & Neviani, 2005). Nevertheless, *Salmonella* spp. is the most important pathogen transmitted by eggs (ICMSF, 1998). The natural defence factors that may affect the egg's infection by microbiological contaminations are:

- *physical factors*: cuticle, shell, shell membranes, viscosity of the albumen and chalazae,

- *chemical factors*: pH of the albumen, lysozyme, avidin, flavoprotein, protease inhibitor protein molecules (ovostatin, ovomucoid, cystatin, etc.).

In addition to the factors mentioned above, we must add the environmental protection factors that are related to hygiene: egg-laying place, litter, surfaces, air, handlings, shell, duration and means of storage. The eggs can, however, be infected transovarianly with *Salmonella* by sick hens or healthy carriers (Cantoni & Ripamonti, 1998). There are many cases reported in the literature in which *Salmonella* was detected in eggs laid by hens with ovarian localization of this pathogen (in this case we speak about "endogenous contamination") (Bozzo, 2008). Through good hygiene practices in breeding facilities, it is possible to limit the number of microorganisms on the shell, as more than 90% of the contaminations of various origins occur after egg laying (Gandini, 1993). These *exogenous contaminations* of the egg can occur at different times: during transport or packaging or during the shelling (Bozzo, 2008). There is evidence (EFSA, 2009b) to indicate that cross-contamination between egg shells may occur during the manufacturing processes (sorting of the eggs, packing, etc.). The probability of this cross-contamination depends on the percentage of eggs contaminated with *Salmonella*, and the prevalence of eggs tested positive for *Salmonella* is also affected by the type of technology used and hygiene practices applied. However, the authors argue that we lack sufficient data to evaluate the occurrence of penetration through the shell and the proliferation of *Salmonella* due to cross- contamination during processing and, therefore, to assess the risks for consumers. The factors that influence the passage of microorganisms into the egg are: dampness, the shell's degree of contamination, the age-related decline in physical defences of the hen and the type of dirt that causes changes in surface tension (Galli & Neviani, 2005). Table eggs are pointed at as a major source of *Salmonella* and egg refrigeration has been recommended as one of many possible measures along the food chain to reduce the incidence of salmonellosis in the human population (EFSA, 2009b). The panel of experts on biological hazards states that refrigerating table eggs to temperatures at or below 7 °C limits the multiplication of pathogens such as *Salmonella*. If the cold chain is maintained, starting the refrigeration already on the farm is the measure with the highest positive effect in order to limit the proliferation of *Salmonella*. Table egg refrigeration is another safety measure together with other steps taken on the farm and during the processing as part of an integrated approach. Interruption of the cold chain is a factor that increases the risk of condensation and this may increase the penetration of bacteria into the egg (Ricci, 2005). The Salmonella infection cycle in poultry farms is summarized in **Table 3**. As stated in the EU Summary Report on trends and sources of zoonoses, zoonotic agents and resistance to antimicrobiotics (EFSA, 2007), the reported cases of human salmonellosis in the EU, respectively amounted to 154,099 and 31.1/100,000 inhabitants. The report also indicates that the prevalence of *Salmonella* in table eggs was 0.8%. According to the opinion of the European Scientific Committee on veterinary measures related to Public Health on *Salmonella* in food products in 2003, eggs and food produced with raw eggs (unpasteurized) are among the food categories most likely to cause cases of human salmonellosis (EFSA 2009). In Sweden, de Jong & Ekdhal (2006) compared the EFSA data on the prevalence of *Salmonella* on European egg-laying hen farms and the prevalence of human salmonellosis, revealing a high linear correlation between the two aspects. The same study analyzed the cases of salmonellosis in travellers returning to Sweden after having been to several European countries with different *Salmonella* prevalence. The research seems to confirm the existence of a clear causal link between the presence of salmonellae in the egg production chain and the human disease. In Spain, Soler Crespo *et al.* (2005) focused on foodborne infections associated with the intake of eggs and egg products between 2002 and 2003. These outbreaks alone would account for 41% of all the episodes of food poisoning recorded throughout the duration of the study. The risk factors most often identified by the authors are the storage of the products at excessively high temperatures, the consumption of raw foods and a too long wait between the preparation and the consumption of the food. **Table 4** shows some events in epidemic proportions observed in recent decades in various parts of the world. These epidemics serve as a constant reminder of the fact that food technology cannot always protect against infectious diseases that may result in large-scale epidemics (multistate outbreaks) (Winn *et al.*, 2009). In the United States, however, the introduction of a program for egg safety and quality (egg quality assurance programs [EQAPs]) plays an important role in reducing disease by *S.* Enteritidis transmitted from eggs (Mumma *et al.*, 2004).

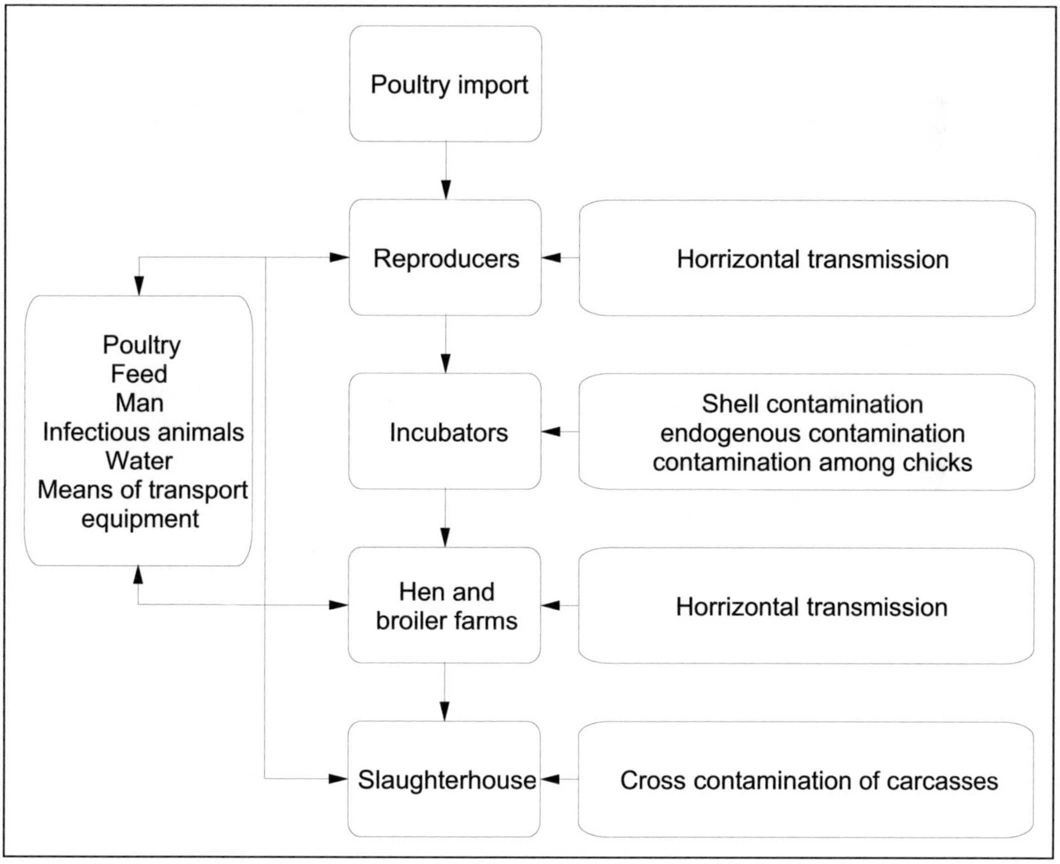


Table 3. *Salmonella* infection cycle in poultry farming.

| Year | Country | Product | Serovar | Cases[a] | Deaths |
|---|---|---|---|---|---|
| 1976 | Spain | Egg salad | Typhimurium | 702 | 6 |
| 1977 | Sweden | Mustard dressing | Enteritidis PT 4 | 2865 | 0 |
| 1987 | People's Republic of China | Egg drink | Typhimurium | 1113 | NS[b] |
| 1988 | Japan | Cooked eggs | *Salmonella* spp. | 10476 | NS |
| 1993 | France | Mayonnaise | Enteritidis | 751 | 0 |
| 2001 | United States | Tuna salad with eggs | Enteritidis | 688 | 0 |
| 2001 | Latvia | Cake/raw egg sauce | Enteritidis PT 4 | 19 | 0 |
| 2002 | Spain | Custard-filled pastry | Enteritidis PT 6 | 1433 | 0 |
| 2002 | England | Bakery products | Enteritidis PT 14 | >150 | 1 |
| 2003 | England, Wales, Scotland | Egg sandwiches | Bareilly | 186 | NS |
| 2003 | Australia | Raw egg mayonnaise | *Salmonella* spp. | >106 | 1 |
| 2003 | United States | Egg salad kit | Typhimurium | 18 | 0 |
| 2004 | People's Republic of China | Cake/raw egg topping | Enteritidis | 197 | NS |
| 2005 | England | Imported shell eggs | Enteritidis PT 6 | 68 | 0 |

[a] Confirmed cases, unless stated otherwise.

[b] Not stated

(Adapted from: D'Aoust. J.Y. & Maurer J., 2007)

Table 4. Examples of outbreaks of human salmonellosis from eggs and egg products

## 6. *Salmonella* in meat and meat products

Meat includes all the edible parts of slaughtered warm-blooded animals, fit for human consumption. According to the EC Regulation 853/2004, this includes domestic ungulates (cattle, pigs, sheep and domestic equines), poultry, farmed lagomorphs (rabbits, hares), farmed game and hunted venison. It is called *fresh* meat if it has not undergone any treatment to extend its shelf life, except for the use of cold (refrigeration, freezing, deep freezing). Vacuum-packed meat and meat packed in a protective atmosphere are also considered fresh. Due to its chemical composition and to its intrinsic characteristics ($A_w$ above 0.99, pH between 5.5 and 5.8), fresh meat is a good substrate for microbial growth. For this reason, cooling after slaughter is a critical point because it determines the microbiological quality of the product and must occur as fast as possible (internal temperature ≤ 7 °C, within 24-30 hours following slaughter). The flesh of healthy and unstrained animals is devoid of microorganisms in depth; but due to stress before slaughter, disease, or weakness, microbial contamination can occur and is defined as endogenous: pathogens, in particular starting from the intestine, spread into the blood due to the failing immune system, and reach the muscles, lymph nodes and internal organs. Among these microorganisms, there may also be *Salmonella*, if it is present in the intestinal contents. In this case, after the analytical laboratory investigations requested by the Veterinary Inspector, carcasses must be confiscated and destroyed, as they represent a potential danger to the consumer. On the other hand, the main microbial contamination occurs during the various stages of butchering and cutting, as well as in the following stages, such as the preparation one (minced meat, sausages, kebabs, etc.) and processing (salami mixture), until the purchase and the preservation of meat products before consumption. This contamination, defined as exogenous, is inevitable, but, by applying good manufacturing practices, it can be successfully controlled. The slaughtering stage which can lead to greater contamination by *Salmonella* is the gutting, where the release of feces even if it is limited (from $10^{10}$ to $10^{12}$ cfu/g microorganisms depending on the animals) results in the contamination of more or less large parts of the carcass. The main animal species that can host *Salmonella* spp. in their intestine, in descending order, are farmed birds, pigs and cattle. Meat is no doubt the food that undergoes the greatest number of tests, imposed by strict rules: on-farm veterinary visits, certificates accompanying the animals during its transport to slaughter, *ante mortem* and *post mortem* inspections, the scalding of the carcass (domestic ungulates and big game) that makes it fit for human consumption; followed by tests in the next stages (butchering facilities, butcher shops, supermarkets, meat-processing facilities, etc.) on meat and internal organs (heart, liver, stomach, etc.). Nevertheless, to restrict the *Salmonella* issue in meat, it is important to act upstream of the chain of production, during primary production. Ever since the 1990s, for poultry, the WHO (1994a) indicated guidelines to follow in order to identify the infected farms, to keep the vectors that carry the infection under control (WHO, 1994b) and to apply prevention methods (WHO, 1994c). In more recent years, the EU has released surveillance systems with specific control programs to significantly reduce the problem of *Salmonella* on farms rearing breeding poultry, egg-laying hens, broilers, turkeys and pigs, both for breeding and for meat (EC Regulation 2160/2003, Appendix 1). In these farming facilities, it is necessary to keep under control the hygienic characteristics of raw materials and animal feed, environmental hygiene, rodents, overcrowding, animal welfare, etc. The contamination of food for animal feed can occur in the factory as well as on the farm by cross contamination (not properly sanitized utensils) or by means of vectors (rodents, insects). Against the spread of *Salmonella* Enteritidis on poultry farms, it is effective to use antimicrobial agents in the feed, such as organic acids; as well as adding to the drinking water mixtures of probiotic bacteria in the early weeks of life, during which the intestinal colonization by potentially pathogenic microorganisms is most likely. Another difficulty resides in the elimination of the pathogen from the environment through cleaning and disinfection carried out after sending the animal to slaughter and before the arrival of the next cycle. Therefore, a good approach for controlling infection on the farm is definitely that of adopting prophylactic measures with serological monitoring and an accurate microbiologic testing of environment and faeces, trying to avoid the overuse of antibiotics in animals, which, on the other hand, can decrease their own organic resistance against *Salmonella*. In pigs, *Salmonella* can also be found very frequently in the tonsils, contaminated orally together with the intake of food. According to Griffith *et al.* (2006), it is possible to detect it in the oropharyngeal secretions and transmission between animals can happen nasally, especially in case of overcrowding on the farm or in transport. In cattle, the increased susceptibility to infection may arise from errors in the formulation of the food that changes the rumen flora, thus favouring the development of *Salmonella*. The EFSA report on

the progress of zoonoses and foodborne diseases (EFSA, 2011) shows that the verification of *Salmonella* in intensive European poultry farming facilities went down in 2009 compared to previous years. Greece (7%), the Czech Republic (11%) and Hungary (32%) were the states where the detections were greater, respectively for roosters, egg-laying hens and broilers. In the first 2 types of farming facilities, the most detected serotypes were: *S.* Enteritidis, *S.* Typhimurium, *S.* Infantis, *S.* Virchow and *S.* Hadar. On pig farms, the data collected among the member states are not homogeneous about sampling time in the production chain (faeces on the farm, lymph nodes in the slaughterhouse): the only countries that submitted full data were Estonia (0.9% on the farm and 8% positive in the slaughterhouse) and Norway (0% in both cases). However, the EU estimated that the presence of *Salmonella* in intensively farmed pigs in 2009 varied from 0 to 64% (on average between 26 and 31%). S. Derby was the most detected serotype. For all other animals, although gathered data are few, the presence of *Salmonella* is low both on the farm and in the slaughterhouse. Finally, *Salmonella* was found in animal feed with a low incidence, ranging on average from 0.4% (for cattle) to 1% (for poultry), and the most contaminated products were meat and bone meal (1.4%). In later farming stages it is necessary to ensure that the animals arrive at the slaughterhouse in the best conditions possible (avoiding overcrowding, dirt on skin and feathers); it is also important to check, in addition to the above, the fasting time before slaughter, the temperature and the renewal of scalding water (poultry, pork) in order to limit the load of organic material and reduce the adhesion of *Salmonella* on the skin; it is also essential to check that the cleaning procedures, the maintenance of facilities and equipment are performed in optimal conditions. These checks should be supported by microbiological tests, in accordance with EC Regulation 2073/2005, to make sure that the slaughter took place in full respect of hygiene conditions and, if not, to review the process. Moreover, EFSA (2006) recommends that swine slaughter monitoring should provide for the research of the pathogen in the ileocaecal lymph nodes or in the meat juice. Decontamination of carcasses after slaughter can be useful for controlling pathogens, including *Salmonella,* but it can absolutely not replace poor hygiene during the slaughter. Some methods put forward, but not always accepted by the regulations, are the use of organic acids, such as acetic acid, which cannot be used for obvious reasons, and lactic acid, which, if used at concentrations of 1% v/v, affects S. Typhimurium well without affecting the colour or the flavour of the meat too much; also ozone mixed with the water used for showering poultry provides excellent results regarding the reduction of microbial load. In the USA, trisodium phosphate (TSP) can be used, an alkaline composite (pH 11) able to diminish the pathogen by 2 logarithmic cycles and bring down the contamination of poultry carcasses to under 5% (Gudmundsdottir *et al.*, 1993), but its disposal after use is a problem.
A very powerful physical method to reduce microbial load is γ-ray irradiation, which is not licensed in Europe. Doses of 3-5 kGy are employed, effective for the decontamination of fresh meat, the Enterobacteriaceae loads ensuing in a fall of 6 logarithmic degrees (WHO, 1994), without causing significant deterioration of the sensory quality of the treated products. As regards the meat of hunted wild game, the microbiological quality depends on where skinning and handling is carried out: on average, it was stated that the total viable count as well as that of fecal coliform are about 2 logarithmic higher in game eviscerated outdoor than the similar value of game eviscerated in slaughterhouse ($10^5$-$10^8$ vs. $10^3$-$10^6$ cfu/g). Anyway, *Salmonella* is rarely found, especially if the wild game does not come into contact with domestic animals. Frogs imported from various countries are frequently contaminated with *Salmonella* (20-30%) belonging to most diverse serotypes and often exotic ones, according to the importing country.

Snails, however, although they are very often contaminated, rarely cause food-poisoning episodes as the way they are cooked ensures they are sanitized; nevertheless, they represent an excellent means for the germ to spread (Tiecco, 2000). Possible contaminations can also occur when the meat is subjected to various types of processing, such as "minced meat", defined as meat meant to be minced and to be sold as such, with the addition of salt up to a maximum of 1%, and "meat preparations", i.e. meat products to which seasonings or permitted food additives have been added or any treatment that does not alter the cellular structure of the core of the meat and does not change its characteristics as fresh meat. In both cases one can easily verify microbial contamination due either to the physical characteristics of the products, or to whether other potentially *Salmonella* carrying ingredients (vegetables, eggs, spices, etc.) are added. It is therefore important to keep the temperature constantly below 4°C, staff hygiene rules must be respected, as some staff members may be asymptomatic carriers of *Salmonella* and, most importantly, cross contamination must be prevented throughout the production chain and after cooking the meat, because this is the major problem for *Salmonella*. The processes of salting, curing, cold smoking, antimicrobial preserving additives and lactic fermentation the meat undergoes for becoming cold cuts are not able to completely eliminate *Salmonella*, but do cause the numbers to fall, sometimes substantially, which protects the consumer from food poisoning (<100 CFU/g). Heat (pasteurization, cooking, hot smoking), on the other hand, if it is done properly, is a good clearing method. But, without respecting basic technological principles, the previous operations will be completely useless. Many researchers agree that *Salmonella* usually contaminates food with a very low charge, mostly <10 cfu/g, but in the case of a human in normal immunological conditions, in order to be effective, an infection requires the ingestion of a fairly large charge, more than $10^4$ cfu/g of food. As a result, it is necessary for the bacteria to find adequate conditions in the substrate to duplicate more or less rapidly. The "hygiene package" regulations introduced the obligation for the owners of manufacturing and processing factories to arrange and implement self-control procedures, to perform microbiological tests on the finished product and to indicate on the label if such meat, other than poultry, is to be subjected to adequate cooking before consumption.

Researches in EU in 2009 (EFSA, 2011) showed that *Salmonella* was found most frequently in raw turkey meat (8.7%), chicken (5.4%), pork (0.7%) and cattle (0.2%). In general, at the pig slaughterhouse, *Salmonella* was detected between 0 and 14%, with a higher incidence in Belgium where a very meticulous sampling method is carried out. According to the EFSA, many episodes of human food-borne illnesses are attributable to pork. Minced meat and meat preparations, especially those intended to be eaten raw, are most often contaminated by bacteria (5.5% positive) and therefore do not meet European sanitary standards. In retail shops *Salmonella* was found in 3.5% of the analyzed samples, a decrease compared with the previous year. Finally, the analysis of the results shows that there is a prevalence of serovars Typhimurium and Enteritidis.

In conclusion, the major risk factors of salmonellosis due to meat are to be found in insufficient cooking, the consumption of raw meat (pork sausages) which was not processed properly (minced horse meat, carpaccio, tartare, etc.), storage at inadequate temperatures, and cross contamination, if the product ready for consumption is in contact with other raw foods or dirty utensils. On the other hand, the staff's role, whether infected or carrier, appears to be less important, as it has been proven that, if Good Manufacturing Practice (GMP) is applied to food, such as careful hand washing, the risk of conveying infection is kept well under control.

## 7. *Salmonella* in raw milk and milk products

Nowadays, according to the EC regulations in force, we can obtain milk for human consumption from all mammalian species, without exception, provided that the animals are reared and milked when they are in good health and nutrition conditions (EC Regulation 853/04). In developed countries the milk that humans use as food is almost always cow's milk; much more seldom we also consume sheep's, goat's and buffalo milk. In poor developing countries, in addition to cow's milk, buffalo, sheep's and goat's milk is also regularly drunk. In different geographical areas and with varying eating habits, along with "traditional" dairy species, man also employs various other animal species (camels, dromedaries, horses, reindeer, etc.) as a source of milk. Thanks to its chemical composition, milk is an almost ideal food for humans and for this reason it is part of the daily ration of most of the world's population. Over time the different peoples on Earth have developed a remarkable range of food products that use milk as raw material: in the world today there are approximately 1,600 different types of cheeses and over 100 different types of fermented dairy products. From raw milk many kind of milk products are obtained, such as pasteurized or UHT milk, cheese, fermented milks and probiotics, ice cream, butter, ricotta and milk drinks or whey. This wide range of food is obtained by subjecting raw milk to one or more technical processes that change the components of milk and its rheological properties to a greater or lesser extent. These "treatments" may be the addition of salt and the removal of water (*seasoning*) or the addition of natural enzymes and/or milk ferments that trigger these complex biochemical processes that we call *ageing* of cheese or fermented milks. *Salmonella,* as well as other pathogenic agents of foodborne disease, can contaminate raw milk: (1) directly inside the mammary gland (very rare event); (2) during milking, because the bacteria are often present in the faeces of milk animals and on their coat; (3) after milking, because salmonellae can contaminate work surfaces with which the raw milk comes into contact; (4) in subsequent phases, still due to the presence of *Salmonella* on work surfaces and/or cross contamination. The fate of salmonellae in milk and milk products widely depends on the antimicrobial effects the different transformation processes may have on the bacteria, as bactericidal effect or more simply bacteriostatic effect. This explains why in developed countries cases of human salmonellosis caused by the consumption of dairy products and milk are much rarer than those caused by the consumption of fresh meat or fish products (Jayarao & Henning, 2001). Raw milk, of course, represents an exception: in recent years it has caused a number of fairly many outbreaks of human salmonellosis (Newkirk *et al.*, 2011). We must not forget that in recent years in many European states the consumption of raw milk purchased directly from the dairy by means of automatic vending machines has greatly increased. The following study will, therefore, give information about the possible presence of *Salmonella* in raw milk and different products that are derived from it, focusing above all on the possibility for *Salmonella* to multiply in different dairy products. According to the epidemiology data of foodborne illnesses provided each year by the EFSA, milk and milk products are not by far the greatest sources of danger for consumers. Like in previous years, in 2009 too there were few cases of *Salmonella* detected in cow's milk. Only three EU Member States conducted specific tests on raw milk sold in vending machines: Austria (71 samples tested), Germany (173 samples) and Hungary (50 samples). *Salmonella* was never detected in any of these samples. On the other hand, as regards pasteurized or UHT milk, seven states reported data: Austria (30 samples), Bulgaria (30 samples), the

Czech Republic (135 samples), Germany (980 samples), Greece (26 samples), Hungary (85 samples) and Romania (57 samples). Again, none of the samples tested contained *Salmonella*. Italy reported that out of a total of 928 samples of cow's milk, 3 were positive for *Salmonella* and that 5 samples out of a total of 5,799 samples of milk from "other unspecified species" also tested positive for the pathogen. 11 member countries supplied EFSA with results of their investigations on cheeses, for a total of 23,023 samples analyzed. In the great majority of cases, the cheese samples proved to be negative for *Salmonella*, with the exception of Spain (4 positive samples out of a total of 424 samples tested), Portugal (2 positive samples out of 181 analyzed) and Italy (2 positive out of a total of 1,879 samples tested). As far as we know from the EFSA report, all the cheeses tested positive were semi-hard cheeses, and only semi-mature, and made from raw or thermised milk (i.e. heated to a temperature between 45 °C and 54 °C, no more). As far as butter is concerned, 7 member states communicated the results of their inspections; no case revealed the presence of *Salmonella*. Besides cheese, the only other product derived from milk which pointed out the presence of *Salmonella* was ice cream. Spain, Hungary and Germany reported the presence of the bacterium respectively in 13 samples out of 305 samples analyzed, 1 out of 140 and 1 in 2,626 samples, always taken in the production facilities. The presence of salmonellae in raw milk is widely documented in the literature, both in the collection tanks on the farms, and in the storage tanks in the food factories (Donaghy *et al.*, 2004; Tondo *et al.*, 2000). *Salmonella* may be present in raw milk ever since milking because the bacterium is present in the mammary gland, but this occurs very rarely. Mastitis due to *Salmonella* is a very rare condition in dairy cows, but it is reported. We know that different *Salmonella* serotypes can colonize the mammary gland and lead to the excretion, at the same time as the milk, of bacterial loads that can extend up to 3.3 log10 cfu/ml (Fontaine *et al.*, 1980). Furthermore, *Salmonella* can pass from animal to animal at the time of milking, both through the milker's hands, and through polluted parts of the milking machines (Bergonier *et al.*, 2003; Vautor *et al.*, 2003; Zadoks *et al.*, 2002; Zschöck *et al.*, 2000). Much more often, however, salmonellae contaminate raw milk in the stages that follow the milking process, because the bacteria may be present on the various surfaces that come into contact with the milk being collected. In particular, *Salmonella* (such as *Listeria monocytogenes* and verotoxigenic strains of *E. coli*) can enter the milk through the traces of animal faeces in the environment (Van Kessel *et al.*, 2004). This factor of pollution, in turn, is influenced by the prevalence among dairy cows of *Salmonella* healthy carriers, which can evacuate various loads of the pathogen more or less frequently. In this regard, it is estimated that the U.S. dairy cows can be healthy carriers of *Salmonella* in their faeces with a prevalence that ranges from a minimum of 2% to a maximum of 27.5% of the animals tested (Kabagambe *et al.*, 2000; Losinger *et al.*, 1995, Wells *et al.*, 2001). What can be the prevalence of a batch of raw milk tested positive for *Salmonella* ever since the milking phase? In view of the data that we can gather from the literature, we can estimate that the batches of raw milk straight after milking can be positive for *Salmonella* from a minimum of 2.6% to a maximum of 25.3% (Jayarao & Henning, 2001; Murinda *et al.*, 2002; Zhao *et al.* 2002). Compared to other pathogenic microorganisms such as *L. monocytogenes*, salmonellae are not very resistant in the outside, so it is not very frequent for the work surfaces in the production plants to transfer salmonellae to the product. Nevertheless, in theory, *Salmonella* can survive for long on any work surface and then pollute the cheese curd which is meant to become cheese. This justifies the episodes of foodborne infection caused by processed dairy products, such as milk powder and cheeses made with pasteurized milk. **Fermented milks** can be divided into two kinds: (i) acid, if their production is based on homolactic fermentation, (ii) acid-alcoholic, if the starter strains used for fermentation are of the heterofermentative type. In case (i) the product will only be acid, while in case (ii) besides the presence of acid there is a fair amount of ethyl alcohol which enhances the food's antimicrobial effect against *Salmonella*. Their production process usually starts from pasteurized milk. Furthermore, milk is caused to coagulate by using acid, by adding selected milk ferments that produce large amounts of lactic acid or other organic acids and possibly ethyl alcohol, with a drastic drop in the substrate's pH which makes the casein coagulate. The presence of high loads of lactic acid bacteria, coupled with low pH levels (4.0 to 4.1 on average) and $A_w$ mean that yogurt and other fermented milk products are a very unfit food matrix for allowing the growth and even the survival of *Salmonella*.

**Cheese** is among the foods which are less likely to cause salmonellosis in humans due to their production process (Little *et al.*, 2008). Nevertheless, in 2008 it was responsible for 0.4% of all episodes of illness reported in the EU (EFSA, 2010). In addition, several cases of salmonellosis caused by the consumption of cheese contaminated with *Salmonella enterica* are reported in the bibliography. The problem is that despite the fact that the production process poses several obstacles to the survival and multiplication of salmonellae, we eat cheese without further heat processing. Moreover, cheese often does not carry pathogenic microorganisms in its inside, but rather on its surface. This may result in the transfer of *Salmonella* and other pathogens to domestic working environments, thus favouring cross contamination, which in turn enables the outbreak of foodborne illnesses (Kousta *et al.*, 2010). The bibliography gives at least a dozen episodes of salmonellosis caused by the consumption of cheeses made not only with raw milk, but also with pasteurized milk. This means that in many cases the milk used to produce cheese is contaminated with *Salmonella* "after" its pasteurization, since this is largely able to inactivate very high loads of the bacteria. Nowadays, HTST pasteurization is often used in the dairy industry (at least 72 °C for at least 15 seconds) and it can produce a drop of about 6 LOG-degrees in the original load of *Salmonella*, as demonstrated by accurate experimental investigations (D'Aoust *et al.*, 1988; D'Aoust *et al.*, 1987; Farber *et al.*, 1988). In particular, these studies showed that *Salmonella* can still be detected in milk heated up to 67.5 °C for 15 seconds, but not at higher temperatures. We need not forget, though, that *Salmonella*, just like *Listeria monocytogenes*, can penetrate into the milk somatic cells that can provide it with a slight protection against the effects of heat. It is not, therefore, possible to exclude *a priori* that in normally pasteurized milk it may still be possible to detect some salmonellae which survived the treatment itself, if it was not carried out at temperatures above 72 °C. In the past decades, salmonellae have caused a series of outbreaks of illness caused by the consumption of various types of cheese. As mentioned before, we can find several references in the literature to outbreaks of salmonellosis caused by foods that contain very low numbers of *Salmonella*. According to D'Aoust (1985) and Ratnam & March (1986), the literature documents cases of salmonellosis caused by Cheddar cheese in which the estimated infectious load proved to be under 10 cfu of *Salmonella*/g of food.

From the data we possess, we can therefore sum up that *Salmonella* may still be present in cheeses for human consumption, but with a prevalence which varies widely depending on several factors:

1. the type of raw material: cheese made with raw milk may contain salmonellae still alive and vital, while it is hard for those made with pasteurized milk to still shelter the pathogen, unless the contamination occurred after the pasteurization process,
2. the duration and type of ageing: in cheeses which mature for a short time, *Salmonella* is more likely to survive, because the maturing biochemical processes that have a good antimicrobial effect against pathogen are not yet established in the substrate. In cheeses that mature for over 60 days, on the contrary, the characteristics of the substrate that are obtained as a result of aging make the product unfit for the reproduction and survival of salmonella,
3. the microbiological quality of milk used to make cheese. Cheeses made with raw milk are not necessarily infected with *Salmonella*, if good hygiene conditions are maintained during the milking process and the ensuing manufacturing process.

As with many other types of foodstuffs, salmonellae can contaminate cheese coming from:

1. raw materials used in production, most likely from raw milk and less likely from other ingredients such as lactic acid starter and salt,
2. salt solutions (brine) used for salting certain products,
3. work surfaces in the cheese factories, including the air that circulates in various environments,
4. packaging materials in which is wrapped the finished product ready for sale (Temelli *et al.*, 2006).

As regards in particular brines used to salt the cheese, Ingham *et al.* (2000) conducted experimental inoculation tests with *Salmonella* ser. Typhimurium to test the viability of the pathogen in the cheeses' brines. The researchers experimentally inoculated two cultures with *S.* Typhimurium and *E. coli* O157, mixed together, in three different brines containing 23% salt, with the addition of 2% of flour. The brines were then stored at 8 °C and 15 °C for 28 days. The same cultures were also inoculated into brines offered for sale, and then stored at 4 °C and 13 °C for 35 days. The load of the two pathogens immediately underwent a gradual decline during storage, but it is significant that the reduction was less noticeable in the brines stored at 4 °C compared to the ones stored at 13 ° or 15 °C. This study shows that *Salmonella* may still survive in saline solutions used for salting cheese, although with very small loads.

Compared to other pathogens such as *L. monocytogenes* and *Staphylococcus aureus*, *Salmonella* is much less often blamed as a source of illness due to the consumption of cheese. As a result, we do not have precise data as to the actual prevalence of *Salmonella* in cheese. We can, however, find some data on the persistence of salmonellae in cheese sold in retail food stores. The pathogen was detected in Turkey in various kind of cheese produced mainly in an artisanal manner with raw cow's, ewe's and/or goat's milk (Colak *et al.*, 2000; Hayaloglu & Kirbag, 2007; Tekinşen & Özdemir, 2006), always in very low prevalence of the samples analyzed. On the other hand, we also have data documenting how salmonellae, potentially present in raw milk and/or in environments where milk and cheese are produced, are not so detectable in the dairy products offered for sale. For example, in Spain Cabedo *et al.* (2008) conducted a large study to test the microbiological quality of the cheeses of their land: they never detected *Salmonella* in any of the samples they analysed. In Britain, two studies conducted by Little *et al.* (2008) first in 2004 and then in 2005, showed that a total of 4,437 samples of various types of cheeses (fresh, semi-mature and mature, made with raw or pasteurized milk) never showed the presence of *Salmonella*.

**Butter** is produced by the mechanical churning of the cream obtained after centrifugation of cheese whey. It can be *sweet* if the cream is used as it is, or *ripened* if it comes from cream that was first matured with the addition of starter enzymes. In most cases, the raw material for butter is subjected to pasteurization in butter before being processed, but in some cases butter is obtained directly from the cream of raw, unpasteurized milk. It is clear that in this second case *Salmonella* may be present in the butter from the start of the making process because the raw material itself was contaminated. In the case of butter made from pasteurized cream, however, a possible contamination with *Salmonella* cannot be excluded, because the pathogen could infect the finished product through a secondary contamination. In the past decades, in fact, several episodes of human salmonellosis caused by butter contaminated with *Salmonella* occurred, but over the years these episodes have registered a sharp decline, due to the fact that producers dedicate more attention to production hygiene and to the fact that butter is now rarely made with unpasteurized cream. The EU has established with EC Regulation 2073/05 that "cheese, butter and cream made from raw milk or milk subjected to heat treatment at sub-pasteurization temperatures" should not contain even one living cell of *Salmonella* in 125 g (25 g in 5 units of the sample) of product throughout its shelf life. **Dried milk products** as a rule, these foods are products obtained after pasteurized milk is nebulized in towers where a very dry and hot air current circulates, but on the market you can find lyophilised products, i.e. put through the cold-removal of water, not involving the use of high temperatures. The sanitary characteristics of milk powders, therefore, is determined by: (i) the microbiological quality of the raw material, (ii) the conditions of the production process (with or without heat treatment), (iii) the possibility of the dehydrated/lyophilised product to be contaminated with salmonellae after its processing. Salmonellae are sensitive to normal temperatures applied in the production process of dried milk products, so it is logical to expect that such products are rarely at risk of containing *Salmonella*, unless they are contaminated after this process, during packaging or storage. In these cases, dried milk products may be a risk to human health, since salmonellae can survive for months in substrates with low water content, such as bone meal and powdered foods. The possible dangers of these products is also enhanced by the fact that such foods are usually meant for very young children, much more sensitive than adults to even minor loads of *Salmonella*. For this reason, the EU has established by law (EC Regulation 2073/05) that "powdered milk and powdered whey" should not contain even one living cell of *Salmonella* in 125 g of product throughout its shelf life. **Ice cream** is a complex food made of various ingredients, including eggs and milk, where water crystallizes, forming a homogeneous creamy mass, thanks to the high amount of fat. As such, also ice cream can be contaminated with *Salmonella*, if it is contained in the raw milk or appears in the manufacturing process. Over the past decades, in fact, many outbreaks of salmonellosis caused by the consumption of ice cream have been documented, but it was not always possible to establish with certainty whether the pollution came from the raw milk or from the eggs, which are also used raw. For several years now, the use of pasteurized milk and eggs has become a habit for producing ice cream, so the risk of *Salmonella* contamination in these products has been greatly reduced. But we must remember that ice cream, due to its almost always neutral or slightly acidic pH levels and to its high amount of free water ($A_w$), can be an excellent substrate for the survival and growth of *Salmonella*, if the latter managed to infect it. The risks to public health may be greater for those who produce ice cream from raw milk. In recent years, in fact, this habit seems to have come back into fashion, under the pressure from consumers who take great pleasure in consuming food products from raw materials treated as little as possible. Regarding ice cream too, the EU has set specific criteria for *Salmonella*, which must be "absent" in 125 g of product. This law does not apply to ice creams "whose manufacturing process or composition properties eliminate the risk of *Salmonella*" as required by Regulation 2073/05.

## 8. Conclusion

All this makes it difficult to control and prevent these toxi-infections; as a result, it is necessary for epidemiologists, clinicians and microbiologists as well as veterinarians to collaborate in order to launch an integrated approach to solve the problem. In order to prevent the occurrence of salmonellosis, it is therefore essential to know which animals and/or which foods most frequently carry the pathogens which have led to sporadic cases or episodes of disease in humans. Epidemiological data should then be given special attention and consideration by meat producers and in general by anyone whose role it is to carry out investigations on food, as they can provide useful information regarding changes or additions to be made to the eradication plans against *Salmonella*.

## 9. References


Berger C. N., Sodha S. V., Shaw R. K., Griffin P M., Pink D., Hand P.& Frankel G. (2010). Fresh fruit and vegetables as vehicles for the transmission of human pathogens. *Environmental Microbiology*, Vol. 12, No.9, pp. 2385-2397

Bergonier D., De Cremoux R., Rupp R., Lagriffoul G.& Berthelot X. (2003). Mastitis of dairy small ruminants, *Veterinary Research*, Vol. 34, No.5, pp. 689-716

Bozzo G. (2008). Uova e ovoprodotti, In: *Igiene e tecnologie degli alimenti di origine animale*, Colavita G., pp. 321-328, Le Point Vétérinaire Italie srl, ISBN 978-88-95995-47-2, Milano, Italy

Cabedo L., Barrot L.P.& Teixidó A.T. (2008). Prevalence of *Listeria monocytogenes* and *Salmonella* in ready-to-eat Food in Catalonia, Spain, *Journal of Food Protection*, Vol. 71, No. 4, pp. 855-859

Cantoni C. & Bersani C. (2010). *E. coli* O157:H7, non O157:H e *Salmonella enterica*. *Qualità e Sicurezza Alimentare*, Vol. 3, No.14, pp. 47-53, ISSN 2038-9760

Cantoni C. & Ripamonti B. (1998). La presenza di *Salmonella* negli alimenti e sua patogenicità. *Tecnologie alimentari*, Vol. 9, No.5, pp. 76-83

Castillo N.A., de Moreno de LeBlanc A., Maldonado Galdeano C. & Perdigón G. (2011). Probiotics: an alternative strategy for combating salmonellosis. Immune mechanisms involved, *Food Research International*, Vol. x, No. x, pp. xxx-xxx.

Catellani P., Giaccone V. & Novelli E. (2005). Studio della flora microbica nei vegetali di IV gamma. Nota preliminare. *Proceedings of S.I.S.Vet*, Viareggio, Italy, 21-24 September, 2005

Colak H., Hampikyan H., Bingol E.B. & Ulusoy B. (2007). Prevalence of *L. monocytogenes* and *Salmonella* spp. in Tulum cheese, *Food Control*, Vol. 18, No.5, pp. 576-579

D'Aoust J.Y. (1985). Infective dose of *Salmonella* typhimurium in Cheddar cheese, *American Journal of Epidemiology*, Vol. 122, No.4, pp. 717-720

D'Aoust J.Y., Emmons D.B., McKellar R., Timbers G.E., Todd E.C.D. & Sewell A.M. (1987). Thermal inactivation of *Salmonella* species in fluid milk, *Journal of Food Protection*, Vol. 50, No.6, pp. 494-501

D'Aoust J.Y., Park C.E., Szabo R.A. & Todd E.C.D. (1988). Thermal inactivation of *Campylobacter* species, *Yersinia enterocolitica*, and hemorrhagic *Escherichia coli* O157:H7 in fluid milk, *Journal of Dairy Science*, Vol. 71, No.12, pp. 3230-3236

D'Aoust J.Y. & Maurer J. (2007). *Salmonella* Species, In: *Food Microbiology. Fundamentals and Frontiers*, Doyle M.P. & Beuchat L.R., pp. 30-33, ASM Press, ISBN: 978-1-55581-407-6, Washington, DC, U.S.A.

D'Aoust J.Y. (2007). *Salmonella*, In: *Food Safety handbook*, Storrs M., pp. 128-141, Biomerieux Editions, ISBN: 9782917162088, Marcy l'Etoile, France

D'Aoust J.Y., Aris B.J., Thisdele P., Durante A., Brisson N., Dragon D., Lachapelle G., Johnston M. & Laidley R. (1975). *Salmonella*-eastbourne outbreak associated with chocolate, *Canadian Institute of Food Science and Technology Journal*, Vol. 8, No. 4 , pp. 181-184

de Jong B. & Ekdhal K. (2006). Human salmonellosis in travellers is highly correlated to the prevalence of salmonella in laying hen flocks, In: *Eurosurveillance*, 02.08.2011, http://www.eurosurveillance.org/ViewArticle.aspx?ArticleId=2993

Donaghy J.A., Totton N.L. & Rowe M.T. (2004). Persistence of *Mycobacterium paratuberculosis* during manufacture and ripening of cheddar cheese, *Applied and Environmental Microbiology*, Vol. 70, No.8, pp. 4899-4905

Duffy G., Cloak O.M., O'Sullivan M.G., Guillet A., Sheridan J.J., Blair I.S.& McDowell D.A. (1999). The incidence and antibiotic resistance profiles of *Salmonella* spp. on Irish retail meat products, *Food Microbiology*, Vol. 16, No.6, pp. 623-631

EFSA (2006) The Community Summary Report on Trends and Sources of Zoonoses, Zoonotic Agents, Antimicrobial Resistance and Foodborne Outbreaks in the European Union in 2005, *The EFSA Journal*, Vol 94, pp. 3-288

EFSA (2007). The Community Summary Report on trends and sources of zoonoses, zoonotic agents, antimicrobial resistance and foodborne outbreaks in the European Union in 2006, *The EFSA Journal*, Vol. 130, pp. 1-352

EFSA (2009a). Analysis of the baseline survey on the prevalence of *Salmonella* in holdings with breeding pigs in the EU, 2008 - Part A: *Salmonella* prevalence estimates, *The EFSA Journal*, Vol. 7, pp. 1-93

EFSA (2009b). Scientific Opinion of the Panel on Biological Hazards on a request from the European Commission on Special measures to reduce the risk for consumers through *Salmonella* in table eggs – e.g. cooling of table eggs, *The EFSA Journal*, Vol. 957, pp. 1-29

EFSA (2010). The Community Summary Report on Trends and Sources of Zoonoses, Zoonotic Agents and food-borne outbreaks in the European Union in 2008, *EFSA Journal*, Vol 8, No. 1, 1496.

EFSA (2011). The European Union Summary Report on Trends and Sources of Zoonoses, Zoonotic Agents and Foodborne Outbreaks in 2009, *EFSA Journal*, Vol. 9, No. 3:2090, pp. 1-378

Farber J.M., Sanders G.W., Speirs J.I., D'Aoust J.Y., Emmons D.B. & McKellar R. (1988). Thermal resistance of *Listeria monocytogenes* in inoculated and naturally contaminated raw milk, *International Journal of Food Microbiology*, Vol. 7, No.4, pp. 277-286

Farkas J. (1997). Physical methods of food preservation, in: *Food Microbiology*, Doyle M.P., Beuchat L.R. & Montville T.J. (Eds), pp. 497–519. Fundamentals and Frontiers ASM Press, Washington, DC.

Fontaine R.E., Cohen M.L., Martin W.T. & Vernon T.M. (1980). Epidemic salmonellosis from cheddar cheese: Surveillance and prevention, *American Journal of Epidemiology*, Vol. 111, No.2, pp. 247-253

Frankel G. (2008). Attachment of *Escherichia coli* O157:H7 and *Salmonella enterica* to Salad Leaves, *Proceedings of International ICFMH Symposium Food Micro 2008*, Aberdeen, Scotland, 1-4 September, 2008

Frankel G. (2009). Microbiologic risk associated with fresh produce: the interaction between foodborne pathogens and vegetables, *Proceedings of XI Congresso Nazionale S.I.Di.L.V.*, Parma, Italy, 30 September-2 October, 2009

Galli A. & Franzetti L. (1998). La sicurezza igienico-sanitaria degli ortaggi di IV gamma, *Informatore agrario*, Vol. 98, No. 19, pp. 46-47

Galli A. & Neviani E. (2005). Analisi microbiologica degli alimenti, In: *Microbiologia degli alimenti*, Galli Volonterio A., pp. 313-317, Casa Editrice Ambrosiana, ISBN 88-408-1321-7, Milano, Italy

Gandini G. (1993). Sistema H.A.C.C.P. applicato all'industria degli ovoprodotti e proposta di procedura ispettiva, *Ingegneria alimentare*, Vol. 3, No. 6, pp. 25-30

Graziani C., Galetta P., Busani L., Dionisi A. M., Filetici E., Ricci A., Caprioli A. & Luzzi I. (27 May 2005). Le infezioni da *Salmonella*: diagnostica, epidemiologia e sorveglianza, In: *Rapporti ISTISAN*, 03.08.2011, http://www.iss.it/binary/publ/publi/05-27.1132583099.pdf

Griffith R.H., Schwartz K.J.& Meyerholz D.K. (2006). *Salmonella* In: *Diseases of Swine*, Straw B.E., Zimmerman J.J., D'Allaire S., Taylor D.J. (Eds.), pp 739-754 Iowa State University Press

Gudmundsdottir K.B., Marin M.L.N., Allen V.M., Corry J.E.L.& Hinton M. (1993). In: *Contamination with Pathogen in Relation to Processing and Marketing of Products*. Loeppe J., Kan C.A., Mulder A.W. (Eds.), pp. 95-100. COVP-DLO Het Sperlderholt.

Hayaloglu A.A. & Kirbag S. (2007). Microbial quality and presence of moulds in Kuflu cheese, *International Journal of Food Microbiology*, Vol. 115, No.3, pp. 376-380

Hennessy T.W., Hedberg C.W., Slutsker L., White K.E., BesserWiek J.M. & Moen M.E. (1996). A national outbreak of *Salmonella* enteritidis infections from ice cream, *New England Journal of Medicine*, Vol. 334, No. 20, pp. 1281-1286

Hopkins K.L., Kirchner M., Guerra B., Granier S.A., Lucarelli C., Porrero M.C., Jakubczak A., Threlfall E.J. & Mevius D.J. (3 June 2010). "Multiresistant *Salmonella enterica* Serovar 4,[5],12:I:- In Europe: A New Pandemic Strain?", In: *Eurosurveillance*, 03.08.2011, http://www.eurosurveillance.org/images/dynamic/EE/V15N22/art19580

ICMSF (1996). Salmonellae, In: *Microorganisms in Foods 5: Characteristics of Microbial Pathogens*, pp. 222-225, Blackie Academic & Professional, London, U.K, ISBN 978-0-412-47350-0

ICMSF (1998). Eggs and egg products, In: *Microrganism in food 6. Microbial ecology of food commodities*, pp. 475-520, Blackie Academic & Professional, London,. U.K, ISBN 0751404306

Ingham S.C., Su Y.-C. & Spangenberg D.S. (2000). Survival of *Salmonella* typhimurium and *Escherichia coli* O157:H7 in cheese brines, *International Journal of Food Microbiology*, Vol. 61, No.1, pp. 73-79

Jasson V., Baert L. & Uyttendaele M. (2011). Detection of low numbers of healthy and sub-lethally injured *Salmonella enterica* in chocolate. *Int J Food Microbiol* Vol 145 No. 2-3, pp. 488-491

Jayarao B.M. & Henning D.R. (2001). Prevalence of foodborne pathogens in bulk tank milk, *Journal of Dairy Science*, Vol. 84, No.10, pp. 2157-2162

Jay J.M. (1996). *Modern Food Microbiology*. (5th Ed.) Chapman & Hall, New York

Kabagambe E.K., Wells S.J., Garber L.P., Salman M.D., Wagner B. & Fedorka-Cray P.J. (2000). Risk factors for fecal shedding of *Salmonella* in 91 US dairy herds in 1996, *Preventive Veterinary Medicine*, Vol. 43, No.3, pp. 177-194

Komitopoulou E. & Penaloza W. (2009). Fate of *Salmonella* in dry confectionery raw materials, *Journal of Applied Microbiology*, Vol. 106, No. 6, pp. 1892-1900

Kousta M., Mataragas M., Skandamis P. & Drosinos E.H. (2010). Prevalence and sources of cheese contamination with pathogens at farm and processing levels, *Food Control*, Vol. 21, No.6, pp. 805-815

Leali L. (2011). La microbiologia della pasta fresca: dalla farina al confezionamento, *Rivista delle tecnologie alimentari*, Vol. 22, No. 3, pp. 30-33

Leyer G.J. & Johnson E.A. (1993). Acid adaptation induces cross-protection against environmental stresses in *Salmonella* typhimurium. *Appl Environ Microbiol*, Vol. 59, No. 6, pp. 1842-1847

Lindhardt C., Schonenbrucher H., Slaghuis J., Bubert A., Ossmer R. & Junge B. (2009). Foodproof salmonella detection kit. Performance tested method 120301, *Journal of AOAC International*, Vol. 92, No. 6, pp. 1876-1884

Little C.L., Rhoades J.R., Sagoo S.K., Harris J., Greenwood M. & Mithani V. (2008). Microbial quality of retail cheese made from raw, thermised or pasteurized milk in UK, *Food Microbiology*, Vol. 25, No.2, pp. 304-312

Liu W.-B., Liu B., Zhu X.-N., Yu S. & Shi X.M. (2011). Diversity of *Salmonella* isolates using serotyping and multilocus sequence typing, *Food Microbiology*, Vol. 28, No. 6, pp. 1182-1189

Losinger W.C., Wells S.J., Garber L.P.& Hurd H.S. (1995). Management factors related to *Salmonella* shedding by dairy heifers, *Journal of Dairy Science*, Vol. 78, No.11, pp. 2464-2472

Manvell P.M. & Ackland M.R. (1986). Rapid detection of microbial growth in vegetable salads at chill and abuse temperatures, *Food Microbiology*, Vol. 3, No. 1, pp. 59-65

Matches & Liston, 1968, as cited in Jay, 1996

Møretrø T., Heir E., Nesse L.L., Vestby L.K. & Langsrud S. (2011). Control of *Salmonella* in food related environments by chemical disinfection, *Food Research International*, Vol. x, No. x, pp. xxx–xxx

Møretrø T., Vestby L.K., Nesse L.L., Storheim S.E., Kotlarz K. & Langsrud S. (2009). Evaluation of efficacy of disinfectants against *Salmonella* from the feed industry. *J Appl Microbiol*, vol 106 No. 3, pp. 1005–1012

Mumma G.A., Griffin P.M., Meltzer M.I., Braden C.R. & Tauxe R.V. (2004). Egg Quality Assurance Programs and Egg-associated *Salmonella* Enteritidis Infections, United States, *Emerging infectious diseases*, Vol. 10, No. 10, pp. 1782-1789

Murinda S.E., Nguyen L.T., Ivey S.J., Gillespie B.E., Almeida R.A. & Draughon F.A. (2002). Prevalence and molecular characterization of *Escherichia coli* O157:H7 in bulk tank milk and fecal samples from cull cows: A 12-month survey of dairy farms in East Tennessee, *Journal of Food Protection*, Vol. 65, No.5, pp. 752-759

Newkirk R., Hedberg C. & Bender J. (2011). Establishing a milkborne disease outbreak profile: Potential food defense implications, *Foodborne Pathogens and Disease*, Vol. 8, No.3, pp. 433-437

Nollet N., Houf K., Dewulf J., De Kruif A., De Zutter L. & Maes D. (2005). *Salmonella* in sows: a longitudinal study in farrow-to-finish pig herds, *Veterinary research*, Vol. 36, No. 4, pp. 645-656

Ramesh N., Joseph S.W., Carr L.E., Douglass L.W. & Wheaton F.W. (2002). Evaluation of chemical disinfectants for the elimination of *Salmonella* biofilms from poultry transport containers. *Poultry Science*, Vol. 81 No. 6, pp. 904-910

Ratnam S. & March S.B. (1986). Laboratory studies on *Salmonella*-contaminated cheese involved in a major outbreak of gastroenteritis, *Journal of Applied Microbiology*, Vol. 61, No.1, pp. 51-56

Ricci A. (2005). Aspetti microbiologici ed epidemiologici delle salmonellosi in medicina veterinaria, In: *Trattato sulle infezioni e tossinfezioni alimentari*, Rondanelli E.G., Fabbi M., Marone P., pp. 283-302, Edizioni Selecta S.r.l, ISBN 9788873321095, Pavia, Italy

Rondanelli M., Bonisio A. & Giocosa A. (2005). Infezioni da *Salmonella* in patologia umana, In: *Trattato sulle infezioni e tossinfezioni alimentari*, Rondanelli E.G., Fabbi M., Marone P., pp. 253-282, Edizioni Selecta S.r.l, ISBN 9788873321095, Pavia, Italy

Ross T. & McMeekin, T.A. (1994). Predictive microbiology - a review, *Int J Food Microbiol* , Vol 23 No. (3-4), pp. 241-264

Rowe B., Hutchinson D.N., Gilbert R.J., Hales B.H., Jepson M. & Begg N.T. (1987). *Salmonella* Ealing infections associated with consumption of infant dried milk, *The Lancet*, Vol. 330, No. 8564, pp. 900-903

Scherer S. & Neuhaus K. (2006). Life at Low Temperatures, in: *The Prokaryotes: A Handbook on the Biology of Bacteria*, Dworkin M. et al. (Eds), 3rd edition, Vol 2: *Ecophysiology and Biochemistry*. Springer, New York.

Schikora A., Carreri A., Charpentier E. & Hirt H. (2008). The dark side of the salad: *Salmonella* typhimurium overcomes the innate immune response of Arabidopsis thaliana and shows an endopathogenic lifestyle. *PLoS ONE*, Vol. 3, No.5, e2279, eISSN-1932-6203

Soler P., Hernández Pezzi G., Echeíta A., Torres A., Ordóñez Banegas P. & Aladueña A. (16 June 2005). Surveillance of foodborne disease outbreaks associated with consumption of eggs and egg products: Spain, 2002-2003, In: *Eurosurveillance*, 02.08.2011, http://www.eurosurveillance.org/ViewArticle.aspx?ArticleId=2726

Tekinşen K.K. & Özdemir Z. (2006). Prevalence of foodborne pathogens in Turkish Van otlu (Herb) cheese, *Food Control*, Vol. 17, No. 9, pp. 707-711

Temelli S., Anar S., Sen C. & Akyuva P. (2006). Determination of microbiological contamination sources during Turkish white cheese production, *Food Control*, Vol. 17, No. 11, pp. 856-861

Tiecco G. (2000). *Microbiologia degli alimenti di origine animale*. Ed. Calderini Edagricole, Bologna, Italy

Tizard I. (2004). Salmonellosis in Wild Birds, *Seminars in Avian and Exotic Pet Medicine*, Vol 13, No 2, pp 50-66

Tondo E.C., Guimaraes M.C., Henriques J.A. & Ayub M.A. (2000). Assessing and analysing contamination of a dairy products processing plant by *Staphylococcus aureus* using antibiotic resistance and PFGE, *Canadian Journal of Microbiology*, Vol. 46, No.12, pp. 1108-1114

Van Kessel J.S., Karns J.S., Gorski L., McCluskey B.J. & Perdue, M.L. (2004). Prevalence of Salmonellae, *Listeria monocytogenes*, and fecal coliforms in bulk tank milk on US dairies, *Journal of Dairy Science*, Vol. 87, No.9, pp. 2822-2830

Vautor E., Abadie G., Guibert J.M., Huard C. & Pepin M. (2003). Genotyping of *Staphylococcus aureus* isolated from various sites on farms with dairy sheep using pulsed-field gel electrophoresis, *Veterinary microbiology*, Vol. 96, No.1, pp. 69-79

Wang Y., Qu L., Uthe J.J., Bearson S.M., Kuhar D., Lunney J.K., Couture O.P., Nettleton D., Dekkers J.C. & Tuggle C.K. (2007). Global transcriptional response of porcine mesenteric lymph nodes to *Salmonella enterica* serovar Typhimurium, *Genomics*, Vol. 90, No. 1, pp. 72-84

Weill F.X. (2009). *Salmonella*: épidémiologie, typage et résistance aux antibiotiques, *Revue Francophone des Laboratoires*, Vol. 39, No. 409bis, pp. 25-35

Wells S.J., Fedorka-Cray P.J., Dargatz D.A., Ferris K. & Green A. (2001). Fecal shedding of *Salmonella* spp. by dairy cows on farm and at cull cow markets, *Journal of Food Protection*, Vol. 64, No.1, pp. 3-11

Werber *et al.*, 2005, as cited in Jasson *et al.*, 2011

World Health Organization (1988). Salmonellosis control: the role of animal and product hygiene, *World Health Organization technical report series*, No. 774, pp. 1-83

World Health Organization (1994a). Guidelines on detection and monitoring of salmonella infected poultry flocks, with particular reference to *Salmonella* enteritidis. *World Health Organization*, Geneva, Switzerland.

World Health Organization (1994b). Guidelines on cleaning, disinfection and vector control in salmonella infected poultry, with particular reference to *Salmonella* enteritidis. *World Health Organization*, Geneva, Switzerland

World Health Organization (1994c). Workshop on competitive exclusion, vaccination and antimicrobials in *Salmonella* control in poultry. Oberkirchen, Germany.

World Health Organization (1994d). Safety and Nutritional Adequacy of Irradiated Food. Geneva, Switzerland

Winn W., Allen S., Janda W., Koneman E., Procop G., Schreckenberger P. & Woods G. (2006). Enterobacteriaceae, In: *Koneman's testo atlante di Microbiologia diagnostica*, Antonio Delfino Editore, pp. 251-302, ISBN: 9788872873960, Roma, Italy

Yan H., Li L., Alam M.J., Shinoda S., Miyoshi S. & Shi L. (2010). Prevalence and antimicrobial resistance of *Salmonella* in retail foods in northern China, *International Journal of Food Microbiology*, Vol. 143, No. 3, pp. 230-234

Zadoks R.N., van Leeuwen W.B., Kreft D., Fox L.K., Barkema H.W., Schukken Y.H. & Van Belkum A. (2002). Comparison of *Staphylococcus aureus* isolates from bovine and human skin, milking equipment, and bovine milk by phage typing, pulsed-field gel electrophoresis, and binary typing, *Journal of Clinical Microbiology*, Vol. 40, No.11, pp. 3894-3902

Zhao C., Ge B., De Villena J., Sudler R., Yeh E., Zhao S., White D.G., Wagner D. & Meng J. (2001). Prevalence of *Campylobacter* spp, *Escherichia coli*, and *Salmonella* serovars in retail chicken, turkey, port and beef from the greater Washington, DC area, *Applied and Environmental Microbiology*, Vol. 67, No.12, pp. 5431-5436

Zhao T., Doyle M.P., Fedorka-Cray P.J., Zhao P. & Ladely S. (2002). Occurrence of *Salmonella enterica* serotype Typhimurium DT104A in retail ground beef, *Journal of Food Protection*, Vol. 65, No.2, pp. 403-407

Zschöck M., Hamann H.P., Kloppert B. & Wolter W. (2000). Shiga-toxin producing *Escherichia coli* in faeces of healthy dairy cows, sheep and goats: Prevalence and virulence properties, *Letters in Applied Microbiology*, Vol. 31, No.3, pp. 203-208

# 4

# The Occurrence of *Salmonella* in Various Marine Environments in Turkey

Gülşen Altuğ
*Istanbul University, Faculty of Fisheries*
*Department of Marine Biology*
*Turkey*

## 1. Introduction

The occurrence and survival of enteric bacteria in marine ecosystems has been of interest to microbial ecology, sustainable usage of aquatic products, and the health of humans and the ecosystem (Barcina et al., 1986; Borrego and Figueras, 1997; Dionisio et al., 2000). Therefore, it is interesting to know and evaluate environmental factors that influence the occurrence of indicator bacteria and *Salmonella* spp. regarding sustainable and economical usage of aquatic products, ecosystem and human health.

The majority of bacteria present in domestic wastewater are comprised of saprophyte bacteria of faecal or terrestrial origin and pathogen bacteria such as *Salmonella, Shigella, Brucella, Mycobacterium, Escherichia coli, Leptospira, Campylobacter* and *Vibrio*. Furthermore, *Adenovirüs, Reovirüs, Rotavirüs* and *Hepatit* viruses as well as prozoons such as *Entamoeba histolytica, Giardia lamblia,* and *Cryptosporidium* may contaminate the sea by means of wastewater (Lynch and Hobbie 1988, Westwood 1994, Black 1996.)

*Salmonella* spp., one of the pathogenic bacteria which enter the sea environment as a result of anthropologic influences and particularly recreational use in coastal areas, continues to be a problem with regard to public health.

In order to define the source of *Salmonella* spp., contamination strains isolated from seawater and rivers were studied by molecular marker methods. Their properties were compared with those of strains originating from possible sources of contamination such as sewage from humans, cattle, and treated sewage water used in watering plants (Graeber et al., 1995).

The perforation of *Salmonella* spp. into sea water is not only from terrestrial originated wastewater but also from ships' ballast water which is imported to and exported from ships to maintain their balance.

The movements of ballast waters, from one continent to another by ships, create a global distribution mechanism for pathogenic and antibiotic-resistant forms and it may be significant in the worldwide distribution of microorganisms, as well as for the epidemiology of waterborne diseases affecting plants and animals (Ruiz et al., 2000). At the same time, most of the pathogens sourcing from sewage have been found to be present in shellfish. Particularly in production areas which are under the heavy influence of contamination, the most frequently found pathogen in shellfish is *Salmonella* spp.

### 1.1 The presence of *Salmonella* spp. and its relationship with primary hydrographic parameters

The presence of *Salmonella* and its relationship with primary hydrographic parameters (temperature, salinity, and dissolved oxygen) and indicator organisms in various marine environments were previously partly documented. It is known that the results of microbiological analysis were influenced by the dynamic structure of the aquatic environments. For instance, estuaries, lagoons, coastal and offshore environments are under variable environmental influences from each other. The hydrodynamic parameters of the estuary, in particular the flow rate, salinity gradient, and tidal cycles, were reported to be possible different relations between faecal-bacterial indicators and pathogens (Mill et al., 2006). Water temperature was positively associated with total *Salmonella* spp. levels. Bradd et. all (2009) reported that the levels of *Salmonella* spp. were correlated with average daily watershed rainfall for the 1 and 2 days preceding each sample collection. Similarly, environmental factors such as seasonal rainfall, salinity, and temperature were also correlated with *Salmonella* spp. abundance and diversity in the environment. (Bradd et. all 2009, Dionisio et al., 2000, Lemarchand and Lebaron, 2003; Martinez-Urtaza et al., 2004).

### 1.2 The presence of *Salmonella* spp. and its relationship with economically important aquatic products

The presence of *Salmonella* spp. and its relationship with aquatic products with respect to food health is one of the important headlines of this issue. Providing quality safety of aquatic products from their catching to their marketing to consumers has great importance in terms of human health as well as economical and ecological aspects.

Shellfish are filter-feeding organisms and because their power of movement is limited, they feed on the organic substances which the sea brings. They can reflect bacterial changes around them because they are capable of accumulating bacteria in high concentrations and the accumulation rate can change depending on microbial species. It was reported that *Chamalea gallina* can accumulate *S. typhimurium, E. coli, Vibrio parahaemolyticus, Aeromonas hydrophyla, Streptococcus faecalis,* and *Staphylococcus aureus* in the first six hours in laboratory conditions (Martinez et al., 1991). Nunes and Parsons (1998) reported that feeding oysters filter the surrounding water at a rate of 2 to 5 liter/hour eventually assimilating all the biotic and abiotic contaminants present in their environment. Due to the sensitivity of organisms and accumulation of environmental contamination, more bacterial contamination can be found in mussels than in the sea samples surrounding them. Because of these characteristics, shellfish have been accepted as bioindicators for detecting bacterial contamination in marine environments.

*Salmonella* spp. infections are one of the primary illnesses caused by the consumption of mussels. Bacterial pollution levels, associated with anthropological factors, are related to the occurrence of pathogenic bacteria in marine environments. *S. typhi* was isolated frequently in bivalve molluscs which were caught from a contaminated sea region. *Salmonella* spp. is one of the most important causes of human gastrointestinal diseases worldwide. Inal et al. (1979) have isolated *S. typhi* in shellfish taken from regions contaminated by slaughterhouse wastewater on the coast of the Aegean Sea, Turkey.

For these reasons, the consumption of shellfish has been generally associated with food-related infective diseases (Cook et al., 2001, Jose 1996). Food borne hazards are still of great concern for human health. Particularly the risks connected with shellfish and seafood consumption continue to be important both in developing and developed countries despite the advances in technology, changes in food processing and packaging (Fedhusen 2000, Huss, et al., 2000, Egli et al., 2002).

### 1.3 The presence of *Salmonella* spp. and its relationship with indicator bacteria

The presence of *Salmonella* spp. and its relationship with indicator bacteria can be variable according to the hydrodynamic characteristics and environmental factors of the studied areas. Some studies have reported that a relation between *Salmonella* spp. and faecal bacterial-indicators was observed only rarely (Polo et al., 1998, 1999).

Because of their better survival in saline waters enterococci have been suggested to be better indicators of microbial risk in coastal and estuarine environments (Dionisio et al., 2000; Kamizoulis and Saliba, 2004; Noble et al., 2003; Polo et al., 1998; Prüss, 1998). Lemarchand and Lebaron (2003) have reported that considering the occurrence of *Salmonella* spp., besides *Giardia* sp. and *Cryptosporidium* sp. and using changes of the levels of indicator organisms, "higher microbiological risk" and "lower microbiological risk" areas can be defined. Additionally, it was reported that fecal indicators do not exactly reflect the presence of pathogens such as *Salmonella* spp. in natural waters and that pathogens and indicators may have different behaviors in the aquatic environment (Lemarchand and Lebaron 2003).

### 1.4 Antibiotic resistance of *Salmonella* spp. in seawater

Beta-lactam antibiotics are widely used for treatment of infections in the world. Domestic waste waters might be an important source of antibiotic-resistant *Enterobacteriaceae*. Resistances to clinically relevant antibiotics are widespread in aquatic bacteria, including potential human pathogens. Since antibiotic resistance related to domestic wastewaters is important for the ecosystem and also for human heath in the aquatic environments, the resistance frequency of some beta-lactam antibiotics to *Salmonella* spp. isolates were investigated in this study.

In this study, the presence of *Salmonella* spp. and its relationship with primary hydrographic parameters and indicator organisms of bacterial pollution (total coliform, feacal coliforms) were investigated in the various marine areas of Turkey. The results were evaluated regarding sustainable and economical usage of aquatic products, the ecosystem and human

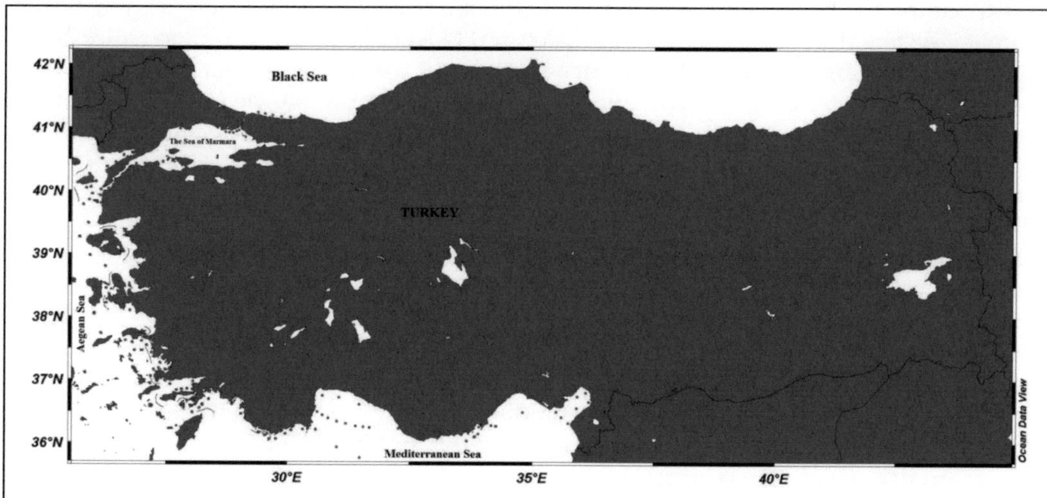


Fig. 1. Location of sampling sites in various marine areas of Turkey

health. Sea water and shellfish samples which were collected from various marine environments were investigated for occurrence of *Salmonella* spp. in different time periods throughout 1998–2010. A total of 832 samples of seawater (495), shellfish (243) and fish (94) were collected from six sites between July 1998 and August 2010.

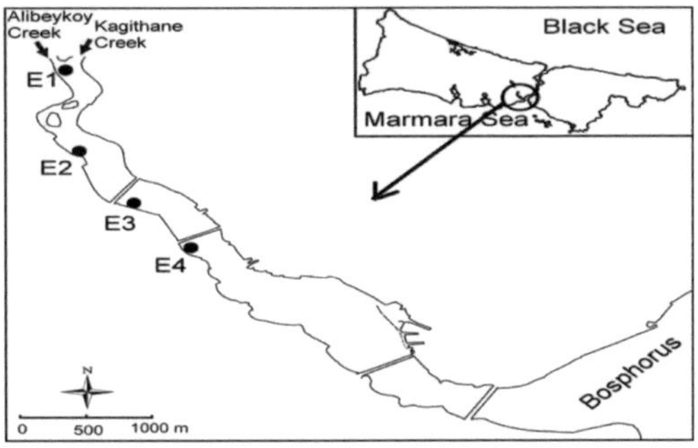


Fig. 2. One of the study areas: Golden Horn Estuary, Istanbul

## 2. *Salmonella* analyses

The presence of *Salmonella* spp. and indicator bacteria with respect to the areas from which they were isolated were investigated in the coastal areas of the Eastern Mediterranean, the Western Black Sea, the Golden Horn Estuary (Istanbul), the Sea of Marmara, the northern part of the Aegean Sea and also in the offshore area extending from the eastern part of Andros Island to the southern parts of Gokceada and Thasos Island, as well as the Mediterranean (Figure 1).

Indicator bacteria and *Salmonella* spp. were investigated in one hundred samples of seawater and 96 groups of *C. gallina* (striped venus) from six stations on the coastline of western Black Sea (Sile), Turkey. Studies were carried out on 15 days from June to December in 1998-1999 (Altuğ and Bayrak 2002).

Indicator bacteria and *Salmonella* spp. were investigated in 75 groups of sea snail (*Rapana venosa*) samples which were collected from the Florya-Ambarlı seashore of the Sea of Marmara, during the period between June 2000 and November 2001 (Altuğ and Güler 2002).

A total of 72 shellfish (*D. trunculus* /wedge-shell and *C. gallina*) were examined (36 groups *C. gallina*, 36 groups *D. trunculus*) which were taken from a site near Tekirdag on the northern coast of the Sea of Marmara, Turkey monthly between November 2005 and October 2006 (Altuğ et al., 2008).

The occurrence of *Salmonella* spp. in the total 44 samples of surface water which were collected from four different areas in the Golden Horn Estuary (Istanbul, Turkey) were tested in the period from November 2002 to December 2003.

The presence of *Salmonella* spp. in the 80 units of seawater samples, which were taken from 22 stations in the Southern part of the Sea of Marmara, was analyzed in 2006-2007 (Altuğ et. al., 2007).

The occurrence of *Salmonella* spp. in the 22 units of seawater samples from coastal areas in the Aegean Sea and 14 units of seawater samples from the Eastern Mediterranean, Turkey were investigated during the months of August in 2007 and 2008.

The occurrence of *Salmonella* spp. was investigated in the 83 units of seawater samples which were taken from various depths ranging from 0-30 cm to 500 m in the northern part of the Aegean Sea in 2006 and 2007. Seven unit samples were taken from the offshore areas extending from the eastern part of Andros Island to the southern part of Gokceada and Thasos Island in 2007 and 2008.

The presence of *Salmonella* spp. in the 136 units of seawater samples which were taken from 68 stations in the eastern and western coastal areas of Istanbul and from around the islands in the Sea of Marmara, Turkey were investigated in 2008 and 2010.

The Sample types, the number of samples and sampling periods were summarized in Table 1.

| **Sample** | **Number of Samples** | **Sampling Areas (Turkey)** | **Sampling Period** |
|---|---|---|---|
| Seawater | 100 | Western Black Sea | 1998-1999 |
| | 44 | Golden Horn Estuary (Istanbul) | 2002-2003 |
| | 22 | Aegean Sea (coastal areas) | 2006-2008 |
| | 83 | Northern Aegean Sea | 2006-2007 |
| | 80 | Southern part of the Sea of Marmara | 2006-2007 |
| | 7 | Northern Aegean Sea (0ffshore) | 2007-2008 |
| | 14 | Eastern Mediterranean | 2007-2008 |
| | 5 | Eastern Mediterranean (offshore) | 2007-2008 |
| | 136 | The Sea of Marmara | 2008-2010 |
| Total Seawater samples | 495 | | |
| *C. gallina* | 96 * | Western Black Sea | 1998-1999 |
| | 36* | The Sea of Marmara (Tekirdağ) | 2005-2006 |
| *D. trunculus* | 36* | The Sea of Marmara (Tekirdağ) | 2005-2006 |
| *R. venosa* | 75* | The Sea of Marmara (Florya-Ambarlı seashore) | 2000-2001 |
| Total Shellfish Samples | 243 | | |
| Fish | | | |
| *Atherina boyeri* | 22 | The Sea of Marmara (Yesilkoy-Avcılar) | 1999-2000 |
| *Scorpaena porcus* | 24 | The Sea of Marmara (Yesilkoy) | 1999-2000 |
| *Spicara smaris* | 31 | The Sea of Marmara (Yesilkoy) | 1999-2000 |
| *Diplodus vulgaris* | 11 | The Sea of Marmara (Tekirdağ) | 1999-2000 |
| *Scophthalmus maeoticus* | 6 | Black Sea (Derekoy-Samsun) | 1999-2000 |
| Total Fish Samples | 94 | | |
| Total number of samples | 835 | Turkey | 1998-2010 |

*A total of 6 individual samples were accepted as a sample group in the analyses

Table 1. The seawater, shellfish and fish samples which were collected from various marine environments, Turkey for bacteriological analyses in different periods.

### 2.1 Sampling areas

#### 2.1.1 Western Black Sea

The Black Sea covers an area that is about one third of the area of continental Europe. The Istanbul Strait connects the Black Sea to the world's oceans. The second largest river of Europe (Danube), also large rivers such as Dnieper, Don and Dniester all flow to the Black Sea. The salinity of the Black Sea is considerably lower (about 22-26 psu) than the Mediterranean. The population in Sile, western Black Sea, the sampling area, rises to 200,000 during the months of July and August due to recreational activities, compared with 50,000 during the other months. The purpose of this study was to determine the effect of the increasing anthropological activity on the bacteriological pollution of the seawater and *C. gallina* samples.

#### 2.1.2 The Golden Horn Estuary (Istanbul)

The Golden Horn Estuary has been heavily polluted by industrial and domestic wastes since 1950. Five million cubic meters of sludge has been removed during the last 10 years of restoration works. After the rehabilitation project, decreases in level of bacteria were reported (Altuğ and Balkıs 2009).

#### 2.1.3 The Sea of Marmara

The Istanbul Strait connects the Sea of Marmara to the Black Sea and the Canakkale Strait to the Aegean Sea. The Sea of Marmara separates Turkey's Asian and European regions. Being an important water route between the Mediterranean and the Black Sea, the Sea of Marmara is under the pressure of heavy marine transportation. The Sea of Marmara is under the influence of various anthropological factors such as dwelling, domestic and industrial wastes. The bacteria which come from ships' ballast water are another effective factor on the composition and abundance of bacteria in the Sea of Marmara. The less saline waters of the Black Sea reach the Mediterranean via upper currents while the concentrated saline waters of the Mediterranean reach the Black Sea via the undercurrents of the Canakkale and Istanbul Straits. These interesting hydrodynamic characteristics of the Sea of Marmara offer us unique opportunities for researching bacterial composition, under different, poorly described conditions.

#### 2.1.4 Eastern Mediterranean

Northeastern Mediterranean is known as a typical example of the world's oligotrophic seas. The salinity of the Mediterranean (38.5-38.6 psu) is considerably higher than the Black Sea. Bacterial composition of these environments have been managed by anthropological activities (Bayındırlı, 2007).

#### 2.1.5 Aegean Sea

The pelagic zones of the northern Aegean Sea and the Sea of Marmara share some main features due to their connection through the Çanakkale Strait. However, because of the anthropological sources, bacterial pollution level of northern part of the Aegean Sea less than the Sea of Marmara (Altuğ et. al., 2007). The population rate rises during the summer season due to recreational activities, compared with the other months in the coastal areas of the Aegean Sea. This situation is inducing the level of bacterial pollution (Altuğ et. all., 2007)

### 2.1.6 Offshore areas

Due to the differences between coastal areas and offshore areas with respect to exposed pollution factors, the offshore areas can be accepted as reference stations for the studies which monitor bacterial contamination.

In this study, seawater samples which were taken from the offshore areas extending from the eastern part of Andros Island to the southern parts of Gokceada and Thasos Island, as well as the Mediterranean were tested for indicator bacteria and *Salmonella* spp.

### 2.2 Sea water sampling

The samples from close stations (western Black Sea, the Sea of Marmara, and the Golden Horn Estuary, western Black Sea) were transported daily to the Aquatic Microbial Ecology Laboratory of Faculty of Fisheries of Istanbul University.

However, because of the long distances (Northern Aegean Sea, Eastern Mediterranean) between the sampling point and the laboratory, some analyses for filtration (indicator bacteria), pre-enrichment, selective enrichment (*Salmonella* spp.) and isolation were carried out during the cruise on the Bacteriology Laboratory of the Research Vessel YUNUS-S.

The numbers of the sea water samples which were collected from various marine areas between the years 1998 and 2010 according to sampling stations were summarized in the Table 1.

### 2.3 Shellfish sampling

C. *gallina* samples were collected by mechanical dredge at approximately 5-10 meters depth from the western Black Sea (Sile) from June to December in 1998-1999 (Altuğ and Bayrak 2002).

*R. venosa* samples were collected by diving from Florya-Ambarlı seashore, (Marmara Sea, Turkey) and with the help of divers during the period between June 2000 and November 2001 (Altuğ and Güler 2002).

*C. gallina* and *D. trunculus* samples were harvested along 500 m of shallow (4–7-m depth) area using a mechanical dredge in a site near Tekirdag (Kumbag), on the northern coast of the Sea of Marmara, Turkey monthly between November 2005 and October 2006. The mechanical dredge used was the standard dredging equipment used in fishing; a net with mesh openings of size 6 mm is attached to the metal dredge; when the dredge is dragged by the fishing vessel, in our case for 8–10 min, those particles equal to or greater than 6-mm size are collected in the net (Altuğ et al. 2008).

All the shellfish samples for the microbiological analyses were immediately transferred to the laboratory sealed in an ice box under aseptic conditions to avoid the possibility of bacterial contamination.

### 2.4 *Salmonella* spp. analyses for seawater samples

*Salmonella* spp. analyses depend on identification with biochemical and serological tests of suspicious colonies from selective solid medium after selective enrichment and unselective prior enrichment at 37 $^{0}$C in liquid medium in the seawater samples (APHA, 2000).

Then the colonies were restreaked several times to obtain pure cultures and the pure isolates of *Salmonella* spp. were identified using GN cards in the automated biochemical identification system VITEK 2 Compact 30 (Biomereux, France). The identification cards are based on established biochemical methods and newly developed substrates. There are biochemical tests (47 tests for GN) measuring carbon source utilization, enzymatic activities, inhibition, and resistance (Pincus, 2005).

### 2.5 *Salmonella* analyses for shellfish samples

In the analyses, 94 groups were used; 6 individuals were accepted as a group, and a total of 10 g (25 g for *Salmonella* spp.) was taken from each of these groups to form a sample group.

In accordance with the purpose of the test, diluted homogenous solutions of samples taken from those parts that are edible, were prepared with 0.1% buffered peptone water: 25:225 for the *Salmonella* spp.

Analyses depend on identification with current biochemical and serologic tests of suspicious colonies from selective solid medium after selective enrichment for 24 h in Selenith cystine broth at a temperature of 35⁰C, and unselective prior enrichment for 18–24 h at 37⁰C in buffered peptone water 25:225 (w/v) (FDA, 1998). To further identify and characterize the strains that were detected and isolated, commercially available API test system (BioMerieux, France) was used. The biochemical reactions tested with API test are: production of indole; utilization of citrate; production of nitrite; fermentations of glucose, mannitol, inositol, sorbitol, rhamnose, sucrose, melibiose, amygdaline, and arabinose; production of $H_2S$; activities of beta-galactosidase, tryptophane desaminase, gelatinase, arginine dihydrolase, lysine decarboxylase, and ornithine decorboxylase; formation of acetoin from pyruvate and oxidase (MacDonell et al.1982, Oberhofer 1983). When there was a need to further identification, the pure isolates of suspicious colonies were identified using GN cards in the automated biochemical identification system VITEK 2 Compact 30 (Biomereux, France).

The identification cards are based on established biochemical methods and newly developed substrates. There are biochemical tests (47 tests for GN) measuring carbon source utilization, enzymatic activities, inhibition, and resistance (Pincus, 2005).

### 2.6 Indicator bacteria analyses

Two different methods were used for indicator bacteria analyses in various sampling periods in 1998-2010.

#### 2.6.1 Membrane filtration method

The water samples were taken from 0-30 cm surface and from various depths ranging from 1 to 50 meters. Water samples were filtered through a 0.45 µm membrane filter with a metal vacuum filtering set (Millipore, Germany) and then the membrane filters were placed on m-Endo, m-FC and Azide-NKS for total coliform, fecal coliform and fecal streptococci. The plates were incubated for 48 h (at 37±0.1°C and 44.5±0.1°C) and the colonies on the plates were evaluated (APHA 1998; EPA 2006). Following the correction tests on suspicious colonies which grew after incubation, the average of three parallel tests was used for the numerical identification (cfu/100 mL: colony formed unit/100 mL). Brown-red colonies which grew on Azide medium were evaluated as fecal streptococci suspicious; blue colonies which grew on m-FC medium were evaluated as fecal coliform suspicious; pink-red colonies with yellow-green metallic shinyness which grew on m-Endo medium were evaluated as coliform suspicious. cytochrome oxidase test (API Strep, BioMereux ) was applied to coliform suspicious colonies and oxidase negative colonies were counted. cytochrome oxidase (API Strep, BioMereux ) and indole (HIMEDIA) tests were applied to fecal coliform suspicious colonies, and oxidase negative and indole positive colonies were counted. (MacFaddin 1980, APHA 2000).

#### 2.6.2 The most probable number method

Diluted homogenous solutions of samples taken from those parts that are edible were prepared with 0.1% buffered peptone water: 10:100 for the *E. coli* total coliform and fecal coliform analyses. Sample dilutions of $10^{-1}$, $10^{-2}$, and $10^{-3}$ with buffered peptone water were transferred to three series of test tubes, each containing 10 mL of Modified Lauryl Sulphate Triptose Broth.

Analyses were done according to the three tube most probable number method (MPN) using Brilliant green bile broth (BGLB), EC broth, Eosin methylene blue agar medium, Plate count agar medium (FDA, 1998).

For characterization of coliform, Endo agar was used.

### 2.7 Antibiotic resistance test

The percentage of bacteria in the samples which exhibited antibiotic resistance was measured on Nutrient agar plates supplemented with Imipenem, Ampicillin, Cefotaxim, Ceftriaxon, Ceftazidim media (NCCLS 1999).

## 3. Occurrence of *Salmonella* spp. in the samples of seawater, shellfish and fish

### 3.1 Seawater

The frequency of *Salmonella* spp. according to their exposure to environmental factors in the areas from which they were isolated were shown in Table 1 in the form of summary data of the level of coliform and fecal coliform bacteria and the occurrence of *Salmonella* spp.

No *Salmonella* spp. was detected in the samples which were taken from the western Black Sea in 1998-1999.

The presence of *Salmonella* spp. in seawater from the four stations was significantly different ($p < 0.05$) in the Golden Horn Estuary, Istanbul from 2002 to 2003. Eleven of 44 seawater samples were found positive for *Salmonella* spp. The number of *Salmonella* spp. positive samples was highest in the inner part of the estuary.

The percentage distribution of the values for the ratio of fecal coliform to fecal streptococci in the surface water of the Aegean Sea and their relation with *Salmonella* spp. was also investigated. The contribution of fecal coliform bacteria to fecal streptococci (FC/FS > 0.7) showed that the sources of fecal contamination were anthropological in this area in 2006-2008. Seven of the 22 unit seawater samples were found positive for *Salmonella* spp. in the sea water samples which were taken from the coastal areas of the Aegean Sea, *Salmonella* spp. positive samples were positive correlated with the indicator bacteria count. In the five stations which have higher number of indicator bacteria than the other stations *Salmonella* spp. were found positive. The percentages of *Salmonella* spp. among the total enteric bacteria were between 25% and 37% in these stations.

*Salmonella* spp. was not isolated in the seawater samples which were taken from the offshore areas.

Four units of 14 seawater samples tested which were taken from coastal areas of eastern Mediterranean were found positive for *Salmonella* spp. in August 2007-2008.

Eight units of 83 seawater samples tested which were taken from 0-30 cm to 500 meters were found positive for *Salmonella* spp. in the samples of 0-30 cm, 50 meters and 100 meters in the June 2006. *Salmonella* spp. was only isolated in the summer period during the study.

Fourteen of 80 seawater samples which were taken from 30 cm to 50 meter were positive for *Salmonella* spp. in July 2006 in southern part of the Sea of Marmara. Also, three seawater samples were found *Salmonella* spp. positive in June 2007. During this study *Salmonella* spp. was isolated only in July 2006 and June 2007.

Sixty four of the 495 unit seawater samples tested was found positive for *Salmonella* spp. (13%) in the stations. Thirty three of the 64 unit *Salmonella* spp. positive samples of seawater (51.5 %) which have been recorded in the stations indicator bacteria were > $10^4$ fecal coliform /100 ml.

Twenty two of 136 unit seawater samples which were taken from 0-30 cm in the Sea of Marmara were found positive for *Salmonella* spp. in the July 2009 and June 2010 period. *S. enterica* ssp. *arizonae, S. enteritidis and S. typhimurium* were the most identified isolates in the samples. *S. typhimurium* represented 64.3% of all *Salmonella* spp. strains and was identified in the seawater samples.

The frequency of *Salmonella* spp. related to fecal coliform bacteria in the seawater samples was summarized in the Table 2. Biochemical details of two of isolated *Salmonella* spp. was summarized in Table 3.

### 3.2 Shellfish

Eight of 243 shellfish samples analyzed were found positive for *Salmonella* spp. (3.29%). Five of eight units of *Salmonella* spp. positive samples of shellfish (83.3%) also had indicator bacteria higher than $10^4$ fecal coliform /100 ml (Table 2).

*Salmonella* spp. was not isolated in the *C. gallina* samples which were collected from the western part of the Black Sea, Turkey in 1998 and 1999.

The highest levels of fecal coliform and *E. coli* within the total of 75 *R. venosa* samples analyzed were found in the samples collected during the months of August 2000 and 2001. In the samples of August 2000, *Salmonella* spp. was found positive in both samples of fecal coliform and *E. coli;* however, *Salmonella* spp. was not isolated in the other samples.

The maximum level of fecal coliform, total coliform, and *E. coli* were recorded in the *D. trunculus* and *C. gallina* samples in July, August, and September, 2006 (Altuğ et al., 2008). *Salmonella* spp. in the *D. trunculus* and *C. gallina* samples was detected only in July and August 2006.

*S. typhimurium, S. enterica* ssp. *arizonae* and *S. enteritidis* also was isolated among the all isolated strains from the shellfish samples.

### 3.3 Fish

Three *(A. boyeri, S. porcus and S.smaris)* of the 94 unit fish samples analyzed were found positive for *Salmonella* spp. in 1999. All of the *Salmonella* spp. positive samples also had indicator bacteria more than $10^4$ fecal coliform /100 ml. All the isolated strains from the fish samples were *S. enterica* ssp. *arizonae*.

The overall prevalence of *Salmonella* spp. was 9.01%, with the highest occurrence in seawater (13%), shellfish (3.29 %), followed by fish (2.13%).

Thirty two of 64 *Salmonella* isolates (50%) showed resistance to Imipenem (21 isolates), Ampicillin (22 isolates), Cefotaxim (19 isolates), Ceftriaxon (11 isolates), and Ceftazidim (18 isolates) acid (9 isolates), with nine of these isolates displaying multiple resistance to four of these antibiotics.

While the highest Multiple Antibiotic Resistance (MAR) was found in the bacteria isolated in seawater which was taken from the Golden Horn Estuary, Istanbul, the bacteria isolated from northern part of the Sea of Marmara and coastal areas of Istanbul respectively followed it.

| Sample Type | F. coliform | Number of *Salmonella* (+) samples | *Relation (%) between the fecal coliform level and the number of Salmonella* (+) samples |
|---|---|---|---|
| Sea Water | 10-<$10^2$ | 0 | 0 |
| | $10^2$-<$10^3$ | 14 | 21.8 |
| | $10^3$-<$10^4$ | 17 | 26.5 |
| | >$10^4$ | 33 | 51.5 |
| Number of seawater samples: 495 | 64 (13% of the 495 samples) | | |
| Shellfish | 10-<$10^2$ | 0 | 0 |
| | $10^2$-<$10^3$ | 1 | 12.5 |
| | $10^3$-<$10^4$ | 2 | 25 |
| | >$10^4$ | 5 | 83.3 |
| Number of shellfish samples: 243 | 8 (3.3% of the 243 samples) | | |
| Fish | 10-<$10^2$ | 0 | 0 |
| | $10^2$-<$10^3$ | 0 | 0 |
| | $10^3$-<$10^4$ | 3 | 100 |
| | >$10^4$ | 0 | 0 |
| Number of fish samples: 94 | 3 (2.13% of the 94 samples) | | |
| Total number of specimens:832 | 75 (9.01% of the 832 samples) | | |

Table 2. The frequency of *Salmonella* spp. (cfu/25 ml; cfu/25 g) and fecal coliform bacteria (cfu/100 ml) in the samples

| TESTS | *Salmonella* spp. | *Salmonella* spp. |
|---|---|---|
| APPA | - | - |
| ADO | - | - |
| PyrA | - | - |
| IARL | - | - |
| dCEL | - | - |
| BGAL | - | - |
| H2S | + | + |
| BNAG | - | - |
| AGLTp | - | - |
| dGLU | + | + |
| GGT | - | - |
| OFF | + | + |
| BGLU | - | - |
| dMAL | - | - |
| dMAN | + | + |
| dMNE | + | + |
| BXYL | - | - |
| BAlap | - | - |
| ProA | - | - |
| LIP | + | + |
| PLE | - | - |
| TyrA | - | - |
| URE | - | - |
| dSOR | - | - |
| SAC | - | - |
| dTAG | + | + |
| dTRE | + | + |
| CIT | - | - |
| MNT | - | - |
| 5KG | - | - |
| ILATk | - | - |
| AGLU | - | - |
| SUCT | - | - |
| NAGA | - | - |
| AGAL | - | + |
| PHOS | + | + |
| GlyA | - | - |
| ODC | + | + |
| LDC | + | + |
| IHISa | - | - |
| CMT | - | - |
| BGUR | - | - |
| O129R | - | + |

| TESTS | *Salmonella* spp. | *Salmonella* spp. |
|---|---|---|
| GGA | - | - |
| IMLTa | - | - |
| ELLM | - | - |
| ILATa | - | - |

***APPA:** Ala-Phe-Pro-ARYLAMIDASE; **ADO:** ADONITOL; **PyrA:** L-Pyrrolydonyl-ARYLAMIDASE; **IARL:** L-ARABITOL; **dCEL:** D-CELLOBIOSE; **BGAL:** BETA-GALACTOSIDASE; **H2S:** H2S PRODUCTION; **BNAG:** BETA-ACETYL-GLUCOSAMINIDASE; **AGLTp:** Glutamyl Arylamidase pNA; **dGLU;** D-GLUCOSE; **GGT:** GAMMA-GLUTAMYL-TRANSFERASE; **OFF:** FERMENTATION/GLUCOSE; **BGLU:** BETA-GLUCOSIDASE; **dMAL:** D-MALTOSE; **dMAN:** D-MANNITOL; **dMNE:** D-MANNOSE; **BXYL:** BETA-XYLOSIDASE; **BAlap:** BETA-Alanine arylamidase pNA; **ProA:** L-Proline ARYLAMIDASE; **LIP:** LIPASE; **PLE:** PALATINOSE; **TyrA:** Tyrosine ARYLAMIDASE; **URE:** UREASE; **dSOR:** D-SORBITOL; **SAC:** SACCHAROSE/SUCROSE; **dTAG:** D-TAGATOSE; **dTRE:** D-TRHALOSE; **CIT:** CITRATE (SODIUM); **MNT:** MALONATE; **5KG:** 5-KETO-D-GLUCONATE; **ILATk:** L-LACTATE alkalinisation; **AGLU:** ALPHA-GLUCOSIDASE; **SUCT:** SUCCINATE alkalinisation; **NAGA:** Beta-N-NCETYL-GALACTOSAMINIDASE; **AGAL:** ALPHA-GALACTOSIDASE; **PHOS:** PHOSPHATASE; **GlyA:** Glycine ARYLAMIDASE; **ODC:** ORNITHINE DECARBOXYLASE; **LDC:** LYSINE DECARBOXYLASE; **IHISa:** L-HISTIDINE assimilation; **CMT:** COUMARATE; **BGUR:** BETA-GLUCORONIDASE; **O129R:** O/129 RESISTANCE (comp.vibrio); **GGAA:** Glu-Gyl-Arg-ARYLAMIDASE; **IMLTa:** L-MALATE assimilation; **ELLM:** ELLMAN; **ILATa:** L-LACTATE assimilation*

Table 3. Biochemical characteristics of some isolated *Salmonella* spp which were identified using GN cards in the automated biochemical identification system VITEK 2 Compact 30 (Biomereux, France)

## 4. Conclusion

The frequency of *Salmonella* spp. according to their exposure to environmental factors in the areas from which they were isolated were different. For instance, higher indicator bacteria and *Salmonella* spp. abundance was found in the coastal stations compared to the offshore areas.
The *Salmonella* spp. prevalence in a total of 832 samples of seawater (495), shellfish (243), and fish (94) which were collected from six sites between 1998 and 2010 exhibited diversity according to geographical areas. The coastal areas which were under the influence of biological pollution with respect to heavy inland population displayed higher levels of *Salmonella* spp. than the offshore areas.
Enteric bacteria of sewage origin undergo a sudden osmotic shock when they enter seawater and may adapt their metabolism to the new medium by means of their osmoregulation systems. This ability of enteric bacteria aids them in gaining resistance to salt in sea environments and increases their probability of survival (Munro et al., 1989). The presence of a negative relationship between salinity concentration and the number of enteric bacteria in sea medium has been determined (Carlucci et al., 1960, APHA 1998, Bitton 2005)
In this study, the influence of salinity on the presence of *Salmonella* spp. associated with water samples was also investigated. In the Sea of Marmara it was possible to isolate *Salmonella* spp. from the under and upper stratification of various localities which possessed salinity values between 24.0 psu and 39.2 psu during the study. The bacteria levels determined in water samples taken from under the halocline layer in the Sea of Marmara were sometimes found to be higher in comparison to sea water samples taken from 0-30 cm. The higher bacteria levels found in the undercurrent were considered to be a result of deep discharge systems carrying domestic waste products. Hydrographic changeable parameters

such as seawater temperature, pH, salinity and dissolved oxygen are significant factors associated with the presence of *Salmonella* spp. In this study, seawater temperature was the only variable showing a linear positive effect on the presence of *Salmonella* in the sea, while the other parameters showed more complex nonlinear effects in the studied areas.

There are many factors such as temperature, salinity, sunlight, grazing by heterotrophic microorganisms affecting the survival of enteric bacteria in marine areas (*Sinton et al 2007:* Harm, 1980, Gameson & Gould 1985, Jagger 1985, Rozen and Belkin 2001, Sinton 2005)

Temperature also seemed to affect efficiently the abundance of indicator bacteria and *Salmonella* spp. in the study areas. *Salmonella* spp. positive samples were mostly recorded in the summer seasons and the indicator bacteria level was also higher during these periods compared to the other sampling seasons in 1998-2010. This situation is directly related to the increase of human activity, especially in coastal areas in summer seasons. However it also shows that despite the salinity stress, occurrences of indicator bacteria and *Salmonella* spp. were possible under these conditions in the seawater.

*C. gallina* and *D. trunculus* are two most common and abundant species in Turkish clam resources. Especially *C. gallina* is very important and valuable species, due to its great export potential, *C. gallina,* which has begun to be gathered since 1986 via mechanical dredge in Turkey, has great importance in terms of economy (Altuğ et. al., 2008).

The mean values of bacterial contamination found in the 75 *R. venosa* samples under bacteriological analysis were between 15x10 and $24 \times 10^3$ and above. It is concluded that the area is under the influence of the waste products of dwellings and naval transportation (Altuğ and Güler 2002).

Beta-lactam antibiotics are widely used for treatment of infections in the world. Domestic waste waters might be an important source of antibiotic-resistant *Enterobacteriaceae.* Resistances to clinically relevant antibiotics are widespread in aquatic bacteria, including potential human pathogens. Because antibiotic resistance related to domestic waste waters is important for the ecosystem and also for human health, the resistance frequency of *Salmonella* spp. isolates to some beta-lactam antibiotics was investigated in this study. The antibiotic derivates which were found to be resistant to bacteria were different in different regions. This situation shows that pollution input and the usage rate of antibiotics have differences related to geographic regions. Further research will help towards setting limits on the prevalence of antibiotic-resistant bacteria and supporting the effectiveness of antimicrobial agents.

It was reported that *Salmonella* spp. presence in marine waters is adequately predicted by total coliforms or fecal coliforms (Efstratiou et al. 2009). In this study, positive correlations were found between the presence of coliform bacteria (especially $>10^3$ cfu/100 ml) and occurrences of *Salmonella* spp. positive isolates. Efstratiou et al.( 2009) reported that the *E. coli* limits set by the EU Directive for defining "good" coastal bathing water quality (500 CFU100 $ml^{-1}$) are much higher than the fecal coliform concentration which would best predict the absence of *Salmonella* spp.

The percentage distribution of the ratio values of Fecal Coliform to Fecal Streptococci in the surface water of the Aegean Sea and the relation of this ratio with the occurrence of *Salmonella* spp. was also investigated (Altuğ et al., 2007). The percentages of *Salmonella* spp. among total enteric bacteria were between 25% and 37%. Positive correlations were observed between the level of indicator bacteria and the presence of *Salmonella,* implying that *Salmonella* spp. occurrence is a part of anthropological pollution input in the investigated areas. The presence of isolates of *Salmonella* spp. in the marine environment is of notable significance with respect to public health due to the potential risk of acquiring infections as a result of the consumption of contaminated aquatic products or ingestion of contaminated seawater.

## 5. Acknowledgment

The author wishes to thank Dr. Mine Cardak, PhD students Sevan Gürün and Pelin S. Çiftçi for their support. The author also thanks the crew of the research vessel Yunus-S for their help in sampling.

## 6. References

Altuğ, G. Bayrak, Y. (2002). Determination of the Levels of Indicator Bacteria and *Salmonella* spp. in *Chamelea gallina*, L. and Seawater on the Coastline of Sile, Turkey. *Journal of the Marine Biology United Kingdom Association (JMBA)*, 82, 4, 673–674.

Altuğ, G., Güler N. (2002). Determination of the Levels of Indicator Bacteria, *Salmonella* spp. and Heavy Metals in Sea Snails (*Rapana venosa*) from the Northern Marmara Sea, Turkey. *Turkish Journal of Fisheries and Aquatic Science*. 2, 2, 141-144.

Altuğ, G., Aktan, Y., Oral, M., Topaloglu, B., Dede, A., Keskin, C., Isinibilir, M., Cardak, M., Ciftci, P.S. (2007). *Evaluation of Biological Diversity related to Physical, Chemical and Biological Data of the Northern Aegean Sea and Southern Marmara Sea*. The Scientific and Technical Research Council of Turkey 105Y039 Technique Report.

Altuğ G., Çardak M., Ciftci P.S. (2007). Kültür Balıkçılığı ve Turistik Faaliyetlerin Besin Tuzları ve Bakteriyolojik Kirlilik Dağılımına Etkisi. *Journal of Fisheries and Aquatic Sciences*, 22, 23, 39-54 (in Turkish).

Altuğ, G., Çardak, M., Çiftçi P. S. (2008). Indicator and Other Bacteria in Striped Venus (*Chamelea Gallina, L*) and Vedge Clam (*Donax Trunculus*) from the Northern Coast of the Sea of Marmara, Turkey. *Journal of Shellfish Research*, 27, 4.

Altuğ, G., Balkıs, N. (2009). Levels of some toxic elements and frequency of bacterial heavy metal resistance in sediment and sea water, Turkey. *Environmental Monitoring and Assessment*, 149, 61–69.

APHA, (1998). *Standard methods for the examination of water and wastewater, 18th Edi.*, American Public Health Association, 8755-3546, Washington, D.C.

APHA, (2000). *Standard Methods for the Examination of Water and Wastewater*. 20th Edition, *In:* Clesceri, L.S., A.E Greenberg and A.D Eaton (eds), American Public Health Association, American Water Works Association and Water Environment Federation. 0875530478, Washington, D.C.

Bayındırlı, C. (2007). *Monthly changes in the abundance and biomass of picoplankton (heterotrophic bacteria & cyanobacteria Synechococcus in the Cilician basin (eastern Mediterranean)*. METU. Institute of Marine Sciences, M.Sc. Thesis. 89 p.

Barcina, I., Arana, I., Iriberri, J., Egea, L. (1986). Influence of light and natural microbiota of the Butron River on E. coli survival. *Antonie van Leeuwenhoek*. 52, 555-566.

Bitton, G. (2005). *Wastewater microbiology*. 3th edi., John Wiley & Sons, Hoboken, doi: 10.1002/0471717967.ch3 New Jersey.

Black, J.G. (1996). *Microbiology: principles and application*, 3rd ed., Prentice-Hall, Oxford,

Borrego, J.J., Figueras, M.J. (1997). Microbiological quality of natural waters. *Microbiol. SEM* 13, 413–426.

Bradd J. Haley Dana J. Cole, Erin K. Lipp. (2009). Distribution, Diversity, and Seasonality of Waterborne Salmonellae in a Rural Watershed. *Applied and Environmental Microbiology,* 75, 5, 1248–1255.

Carlucci, A. F., Scarpino, P. V., Pramer, D. (1960). Evaluation of factors affecting survival of *Escherichia coli* in sea water studies with heat and filter-sterilized sea water. *Applied Microbiology.* 5, 9, 400–404.

Cook, D. W., Burkhardt, W. III, A. DePaola, S. A., McCarthy K., Calci, R. (2001). *Molluscan shellfish: oyster, mussels and clams.* In: F. P. Downes & K. Ito, editors. Compendium of methods for the microbiological examination of foods. 4th ed. APHA, Washington.

Dionisio, L.P.C., Joao, M., Ferreiro, V.S., Fidalgo, M.L., Garcia Rosado, M.E., Borrego, J.J. (2000). Occurrence of Salmonella spp in estuarine and coastal waters of Portugal. *Antonie van Leewenhoek.* 78, 99–106.

Efstratiou, M.A., Mavridou, A., Richardson, C. (2009). Prediction of Salmonella in seawater by total an faecal coliforms and Enterococci. *Marine Pollution Bulletin,* 58, 201-205.Egli, T., Koster, W., Meile, L. (2002). Pathogenic microbes in water and food: changes and challenges. *FEMS Microbiology Reviews* 26, 111- 112.

EPA, (1986*). U.S.Environmental Protection Agency. Ambient Water Quality Criteria for Bacteria-1986.* U.S.Environmental Protection Agency, EPA-440/5-84-002, Washington, D.C

FDA. (1998). *Bacterial analytical manual,* 8th ed. Revision A. AOAC International, Washington, DC.

Feldhusen, F. (2000). The role of seafood in bacterial foodborne diseases. *Microbes Infection,* 2, 1651–1660.

Gameson, A. L. H., Gould, D. J. (1985). Bacterial mortality, Part 2. In Investigations of sewage discharges to some British coastal waters. WRc Techn. Rep. TR 222. WRc Environment, Medmenham, UK.

Graeber, I., Montenegro, M.A., Bunge, C., Boettcher, U. (1995). Molecular marker analysis of *Salmonella typhimurium* from surface water, humans, and animals. *Europan Journal Epidemioogy.* 11, 325-33.

Harm, W. (1980). Biological Effects of Ultraviolet Radiation. Cambridge University Press, London, England.

Huss, H. H., Reilly, A., Embarek, P.K.B. (2000). Prevention and control of hazards in seafood. *Food Control,* 11, 149–156.

Inal, T., Bese, M., Ugur, M., Tantas, A. (1979). Izmir seaport waters and Salmonella contamination. *Research Bulletin TUBITAK,* Ankara 293, 20.

Jagger, J. (1985). Solar-UV Actions on Living Cells. Praeger, New York, USA.

José,V.F. (1996). Bivalves e a segurança do consumidor. Dissertação de Mestrado. Ciência Ambiental, São Paulo, USP.

Kamizoulis, G., Saliba, L. (2004). Development of coastal recreational water quality standards in the Mediterranean, *Environment International,* 30, 841–854.

Lemarchand, K., Lebaron P. (2003). Occurrence of Salmonella spp. and Cryptosporidium spp. in a French coastal watershed: relationship with fecal indicators. *FEMS Microbiology Letters.* 218, 203-209.

Lynch, E., Hobbie, J.E. (1988). *Principles of microbial behaviour in ecosystems,* Blackwell, Oxford,

Martinez-Urtaza, M. Saco, J. de Novoa, Perez-Pieiro, P., Peiteado, J., Lozano-Leon, A. (2004). Influence of environmental factors and human activity on the presence of *Salmonella* serovars in a marine environment. *Journal of Applied and Environmental Microbiology* 70, 2089–2097.

Martinez, M. E., Egea, F., Castro, D., Morinigo, M.A., Romero, P., Borrego, J.J. (1991). Accumulation and depuration of pathogenic and indicator microorganisms by the bivalve mollusc, Chamelea gallina L, under laboratory. *Journal of Food Protection. USA* 54, 612–618.

MacDonell, M.T., Singleton, F. L., Hood, M.A. (1982). Diluent composition for use of API 20E in characterizing marine and estuarine bacteria. *Applied Environmental Microbiology,* 44, 423–427.

MacFaddin, J.F. (1980). Biochemical Tests for Identification of Medical Bacteria, 2nd ed., Williams and Wilkins, Baltimore MD. 249-260.

Mill, A., Schlacher, T., Katouli, M. (2006). Tidal and longitudinal variation of faecal indicator bacteria in an estuarine creek in southeast Queensland, Australia. *Marine Pollution Bulletin,* 52, 881–891.

Munro, P.M., Gauthier, M.J., Breittmayer, V.A., Bongiovanni, J. (1989). Influence of some osmoregulaiton processes on starvation of *Escherichia coli* in seawater. *Applied and enviromental microbiology,* 55, 2017- 2014.

National Comittee for Clinical Laboratory Standards. (1999). (NCCLS) Performance standards for antimicrobial susceptibility testing, Ninth Informational Supplement, M100-S9, Wayne.

Noble, R.T., Moore, D.F., Leecaster, M.K., McGee, M.K., Weisberg, S.B. (2003). Comparison of total coliform, fecal coliform, and enterococcus bacterial indicator response for ocean recreational water quality testing, *Water Research,* 37, 1637–1643.

Nunes, A.J.P., Parsons, G. J. (1998). Dynamics of tropical coastal aquaculture systems and the consequences to waste production. *Journal of the World Aquaculture Society,* 29, 27–37.

Pincus, D. H. (2005). Encyclopedia of Rapid Microbiological Methods Volume 1. Ed. Miller, M. J. Chapter 1 *Microbial Identification using the Biomérieux VITEK® 2 System Biomérieux,* Inc. Hazelwood, MO USA PDA/DHI 1-32.

Polo, F., Figueras, M., Inza, I., Sala, J., Fleisher, J., Guarro, J. (1998). Relationship between presence of *Salmonella* and indicators of faecal pollution in aquatic habitats, *FEMS Microbiology Letters,* 160, 253–256.

Prüss, A. (1998). Review of epidemiological studies on health effects from exposure to recreational water, *International Journal of Epidemiology,* 27, 1.

Rozen, Y., Belkin, S. (2001). Survival of enteric bacteria in seawater. *FEMS Microbiology Reviews,* 25, 513–529.

Ruiz, G. M., Rawlings, T. K., Dobbs, F. C., Drake, L. A., Mullady T., Huq, A., Colwell, R. R. (2000). Global spread of microorganisms by ships. *Nature,* 408, 49-50.

Sinton, L. W. (2005). Survival of enteric bacteria in seawater: biotic and abiotic effects. In Oceans and Health: Pathogens in the Marine Environment (ed. R. R. Colwell & S. Belkin). Kluwer Academic/Plenum Publishers, USA.

Sinton, L., Hall, C., Braithwaite, R. (2007). Sunlight inactivation of Campylobacter jejuni and Salmonella enterica, compared with Escherichia coli, in seawater and river water. *Journal of water and health*, 5, 3, 357-65.

Westwood, D. (1994). *The microbiology of water, methods for the examination and association materials, report on public health and medical subjects* No:71, HMSO, London.

# 5

# *Salmonella* in Fish and Fishery Products

İlkan Ali Olgunoğlu
*University of Adiyaman*
*Vocational School of Kahta*
*Turkey*

## 1. Introduction

With more than 30.000 known species, fish form the biggest group in the animal kingdom that is used for the production of animal-based foods. About 700 of these species are commercially fished and used for food production. Further, some 100 crustacean and 100 molluscan species (for example mussels, snails and cephalopods) are processed as food for humans in fish industry (Oehlenschläger & Rehbein, 2009). However, some fishery product is processed in a modern fish industry which is a technologically advanced and complicated industry in line with any other food industry, and with the same risk of product being contaminated with pathogenic organisms (Huss, 1994).

The vast majority of outbreaks of food-related illness are due to pathogenic microorganisms, rather than to chemical or physical contaminants. As they are generally undetectable by the unaided human senses (i.e.they do not usually cause colour changes or produce off-flavours or taints in the food) and they are capable of rapid growth under favourable storage conditions (Lelieveld et al. 2003). The United States Centers for Disease Control and Prevention reported that fish and shellfish account for 5% of the individual cases and 10% of all foodborne illness outbreaks, with most of the outbreaks resulting from the consumption of raw molluscan shellfish (Flick, 2008).

*Salmonella* is responsible for more than 40.000 cases of food-borne illness every year. The incidence of *Salmonella* infections has risen dramatically since the 1980s, leading to high medical costs, a loss of wages for workers who become ill, and a loss of productivity for the companies whose workers do become ill. In all, these financial losses can cost more than $3.6 billion each year. *Salmonella* infections have long been a concern to scientists, doctors, and the U.S. Food and Drug Administration (FDA) (Brands, 2006). *Salmonella* is causing a public health problem associated with fish and fishery products. A monitoring of *Salmonella* has been suggested as a measure of fish quality. Also, risk management decisions should take into account the whole food chain from primary production to consumption, and should be implemented in the context of appropriate food safety infrastructures, for instance regulatory enforcement, food product tracing and traceability systems. In the fish processing chain managing risks should be based on scientific knowledge of the microbiological hazards and the understanding of the primary production, processing and manufacturing technologies and handling during food preparation, storage and transport, retail and catering (Popovic et al., 2010). Their presence in fish and fishery product is therefore seen as a sign of poor standards of process hygiene and sanitation (Dalsgaard, 1998).

## 2. Description of *Salmonella*

*Salmonella* is a member of the Enterobacteriaceace, Gram negative, motile, with peritrichous flagella and nonsporeforming rods (the rods are typically 0.7-1.5 µm x 2.5 µm in size). *Salmonella* is a facultatively anaerobic (can grow with or without oxygen) catalase positive and oxidase negative bacteria. However, *Salmonella* is not included in the group of organisms referred to as coliforms (Huss & Gram, 2003; Adams & Moss, 2005; Erkmen, 2007; Lawley et al., 2008). These mesophilic organisms are distrubuted geographically all over the world, but principally occurring in the gastrointestinal tracts of mammals, reptiles, birds, and insects and environments polluted with human or animal excreta (Huss, 1994, Huss & Gram, 2003; Saeed & Naji 2007). Survival in water depends on many parameters such as biological (interaction with other bacteria) and physical factors (temperature). More than 2,500 different types of *Salmonella* exist, some of which cause illness in both animals and people. Some types cause illness in animals but not in people. The various forms of *Salmonella* that can infect people are referred to as serotypes, which are very closely related microorganisms that share certain structural features. Some serotypes are only present in certain parts of the world (Brands, 2006). For over 100 years *Salmonella* have been known to cause illness. The bacterium was first isolated from pigs suffering hog cholera by an American scientist, Dr. Daniel Elmer Salmon, in 1885 (Bremer et al., 2003).

## 3. Sources of *Salmonella* contamination in fish and fishery products

Aquatic environments are the major reservoirs of *Salmonella*. Therefore, fishery products have been recognized as a major carrier of food-borne pathogens (Kamat et al., 2005; Upadhyay et al., 2010).

Pathogenic bacteria associated with fish and fishery product can be categorised into three general groups: (1) bacteria (indigenous bacteria) that belong to the natural microflora of fish (*Clostridium botulinum*, pathogenic *Vibrio* spp., *Aeromonas hydrophila*); (2) enteric bacteria (non-indigenous bacteria) that are present due to fecal contamination (*Salmonella* spp., *Shigella* spp., pathogenic *Escherichia coli*, *Staphylococcus aureus*); and (3) bacterial contamination during processing, storage or preparation for consumption (*Bacillus cereus, Listeria monocytogenes, Staphylococcus aureus, Clostridium perfringens, Salmonella* spp.) (Lyhs 2009).

Information from literature indicates that fresh fish, fish meal, oysters, farmed and imported frozen shrimp and froglegs can carry *Salmonella* sp., particularly if they are caught in areas contaminated with faecal pollution (prior to harvest and during harvest) or processed, packed, stored, distributed under unsanitary conditions and consumed raw or slightly cooked (Kumar et al., 2003; Kamat et al., 2005, Mol et al., 2010; Norhana et al., 2010).

There are some pathways of contamination of aquaculture systems with *Salmonella*.

**Non-point water run-off**

During rainfall events, increased run off of organic matter into ponds may occur and can contaminate the aquaculture system.

**Animals (domestic animals, frogs, rodents, birds, insects, reptiles, etc.)**

A variety of animal waste has been shown to be potential sources of *Salmonella*. Animal waste can be introduced directly through bird droppings or frogs living in ponds or indirectly through runoff.

**Fertilization of ponds**

In some aquaculture systems animal manures are used in ponds to stimulate the production of algae. The use of non-composted manures can lead to production systems being contaminated with *Salmonella*.

**Contaminated feed**

Improperly stored feed or feed prepared on a farm under poor hygienic conditions can be a source of *Salmonella*.

**Contaminated source water**

The water used in growout ponds, cages or tanks can be contaminated with *Salmonella* through wildlife runoff, untreated domestic sewage, discharge from animal farms, etc.

**On farm primary processing**

Aquaculture products can become contaminated with *Salmonella* through the use of unsanitary ice, water, containers, and poor hygienic handling practices (FAO, 2010).

For example, for shrimp processing industry the information from literature indicates that the principal sources of *Salmonella* contamination are culture ponds, coastal water used for handling and processing of seafood (Hariyadi et al., 2005; Shabarinath et al., 2007; Upadhyay et al., 2010). Similarly, Pal and Marshall (2009) reported that the potential source of *Salmonella* contamination in farm-raised catfish is likely due to poor water quality, farm runoff, fecal contamination from wild animals or livestock, feed processing under poor sanitary conditions or distribution, retail marketing, and handling/preparation practices.

Ray et al.,(1976) reported that the potential hazard in cooked fishery product is cross contamination of the cooked products with raw fishery product which might occur under commercial processing condition. Thus, good sanitation practices on the unloading docks and during transport to the processing facility are essential for preventing product contamination. The use of contaminated ice or uncleaned holding facilities may also contribute to the product contaminant load (Gecan et al., 1988). As a result, many factors including inadequate supplies of clean water, inadequate sanitary measures, lack of food hygiene and food safety measures have been responsible for increased incidence of foodborne salmonellosis (Shabarinath et al., 2007).

Deep-sea fish are generally *Salmonella* sp. free but susceptible to contamination post-catch. Water temperature has been

proposed as playing an important role in the long-term survival of *Salmonella* in the environment (FAO, 2010). In raw seafood products mainly from tropical climates, there is a high prevalence of *Salmonella* whereas low prevalence or absence can be common in temperate regions (Millard and Rocklif, 2004).

## 4. Occurrence in fish and fishery product

*Salmonella* has been isolated from fish and fishery product, though it is not psychrotrophic or indigenous to the aquatic environment (Mol et al., 2010). The relationship between fish and *Salmonella* has been described by several scientists; some believe that fish are possible carriers of *Salmonella* which are harbored in their intestines for relatively short periods of time and some believe that fish get actively infected by *Salmonella*. The organism was never recovered from the flesh of the fish, but was isolated from viscera and epithelium (Pullela, 1997). Most outbreaks of food poisoning associated with fish derive from the consumption of raw or insufficiently heat treated fish and cross-contamination during processing and about 12% of the foodborne outbreaks related to consumption of fish are caused by bacteria including *Salmonella* (Huss et al., 2000; Aberoumand, 2010). Similarly, The U.S. Food and Drug Administration's (FDA) data showed that *Salmonella* was the most common contaminant of fish and fishery products (Allshouse et al., 2004). Up to 10-15% of fish samples from India and Mexico were positive of *Salmonella* which has also been detected in several crustacean and molluscan products from India and Malaysia (Huss & Gram 2003). *Salmonella* contamination in fish and fishery products has also been reported from other countries like Thailand, Hong Kong, Spain and Turkey (Herrera et al., 2006; Kumar et al., 2009; Pamuk et al, 2011). The highest *Salmonella* incidence in fishery products was determined in Central Pacific and African countries while it was lower in Europe and including Russia, and North America (Heinitz et al. 2000). For example, Davies et al. (2001) reported the absence of *Salmonella* in fish from European Countries such as France, Great Britain, Greece and Portugal. However, Novotny et al., (2004), reported an outbreak of *Salmonella* blockley infections following smoked eel consumption in Germany. *Salmonella* paratyphi B infections were also reported associated with consumption of smoked halibut in Germany (Da Silva, 2002). Besides, consumption of dried anchovy was found to be the cause of *Salmonella* infection (Ling et al., 2002).

Table 1 shows the incidence of salmonellosis associated with all food vehicles, and with separately seafood, for the European Union in 2007 (FAO,2010).

| **Food vehicle** | **Number of outbreaks** | **Number of *Salmonella* outbreaks** | **% of outbreaks associated with *Salmonella*** |
|---|---|---|---|
| Fish and fishery products | 130 | 3 | 2.3 |
| Crustaceans, shellfish, molluscs, and products | 75 | 2 | 2.7 |
| All food vehicles | 2025 | 590 | 29.1 |

Table 1. Fishery product associated outbreaks in the European Union, 2007 (Data from FAO,2010)

*Salmonella* has also been detected in US market oysters and in other US imported seafood from different countries (Heinitz et al. 2000; Ponce et al., 2008). For the 9-year period 1990–1999, the FDA in the United States examined imported and domestic fish and seafoods for *Salmonella*. Of the 11.312 imported samples, 7.2% were positive while only 1.3% of the 768 domestic samples were positive.

The most common serovar found in the world was *S. Weltvreden* (Heinitz et al. 2000; Jay et al., 2005). In seafood the commonest serotype encountered was S. Worthington followed by S. Weltevreden. The diversity of serovars associated with fish and fishery product was highest in Southeast Asia and next highest in South America (FAO, 2010). Most *Salmonella* contamination problems in fishery product associated with shrimp. Almost one-quarter of all detentions, and more than half of the violations for *Salmonella*, were for shrimp and prawns (farm raised and wild caught).

| *Salmonella* Serotype | India/ SE Asia | Africa | Central America | Central pacific | Eastern Caribbean | Europe and Russia | Mexico | Middle East | North America/ Multiple | South America |
|---|---|---|---|---|---|---|---|---|---|---|
| *S.* Abaetetu | | | + | | | | | | | + |
| *S.* Aberdeen | + | | | | | | | | | |
| *S.* Agona | + | | | | | | + | | | + |
| *S.* Ahepe | | + | | | | | | | | |
| *S.* Albany | + | | | | | | | | | |
| *S.* Anatum | + | | | + | + | + | + | | | + |
| *S.* Anfo | + | | | | | | | | | |
| *S.* Arizonae | + | | | + | | | + | | | + |
| *S.* Atakpam | + | | | | | | | | | |
| *S.* Augusten | + | | | | | | | | | |
| *S.* Baguida | | | | | | | | | | + |
| *S.* Bareilly | + | | | | | | + | | | |
| *S.* Biafra | + | | | | | | | | | |
| *S.* Blockley | + | | | | | | | | | |
| *S.* Bovis-mobificans | + | | | + | | | | | | |
| *S.* Bradford | + | | | | | | | | | |
| *S.* Braender | + | | | | | | | | | |
| *S.* Brancast | + | | | | | | | | | |
| *S.* Bredeney | | | | | | | | | | + |
| *S.* Brunei | + | | | | | | | | | |
| *S.* Bullbay | | | | | | | | | | + |
| *S.* Cannstat | | | | | | | + | | | |
| *S.* Carrau | | | + | | | | | | | |
| *S.* Cerro | + | | | | | | | | | + |
| *S.* Derby | + | | | + | | | | | | |
| *S.* Drypool | + | | | | | | | | | |
| *S.* Dublin | + | | | | | | | | | |
| *S.* Duesseldorf | | | | + | | | | | | |
| *S.* Emek | + | | | | | | | | | |
| *S.* Emek | + | | | | | | | | | |
| *S.* Enteritidis | + | + | | + | | | + | | + | + |
| *S.* Farmsen | + | | | | | | | | | |
| *S.* Gallinaru | + | | | | | | | | | |
| *S.* Georgia | + | | | | | | | | | |
| *S.* Gwaai | | | | | + | | | | | |
| *S.* Hadar | + | | | + | | | + | + | | |
| *S.* Harmelen | | | + | | | | | | | |
| *S.* Havana | + | | | | + | | | | | |
| *S.* Havana | | | | | | | | | | |

| *Salmonella* Serotype | India/ SE Asia | Africa | Central America | Central pacific | Eastern Caribbean | Europe and Russia | Mexico | Middle East | North America/ Multiple | South America |
|---|---|---|---|---|---|---|---|---|---|---|
| *S.* Heidelber | + | | | + | | | | | | + |
| *S.* Hilversum | | | | + | | | | | | |
| *S.* Houten | | | + | + | | | | | | + |
| *S.* Houten | + | | | | | | | | | |
| *S.* Hull | | + | | | | | | | | |
| *S.* Hvittingfoss | + | | | | | | | | | |
| *S.* Idikan | + | | | | | | | | | |
| *S.* Infantis | + | | + | | + | | | | | |
| *S.* Irumu | + | | | | | | | | | |
| *S.* Isangi | + | | | | | | | | | |
| *S.* Javiana | + | | | + | | | | | | + |
| *S.* Kentucky | + | | | + | | | + | | | + |
| *S.* Kirkee | + | | | | | | | | | |
| *S.* Kottbus | + | | | | | | | | | |
| *S.* Krefeld | + | | | | | | | | | |
| *S.* Kumasi | + | | | | | | | | | |
| *S.* Lanka | + | | | | | | + | | | |
| *S.* Lansing | + | | | | | | | | | |
| *S.* Lexington | + | | | | | | | | | |
| *S.* Liandoff | | | | | | | + | | | |
| *S.* Lindenburg | + | | | | | | | | | |
| *S.* Litchfield | | | | | | | | | | + |
| *S.* Liverpool | + | | | | | | | | | |
| *S.* London | + | | | + | | | | | | |
| *S.* Manila | | | | + | | | | | | |
| *S.* Marina | | | | | | | | | | + |
| *S.* Mbandaka | + | | + | | | | | | | |
| *S.* Meleagridis | + | | | | | | + | | | |
| *S.* Mendoza | | | | | | | | | | + |
| *S.* Mgutani | + | | | | | | | | | |
| *S.* Miami | | + | | | | | | | | |
| *S.* Michigan | | | | | | | + | | | |
| *S.* Minnesota | + | | | | | | + | | | |
| *S.* Montevideo | + | | | | | | | | | |
| *S.* Morehead | + | | | | | | | | | |
| *S.* Mosselbay | | | | | | | | | | + |
| *S.* Muenchen | + | | | | | | + | | | |
| *S.* Muenster | + | | | | + | | | | | |
| *S.* Nairobi | | + | | | | | | | | + |

| *Salmonella* Serotype | India/ SE Asia | Africa | Central America | Central pacific | Eastern Caribbean | Europe and Russia | Mexico | Middle East | North America/ Multiple | South America |
|---|---|---|---|---|---|---|---|---|---|---|
| *S.* Nchanga | + | | | | | | | | | |
| *S.* Newbrunswick | | | | | | | + | | | |
| *S.* Newington | | | | | | | | | | + |
| *S.* Newport | + | | + | + | | | | | + | + |
| *S.* Ohio | + | | | | | | + | | | |
| *S.* Onireke | | + | | | | | | | | |
| *S.* Oranienburg | + | | | | + | | + | | | + |
| *S.* Orientalis | | | | + | | | | | | |
| *S.* Oslo | + | | + | | | | | | | |
| *S.* Othmarschen | + | | | | | | | | | |
| *S.* Panama | | | | | | | | | | + |
| *S.* Paratyphi B | + | | | + | | | | | | |
| *S.* Paratyphi B Java | + | | | | | | | | | |
| *S.* Parera | | + | | | | | | | | |
| *S.* Phoneix | | | | | | | | | | + |
| *S.* Pomana | | | + | | | | + | | | |
| *S.* Poona | + | | + | | | | + | | | |
| *S.* Potsdam | + | | | | | | | | | |
| *S.* Pullorum | | | | + | | | | | | |
| *S.* Reading | + | | | | | | | | | |
| *S.* Redba | | + | | | | | | | | |
| *S.* Reinikendorf | + | | | | | | | | | |
| *S.* Riggil | + | | | | | | | | | |
| *S.* Rissen | + | | | | | | | | | |
| *S.* Rubislaw | | + | + | | | | + | | | |
| *S.* Saintpaul | + | | | + | | | + | + | + | + |
| *S.* Saka | | + | | | | | | | | + |
| *S.* Sandiego | + | | | | | | | | | |
| *S.* Saphra | | | | | | | + | | | |
| *S.* Sarajane | + | | | | | | | | | |
| *S.* Schleisshein | + | | | | | | | | | |
| *S.* Schwarzengrun | | | | | | | | | | |
| *S.* Senftenberg | + | | + | | + | | + | + | | |
| *S.* Singapore | + | | | | | | | | | |
| *S.* Srinagar | + | | | | | | | | | |
| *S.* Stanley | + | | | + | | | | | | |
| *S.* Takoradi | + | | | | | | | | | |

| *Salmonella* Serotype | India/ SE Asia | Africa | Central America | Central pacific | Eastern Caribbean | Europe and Russia | Mexico | Middle East | North America/ Multiple | South America |
|---|---|---|---|---|---|---|---|---|---|---|
| *S.* Tananarive | + | | | | | | | | | |
| *S.* Telelkebir | | + | | | | | | | | |
| *S.* Tennessee | + | | | | | | + | | | |
| *S.* Thompson | + | | | + | | | + | | + | |
| *S.* Tornow | | | | + | | | | | | + |
| *S.* Typhi | + | | | | | | | | | |
| *S.* Typhimurium | + | | + | | + | | + | | + | + |
| *S.* Uganda | | | | | + | | | | | |
| *S.* Urbana | + | | | | | | | | | |
| *S.* Virchow | + | | | + | | | | | + | |
| *S.* Wandsworth | + | | | | | | | | | |
| *S.* Washington | + | | | | | | | | | |
| *S.* Weltevreden | + | | + | + | | + | + | | | + |
| *S.* Weston | + | | | | | | | | | |
| *S.* Worthington | + | | | | | | | | | |

Table 2. *Salmonella* serotype reported in fish and fishery products (Data from FAO, 2010)

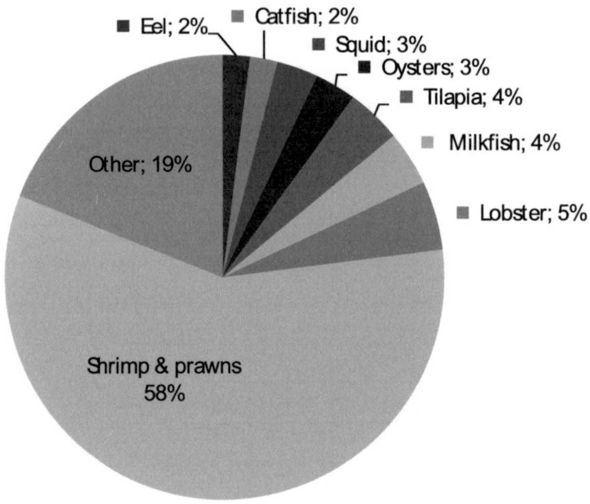


Fig. 1. Share of FDA violations for *Salmonella*, by fishery product, 2001 (data from Allshouse et al., 2004).

## 5. Survival and growth parameters

*Salmonella* sp. can multiply and survive in the estuarine environments and tropical freshwater environments for weeks although open marine waters are free from *Salmonella* (Huss,1994; Huss & Gram 2003). *Salmonella* prefers to grow at 37°C. Compared to other Gram-negative bacteria, *Salmonella* are relatively resistant to various environmental factors. They grow at temperatures between 5°C and 47°C. There are reports that they survive for longer than *E. coli* in sea and freshwater environments (Huss, 1994; Sugumar & Mariappan, 2003; Marriot & Gravani, 2006). *Salmonella* have been also reported to be able to grow within the temperature range of 2-54°C, although growth below 7°C has largely been observed only in microbiological culture media and growth above 48°C is confined to mutants or tempered strains (Bremer et al. 2003). A few *Salmonella* serotypes can grow over a pH range of 3.6–9.6, which is mildly basic to strongly acidic. Optimum growth occurs at a pH of 6.5–7.5, which is close to neutral. Other factors such as temperature, the type of acid present and the presence of antimicrobials can effect the minimum pH for growth (Brands, 2006; Marriot & Gravani, 2006; Lawley et al., 2008). It requires a minimum Aw of 0.94 (and possibly 0.93) with a maximum salt content of 4.0% to 5.0% (Huss, 1994; Lawley et al., 2008). A study by Basti et al., (2006), for example, showed complete elimination of *Salmonella* on heavy salted fish and heavy salted cold smoked fish due to the high concentration levels of NaCl (>7%). Limiting conditions were summarized for *Salmonella* in Table 3.

| Pathogen | min. Aw (using salt) | min. pH | max. pH | max.% water phase salt | min. temp | max. temp | Oxygen requirement |
|---|---|---|---|---|---|---|---|
| *Salmonell a* spp. | 0.94 | 3.7 | 9.5 | 5 | 5 °C | 47 °C | facultative anaerobe |

Table 3. Limiting Conditions for *Salmonella* Growth

## 6. Control of *Salmonella* in fish and fishery products

Since most of fish products, with the exception of coldsmoked fish, sushi, and a few specialty products such as spiced, salted, or pickled fish, are expected to be cooked prior to consumption, the presence of microbiological pathogens should not present a human health hazard (Flick, 2008).

The aquaculture farm is the first link in the food safety continuum and controls must be in place and implemented throughout the food safety chain. The experts agreed that good hygienic practices during aquaculture production and biosecurity measures can minimize but not eliminate *Salmonella* in products of aquaculture.

**Some important control measures to minimize the risk of *Salmonella* contamination of aquaculture products according to FAO (2011)**

**Farm location**

- Farms should be secured from the entry of wild and domestic animals that may lead to the contamination of aquaculture products with *Salmonella.*

**Farm layout, equipment and design**

- Farm design and layout should be such that prevents cross contamination

- Equipment such as cages, nets and containers should be designed and constructed to allow for adequate cleaning and disinfection
- Septic tanks, toilet facilities and bathrooms/showers should be constructed and placed so drainage does not pose a risk of contamination of farm facilities.

**Source water**

- Farm source water should be free from sewage contamination and suitable for aquaculture production
- Farms should have settling ponds or waste water treatment in place to condition the output water prior to discharge

**Ice and Water Supply**

- Potable or clean water is available and used in sufficient amount for harvest, handling and cleaning operations
- Ice should be manufactured using potable water and produced under sanitary conditions
- Ice should be handled and stored under good sanitary conditions which precludes the risk for contamination.

**Harvesting**

Harvesting equipment and utensils easy to clean and disinfect and kept in clean condition.

- Harvesting is planned in advance to avoid time/temperature abuse.
- Aquaculture products should be hygienically handled.
- Records on harvesting are maintained for traceability.

**On farm post-harvest handling**

- Utensils and equipment for handling and holding of aquaculture products is maintained in a clean condition.
- Aquaculture products are cooled down quickly and maintained at temperatures approaching that of melting ice.
- Operations such as sorting, weighing, washing, drainage, etc., are carried out quickly and hygienically.
- All additives and chemicals (disinfectants, cleaning agents, etc) used in post-harvest aquaculture products should be approved by the national competent authority.

**Transport of aquaculture products from farm**

- Transport is carried out in easy to clean and clean facilities (boxes, containers, etc.).
- Conditions of transport should not allow contamination from surroundings (e.g. dust, soil, water, oil, chemicals, etc.).
- Aquaculture products are transported in containers with ice or with, in sufficient amounts to ensure temperature around 0ºC (approaching that of melting ice) in all products and during the whole period of transport.

**Employee health**

- Staff should be medically fit to work and should be screened regularly to determine carriers of *Salmonella*.

On the other hand, a number of studies have been carried out to develop methods to control contamination of proceed fishery products. They are sub-divided into physical or chemical approaches (Norhana et al., 2010).

## 7. Physical approaches

### 7.1 Cooking

Application of heat is one of the simplest and most effective methods of eliminating pathogens from food. Heat application of 90°C for 1.5 min. in the center for mollusc and 99–100°C for 3–4 min. for shellfish are accepted as safe processes before consumption. These temperatures are sufficient for the destruction of vegetative forms of the pathogens (Olgunoglu, 2010). Ray et al. (1976) reported that the processing of blue crabs involving steam cooking with pressure of approximately 15 psi (121°C) for 10 min. is sufficent to kill pathogens on the raw crab. Vegetative, unstressed *Salmonella* cells are heat-sensitive and are easily destroyed at pasteurisation (hot-smoking) temperatures. D-values (Decimal reduction time) at 60°C are typically 1-3 minutes (Huss & Gram 2003). Time/Temperature Guidance for Controlling *Salmonella* growth in Fishery Products were given Table 4.

| Potentially Hazardous | Product Temperature | Maximum Cumulative Exposure Time |
|---|---|---|
| Growth of *Salmonella* species | 5.2-10˚C<br>11-21˚C<br>above 21˚C | 2 days<br>5 hours<br>2 hours |

Table 4. Time/Temperature Guidance for Controlling *Salmonella* Growth inFih and Fishery Products (FDA, 2011)

### 7.2 Refrigeration

Refrigeration and freezing are well-known techniques for extending the shelf-life of food products. These processes lower the temperature to levels at which bacterial metabolic processes are stopped and the rates of chemical and biochemical reactions reduced (Norhana et al., 2010). Although most *Salmonella* serotypes are unable to grow at refrigeration temperatures, the organismis can be prevented holding chilled fishery products below 4.4°C (Ward &Hart, 1997). Worldwide, the most common cause of foodborne salmonellosis is *Salmonella typhimurium*. The minimum growth temperature reported for this species is 6.2°C (A study by Ingham et al., (1990), indicate that the temperature preventing growth of S. typhimurium in picked crab meat is at or below 7°C). Thus, proper refrigeration will prevent growth of S. Typhimurium. However, maintenance of optimal refrigeration temperatures often cannot be guaranteed at all times prior to food consumption (Ingham et al., 1990). Thus, good sanitation after refrigeration process of fishery products such as cooked crabs or cooked shrimp are very important in maintainning product quality(Ray et al., 1976).

### 7.3 Irradiation

The irradiation of fishery products is a physical treatment involving direct exposure to electron or electromagnetic rays, for their long time preservation and improvement of quality and safety (Oraei et al., 2011; Özden & Erkan, 2010). Irradiation of food has been legally allowed in many countries and the WHO has sanctioned radiation of up to 7.0 kilo Gray (kGy) as safe. This process is one of the most effective methods for decontaminating both the surface and deep muscle of fresh meat. There is substantial literature on the effects of irradiation in reducing *Salmonella* on some fishery product such as shrimp (Norhana et al., 2010). The alteration in pathogen population as a result of irradiation depends on the dose of irradiation, storage temperature, packaging conditions and fish species (Özden et al., 2007). For example a study, showed complete elimination of *Salmonella* on frozen shrimp when irradiated at 4.0 kGy. Similarly it is also reported that doses of 4.0–5.0 kGy were required to reduce the numbers of *S. typhimurium* on shrimp by 6.0 log cycles. According to Oraei et al., (2011), low-dose gamma irradiation (especially 3 kGy) can be applied for microbial control and the safety of rainbow trout and shelf life extension in frozen state. Gamma irradiation at 3 kGy was more effective than irradiation at 1 and 5 kGy in eliminating microorganisms of rainbow trout fillets. The irridation doses are also reported in the range 1.5–2.0 kGy effectively control all pathogenic bacteria tested in shellfish except *Salmonella* spp., particularly, *S. enteritidis*, which requires 3.0 kGy (IAEA,2001). Similarly to achieve safety levels against *Salmonella* spp., particularly *S. enteritidis*, in raw oysters, a dose of 3.0 kGy is recommended by Gelli (2001). As a results although irradiation appears to be effective in eliminating pathogens in fishery product, there is an unsubstantiated view amongst the public that food irradiation is unsafe and undesirable. There is also evidence some that irradiation may reduce the nutritional value of some foods by the destruction of aromatic amino acids and producing rancidity and off-odours (Norhana et al., 2010).

## 8. Modified atmosphere packaging (MAP)

Modifed atmosphere packaging (MAP) has been widely used for extending the shelf life of a wide variety of food, including fish and fish products since 1980. Packages are injected with carbon dioxide, nitrogen, and very small (0.4 percent) amounts of carbon monoxide. The effciency of MAP in eliminating pathogens from fish depends on the gas mixture in MAP and, most importantly, the storage temperature (Redman, 2007; Hudecová et al., 2010). There is limited information on the effect of MAP with elevated $O_2$ level on *Salmonella* in the literature. A study by Hudecová et al., (2010), for example, showed a signifcant decrease in the microbial growth rate on fresh chilled common carp (Cyprinus carpio) during storage at +4 ± 0.5 °C in two different MAP (70% $N_2$/30% $CO_2$ and 80% $O_2$/20% $CO_2$) for 10 days when compared to air packaging and no *Salmonella* was reported in these conditions. Ingham et al., (1990) reported that modified atmosphere storage using 50% $CO_2$/10% $O_2$ dose effectively reduce the growth rate of *S. typhimurium*, but it cannot, in the absence of proper refrigeration, be relied upon to prevent salmonellosis.

## 9. High-pressure processing (HPP) and superheated steam drying (SSD)

High-pressure processing is an emerging non-thermal process that can be used to destroy pathogenic microorganisms in seafood without greatly affecting the quality of the product. In addition to improving the safety of shrimp, HPP has also been demonstrated to extend shrimp shelf-life. Shrimp are generally spoiled by Gram-negative bacteria, which tend to be relatively pressure sensitive due to their cell wall structure and HPP may therefore prove to be a valuable processing technology for shrimp. Although research has demonstrated the benefit of using HPP on shrimp and shrimp products, limited studies have been carried out specifically to eliminate or reduce *Salmonella* in fishery product using this technology.

Superheated steam drying (SSD) is a promising drying technology to a variety of industries. Superheated steam is steam heated to a temperature higher than the boiling point corresponding to its pressure (Norhana et al., 2010).

## 10. Chemical approaches

### 10.1 The use of antimicrobial agents

Chlorine is the decontaminating agent most widely used to kill pathogenic microorganisms in the seafood industry. It is used to disinfect water used in the process (such as thawing frozen products), washing raw materials and in making ice for chilling fishery products. Commonly used chlorine compounds are liquid chlorine solution (HOCl) and hypochlorite ($OCl^-$). More recently chlorine dioxide ($ClO_2$) and electrolyzed oxidizing (EO) water have also been used for this purpose. Specifically, $ClO_2$ has been recognized as a bactericidal, viricidal and fungicidal agent and is widely used in Europe and US as an alternative to chlorine and hypochlorite. In addition, EO water has also been shown to possess strong bactericidal activity against various foodborne pathogens.

Both gaseous and dissolved forms of ozone are approved to be used as antimicrobial agents by the food industry, including the seafood industry. There are investigations on the effect of 2% ozonated saline (5.2 mg ozone/L, 5°C) on the inactivation of nine bacterial strains (including *S. typhimurium*) in shrimp meat. Findings showed that *S. typhimurium* was the most resistant of the species tested, with only 0.1 log cycle reductions (Norhana et al., 2010).

Lactate is considered to be an effective additional hurdle against the growth of contamination flora and pathogens such as *Salmonella* and it is used in the further processed fish industry (fish cakes, smoked salmon, injected fillets, marinated fish). Studies on the specific action of lactates indicate they stimulate mechanisms that interfere with the metabolism of the bacteria, such as intercellular acidification and interfere with proton transfer across the cell membrane and feedback inhibition. Lactate also lowers water activity. Since lactate does not kill bacteria, it cannot be used to mask poor sanitation practices (Da Silva 2002).

## 11. International commision on microbiological specification for food (ICMSF) recommended microbial limits

| Product | n[1] | c[2] | Bacteria/gram or $cm^2$ | |
|---|---|---|---|---|
| | | | m[3] | M[4] |
| Fresh and frozen fish and cold-smoked fish | 5 | 0 | 0 | - |
| Frozen raw crustaceans | 5 | 0 | 0 | - |
| Frozen cooked crustaceans | 10 | 0 | 0 | - |
| Fresh and frozen bivalve molluscs | 20 | 0 | 0 | - |

[1]Number of representative sample units.
[2]Maximum number of acceptable sample units with bacterial counts between m and M.
[3]Maximum recommended bacterial counts for good quality products.
[4]Maximum recommended bacterial counts for marginally acceptable quality products. Plate counts below "m" are considered good quality. Plate counts between "m" and "M" are considered marginally acceptable quality, but can be accepted if the number of samples does not exceed "c." Plate counts at or above "M" are considered unacceptable quality (SeafoodNIC; http://seafood.ucdavis.edu/haccp/compendium/chapt17.htm)

Table 5. Recommended microbiological limits for *Salmonella* spp. in fish and fishery products

## 12. Conclusions

Significant numbers of detections of *Salmonella* in fish and fishery products indicate that current strategies for *Salmonella* control in the aquaculture production and processing sectors are not adequate. While some marine fish caught offshore and handled hygienically and at low temperature according to the Codex Code of Practice for fish and fishery products (CAC/RCP/52-2003) may be suitable for raw consumption, it would be advisable to consume products of aquaculture only after cooking. The *Salmonella* problem should be resolved by the use of good manufacturing procedures and the strict application of sanitary practices. On the other hand, Hazard analysis and critical control point (HACCP) systems should be implemented increasingly by private industry for seafood, sometimes voluntarily and sometimes as mandated by Federal governments. These must be rigidly enforced throughout the processing line and require the full understanding and cooperation of plant management and every employee. Investment in new technologies and equipment will also improve the seafood safety.

## 13. References


Aberoumand, A. (2010). Estimation of Microbiological Variations in Minced Lean Fish Products. *World Journal of Fish and Marine Sciences*, 2 (3): 204-207.

Adams M.R. & Moss M.O. (2005). Food Microbiology Second Edition University of Surrey, Cuildford, UK. 475

Allshouse J., Buzby J., Harvey,D., Zorn D., (2004). United States Department of Agriculture Economic Research Service, Seafood Safety and Trade, *Agriculture Information Bulletin,* Number 789-7.

Basti, A. A.; Misaghi, A.; Salehi, T. Z. & Kamkar A.,(2006). Bacterial pathogens in fresh ,smoked and salted Iranian fish *Food Control* 17: 183–188.

Brands D. A. (2006). Deadly Diseases and Epidemics *Salmonella,* Chelsea House Publishers, a subsidiary of Haights Cross Communications. 102p.

Bremer, P. J.; Fletcher G. C. & Osborne, C. (2003). *Salmonella* in seafood. New Zealand Institute for Crop & Food Research Limited A Crown Research Institute 4p.

CAC/RCP 52-2003 Code of Practice For Fish and Fishery Products.

Da Silva, Antonia L. V. (2002). Hazard Analysis Critical Control Point (HACCP), Microbial Safety, and Shelf Life of Smoked Blue Catfish (Ictalurus furcatus). Master of Science (M.S.) The Department of Food Science, 100p.

Dalsgaard, A. (1998). The occurrence of human pathogenic Vibrio spp. and *Salmonella* in aquaculture International *Journal of Food Science and Technology,* Volume: 33 Issue: 2 Pages: 127-138.

Davies, A. R.; Capell, C.; Jehanno, D; Nychas, G. J. E. & Kirby, R. M. (2001). Incidence of foodborne pathogens on *European fish Food Control,* Volume 12, Issue 2, Pages 67-71.

Erkmen O. (2007). Basic Methods for the Microbiological Analysis of Foods. Nobel Publishing, Scinece and Biology Publishing Series Publishing No:1069, Series: 29, 564 p.

FAO (2010). Expert Workshop on the application of biosecurity Measures to control *Salmonella* Contamınatıon in Sustainable aquaculture FAO Fisheries and Aquaculture Report No. 937 ISSN 2070-6987, Mangalore, India, 19–21 January 2010.

FDA. (2011). Fish&Fisheries Products Hazards&Control Guidance: Fourth Edition. Center for Food Safety and Applied Nutrition. Office of Seafood. 317p.

Flick, G. J.(2008). Microbiological Safety of Farmed Fish Food Safety and Technology Global Aquaculture Advocate 33-34.

Gecan, J. S.; Bandler, R. & Atkinson J.C. (1988). Microanalytical quality of canned crabmeat, sardines and tuna. Journal of Food protection 51:12 979-981.

Gelli, D. S., Mastro, del N., Rodrigues, de M. I. & Jakabi, M. (2001). Study on the radiation sensitivity of pathogenic Vibrionaceae and Enterobacteriaceae in vitro and after inoculation into oysters (Cassostrea brasiliana) Irradıatıon to control Vibrio Infection from Consumptıon of Raw Seafood and fresh produce Printed by the IAEA in Austria. 77p.

Hariyadi, R. D.; Nuraida, S. L. & Fardiaz S. (2005). Determination of contamination profiles of human bacterial pathogens in shrimp obtained from Java, Indonesia. Determination of human pathogen profiles in food by quality assured microbial assays. Proceedings of a final Research Coordination Meeting held in Mexico City, Mexico, 22–26 July 2002.

Heinitz, M. L.; Ruble, R. D.; Wagner, D. E. & Tatini, S.R. (2000). Incidence of *Salmonella* in fish and seafood. Journal of Food Protection 63 (5), 579–592.

Herrera, F. C.; Santos, J.A.; Oteroand, A. & Lopez M. L. G. (2006). Occurrence of foodborne pathogenic bacteria in retail prepackaged portions of marine fish in Spain. The Society for Applied Microbiology, Journal o fApplied Microbiology 100, 527–536.

Huss, H. H. (1994). Assurance of Seafood Quality FAO Fisheries Technical Paper 334 169p.

Huss, H. H.; Reilly, A. & Embarek, P. K. B. (2000). Prevention and control of hazard in seafood. Food Control 11, 149–156.

Hudecová, K., Buchtová, H. & Steinhauserová I. (2010). The Effects of Modifed Atmosphere Packaging on the Microbiological Properties of Fresh Common Carp (*Cyprinus carpio* L.) *ACTA VET*. BRNO 79: 93–100.

Huss, H. H. & Gram, L. (2004). Characterization of Hazards in Seafood Assurance of Seafood Quality FAO Fisheries Technical Paper 444 227p.

IAEA (International atomic Energy) (2001). Irradiation to control vibrio infection from consumption of raw seafood and fresh produce IAEA-TECDOC-1213 Printed by the IAEA in Austria. 77p.

Ingham, S. C.; Alford, R. & Mccown, P. (1990). Comparative growth rates of *salmonella* typhimurium and Pseudomonas fragi on cooked Crab meat Stored Under air and modified atmosphere. *Journal of Food Protection,* 53:7, 566-567.

Jay, J. M.; Loessner, M. J. & Golden D.A. (2005). Modern Food Microbiology. Seventh Edition. Food Science Text Series. 751p.

Kamat, A. S.; Bandekar, J. R. M.; Karani, S.; Jadhav, R.; Shashidhar, A.; Kakatkar, S.; Pingulkar, K.; Ghadge, N.; Warrier S. B. R. & Venugopal, V. (2005). Microbiological qualıty of some major fishery products Exported from India. Determination of human pathogen profiles in food by quality assured microbial assays. *Proceedings of a final Research Coordination Meeting held in Mexico City*, Mexico, 22–26 July 2002

Kumar, S. H.; Sunil, R.; Venugopal, M. N.; Karunasagar, I. & Karunasagar I. (2003). Detection of *Salmonella* spp. in tropical seafood by polymerase chain reaction. International Journal of Food Microbiology 88. 91- 95.

Kumar, R.; Surendran P. K. &Thampuran N. (2009). Detection and characterization of virulence factors in lactose positive and lactose negative *Salmonella* serovars isolated from seafood. Food Control 20: 4, 376-380.

Lelieveld, H. L. M.; Unilever, R. & Vlaardingen, D. (2009). Chaper 5. The Netherlands Sources of contamination 61-72.

Ling, M. L.; Goh, K. T.; Wang, G. C. Y.; Neo, K. S. & Chua, T. (2002). An outbreak of multidrugresistant *Salmonella* enterica subsp. enterica serotype Typhimurium. *Epidemiology and Infection*, 128, 1–5.

Lyhs, U. (2009). Microbiological Methods, Chapter 15. Fishery Products Quality, safety and authenticity Edited by Hartmut Rehbein and Jörg Oehlenschläger (318-348).

Lawley, R., Curtis, L. & Davis, J. (2008). The Food Safety Hazard Guidebook. Food Safety Info, London, UK RSC Publishing ISBN: 978-0-85404-460-3 422 p.

Marriot, N. G., Gravani R. B.,(2006). Principles of Food Sanitation Fifth Edition Printed in the United States of America. 413 p.

Millard, G. & Rockliff, S. (2004). Incidence of *Salmonella* in Raw Fish Fillets ACT Health Protection Service

Mol, S.; Cosansu, S.; Alakavuk, D. U. & Ozturan, S. (2010). Survivalof *Salmonella enteritidis* during salting and drying of horse mackerel (*Trachurus trachurus*) fillets. *International Journal of Food Microbiology*, 139: 36–40.

Norhana, M. N.W.; Poolec, S. E.; Deethah, C. & Dykesd, G. A. (2010). Prevalence, persistence and control of *Salmonella* and Listeria in shrimp and shrimp products. *Food Control*, 21:4, 343-361.

Novotny, L.; Dvorska, L.; Lorencova, A.; Beran V. & Pavlik I. (2004). Fish: a potential source of bacterila pathogens for human beings. *Vet. Med.-Czech* 49, (9): 343-358.

Oehlenschläger, J. & Rehbein, H. (2009). Basic facts and figures, Chapter 1. Fishery Products Quality, safety and authenticity Edited by Hartmut Rehbein and Jörg Oehlenschläger (1-18).

Olgunoglu, I. A. (2010). Determination of Microbiological Contamination Sources of Blue Crabmeat (Callinectes sapidus Rathbun, 1896) During Pasteurization Process. *Pakistan J. Zool.*, vol. 42(5), pp. 545-550.

Oraei, M., Motalebi, A. A., Hoseini, E., Javan, S. 2011. Effect of Gamma irradiation and frozen storage on microbial quality of Rainbow trout (*Oncorhynchus mykiss*) filet. *Iranian Journal of Fisheries Sciences*, 10(1) 75-84.

Özden, Ö.; Inugur, M. & Erkan, N.( 2007). Effect of different dose gamma radiation and refrigeration on the chemical and sensory properties and microbiological status of aqua cultured sea bass (*Dicentrarchus labrax*). *Radiation Physics and Chemistry*, 76, 1169–1178.

Özden, Ö. and Erkan, N., (2010). Impacts of gamma radiation on nutritional components of minimal processed cultured sea bass (*Dicentrarchus labrax*). *Iranian Journal of Fisheries Sciences*, 9(2), 265-278.

Pal, A. & Marshall D. L. (2009). Comparison of culture media for enrichment and isolation of *Salmonella* spp. from frozen Channel catfish and Vietnamese basa fillets. *Food Microbiology*. 26: 3, 317-319.

Pamuk, S.; Gurler, Z.; Yıldırım, Y. & Siriken B., (2011). Detection of Microbiological Quality of common Carp (Cyprinus carpio) Sold in Public Baazar in Afyonkarahisar. *Journal of Animal and Veterinary Advances*, 10(8):1012-1018.

Ponce, E.; Khan, A. A.; Chorng-Ming, C.; Summage-West, C. & Cerniglia, C. E. (2008). Prevalence and characterization of *Salmonella enterica* serovar Weltevreden from imported seafood. *Food Microbiology*, Volume 25, Issue 1, 29-35.

Popovic, N. T, Benussi, S. A.; Dzidara, P.; Coz-Rakovac, R.; Strunjak-Perovic, I.; Kozacinski, L.; Jadan, M. & Brlek-Gorski, D. (2010). Microbiological quality of marketed fresh and frozen seafood caught off the Adriatic coast of Croatia. *Veterinarni Medicina*, 55, (5): 233–241.

Pullela, S. V. S. (1997). Aquaculture of Pacu (Piaractus mesopotamicus) and a compariıson of its qualıty: mıcrobıologıcal, sensory and proximate composıtıon. Master Of Scıence in Food Science and Technology. Virginia Polytechnic Institute and State University 191 p.

Ray, B., Webb, N. B. & Speck M.L. (1976). Microbiological Evaluation of Blue crab processing operations. *Journal of Food Science* Volume 41, 398-402.

Redman, N. E. (2007). Food Safety, Reference Handbook Second Edition. Contemporary World Issues Series 331p.

Saeed, A. M. & Naji, R., (2007). Infection Agents. Epidemiologic Principles and Food Safety, Edited by Tamar Lasky Oxford University Press 18-40.

SeafoodNIC (Seafood Network Information Center) (2011). Chapter 17: *Salmonella*, Updated: 07/18/07
http://seafood.ucdavis.edu/haccp/compendium/chapt17.htm 06.06.2011

Shabarinath, S.; Kumar, H. S.; Khushiramani, R.; Karunasagar, I. & Karunasagar, I. (2007). Detection and Characterization of *Salmonella* Associated with Tropical Seafood. *International Journal of Food Microbiology*, 114:2 227-233.

Sugumar, G. & Mariappan, S. (2003). Survival of *Salmonella* sp. in Freshwater and Seawater Microcosms Under Starvation. *Asian Fisheries Science*, 16:247-255.

Upadhyay, B. P.; Utrarachkij, F.; Thongshoob, J.; Mahakunkijcharoen, Y.; Wongchinda, N.; Suthienkul, O. & Khusmith S., (2010). Detection Of *Salmonella* inva Gene in Shrimp Enrichment Culture By Polymerase Chain Reaction. *Southeast Asian J. Trop Med. Public Healt*. 41: 2, 426-435.

Ward, D. & Hart, K. (1997). HACCP: Hazard Analysis and Critical Control Point Training Cirriculum. p. 168. Publication UNC-SG-96-02, North Carolina Sea Grant, N.C. State University, Raleigh, NC

6

# Occurrence of *Salmonella* in Minimally Processed Vegetables

Silvana Mariana Srebernich[1,*], Rita de Cássia Salvucci Celeste Ormenese[2], Cristiane Rodrigues Gomes Ruffi[2], Gisele Mara Silva Gonçalves[1]
[1]*Catholic University of Campinas, Campinas-SP*
[2]*Institute of Food Technology, Campinas-SP*
*Brazil*

## 1. Introduction

Vegetables that have been physically altered from its original state but remain in its fresh state are considered minimally processed. These vegetables are subjected to one or more physical changes (processes of washing, peeling, slicing and cutting), which make them ready for consumption. However, in the dicing step occurs the release of internal cellular fluids, rich in nutrients, which allow microorganisms to multiply rapidly increasing the initial microbial load and thus reducing considerably the shelf life of these products (FARBER, 1999). Therefore, the sanitization step aiming the reduction or destruction of pathogenic and spoilage microorganisms to acceptable levels is critical for these products (BACHELLI, 2010) since food poisoning outbreaks associated with contamination of vegetables continue to exist despite the technological advances. Leafy vegetables have been identified as significant vehicles of pathogens relevant to public health, including enterohaemorrhagic *Escherichia coli* (O157: H7), *Listeria* sp., *Salmonella* sp. and *Shigella* spp. (FRANK & TAKEUSHI, 1999) especially if proper care is not met on the steps of growing, harvesting and processing (GARG et al., 1990). Thus, a minimally processed product should be consistent, to have fresh look, be of acceptable color, free from defects and safe from a microbiological standpoint.

## 2. *Salmonella* sp. as a pontential contamination microorganism of minimally processed vegetables

### 2.1 Taxonomy

*Salmonella* is a genus of Rod-shaped gram negative bacteria that belong to the family *Enterobacteriaceae*. Their species are motile, oxidase-negative, catalase positive and utilize glucose and other carbohydrates with the production of acid and gas.

Officially the genus is composed of a single species, *Salmonella choleraesuis,* divided into seven subspecies, which are also known by Roman numerals: I. *choleraesuis,* II. *salamae,* IIIa. *arizonae,* IIIb. *diarizonae,* IV. *houtenae,* V. *bongori* and VI. *indicates*. In 1987 a proposal was made to change the name *Salmonella choleraesuis* for *Salmonella enterica* and in 1989 the

* Corresponding author

proposed elevation of the subspecies to the species category bongori. This proposal received unanimous support of the Subcommittee on *Enterobacteriaceae* of the International Committee on Systematic Bacteriology at the Fourteenth International Congress of Microbiology, but was not made official by the International Committee of Nomenclature of Bacteria. Still, it was adopted and used by the CDC (U.S. Center for Disease Control and Prevention), ASM (American Society for Microbiology) and WHO (World Health Organization). The strains most frequently involved in human disease are *S. enterica* subsp. *enterica,* which is the habitat for warm-blooded animals and are responsible for 99% of human salmonellosis. *S. enterica* subsp. *salamae* subsp. arizonae and subsp. diarizonae, are often isolated from the intestinal contents of cold-blooded animals and rarely humans or warm-blooded animals. *S. enterica* subsp. *houtenae* and *S. bongori* are predominantly isolated from the environment and are rarely pathogenic to humans (SILVA et al., 2010).
More than 50% of the serotypes of *Salmonella* belong to the *Salmonella enterica* subsp. *enterica,* and the most common somatic serogroups are; A, B, C1, C2, D, E1, and E4. Approximately, 99% of *Salmonella* infections in humans and warm-blooded animals, are due these serogroups, including widely known serotypes Parathyphi A (A group), Paratyphi B and Thyphimurium (B group), Paratyphi C and cholerasuis (C group), Typhi, Enteritidis and Gallinarum (D group) (SILVA et al., 2010).

### 2.2 Growth and survival

*Salmonella* sp. has the ability to growth in the temperature range of 2-45°C, with the optimum at 35-37°C. The psychotropic attribute of *Salmonellae* and ability to growth slowly at cold temperature raises concerns on cold-induced bacteriostasis as a food safety measure. *Salmonellae* can growth in the pH range with an optimum pH range of 6.5-7.5 for growth. The water activity for this genus is 0.93 or greater (SILVA et al., 2010).
The propensity of *Salmonella* sp. to survive bactericidal food process and to persist for years in frozen foods and in dry foods stores at ambient temperature is a food safety concern. The thermal process in food industry widely used to eliminated bacterial human pathogens is a challenge concerning to *Salmonella* sp., because of its heat resistance in foods with low water activity. The classical study on solute dependent thermal resistance showed that heating of *Salmonella* sp. at 57.2°C in aqueous solutions of sucrose and glycerol adjust the AW = 0.90 yields D value of 40-55 minutes and 1.8-8.3 min. respectively (GOEPFERT et al., 1970).

### 2.3 Detection methods

The traditional technique for detecting *Salmonella* sp. in food is a classic culture method for presence/absence, developed in order to ensure detection even under extremely unfavorable conditions. This is the case of food microbiology with a competitor microbiota much larger than the population of *Salmonella* and / or food in which the cells of *Salmonella* sp. are very few in number and/or foods in which the cells are injured by the process of preservation (application of heat, freezing, drying) (SILVA et al., 2010).
The procedures recommended by different regulatory bodies, although they present some variations in the selection of culture media and method of sample preparation basically follow five steps: pre-enrichment, selective enrichment, plating, biochemical and serological confirmation (DÁOUST, 1994). All samples should be pre-enriched in a non-selective broth medium for 18-24h at 35-37°C. The aim of this step is to resuscitate the few injured or stressed cells of *Salmonella* sp. By the method ISO 6579 (2007), one of the most recommended

for minimally processed vegetables, a portion of 25 g or 25 mL of the sample, is taken and placed in 225 ml of buffered peptone water (BPW). Incubate for 18 hours at 37°C (SILVA et al., 2010).

Selective enrichment of portion of pre-enriched culture in nine volumes of tetrathionate brilliant green (TBG), selenite cistine (SC) or Rappaport-Vassilads (RV) broth medium for 18-24h represses the growth of competitive microflora and makes easy the recovery in different plating media.

Selective differential plating objectives to promote the preferential development of colonies with typical *Salmonella* sp. It is recommended to be done in one or more culture media. The most common are the Hectoen Enteric Agar (HE), Xylose Lysine Desicolato Agar (XLD) agar and Xylose Lysine tergitol4 (XLT4) (Silva et al., 2010). Each culture purview a streak SVR (depletion) in the differential media recommended. Repeat this procedure with the broth MKTTn. Incubate plates inverted XLD 37°C/24 hours. Follow the incubation plates of the others differential culture media, according to the manufacturer.

Confirmation is a step that aims to verify whether the colonies obtained in the typical differential plating are actually colonies of *Salmonella* sp. is carried out through biochemical and serological tests.

In the XLD medium, typical colonies are dark pink in color with black center and a reddish zone, slightly transparent around. In the second chosen medium, after plating, following the manufacturer's guidelines for evaluating features of typical colonies of *Salmonella* sp. Select at least two colonies of each medium for further confirmation.

Confirmation checks the biochemical profile biochemical characteristics of strains of *Salmonella enterica* subsp. enterica. Miniaturized kits are also recommended for this aim.

Series recommended for biochemical analysis method for *Salmonella* sp.: Incubation of all tests: 37C/24 hours (SILVA et al., 2010).

- Growth test Agar Triple Sugar Iron-TSI: Initial color: orange. Positive test: ramp alkaline (red), background acid (yellow) with production of gas (bubbles) with or without H2S production.
- Urease test: deep pink colour. Negative for *Salmonella* sp. The medium maintains its original color.
- Test Lysine Carboxylase: Most lysine-positive strains. Serotype Parathypi are negative.
- Voges-Proskauer test: tubes with 3 mL of methyl red (VM)-VP, Voges-Proskauer. *Salmonella* sp. are negative.
- Indole: indole-negative: the most of them.
- Beta-galactosidase test. Most strains of *Salmonella enterica* subsp. *enterica* are negative.

A serological confirmation checks for the presence of antigens "O", "Vi" and "H" for tests agglutination polyvalent antisera. The results for confirmed positive *Salmonella* sp. by the ISO 6579 method (2007) are: typical for biochemical tests, no self-agglutination and antibody positive serological test for O, Vi, or H. The methods of analysis of food end up confirming this stage, since the full characterization of *Salmonella* sp. is usually done by reference laboratories in each specific country (SILVA et al., 2010).

Over the past ten years there was a breakthrough in developing new methods, especially immunological methods and to a lesser extent, methods based on nucleic acids. These methods follow the current trend of development kits analytical trademarked defined by AOAC (Association of Official Analytical Chemists) as "a system containing all key components to the analysis of one or more microorganisms, one or more types of food, according to a particular method" (ANDREWS, 1997). The great advantage of the kits is that the material required for tests (all or part of it) is sold together, eliminating the preparation in the laboratory (SILVA et al., 2010).

The polymerase chain reaction (PCR) detection of *Salmonella* spp is based on the amplification of bacterial DNA sequence that is unique to salmonellae. The PCR assay consists of three different steps: denaturation of duplex bacterial DNA into single strands (94ºC), annealing of synthetic oligonucleotide primers (45-65ºC) that are highly- specific to *Salmonella* sp. DNA sequences that flank the *Salmonella*-specific DNA targed, and a polymerase-dependent extension (72ºC) of the single-stranded DNA starting at the primer site where elongation progress from 3min to 5min end of template DNA strand. The commonly targeted sequence for amplification lies within the inVA gene of *Salmonella* sp. (DÁOUST, 1994).

Related to the minimally processed vegetables, the main method used is the traditional technique described in this chapter together with the use of miniaturized kits for biochemical bacteria identification.

## 3. Foods involved in *Salmonella* sp. outbreaks

*Salmonella* is a bacteria with wide occurrence in animals and in environment, and the main sources are water, soil, animal feces, insects and surfaces of factory's equipment and kitchen utensils. A disease is generally contracted mainly through consumption of contaminated food of animal origin. It is commonly accepted that at between 1 million to 1 billion bacteria are needed to cause infection although some investigators suggest some people may be infected by far fewer bacteria. Other authors mention that the infectious dose is 15 to 20 cells and can reach any age range, with the elderly and children under seven years the more susceptible to get ill (SILVA et al., 2010). Nevertheless, most data suggest food, water, or other sources of contamination contain large amounts of bacteria. Although human stomach acid can reduce and sometimes eliminate *Salmonella* spp., occasionally some bacteria get through to the intestine and then attach and penetrate the cells. Symptoms may include headache, muscle aches, diarrhea, vomiting, abdominal cramping, chills, fever, nausea and dehydration. According to the Illinois Department of Public Health, most persons infected with *Salmonella* bacteria develop diarrhea, fever and abdominal cramps 12 to 72 hours after infection. The illness usually lasts 4 to 7 days, and most persons recover without treatment. However, in some persons, the diarrhea may be so severe that the patient needs to be hospitalized. *Salmonella* sp. infection may spread from the intestines to the bloodstream, and then to other body sites and can cause death unless the person is treated promptly with antibiotics. On the other hand, persons can be infected with the bacteria without having symptoms. Persons with and without symptoms shed the bacteria in their stool, which is why proper handwashing after toileting and before handling food is so important. Children younger than 1 year old, people who have had ulcer surgery or take antacids, the elderly, infants and those with impaired immune systems are more likely to have a severe illness from *Salmonella* sp. which can contaminate a wide variety of foods. These include raw foods derived from animals like eggs and egg products, meat and meat products, unpasteurized milk and other dairy products, and raw poultry. Shell eggs and eggs products figured as prominently in recent years as a human salmonellosis. More recently, *Salmonella* sp. outbreaks have been tied to a variety of fresh produce like lettuce, salad mixes, sprouts, melons, tomatoes and even peanut butter. Minimally processed vegetables have risen, since the 90"s, as a new source of *Salmonella* sp. in food industry. Fresh cut vegetables are by definition, perishables. The process of cutting, slicing, chopping, breaks the protective skin of fresh vegetables and increases their vulnerability to biological contamination. A poor hygiene in minimally processed vegetables, especially in developing countries are the main cause of food borne disease associated to this product. The minimally processed vegetables are products that have suffered some manipulation, thus, the useful life, compared to fresh produce is much lower (BOONER et al., 2003). Microorganisms that cause disease in humans as bacteria, protozoa, virus, has been the focus of many studies of minimally processed vegetables. *Salmonella* sp. serotypes however are estimated to be responsible for most cases of food poisoning due the consumption of this kind of product worldwide (MEAD et al., 1999).

According to Francys et al. (1999) *Salmonella* is the organism that are relevant to public health more commonly associated with food poisoning outbreaks involving vegetables ready for consumption. An outbreak of salmonellosis occurred in the UK in 1988, involved the consumption of green beans. Epidemiological studies in England and Wales between 1992 and 1996 linked the consumption of coleslaw with *Salmonella* outbreaks that occurred during this period.

Machado et al. (2009), in a research for microbiological evaluation of some minimally processed vegetables in Brazil, evaluated samples of watercress, lettuce, grated carrot, spinach, green cabbage and rocket minimally processed for some pathogens, including *Salmonella* sp. The vegetables were stored at a temperature of 5°C. *Salmonella* sp. was detected in 12.7% of the samples.

Bruno et al. (2005), evaluating the microbiological quality of 15 samples of vegetables including carrots, cabbage, chayote, all minimally processed and marketed in the north part of Brazil verified that *Salmonella* sp. was present in 66% of the samples.

Santana et al. (2011) tested 512 samples of minimally processed vegetables in São Paulo, Brazil, and obtained that *Salmonella* sp. was detected in four samples. The serovars were *Salmonella* Typhimurium (three samples) and *Salmonella enterica* subsp. *enterica* (one sample).

A small outbreak of *Salmonella* sp happened in five states of United States of America, in June, 2011. A total of 21 persons with the outbreak strain of *Salmonella enteritidis* have been reported from 5 states: Idaho (3), Montana (7), North Dakota (1), New Jersey (1) and Washington (9). Among persons for whom information is available, ill persons range in age from 12 years to 77 years old, with a median age of 35 years old. Seventy-one percent are female. Among the 10 ill persons with available information, 3 (30%) persons have been hospitalized. No deaths have been reported. It was announced by Los Angeles Times. The outbreak was linked with the consumption of alfafa sprouts (http:// articles.latimes.com/ 2011). In USA, a total of 99 individuals infected with the outbreak strain of *Salmonella* Agona have been reported from 23 states, late July, 2011. Epidemiologic, traceback, and laboratory investigations have linked this outbreak to eating fresh, whole papayas imported from Mexico (CDC, 2011). According to the Center for Disease Control (CDC), in the United States, food poisoning causes nearly 76 million illness cases with about 325,000 hospitalizations, and approximately 5,000 deaths yearly. The *Salmonellae* organisms are reportedly responsible for as much as $1 billion in medical costs and lost time from work.

Concerning to salmonellosis preventions, it is important to say that *Salmonella* bacteria are killed when food is thoroughly cooked properly. Once cooked, any food held in a buffet should be kept hotter than 55°C. Cross contamination, may be avoided using different utensils, plates, cutting boards and count tops before and after cooking. Cooking food stands at room temperature for a long time, such as two hours, is also at risk. It is important to assent that vegetables, now identified as a source of *Salmonella* sp., must be thoroughly washed in treated or healthy running water before they are eaten, as basic operations of food borne disease. In food industry, internal systems of quality control are essential to prevent occurrence of foodborne illness to consumer. As an example, the HACCP (Hazards Analysis and Control of Critical Points) system, adopted by major international markets, basically ensures that the manufactured products are developed without risk to public health, and also have uniform standards of identity and quality (SILVA, 1999).

## 4. Sanitizers as a control measure

Minimally processed vegetables are products ready for consumption and must be free of pathogenic microorganisms. Its washing step must be done with good quality water followed by the addition of sanitizer solution aiming to reduce the microbial counting and increasing microbial safety and the product preservation. Thus, the sanitation plays an important role in reducing decay and maintaining quality. Therefore, the types of sanitizers, the forms of application, generally a function of time and concentration, will depend on the accompanying microbiota and characteristics of raw material processing.

Chlorine, in its various forms, is the group of most commonly used compound sanitizers because of its efficiency and low cost. They are compounds of broad-spectrum germicidal action by reacting with membrane proteins of the microorganism. Sodium hypochlorite is the most widely used chemical sanitizer because of its complete dissociation in water, easy application and quick action being effective in reducing populations of bacteria, fungi, viruses and nematodes. In water, produces sodium hydroxide (NaOH) and hypochlorous acid (HOCl), the latter being the germicidal agent, which dissociates into $H^+$ and $OCl^-$ ion according to the following reactions:

$$NaOCl + H_2O \leftrightarrows NaOH + HOCl$$

$$HOCl \rightarrow H^+ + OCl^-$$

It is proved that the hypochlorous acid (HOCl) has greater disinfecting action (about 80 times more) than the same concentration of hypochlorite ion ($OCl^-$). The amount of HOCl formed depends on the pH of the solution and its concentration is considerably higher at pH 4.0 decreasing as pH increases. Thus, at pH above 5.0 occurs an increase of the hypochlorite ion ($OCl^-$). The sanitizing step is usually performed at pH between 6.5 and 7.0 because in this range there is still considerable amount of hypochlorous acid. The greatest disinfecting power of the hypochlorous acid is explained by the fact that being a small, neutral molecule has a greater ease of penetration through the cell wall. In turn, the hypochlorite ion due to its negative charge is more difficult to cross the cell wall and reach the enzyme system. It is therefore possible that the greatest difficulty in the elimination of sporulated forms is related to the penetration of the disinfecting agent as this may be hampered by the protective mantle of the microorganism.

A study carried out by Berbari et al. (2001) showed that soaking for 15 minutes in a solution containing a chlorine $70mg.L^{-1}$ enables a shelf-life of up to 6 days for minimally processed lettuce stored at 2°C, increasing to 9 days if treated with a solution containing 100 to $130mg.L^{-1}$ of chlorine. On the other hand, a study by Nunes et al. (2010) with Peruvian carrot minimally processed, showed that soaking for 10 minutes in a solution containing $100mg.L^{-1}$ of chlorine allowed a shelf-life of 6 days when stored at a temperature of 5°C ± 1°C. Nascimento (2002) showed that vegetables washed with a solution containing 50 ppm of free chlorine showed a significant reduction in the total count of aerobic and that fecal coliforms were even more sensitive to chlorine, not being more detected in vegetables after washing. Therefore, chlorine and its salts, especially hypochlorite, are effective and of low cost, and widely applied as a spray for bacteriological control in industries working with vegetables (KIM et al., 1999). However, in recent years there has been some concern in the use of chlorine due to the inconvenience of toxic compounds that can be formed and leave residual taste in food (OLIVEIRA & VALLE, 2000). Among these compounds, there are the trihalomethanes (THM), aldehydes, halocetonas and chloramines, which when hydrolyzed proved related to some types of cancer according to epidemiological studies of Meyer (1994). Depending on the toxicity of these compounds, there is a recognized need to find alternative sanitizers for hygiene and sanitization procedures for vegetables. Thus, chlorine dioxide ($ClO_2$) has received special attention (ARENSTEIN, 2003) for, although it is a derivative of chlorine, generates negligible amount of by-products (trihalomethanes), characterized as a product of low carcinogenic potential (ANDRADE & MACEDO, 1999). In addition, chlorine dioxide is a strong oxidizing agent that reacts mostly through a mechanism of electron transfer by attacking the cell membrane, penetrating, dehydrating, and lastly, oxidizing the internal components of the microbial cell without however causing toxic effects, as most of the chlorine compounds do. It also has the advantage of being effective against gram negative and positive. Still, by the fact that hydrolyzes the phenolic compounds it reduces the possibility of formation of tastes and odors.

Another important aspect of chlorine dioxide is its sharp and sporicidal disinfectant action in lower concentrations than that of chlorine. The explanation of its high bactericidal action is due to the fact that it is soluble in oils, greases and substances of mixed composition, such as cells of virus and bacteria, whose membranes easily penetrates in, as opposed to other disinfectants of polar nature.

Chlorine dioxide is stable under a wide pH range (6-10) and its decomposition are first formed chlorite ($ClO_3$) and then chlorate ($ClO_2$) which can be seen in the equations:

$$2\,NaClO_2 + Cl_2 \leftrightarrows 2\,ClO_2 + 2\,NaCl$$

$$2\,ClO_2 + H_2O \leftrightarrows ClO^-_2 + ClO^-_3 + 2\,H^+$$

$$4\,ClO_2^- + H_2^+ \leftrightarrows 2\,ClO^-_2 + ClO^-_3 + 2\,H_2O$$

However, the major disadvantages of chlorine dioxide are its cost and its sensitivity to high temperatures.

Currently, several studies are being conducted with chlorine dioxide in different countries. Felkey et al. (2003) and Rash (2003) showed in their studies the efficiency of chlorine dioxide in reducing *Salmonella* on the surface of tomato and melon, respectively. Another sanitizing agent that has been used quite successfully is peracetic acid, also known as peroxide of acetic acid or peroxyacetic acid. It is obtained by the reaction of acetic acid or acetic anhydride with hydrogen peroxide in the presence of sulfuric acid, which has the function of catalyst. The decomposition products are acetic acid, hydrogen peroxide and water.

The peroxyacetic acid has currently one of the largest application as disinfectants in the food industry and its efficiency is similar or superior to sodium hypochlorite (NASCIMENTO, 2002), but more potent than hydrogen peroxide. It is an excellent sanitizer for the great

oxidation capacity of the cellular components of microorganisms having a rapid action at low concentrations and still effective in the presence of organic material and therefore being an effective biocide.
Its biocide action is influenced by the concentration, shape and type of microorganism. It degrades rapidly in biodegradable and harmless substances such as acetic acid and active oxygen, which pose no risk of toxicity and does not affect the taste and odor of food. Do not have mutagenic or carcinogenic effects (COSTA, 2007). However peroxyacetic acid has low stability during storage and handling must be done carefully. A study performed by Hilgren & Salverda (2000) showed a significant reduction in the total count of bacteria and fungi in vegetables treated with peroxyacetic acid. Alvarenga et al. (1991) found that after 1, 3 and 5 minutes of contact with peracetic acid at a concentration of 300mg.L$^{-1}$ reached respectively 0.43, 1.2 and 2.8 decimal reductions in the population of spores of *Bacillus subtilis*.
Also according to Nascimento (2002), there was no significant difference to the performances of the peracetic acid compared to sodium hypochlorite. Similar results were reported by Farrell et al. (1998), Sapers et al. (1999) and Wisniewsky et al. (2000). However other authors have demonstrated the superiority of peracetic acid when compared to the sodium hypochlorite in the presence of organic matter. Jones et al. (1992) got a reduction of 3 log cycle for *Vibrio cholerae* and *E. coli* using peracetic acid (25ppm) when compared to sodium hypochlorite (25 ppm). Thus, although there are a number of studies reported in the international literature, most of the time these were carried out under different conditions not allowing comparisons. Therefore, further studies are needed to know the effectiveness of sanitizers in the real conditions of use, working with vegetables available in the local market, with its natural contaminant microbiota unchanged. It is also interesting the implementation in the food sector, of a rotation between different sanitizers thereby preventing the development of resistance by microorganisms to the active principles of the same.

## 5. Chlorine dioxide and peracetic acid as sanitizers to control microorganisms presents in minimally processed chicory (*cichorium endivia* l.) and rocket (*eruca vesicaria sativa*)

### Combined effect of type, concentration and action time of sanitizer in the microbial control of minimally processed chicory and rocket. An observation.

Sodium hypochloride has been the sanitizer usually used to reduce the microbial counting in minimally processed vegetables, although its use is questioned due to be precursor in the formation of organic chloramines, compounds of high carcinogenic potential. As a consequence of this fact, other sanitizers have been proposed to replace it, among them chlorine dioxide and peracetic acid. Therefore in this work chlorine dioxide (10, 25 and 50ppm/2, 5 and 10min) and peracetic acid (50, 75 and 100ppm/4, 7 and 10min) were compared with sodium hypochloride (120ppm/15min) in the control of natural microbiota of minimally processed rocket and chicory.
In green leafy vegetables, the physical form of the vegetable being processed is very important because certain types of leaves are difficult to be washed and sanitized requiring greater care. The leafy vegetables, rocket and chicory, present this kind of difficulty, which by being consumed as salad, so fresh, are potentially risk factors, that's why they were chosen for the work associated with their high consumption.

The microbial counts on fresh materials rocket and chicory after washing followed by immersion in water for 15 min. showed high contamination of molds and yeasts (5.90 and 5.62 log $CFU.g^{-1}$), total coliforms (6.22 and 5.59 log $CFU.g^{-1}$) and *Escherichia coli* (2.61 and 2.37 log $CFU.g^{-1}$).
It has also been seen that the samples of rocket showed initial contamination superior to the chicory for the same tests, which may be a consequence of the type of rocket leaf that by being rough ends up retaining contaminants on its surface, unlike the chicory which has the smooth leaf.
Data regarding to the effects of chlorine dioxide and peracetic acid in the population of yeasts and molds in minimally processed chicory (Table 1) showed that the variables concentration and contact time influenced significantly (at 5%), and both concentrations as the contact times studied was inversely proportional to the population of yeasts and molds naturally present in chicory minimally processed.

| Time* | Treatment with chlorine dioxide ($ClO_2$) | | | |
|---|---|---|---|---|
| (Min) | 10ppm | 25ppm | 50ppm | MSD[1] |
| 2 | 3.312 ± 0.212 [a, A] | 2.871 ± 0.157 [b, A] | 2.436 ± 0.120 [c, A] | 0.419 |
| 5 | 3.026 ± 0.266 [a, A, B] | 2.598 ± 0.182 [a, b, A] | 2.242 ± 0.084 [b, A] | 0.482 |
| 10 | 2.541 ± 0.278 [a, B] | 2.026 ± 0.046 [b, B] | 2.000 ± 0.000 [b, B] | 0.407 |
| DMS[2] | 0.635 | 0.353 | 0.212 | ---- |
| Time* | Treatment with peracetic acid ($CH_3$-COOOH) | | | |
| (Min) | 50ppm | 75ppm | 100ppm | MSD[1] |
| 4 | 3.445 ± 0.279 [a, A] | 3.247 ± 0.185 [a, A] | 2.716 ± 0.119 [b, A] | 0.514 |
| 7 | 3.131 ± 0.174 [a, A, B] | 2.785 ± 0.094 [b, B] | 2.452 ± 0.119 [b, B] | 0.334 |
| 10 | 2.902 ± 0.139 [a, B] | 2.308 ± 0.166 [b, C] | 2.000 ± 0.000 [b, C] | 0.313 |
| MSD[2] | 0.517 | 0.384 | 0.243 | ---- |
| Blank (washing and immersion in tap water for 15 minutes) ** .(log $CFU.g^{-1}$) | | | | 5.616 |
| Standard (washing with water and immersion in a solution of sodium hypochlorite: 120ppm/15min) ** ........................................(log $CFU.g^{-1}$) | | | | <2.000 |

MSD[1] = for the data on the lines; MSD[2] = for the data on the columns; small letter compares averages on the same line, capital letters compare means in the same column, different letters indicate that the data differ significantly at 5% probability; * Time of contact with the sanitizer product; ** reference treatments.

Table 1. Yeast and mold count (log $CFU.g^{-1}$) observed in samples of minimally processed chicory.

In the case of chlorine dioxide, the treatments performed with 25ppm/10min and 50ppm/10min were statistically superior to the others and there wasn't, however, significant differences between the two. Both treatments showed a reduction equivalent to 3 logarithmic cycles in the population of yeasts and molds when compared with the treatment by washing followed by immersion in water for 15 minutes. On the other hand, regarding the effect of peracetic acid in the population of yeasts and molds, the treatments carried out at concentrations of 75ppm/10min and 100ppm/10min proved to be statically superior to others, but without showing any significant difference between them. Just as in the treatments with chlorine dioxide, peracetic acid treatments had reduced to the equivalent of 3 logarithmic cycles in the population of yeasts and molds when compared with the treatment by washing followed by immersion in water for 15 minutes (blank). Treatment with chlorine dioxide and peracetic acid, described above as having showed the best results in terms of population control of yeasts and molds in chicory, showed the same level of standard treatment (2 log $CFU.g^{-1}$). When the same treatments were performed using minimally processed rocket (Table 2), the counts were higher and showed no significant differences between them, as much for the treatments with chlorine dioxide as for treatment with peracetic acid. However, even with no significant difference between them, the greatest reductions in populations of yeasts and molds were obtained in the case of peracetic acid treatments, with 100ppm/10min and in the case of chlorine dioxide with 50ppm/10min.

| Time* | Treatment with chlorine dioxide ($ClO_2$) | | | |
|---|---|---|---|---|
| (Min) | 10ppm | 25ppm | 50ppm | MSD[1] |
| 2 | 5.149 ± 0.544 $^{a, A}$ | 4.433 ± 0.538 $^{a, A}$ | 4.078 ± 0.479 $^{a, A}$ | 1.305 |
| 5 | 4.839 ± 0.504 $^{a, A}$ | 4.127 ± 0.463 $^{a, A}$ | 3.709 ± 0.387 $^{a, A}$ | 1.138 |
| 10 | 4.327 ± 0.375 $^{a, A}$ | 3.797 ± 0.439 $^{a, A}$ | 3.371 ± 0.370 $^{a, A}$ | 0.992 |
| MSD[2] | 1.202 | 1.207 | 1.039 | ---- |
| Time* | Treatment with peracetic acid ($CH_3$-COOOH) | | | |
| (Min) | 50ppm | 75ppm | 100ppm | MSD[1] |
| 4 | 4.314 ± 0.425 $^{a, A}$ | 3.869 ± 0.577 $^{a, A}$ | 3.400 ± 0.593 $^{a, A}$ | 1.345 |
| 7 | 3.998 ± 0.472 $^{a, A}$ | 3.563 ± 0.640 $^{a, A}$ | 3.020 ± 0.692 $^{a, A}$ | 1.525 |
| 10 | 3.594 ± 0.468 $^{a, A}$ | 3.160 ± 0.690 $^{a, A}$ | 2.644 ± 0.673 $^{a, A}$ | 1.549 |
| MSD[2] | 1.141 | 1.596 | 1.638 | ---- |
| Blank (washing and immersion in tap water for 15 minutes) ** (log $CFU.g^{-1}$) | | | | 5.896 |
| Standard (washing with water and immersion in a solution of sodium hypochlorite: 120ppm/15min) ** .......................................(log $CFU.g^{-1}$) | | | | 2.400 |

MSD[1] = for the data on the lines; MSD[2] = for the data on the columns; small letter compares averages on the same line, capital letters compare means in the same column, different letters indicate that the data differ significantly at 5% probability; * Time of contact with the sanitizer product; ** reference treatments.

Table 2. Yeast and mold count (log $CFU.g^{-1}$) observed in samples of minimally processed rocket.

As for the action of these sanitizers in counts of total coliform in chicory (Table 3) and rocket (Table 4), minimally processed, the response was almost linear and inversely proportional, that is, when the concentration of sanitizers or their periods of contact were increased, the population of total coliforms also decreased.

Referring to the action of chlorine dioxide on the total coliform in chicory only the treatment with 50ppm/10min showed the same log cycle (1.34 log $CFU.g^{-1}$) of the standard treatment

(1.48 log CFU.g$^{-1}$) and statistically different from the others. In the case of peracetic acid, 2 treatments were better: 100ppm/10min (1.10 log CFU.g$^{-1}$) and 100ppm/7min (1.44 log CFU.g$^{-1}$) and they were statistically different from the others, however not different from each other. Therefore, as far as the control of total coliform in minimally processed chicory under the conditions of the treatments performed peracetic acid was more effective than chlorine dioxide.

In the case of the action of chlorine dioxide on the total coliform in minimally processed rocket only one treatment (50ppm/10min) provided results (3.85 log CFU.g$^{-1}$) in the same logarithmic cycle of the standard treatment (3.52 log CFU.g$^{-1}$) being statistically different from the others. When peracetic acid was used as sanitizer, only one treatment (100ppm/10min) was able to reduce the count of total coliforms to below the standard, respectively 2.87 x 3.52 log CFU.g$^{-1}$. Other 3 treatments (100ppm/4min, and 100ppm/7min 75ppm/10min) provided counts (3.65 log CFU.g$^{-1}$, 3.33 log CFU.g$^{-1}$ and 3.45 log CFU.g$^{-1}$) similar to the standard (3.52 log CFU.g$^{-1}$) being in the same log cycle.

| Time* | Treatment with chlorine dioxide ($ClO_2$) | | | |
|---|---|---|---|---|
| (Min) | 10ppm | 25ppm | 50ppm | MSD[1] |
| 2 | 3.088 ± 0.647 $^{a, A}$ | 2.944 ± 0.613 $^{a, A}$ | 2.302 ± 0.424 $^{a, A}$ | 1.428 |
| 5 | 2.820 ± 0.535 $^{a, A}$ | 2.578 ± 0.561 $^{a, A}$ | 2.014 ± 0.399 $^{a, A, B}$ | 1.213 |
| 10 | 2.544 ± 0.561 $^{a, A}$ | 2.423 ± 0.515 $^{a,b, A}$ | 1.339 ± 0.308 $^{b, B}$ | 1.883 |
| MSD[2] | 1.460 | 1.415 | 0.953 | ---- |
| Time* | Treatment with peracetic acid ($CH_3$-COOOH) | | | |
| (Min) | 50ppm | 75ppm | 100ppm | MSD[1] |
| 4 | 3.446 ± 0.143 $^{a, A}$ | 3.256 ± 0.194 $^{a, A}$ | 2.344 ± 0.292 $^{b, A}$ | 0.547 |
| 7 | 2.806 ± 0.412 $^{a, A, B}$ | 2.681 ± 0.397 $^{a, A, B}$ | 1.440 ± 0.095 $^{b, B}$ | 0.839 |
| 10 | 2.310 ± 0.544 $^{a, B}$ | 2.170 ± 0.492 $^{a,b, B}$ | 1.100 ± 0.174 $^{b, B}$ | 1.090 |
| MSD[2] | 1.008 | 0.957 | 0.510 | ---- |
| Blank (washing and immersion in tap water for 15 minutes) ** .(log CFU.g$^{-1}$) | | | | 5.587 |
| Standard (washing with water and immersion in a solution of sodium hypochlorite: 120ppm/15min) ** .....................................(log CFU.g$^{-1}$) | | | | 1.480 |

MSD[1] = for the data on the lines; MSD[2] = for the data on the columns; small letter compares averages on the same line, capital letters compare means in the same column, different letters indicate that the data differ significantly at 5% probability; * Time of contact with the sanitizer product; ** reference treatments.

Table 3. Total coliform count (log CFU.g$^{-1}$) observed in samples of minimally processed chicory.

All samples of minimally processed chicory and rocket, treated with chlorine dioxide and peracetic acid were reduced by two logarithmic cycles for *Escherichia coli,* ie, an initial count of 2.86 log CFU.g$^{-1}$ in the treatment by washing and immersion in water to less than 1.00 log CFU.g$^{-1}$. However, in the sample of standard treatment there was a total control, that is, no growth.

There was no *Salmonella* sp./25g in all samples analyzed.

Therefore, when the results of the best treatments were considered, the two sanitizers tested proved to be as effective as treatment with sodium hypochlorite. Thus, both chlorine dioxide and peracetic acid are able to replace the sodium hypochlorite in concentrations and times considered (50ppm/10min chlorine dioxide, peracetic acid and the 100ppm/10min 120ppm/15min sodium hypochlorite). On the other hand, none of the sanitizers caused any kind of physical or unfavorable organoleptic product changes (wilting, darkening, strong odor, color change etc.) at the concentration levels studied.

| Time* | Treatment with chlorine dioxide ($ClO_2$) | | | |
|---|---|---|---|---|
| (Min) | 10ppm | 25ppm | 50ppm | MSD[1] |
| 2 | 5.132 ± 0.064 [a, A] | 4.732 ± 0.047 [b, A] | 4.487 ± 0.106 [c, A] | 0.191 |
| 5 | 4.896 ± 0.138 [a, A, B] | 4.530 ± 0.157 [b, A] | 4.215 ± 0.094 [b, B] | 0.331 |
| 10 | 4.570 ± 0.177 [a, B] | 4.136 ± 0.187 [b, B] | 3.847 ± 0.114 [b, C] | 0.407 |
| MSD[2] | 0.338 | 0.359 | 0.263 | ---- |
| Time* | Treatment with peracetic acid ($CH_3$-COOOH) | | | |
| (Min) | 50ppm | 75ppm | 100ppm | MSD[1] |
| 4 | 5.031 ± 0.324 [a, A] | 4.415 ± 0.341 [a, A] | 3.652 ± 0.207 [b, A] | 0.744 |
| 7 | 4.680 ± 0.320 [a, A] | 4.078 ± 0.283 [a, A, B] | 3.334 ± 0.100 [b, A] | 0.634 |
| 10 | 4.283 ± 0.353 [a, A] | 3.451 ± 0.167 [b, B] | 2.869 ± 0.158 [b, B] | 0.609 |
| MSD[2] | 0.833 | 0.685 | 0.403 | ---- |
| Blank (washing and immersion in tap water for 15 minutes) ** .(log $CFU.g^{-1}$) | | | | 6.224 |
| Standard (washing with water and immersion in a solution of sodium hypochlorite: 120ppm/15min) ** .......................................(log $CFU.g^{-1}$) | | | | 3.517 |

MSD[1] = for the data on the lines; MSD[2] = for the data on the columns; small letter compares averages on the same line, capital letters compare means in the same column, different letters indicate that the data differ significantly at 5% probability; * Time of contact with the sanitizer product; ** reference treatments.

Table 4. Total coliform count (log $CFU.g^{-1}$) observed in samples of minimally processed rocket.

## 6. References

Andrade, J.N.; J.A.B. Macedo. Higienização na Indústria de Alimentos. São Paulo, Varela, 182p., 1996.

Andrews, D.H. New trends in food microbiology: an AOAC International perspective. Journal of AOAC International. v.80, n.4, p.908-912, 1997.

Arenstein, I.R. Dióxido de cloro estabilizado em solução aquosa: coadjuvante tecnológico de alimentos. Higiene Alimentar, São Paulo v.17, n.107, p.32-33, 2003.

Bachelli, M.L.B. Sanitização para alface minimamente processada em comparação ao hipoclorito de sódio. Dissertação de mestrado. Feagri, UNICAMP, Campinas, 2010.

Berbari, S.A.G.; J.E. Paschoalino; N.F.A. Silveira. Efeito do cloro na água de lavagem para desinfecção de alface minimamente processada. Ciência e Tecnologia de Alimentos, Campinas, v.21, n.2, p.197-201, maio-ago., 2001.

Beuchat, L.R. Standardization of methods to determine the efficacy of disinfectants for raw fruits and vegetables. *In:* TUIJTELAARS et al., (eds.) Food Microbiology and Food Safety into the next millenium. Proceedings of 17th International Conference of International Committee on Food Microbiology and Hygiene (ICFMH), Vendhoven, The Netherlands, 13-17, September, 1999, p.785-786, 1999.

Bruno, L.M.; A.A.M. Queiroz; A.P.C. Andrade; N.M. Vasconcelos; M.F. BORGES. Avaliação microbiológica de hortaliças e frutas minimamente processadas comercializadas em Fortaleza (CE). B. CEPPA, Curitiba, v.23, n.1, p.75-84, jan./jun., 2005.

CDC (Center for Disease Control and Prevention). Salmonellosis. National Center for Infectious Desease. Site: http;//www.salmonelosis. Acess in 27th July, 2011.

Costa, J.B. Avaliação ecotoxicológica de efluente de tratamento secundário de esgoto sanitário após desinfecção com acido peracético, cloro, ozônio e radiação ultravioleta. 180f. Tese (Doutorado em Ciências de Engenharia Ambiental) Escola de Engenharia de São Carlos, Universidade de São Paulo, São Carlos. 2007.

Dáoust, J.Y. *Salmonella* and International Trade. International Journal of Microbiology. v.5, n.2-3, p.85-94, 1994.

Farber, J. Microbiological issues surrounding the safety of fresh cut produce. 10th World Congress of Food Science and Technology. Abstract Book, Sydney, Australia; p.11, 1999.

Farrel, B. L. et al. Attachment of *E. coli* O157:H7 in ground beef to meat grinders and survival after sanitation with chlorine and peroxyacetic acid. Journal of Food Protection. v.61, n.7, p.817-22, 1998.

Felkey, K.D. et al. Optimization of chlorine treatments and the effects on survival of *Salmonella* spp. on tomato surfaces. In: Program and Abstract Book, 90th Annual Meeting of IAFP (International Association for Food Protection), New Orleans, August 10-13, 2003, Abstract P212, p.132, 2003.

Franco, B.D.G.M.; M. Landgraf. Microbiologia dos Alimentos. São Paulo: Editora Atheneu, 2005.

Francys, G.A; C. Thomas; D. O´Beirne. The microbiological safety of minimally processed vegetables. International Journal Food Science and Technology. v.34, p.1-22, 1999.

Frank, J. F.; K. Takeushi. Direct observation of *Escherichia coli* O157:H7 inactivation on lettuce leaf using confocal scanning laser microscopy. *In:* TUIJTELAARS et al., (eds) Food Microbiology and Food safety into the next millennium. Proceedings of 17th International Conference of International Committee on Food Microbiology and Hygiene (ICFMH), Vendhoven, The Netherlands, 13-17, September, 1999, p.795-797, 1999.

Garg, N.; J.J. Churey; D.F. Splitistoesser. Effect of processing conditions on the microflora of fresh cut vegetables. Journal of Food Protection, v.53, n.8, p.701-703, 1990.

Gopal, A.; S. Ajlonni; H. Roginskif; J. Coventry; J. Wan. Application of non-conventional disinfection techniques to extend the shelf-life of Minimally processed foods. 10th, World Congress of Food Science and Technology. Abstract Book, Sydney, Australia, 1999.

Hilgren, J.D.; J.A. Salverda. Antimicrobial efficacy of a peroxyacetic/octanoic acid mixture in fresh-cut-vegetable process waters. Journal of Food Science, v.65, n.8, p.1376-1379, 2000.

ISO 6579. Microbiology of food and animal feeding stuffs- Horizontal Method for detection of *Salmonella* spp., 4th ed.2002. The International Organization for Standardization, amendment 1: 15/07/2007.

Jones, M. V. et al. Comparative sensitive of *Vibrio cholerae* O1 EL TOR and *E. coli* to disinfectants. Letters Appl. Microb., v.14, p.51-3, 1992.

Kim, J.G; A.E. Yousef; S. Dave. Application of ozone for enhancing the microbiological safety and quality of foods: a review. Journal of Food Protection, v.62, n.9, p.1071-1087, 1999.

Machado, T.F; C.M. Delfino; P.H.M. Sousa. Microbiological quality evaluation minimally processed vegetables. In Tressler, J.F.M et al., 1722. Cienc. Agrotec., Lavras, v. 3. Edição Especial, p.1722-1727, 2009.

Maistro, L.C. Alface minimamente processada: uma revisão. Revista de Nutrição, Campinas, v.14, n.3, p.219-224, set./ - dez., 2001.

Mead, P.S. et al. Food-related illness and Death in the United States. Emerging Infection Desease. v.5, p.607-625, 1999.

Meyer, S.T. O uso de cloro na desinfecção de águas, a formação de trihalometanos e os riscos potenciais à saúde pública. Caderno de Saúde Pública, Rio de Janeiro, v.10, n.1, p.99-110, 1994.

Nascimento, M.S. Avaliação comparativa de tratamentos químicos na sanitização de frutas e verduras. 2002, 74f. Tese (mestrado em Ciência dos Alimentos) - Faculdade de Ciências Farmacêuticas, Universidade Estadual Paulista "Júlio de Mesquita Filho", Araraquara/SP.

Nascimento, H.M.; D.A. Delado; I.F. Barbaric. Avaliação da aplicação de agentes sanitizantes como controladores do crescimento microbiano na indústria alimentícia. Revista Ceciliana, Santos, v.2, n.2, p.11-13, 2010.

Nunes, E.E.; E.V.B. Vilas Boas; A.L.R.P. Xisto; S.C. Leme; M.C. Botelho. Avaliação de diferentes sanitizantes na qualidade microbiológica de mandioquinha-salsa minimamente processada. Ciência agrotec., Lavras, v.34, n.4, p.990-994, jul./ago., 2010.

Oliveira, E.C.M.; R.H.P. do Valle. Aspectos microbiológicos dos produtos hortícolas minimamente processados. Higiene Alimentar, São Paulo, v.11, n.78/79, p.50-54, 2000.

Rash, V.A. Physical and chemical treatments for control of *Salmonella* on cantaloupe rinds, In: Program and Abstract Book, 90th Annual Meeting of IAFP (International Association for Food Protection), New Orleans, August 10-13, 2003, Abstract P240, p.142, 2003.

Sapers, G.M. et al. Effectiveness of sanitizing agents in inactivating *E. coli* in Golden Delicious apples. Journal of Food Science, v.64, n.4, p.734-737, 1999.

Santána, A.S; M. Landgraf; M.T Destro; B.D.G.M Franco. Prevalence and counts of *Salmonella* spp. in minimally processed vegetables in São Paulo, Brazil. Food Microbiology, 28, 2011. (available online, 15 April, 2011).

Silva, E.A.J. Manual de Controle Higiênico-Sanitário em Alimentos. 3.ed. São Paulo: Ed. Varela, 1999.

Silva, N. et al. Manual de Métodos de Análise Microbiológica de Alimentos e Água. São Paulo: Ed. Varela, 2010.

Wisniewsky, M.A. et al. Reduction of *E. coli* O157:H7 counts on whole fresh apples by treatment with sanitizers. Journal of Food Protection, v.63, n.6, p.703-708, 2000.

# 7

# Isolation and Identification of *Salmonellas* from Different Samples

Birol Özkalp
*Department of Medicinal Laboratory*
*Vocational School of Health Services of Selçuk University, Konya*
*Turkey*

## 1. Introduction

*Salmonella* causes various infections in humans. Contamination of people by *Salmonella* may be caused by infected persons, animals and direct contact of those with fluids *Salmonella* also has an important role in producing pathogens that cause food posinoning. *Salmonellas* act as primary reservoir for foods such as chicken meat, milk and milk products, eggs and meat products etc. Some of microorganisms lsuch as Coliform bacteria have same features with *Salmonella*. For that reason, isolation and identification of *Salmonella* from clinical and other samples are important.

## 2. *Salmonella*

Efforts related with classification of these bacteria since first *Salmonellas* has been found also continues recently. When *Salmonella* bacteria are examined by DNA/DNA hybridization trials which are performed among bacteria, all *Salmonellas* should be accepted as one species including Arizona species added to them. According to this, subgenuses that Kauffman has created among *Salmonellas* according to genetic and other characteristics (subgenus 1, subgenus 2, subgenus 3= Arizona and subgenus 4) and subgenus 5 which was added by Le Minor should be accepted as sub-species instead of subgenus.

Up to the present, *Salmonella* bacteria were named according to their pathology, their host and the city where they have been found first and an attention was paid to use an individual name for every bacteria within the same antigen structure in Kauffman-White classification. These bacteria which were accepted as individual serovars were classified as separate species. It is known that these characteristics of bacteria are not appropriate and sufficient to determine a species and none of the methods that has been used up to the present is scientific in terms of taxonomy. Furthermore, international enterobacteriaceae subcommittee which is the most reliable organization about this subject have not performed a scientific guidance about various *Salmonellas* erovars classification. While studies continue, this committee has suggested as follows:

To protect validity of Kauffman white classification without having a bias related with definition of this species; to keep names of bacteria in *Salmonellas* ubgenus 1 (like individual species names) by continuing a normal tradition in medicine, cliniz and microbiology up to the present; when new bacteria which comply to this subgenus is found, to classify them

individually; to keep names of bacteria which have been found up to the present in other subgenus similarly, but in case of finding new bacteria which comply to this genus, to classify them only by antigenic formulas.
The idea which has arisen lately is that all *Salmonellas* including Arizona are single species and to classify this species as *Salmonella* enterica. Discriminations related with antigenic, biochemical, host and geographical distribution which are seen among bacteria has been depended on differentiation of this single species. Six subgroups were detected as a result of researches performed by DNA hybridization methods.
These are; *Salmonella*: 1 subgroup including s. enterica subspecies; *Salmonella* : 2 subgroup including salamae subgroup; *Salmonella*: 3a and *Salmonella*: 3b subgroups including arizonae and diarizonae subspecies; *Salmonella*: 4 subgroup including hautenae; *Salmonella*: 5 subgroup including bongori subspecies and *Salmonella*: 6 subgroup including indica subspecies.
In practice, bacteria are named as serovar names and for example, to use only *Salmonellas* erovar typhimurium, even *Salmonellas* erovar typhimurium name is preferred instead of long names such as *Salmonella* enterica subsp., Enterica serovar typhimurium.

### 2.1 Appearance and staining characteristics

*Salmonella* bacteria are asporogenic, capsule-free, motile via peritrichous cilium (*Salmonella* gallinarium or *Salmonella* pulorum are immotile), rod-shaped bacteria with an approximate length of 2,0-5,0 µm, width of 0,7-1,5 µm. They are stained well with bacteriologic stains and they are gram-negative *(Figure 1)*. Most of them have type 1 (mannose sensitive (ms), hemagglutinating); S. Gallinarium and some origins have type 2 fimbriae. S. paratyphi As do not have fimbriae.

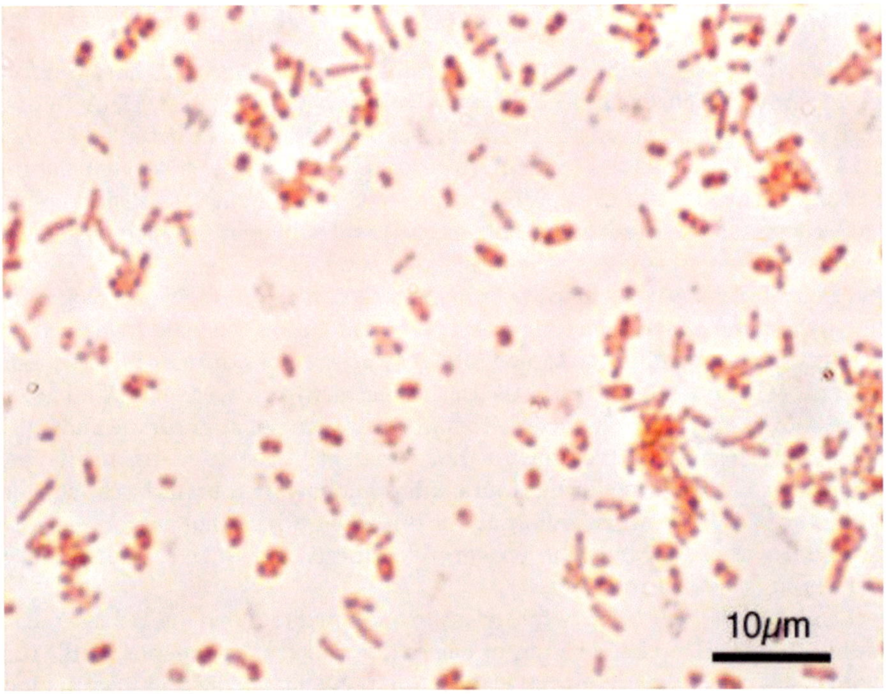


Fig. 1. Microscopic View of *Salmonella*

### 2.2 Reproduction and biochemical characteristics

*Salmonella* bacteria reproduce in many ordinary mediums. They are aerobe and facultative anaerobe. Their reproduction temperature limit is very wide even they reproduce at 37° C best. (20°C- 42°C). This is extremely important for reproduction of *Salmonellas* which cause food intoxication at room temperature. They like to produce at average pH of 7,2. They make homogenous turbidity in bouillon and similar liquid medium. They make round, slab sided, mostly tumescent colonies with a diameter of 2-3 mm, regular surface. In colonies of various *Salmonellas* , some differences may exist in terms of size, protuberance, surface and side. *Salmonella* typhi may also make gnome colonies which may reach to 0,2-0,3 mm diameter within the first 24 hours. Biochemical characteristics of bacteria which are obtained from these colonies are same as normal colonies; and they are agglutinated with O serums only antigenically and they differ from bacteria in S colonies in terms of not reacting with anti H, anti Vi serums. If they are reproduced in mediums including sulfurous compounds, sulfates and tiosulfates which may be assimilated, normal colonies occur from bacteria that make gnome colonies.

Some of *Salmonellas* , S. Schottemuelleri (s. paratyphi) in particular and some others form M colonies in appropriate mediums. It is detected that these bacteria have M antigens and agglutination is prevented by anti O and anti H serums. Furthermore, R colonies are formed by *Salmonella* which reproduce in inappropriate mediums (*Figure* 2).

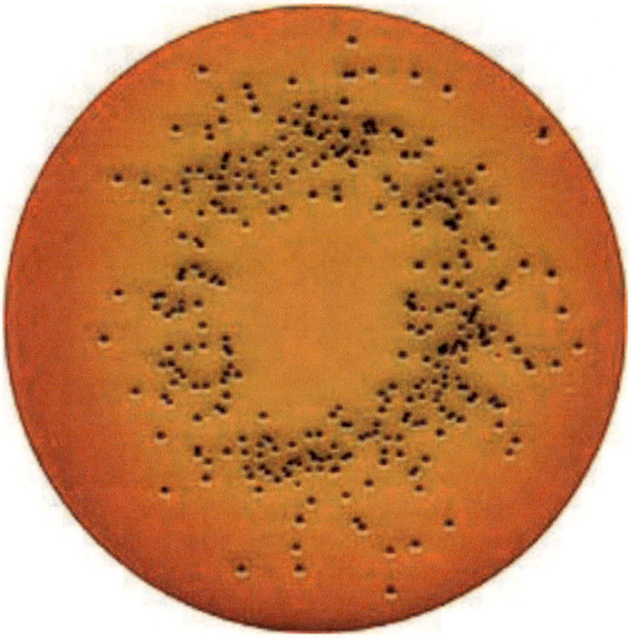

Fig. 2. *Salmonella* colonies

*Salmonellas* are not effective on lactose. This characteristics is important in first differentiation from Escherichias. As these bacteria which are planted in a separator plaque medium (endo, EMB) including lactose and an appropriate reagent are not effective on lactose, they make colorless colonies; however those effective on lactose make dark red, black, greenish bright colonies (*Figure 3*).

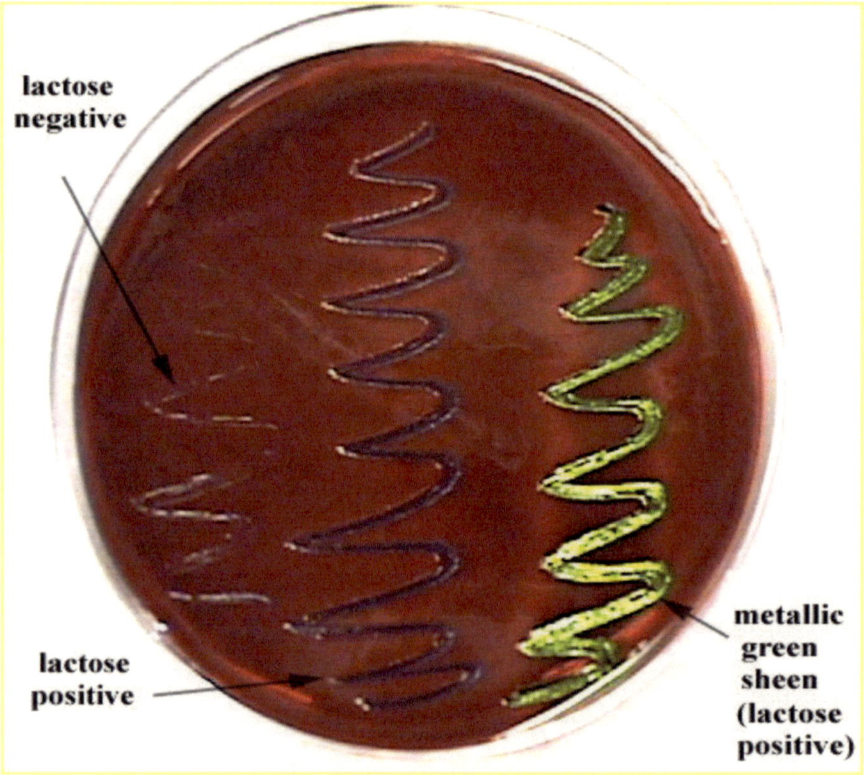


Fig. 3. View of *Salmonella* and Lactose Positive Colonies

*Salmonellas* do not effect on sucrose, adonitole and salicin in usual other than lactose. They digest glucose, mannite and maltose by producing acid and gas except *Salmonella* typhi and S. gallinarum; and *Salmonella* typhi and gallinarum digest them by producind acid only. They produce H2S in general (except S. paratyphi A); they are indole negative, methyl red positive, Vogesproskauter negative and they reproduce in citrated mediums (Simmon), they do not digest urea. They could not be produced in KCN (potassium cyanide 0,5%) mediums. ONPG (orthonitro phenyl galactopyranoside) assay is negative. (They do not have beta galactosidase enzymes that may digest lactose). This assay is positive in Arizona. Biochemical characteristics of *Salmonellas* were shown in *Table 1*.

| | |
|---|---|
| Motility | + |
| Indole | - |
| H2S | + |
| Oxidase | - |
| Urease | - |
| Nitrate reduction | + |
| Citrate Utilization | + |
| MR | + |
| VP | - |
| Lysine decarboxilation | + |
| Ornithine decarboxilation | + |
| Phenylalanine deamination | - |
| Malonate Utilization | - |
| Lactose | - |
| Sucrose | - |
| Salicine | - |
| Inositol | - |
| Amygdalin | - |
| Gas Production from glucose | + |
| β-galaktosidase (ONPG Test) | - |
| Reproduction in KCN | - |
| | (-) Negative (+) Positive |

Table 1. Biochemical characteristics of *Salmonellas*

## 3. Important terms ın takıng examınatıon sample

As delay in the diagnosis of acute infection is unhealthful in terms of delay in the treatment and it is also dangerous that other persons may be infected due to more contact. To obtain rapid and correct etiological diagnosis is possible to take the examination material appropriately, to send it to the laboratory rapidly and to examine them in the laboratory well. Inability to produce the active germ is due to faulty examination material taking in general. Examination material should be taken by persons who know the purpose of such procedure and by being careful in the following subjects.

It should be especially noted that examination material should be taken before administration of any antibiotics or other chemotherapeutic medications. Pathogen bacteria may not exist in the purulence even 24 hours after antibiotic administration. If bacteria that chemotherapeutic substance inhibit can not be produced from the examination material during the administration, it may be produced several days after discontinuation of the medication.

Examination material should be taken from the place where suspicious germ may exist. While taking sterile materials in normal such as urine, cerebrospinal fluid, special attention should be paid for contamination with outer germs. Sometimes, falling of several bacteria from outside causes not to obtain a result from the culture. The orifice of the tube or bottle should be singed when it is opened or before closing after material is put. The cap or seal of the tube or the bottle should be closed after removal without contacting any where. Although an extreme care is not necessary for materials including normal flora such as phlegm and stool, it is appropriate to take materials carefully by avoiding contamination from outside.
To obtain a successful result from the culture of the examination material, it should be taken within an appropriate period of the disease. In intestinal infections, bacteria may exist more in diarrhea period. It is more possible to isolate them within this period.
Furthermore, to take the examination material within certain times of the day may be important. To obtain a positive result by a culture made with the blood which was taken in febrile period is more likely. To obtain the phlegm in the morning is easier. The patient may expectorate more with a less effort.
No disinfecting or antiseptic are added into the examination material. If upper surface of the lesion is desired to be cleaned, a swam immersed into sterile saline or sterile cotton which is hold by a sterile holder is used. The material is taken after cleaned area dried.
Examination material should be sufficient to perform the examinations completely. It is not necessary to take excessive material. For example, when materials such as phlegm or stool are put more, they smear outside of the container. Particularly, a janitor who does not know the importance of the procedure may be infected by touching these containers. This should be prevented by continuous warnings and trainings.
The examination material should be sent to the laboratory as soon as possible and examined. Sensitive bacteria in the material of which examination is delayed die due to low temperature, effect of enzymes, drying or not being nourished. Saprophyte bacteria which may be present in the examination material reproduce at room temperature; to produce pathogenic bacteria is not possible as their count increases. Therefore, the material is stored in the refrigerator until the examination time when germs which are effected from cold are not searched. By this procedure, saprophytes do not reproduce and pathogens continue their vitality. Sometimes, mediums and required tools are carried near to the patient's bed and examination material is added immediately when taken.
Examination material should be sent to the laboratory early in the day. By this means, examination is possible within working hours of the laboratory. Laboratory should be notified one hour earlier for immediate examination.

### 3.1 Taking examination material and putting in a suitable container

It is extremely important not to contaminate with external germs for the material of which microbiological examination will be performed. The material which is taken in aseptic conditions should be put in a sterile container immediately and the cap should be closed. When germs in the examination material kept in hot conditions, they may reproduce and die in the cold. Therefore, the material which is taken to a sterile container should be implanted to the medium as soon as possible.

### 3.2 Stool

The stool that culture will be performed should be taken into a sterile container. By this means, contamination with bacteria in containers that stool was put before. There are special containers to put stool. These are tubes made of glass which were closed by cork. A small spoon made of metal was put on the edge of cork seal. Purulence or mucous parts of stool is taken by this spoon and put into the tube and cork of the tube is closed. To send to far distances, this special tube is put into a cylinder shaped box and this box is put into a wooden box. Also, scoop shaped small spoons made of metal are used to take stool. The stool is taken by deep side of this spoon which is sterilized by wrapping to a paper and the spoon is put into a screw cap bottle. Especially, bottles with wider orifices are suitable to put stool. Stool may be taken into glass like cardboards directly.

If culture of the stool will delay for several hours after taking, 1 g stool is mixed with 10 $cm^3$ 30% neutral glycerol solution in 6% saline buffer. It is seen that reaction is alkaline by pink-violet color after addition of phenol red. If this mixture is kept for a period, reaction becomes acid and indicator shows yellow color; so this mixture is not used anymore. Glycerol solution prevents saprophyte bacteria to reproduce and mask pathogen bacteria.

The solution is prepared as follows:

| | |
|---|---|
| 6% saltwater | 70 $cm^3$ |
| Glycerol | 30 $cm^3$ |
| $Na_2HPO_4$ | 1 g |

0,02% phenol red is added into this.

Prepared solution is divided into bottles as 10 cm3. The stool is taken into this bottle.

Stool may be sent to a far laboratory by a filter paper to search *Salmonella* bacteria. For this, stool is applied on a filter or blotter as a thin layer and left for drying in the room. Two edges of the paper is folded by superimposing by a holder, stool is kept between the folded part. The paper is placed into a plastic envelope. Various samples which were prepared by this manner may be sent with a package prepared accordingly for mail. Such paper is cut into three parts in the laboratory. Suspension is made with salt water and it is smeared on appropriate medium in petri plate. Other parts are put into selenite and tetra thionate bouillon, they are smeared on the petri plate after reproduction.

Stool sample which was taken into sterile containers or stool sample which was taken by swab rectally, the sample taken from bedpan or diaper of unconscious patient, and stool sample taken from baby diapers should be examined within at least one hour. If the sample is not examined within one hour, it may be stored in the refrigerator for three to four hours. Because, coliform bacteria which are dominant on the stool reproduce more in the room temperature and acidize the environment. This prevents reproduction of *Salmonella* bacteria as well as causes death.

Bean sized sample is taken into any of selenite or tetra thionate bouillon mediums and processed to pre-enrichment at 37°C for 3 to 4 hours in the incubator, then it is planted on SS, EMB, endoagar plates according to dilution planting technique and identification process is started by considering lactose negative colonies.

### 3.3 Microbiological examination of the urine

Kidneys, ureter, bladder and most of the urethra are sterile areas in healthy human. Urethra includes a bacteria flora as far as 1,5-2 cm inside from the orifice both in women and men. In normal, the urine coming from upper sterile areas always contaminates more or less while passing from this region of the urethra. But this contamination is not over a certain bacteria count in a healthy person. By considering this feature of the urinary system and the urine, some criteria should be followed before taking the urine sample, while taking the sample and sending it to the laboratory for microbiological examinations.

Generally, urinary antiseptics and antibiotic drugs and excessive water should not be given to persons before taking the sample.

The form so called middle flow is the most common method applied in all hospitalized and polyclinic patients who are cooperated for taking urine sample. The most important subject that patients should know and should be informed in this method is genital region cleaning which is required to be performed before taking the urine sample. Because, bacteria reproduce over $10^5$ criteria in urine samples taken from persons who do not care about genital area hygiene and cleaning, frequently in women and urinary infection is diagnosed inaccurately. No infection is found in urine samples of these persons after a well cleaning is performed. Soap and water are sufficient for cleaning. Persons should wash their hands first, and clean glans penis and orifice in men and genital areas, labias and the orifice of women from front to back and from up to down. The person will start to urinate just after this cleaning and take the urine which is in the middle of the urination stage, not the first or the last urine into a sterile tube or sterile bottle with a wide opening (as 5 to 10 ml) and close the cap immediately. The urine taken should be transmitted to the laboratory as soon as possible. If this is not possible, the urine should be stored in the refrigerator for a certain period.

The urine sample brought to the laboratory should be stored in the refrigerator or examined within 1 hour.

The other process that will be done with the urine sample is culturing.

The method used in almost every microbiology laboratory is to plant with a washing bottle or loop. Loops used for planting are fabrication products which are calibrated and they are expensive. Apart from this, they should be controlled whether their calibration was deteriorated by special methods. The most suitable for us is 1 ml serological pipettes with 0,1 calibrated.

The urine brought is planted as 0,1 ml on every petri plate (blood agar- EMB, endo, Mac Conkey etc.) by a pipette after mixing well and smeared to the plate by a sterile glass rod.

Plates put into the incubator (35-37°C) are removed after an incubation of 18 to 24 hours, and colony count is performed. The colony amount which is counted in every plate is multiplied with 10 and it is expressed as colony amount in ml. According to the values obtained, colony count between -10,000 is accepted as NORMAL, between 10,000-100,000 as SUSPICIOUS and over 100,000 as URINARY INFECTION.

Except these criteria, lactose negative colonies are evaluated and identified in EMB or ENDO AGAR; and *Salmonella* is diagnosed. In this case, this is accepted as an infectious agent without considering 100,000 ml/cfu bacteria count as we accepted as infectious agent.

### 3.4 Cerebrospinal fluid

Bacteriological examination of cerebrospinal fluid is performed in cases that meningitis is suspected. Examination material taken under sterile conditions is sent to the laboratory as soon as possible. If the material will not be examined instantly, it is stored in the incubator to examine within one hour. Germs obtained from cerebrospinal fluid most:

Neisseria meningitidis, Diplococcus pneumoniae, Haemophilus influenzae, Mycobacterium tuberculosis, Staphylococcus aureus, Streptococcus pyogenes, *Salmonella* escherichia,

Proteus, Pseudomonas, Mimeae, Flavobacterium, Bacteroides, Listeria monocytogenes, Pasteurella multocida, Leptospira, Cryptococcus, Neoformans viruses.
While CSF is taken, the area where puncture will be performed should be cleaned with iodine and alcohol to avoid contamination with flora bacteria on the skin. Sufficient material should be taken to be able to perform cellular, chemical and microbiological examinations. To take material, to put sterile screw cap tubes in lumbar puncture sets is more appropriate instead of cotton or plastic seal tubes. In cases that sufficient CSF can not be obtained, only required examinations should be requested first from the laboratory. CSF should be transmitted to the laboratory immediately and examined instantly. As CSF is regarded as materials that planting should be performed near the patient, if examinations can not be done within a very short period it should be stored in the incubator. The sample taken to isolate *Salmonellas* hould be taken into selenite f medium and it is kept under pre-incubation at 37°C for 3 to 4 hours, then planted on mediums such as SS, EMB, MAC KONKEY by dilution planting technique and lactose negative colonies are identified.

### 3.5 Autopsy material

Examination material is taken from ileum in suspicion of typhoid fever. Intestinal wall is cauterized by superheated spatula. A sterile swab is inserted from the hole opened and moved on the mucosa by rotating. The swab is removed and immersed into tetrahionate bouillon or selenite bouillon. The swab is rotated by pressing on the wall of the tube and a clouded fluid is obtained. Planting is performed from this fluid to Endo, SS, bismuth sulphite agar mediums which are used to produce *Salmonella* bacteria. Material is taken from the bladder by the same way.

### 3.6 Purulence

The infectious agent from lesions such as abscess, wound and fistula are searched by bacteriological examination.
Taking Examination material:

- The purulence is taken from open lesions by a swab or a loop which is superheated and cooled.
- If there is a closed abscess, upper surface is cleaned with tincture of iodine and alcohol and drying is waited. Abscess is opened, the first purulence is removed, the purulence appeared is taken by a swab, it is put into the tube without contacting the skin. Or, purulence is taken from the abscess by a sterile syringe or a Pasteur pipette and put into a sterile tube. Small pustules are pierced with a sterile needle after the upper surface is cleaned and the fluid appeared is taken by a Pasteur pipette, swab or a loop and examined.

### 3.7 Serous liquids

Liquids accumulated in cavities of pleura, pericardium and peritoneum and synovial and hydrocele liquids are sent to the laboratory to search for the bacteriological agent in case of infection.
Serous liquids should be taken under sterile conditions and out into a sterile container. To prevent the coagulation by putting some of the liquid into a citrate solution or a beaded bottle is appropriate.

### 3.8 Microbiological examination of wound and abscess materials

Wound infections and abscess appear as a complication of surgical interventions and traumas or contamination of any infectious disease to the skin, mucosa, tissues and organs. In general, agents in the wound and abscesses are closely associated with the flora in the region. However, open wounds, ulcers and fistulas are contaminated from the flora or air and microorganisms coming from objects according to their region. Therefore, a cleaning should be performed before taking a material from these lesions. To take material from dry lesions is impossible and useless many times.
To isolate the agent in acute wounds is easy, however, to isolate the agent is quite difficult as number of microorganisms in chronic wounds decreased very much.

### 3.9 Vomitus

The vomit is examined when food poisoning occurs. Bacteria such as *Salmonella* , shigella, Staphylococcus aureus and Clostridium perfringens (welchii) are searched. Food poisoning also occurs when food contaminated with many other bacteria is eaten. In case of epidemic, the type of pathogen bacteria which is reproduced too many should be thought as the agent.
Examination substances are planted into 2 blood agar and put into aerobe and anaerobe conditions. Selective medium is used for *Salmonella* bacteria. It is possible to obtain *Salmonellas* from the stool in food poisonings. Negative culture does not remove possibility of food poisoning with bacteria.

## 4. *Salmonella* isolation from non-clinical samples

Bacteria are present everywhere in the nature. Many of them are harmless. Some of them may infect humans and animals. These bacteria may reproduce only under certain circumstances. Dissemination may be from human to human, from animal to human or from human to animal. Dissemination may be either directly or indirectly. Dissemination via food takes an important place. Bacteria which cause disease by food may pass to human as well as some bacteria which may reproduce on food may cause food poisoning.
*Salmonella* and Shigella bacteria are present in stools of sick human, animal and porters. These bacteria may pass from person to person by contact when hygiene rules are ignored and *Salmonella* bacteria which causes food poisoning may pass to food.
Also, cats and dogs kept at homes may reveal *Salmonella* without any symptom. Livestocks also may be infected with *Salmonellas* and spread them to the environment.
*Salmonellas* appeared with stools of pets and livestock may directly contaminate to food. However, if hygiene rules are ignored in places where livestock is kept, everything belonging to the animal may cause contamination.
In some places, flies play an important role in spreading of the infection. In case of spoiling of stools on the road in settlements where humans and animals live together, flies are effective in spreading if they were not controlled. If bacteria such as typhoid, dysentery etc. are endemic in these regions, flies create a big problem.
With less possibility, bees, spiders and ants play role for spreading harmful bacteria in places where environmental conditions are not hygienic.
Inorganic objects such as towels, pens, door handles, toilet (WC) equipment, containers may play a role in spreading of the infection from human to human or from human to food.

**Reservoirs of microorganisms that cause food poisoning**

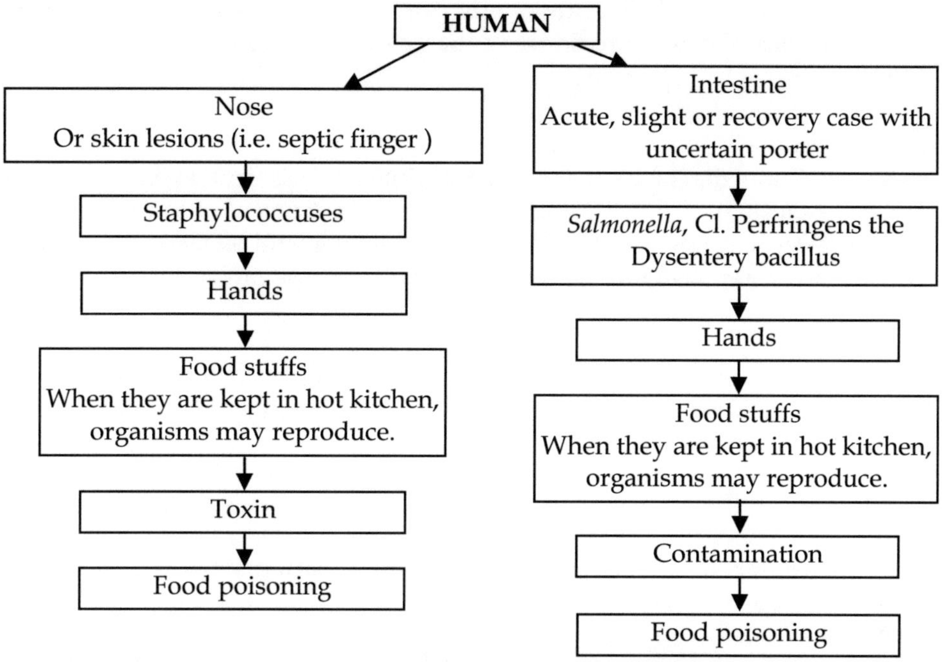


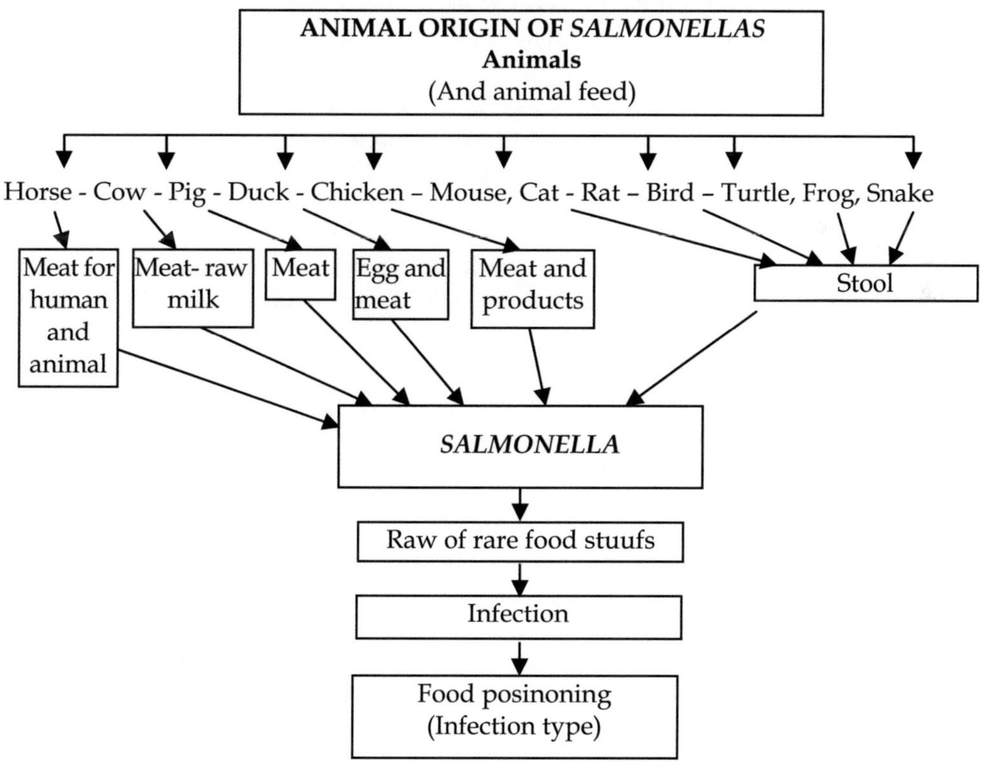

Methods which is being used to detect pathogen microorganisms in the food are ineffective if such pathogenic microorganisms diffused rarely or the food is severely contaminated with other microorganisms. For these reasons, various indicator microorganisms are used for various purposes.

### 4.1 Sample taking

To take samples from the foods for microbiological analysis and to bring this to the laboratory by "protecting all microbiological criteria at the moment of sampling" are quite difficult. Subjects such as how much and how many sample will be taken, bringing to the laboratory, opening and preparation for planting should be overemphasized.

### 4.2 Sample amount

Many national and international standards give the food quantity to be analyzed as 10 g (mL). This value is valid for quantitative analyses only. Pathogens are usually analyzed by present/absent test in 25 grams of food.

While 10 grams of sample is sufficient for a standard analysis, usually 25 grams of food is required for every additional pathogen test in accordance with special homogenization requirements as mentioned above. According to this, at least 60 grams of sample including10 grams for total bacteria, coliform group bacteria, yeast and mold and staphylococcus and 25 grams of each for *Salmonella* and Lysteria analysis should be brought to the laboratory.

The requirement that how many items should be taken from a sample mostly causes confusion. In daily controls performed in food industry, only 1 sample is sufficient.

More samples should be taken from foods that have high pathogenic risk such as *Salmonella*, Lysteria etc.

### 4.3 Bringing the sample to the laboratory and acceptance

The sample taken from the enterprise should be brought to the laboratory as cleared from all conditions that will increase or decrease the single microorganism count as soon as possible and analyzed.

In microbiologically stable products such as sterile, dry and humid resistant packages, no cooling is required during transportation. On the other hand, unprocessed, cooled, pasteurized, spoiled foods should be transported between 0°C and +4°C and frozen products should be transported at -18°C and those bulged (or having a risk of bulge) should be packaged separately against explosion and leakage and brought to the laboratory.

First, the sample should be accepted to be analyzed by the laboratory. For this acceptance, laboratory personnel should control whether the sample is brought to the laboratory under required conditions; if such personnel is sure that the sample was brought under standard conditions, she/he should accept the sample for the analysis; otherwise she/he should either reject or write all negativities related with this to the acceptance form.

For the sample which has come to the laboratory and accepted, date of acceptance, time of acceptance, all information related with the product (date of production, package features, batch number, shift number, time of sampling, temperature of sampling, temperature of arrival etc. if required) should be recorded according to the features of the laboratory.

Frozen liquid products are not accepted for microbiological or somatic cell analysis. If chemical tests will be performed, sub-samples should be separated for microbiological analysis first.

### 4.4 Opening the sample

The sample which has come for analysis should be analyzed within the shortest period. If there is a necessity to wait for a while;

- Microbiologically stable products should be analyzed before the expiry date and as soon as possible.
- Fresh and cooled products should be analyzed within 24 hours after the acceptance. If a longer storage period is necessary, the product should be frozen immediately and stored under -18°C. As the frosting process will affect the microbial flora in the product, this situation should be specified in the analysis report exactly.

Frozen products should be thawed in +4°C refrigerator temperature. It should be considered that big particle products will thaw within a longer period than small particle products and psycrophile bacteria may develop within the thawing period, therefore the food should be frozen with portions not more than 50 grams within bounds of possibility. If the sample is frozen by weighing before, it may be thawed by transferring into homogenization solution directly.

Parallel of the sample which has come to the laboratory and accepted should be protected as witness of which features will not change until the termanitaion of the analysis.

Before opening the closed package, the place and its surroundings should be disinfected via 76% (v/v) alcohol or any appropriate chemical agent and if the package is appropriate, it should be singed. Packages that can not be singed (paper etc.) should be removed by cleaning with disinfecting sterile water after chemical disinfection and such disinfection should not be contacted with the food sample anyhow. Otherwise, negative result may be taken. Materials which will be used to open the sample such as scissors, tin opener, bottle opener etc. should have been disinfected or sterilized in the drying oven or autoclave by wrapping to an appropriate package (paper, kitchen type aluminum folio).

Liquid samples may be analyzed directly. Solid foods should be pre-processed such as weighing, homogenization etc.

Weighing to a certain weight (10 g, 25 g, etc.) in solid sample should be performed under aseptic conditions. To weight in vertical type planting cabinet is the most reliable method. The container that weighing will be performed should have been sterilized and should be in the size to take pre-enrichment medium like *Salmonella*.

If solid food consists of particles which may create a problem during weighing in terms of size and qualification, it should be divided into suitable sizes.

It should be remembered that this application is valid for weighing which is more than aimed weight and weighing over 5% should not be performed as far as possible. If microorganisms such as *Salmonella* was weighed as 26 grams instead of 25 grams in present/absent tests, to use a 234 (=225+9) mL medium instead of 225 mL of pre-enrichment medium is not a condition. Because, the process performed here by using 25 grams of food + 225 mL medium is not a dilution, but using 9 mL medium per 1 gram food. Tolerence of +/- 5% is always accepted. The deviation in this sample is only 4%.

Generally, it is the process to make solid and semi-solid foods homogenous in a homogenization solution. Liquid foods show a homogenous distribution in anyway. The purpose of homogeneity here is to distribute all microorganisms in the food to all mass to be analyzed. Homogenization process is performed as 1:9 in general whether it is used for counting or present/absent tests. According to this, 1 part food is homogenizated by 9 part solution. In present/absent tests, 1 part food is homogenizated by 9 parts of medium. If counting will be performed, 1:9 homogenization is also used as $10^{-1}$ dilution. Therefore, amount of the food and homogenization solution should be cared about.

### 4.5 Homogenization and dilution solutions

Although "normal saline" (0.85% NaCl; Merck 1.06404) has been used as diluting solution for general purpose, "Maximum Recovery Diluent (Merck 1.12535) which has the formula of Normal Saline (0,85%) + Peptone (0,1%) in accordance with ISO 6887 is used recently. This solution is also referred as "peptone-saline". Furthermore, 0.1% peptone solution (Merck 1.07214) and "Buffered Peptone Water" (Merck 1.07228) which is used in *Salmonella* analysis are used for dilution in accordance with ISO 6887.

### 4.6 Water

To drink and to use waters contaminated with stool or sewage leakages is very important because they may cause infections such as typhoid, dysentery, cholera. In contaminated water, typhoid germ may exist together with intestinal bacteria. However, number of these bacteria is very less in general and it is impossible to obtain. On the other hand, commensal bacteria such as coliform bacteria, Streptococcus faecalis and Clostridium perfringens (welchii) are always obtained in contaminated water easily. Such water containing these bacteria means that the water was contaminated with the stool an this may contain typhoid germ. Coliform bacteria shows the contamination with the stool with the safest manner. The most important of them is Escherichia coli which is main commensal bacteria of the intestine. Existence of spore forming anaerobe bacteria in the absence of other bacteria shows an old contamination with the stool.

Colifrom bacteria also exists in water contaminated with stool of various animals. But they are less. More bacteria are present in the water contaminated with sewage water. It is important to detect the bacteria count in the water to determine the level of the contamination.

Detection of alive bacteria count gives information about quantity and type of organic substances. The trial is performed both at 37°C and 22°C. Bacteria which mix from human and animal origin organic substances reproduce at 37°C in particular. Those which reproduce in lower temperature are saprophyte bacteria that mix from the soil and plants or exist in the water normally.

#### 4.6.1 Taking the water sample

The water to be examined should be taken into colorless, preferably glass cap bottles with a volume of 250 $cm^3$ . Orifice and cap of the bottle are wrapped with separate papers and sterilized in the autoclave. If water will be taken from running water, the orifice of the tap is burned with spirit flame and the water is put into the bottle after leaving the water run for five minutes. The cap of the bottle is closed by caring the sterility conditions. To take water from the creek or river, the bottle is hold from the bottom, it is immersed into the water upside down to 30 cm deep. The orifice of the bottle is turned to the flow direction and water is filled with water without touching. To take water from dead water, lakes and depots, the bottle that a ballast was hung to the bottom and bounded with ropes from the neck and the cap is immersed into the water with a desired depth. The rope is pulled and the cap is opened, after the bottle is filled with water, it is pulled to up and the cap is closed.

If a period more than 3 hours will pass from taking the water sample until the examination, the bottle should be kept in ice. It may be sent to far places only in ice.

If sample will be taken from chlorinated water, chlorine should be neutralized immediately. For this, one sodium thiosulphate crystal is put into the bottle or 0,2 cm3 from 1 g of crystallized sodium thiosulphate solution which was dissolved in 100 cm3 sterile water before sterilization.

To mix the water well before the assay, the bottle that water sample is taken is shaken.

#### 4.6.2 Approximate assay for coliform bacteria count

To produce coliform bacteria, water is planted into Durham tubes including 2% peptone, 0,5% sodium taurocholate, 1% lactose and bromthymol blue (or bromeresol purple) as indicator. Amount of the water planted varies between 0,1 cm3 and 50 cm3. Concentrated medium is used if more water will be planted. The least water amount including coliform bacteria is detected by assays and contamination degree of the water is determined. Generally, 20 cm of 15 tubes included medium is taken. 0,1-1 cm3 water is put into 5 tubes; 1 cm3 water is put into 5 tubes; and 10 cm3 water is put into 5 tubes. Tubes are left at 37°C for 48 hours. After 24 and 48 hours, tubes are controlled and acid and gas formation is controlled. If gas is produced, it is examined that such gas has filled 1/10 of the small tube in Durham tube. Formation of gas which will occupy 1/10 of the tube after 24 hours shows possibility of Eschericihia coli reproduction. If no gas has formed within 24 hours or the gas occurred is less than 1/10 of the small tube, tubes are left at 37°C for 48 hours. Any gas formation is considered as suspicious. No gas formation after 48 hours shows no reproduction of Eschericihia coli.

To confirm whether reproduced bacteria are Eschericihia coli, planting is performed from tubes with least amount of water that reproduction was observed to eosine-methylene blue agar by decreasing method. Petri dishes are left at 37°C for 24 hours and examined and it controlled whether the bacteria reproduced is Eschericihia coli.

#### 4.6.3 Searching for *Salmonella* bacteria

Same amount of water is added into tubes including selenite f medium which was prepared with one portion concentrate. After waiting at 37°C for 24 hours, planting is performed from every tube to SS agar. Furthermore, one cm3 each from tubes are taken and mixed with bismuth sulphite agar and poured into petri plates. When reproduction occurs, it is searched whether it is from *Salmonella* group. (551,602,611)

### 4.7 Meat

Meat may include many germ types such as bacillus suptilis, Escherichia, proteus, *Salmonella* , staphylococcus species and fungus and especially anerobe spore forming bacteria show fundamental change. These bacteria cause formation of bad odor by making putrefaction in proteins. It is not very possible to decide on the status of the meat by bacteria on it.

To detect bacteria, one gram is weighed, it is meshed in mortar with sand. 1000, 10.000, 100.000 dilutions are prepared. Colony count is performed with these in the petri plate. Diagnose of bacteria is performed if required.

### 4.8 Egg

Fresh egg is not always sterile. Gran (+) coccus, gram (-) bacillus and some fungus species may be present in the egg. Sometimes, egg may include *Salmonella* bacteria. (617, 618)

The shell of the egg has a porous structure. Gases and microscopic particles may pass through these pores. Bacteria always exist on the shell of the egg. Escherichia coli is present almost on all shells. Humidity causes bacteria to pass through pores in humid and dirty eggs. Therefore, eggs which sill be stored for a while must not be washed.

The egg which will be examined is cleaned well by washing with brush, water and soap. It is kept in 0,1% sublimated solution for 30 minutes. It is taken from here by a sterile spoon and put into 200 $cm^3$ of sterile water. It is kept in the water for 10 minutes and put into 95% alcohol and left for 5 minutes. The egg is taken from the alcohol and left for drying and broken from the wide edge by a sterile holder. The content is transferred into a sterile beaded jar. Egg white and yolk are mixed by shaking well. Microorganisms are searched by planting into various mediums.

### 4.9 Milk

There are various methods for bacterial analysis in the milk. The most used methods include alive bacteria count in petri plate, direct microscope count, coliform bacteria detection, methylene blue assay, phosphatase assay, turbidity assay and assay for special bacteria search. These methods are applied to various milks.

The milk which will be drunk should not include bacteria more than 30,000 and coliform bacteria in 0,1 cm3. 0,01 cm3 of pasteurized milk should not include any coliform bacteria and its pasteurization should be understood by phosphatase assay. Turbidity assay should be positive in sterilized milk.

The milk which was milked in the morning is kept waiting 9 to 11 hours in the shadow and the milk which was milked at night is kept waiting until the next day. Other samples are tried immediately when they come to the laboratory. Milk that analysis is not performed immediately may be stored at refrigerator for 24 hours at most.

### 4.10 Microbiological examination of fruit juices and other soft drinks

Main soft drink is water. These beverages may be classified as follows.

1. Water (mineral water etc.)
2. Fruit juices ( fruit juices including alcohol less than 5 g/1 and $SO_2$ less than 10 mg/1)
3. Fruit juice concentrates (concentrates which were condensed and partially canned and is drunk by diluting, basic substances and essence)
4. Beverages including carbonic acid (lemonades, soda pops, cokes)

Mineral water including carbonic acid is microbiologically safe water. They lat for a long time. Some microorganisms may exist in them.

As fruit juices are acidic and sugared foods; yeasts, molds and milk acid bacteria cause spoiling. Microbiological spoiling in fruit juice concentrates is very less. Abovementioned microorganisms also spoil concentrates. Yeasts (Candida saccharomyces, torolopsis species), milk acid bacteria (leuconostoc, lactobacillus species) in lemonades, sodas and cokes cause spoiling.

Examination of the samples are performed according to the following steps.

PROCESS

1. BEVERAGE BOTTLES ARE TAKEN UNDER ASEPTIC CONDITIONS. Bottle of beverages with carbonic acid is opened 1 hour before, it is heated slightly and the gas moves out.
2. Dilutions are prepared if necessary. (from intense textured beverages and concentrates)
3. Samples are planted into or on the medium as 1,0 ml or 0,1 ml.
4. If there are membrane filters, 100 ml of sample is filtered via water squinch and the membrane filter is placed on the medium.
5. Plates are incubated at 30-32°C for 3 to 5 days and evaluated.
6. Same amount of sample is added into tubes including selenite f medium which was prepared with one portion concentrate. After waiting at 37°C for 24 hours, planting is performed from every tube to SS agar. Furthermore, one cm3 each from tubes are taken and mixed with bismuth sulphide agar and poured into petri plates. When reproduction occurs, it is searched whether it is from *Salmonella* group. (551,602,611)

## 5. Culture and identification methods of *Salmonellas*

For identification of various samples, methods which alternate and support each other. These are:

- Culture methods
- Invic test
- Triple tube method
- Api method
- Full automatic bacteria identification device
- Serological tests
- Grubul Widel

### 5.1 Culture methods

Culture method in identification of *Salmonellas* is conducted with pre-enrichment and selective medium planting.

Identification studies are same regardless from the source of the culture. Variety of mediums used in the culture may depend on characteristics of the sample examined. Especially when number of *Salmonellas* are less and other organisms are more, very careful study is required. If extra clinical samples are processed such as heating, drying and radiation or they are frozen or kept for a long time or pH level is low although clinical samples are examined as fresh, non-selective pre-enrichment culture is applied. Because these processes weakened *Salmonellas* and made them semi-selective. The purpose is to provide this kind of bacteria to their normal reproduction period before contacting inhibitor substances. Because selective substances may make a toxic effect for "weakened" *Salmonellas* . While enrichment bouillon culture facilitates reproduction of *Salmonellas* , it also provides inhibiting or decreasing effect for reproduction of other organisms. Accompaniment organisms mainly include coliforms, proteus species and pseudomonas. As the proportion of these organisms is more than *Salmonellas* in particular, selective enrichment process gains importance. However, there are differences between *Salmonella* types in terms of inhibitor substance sensitivity. Therefore, it is impossible to say which selective enrichment bouillon is the most suitable definitely for today. Selective agar mediums generally include inhibitor substances and an inhibitor system. Indicator system either changes the color of colonies or the color of agar area around the colony changes. Thus, it helps to identify suspicious *Salmonella* colonies.

The following Agar Mediums are used in various countries.

Brillant green agar Brillantgreen Sulphadiazine agar Brillant Green Mac Conkey agar Desoksicholate Citrate agar *Salmonella* -Shigella Agar,(SS) Bismuth Sulphite agar EMB AGAR ENDO AGAR

Samples are taken into non-selective enrichment medium (lactone bouillon) according to their clinical or extra clinical sample characteristics and incubates at 35-37 °C for 24 to 48 hours, then 1 ml from them is taken and taken into selective enrichment medium and (Selenite F, tetrathionate bouillon) A and incubated at 35-37 °C for 24 hours.

#### 5.1.1 Non selective enrichment

1. Clinical and other samples are taken into lactose bouillon with appropriate amounts. If the sample food is also solid, it is mixed in the blender. Ot is transferred into 500 ml of erlenmayer flask or flasks.
2. It is incubated at 35-37°C for 48 hours and passed to selective enrichment.

3. At this time, a loop full of the sample is taken and planting to selective agar medium is performed.

### 5.1.2 Selective enrichment

1. 1 ml of non selective enrichment medium culture is taken and it is transferred into a tube including 10 ml of selenite cystine. 1 ml is planted into one of 5 tetrathionate medium of 10 ml.
2. Tubes are incubated at 35-37 °C for 24 hours.

### 5.1.3 Planting to selective agar medium

1. Two selective agar medium plate is prepared by drying. One of them may be enrichment and the other may be selective medium.
2. A loop from every enrichment culture with a diameter of 5 mm is taken and planted to provide single colony.
3. Plates are incubated by reversing at 35-37°C for 24 hours. If typical colonies are not observed at the end of 24 hours, incubation is extended to 48 hours.
4. Suspicious two colonies are selected from every selective agar medium and identification is directed.
5. If agar plates are completely full of coliforms, 1/1000 dilution of enrichment culture is prepared and kept at the room temperature or in the refrigerator.
6. Selective agar plates are kept at 5-8°C until completion of identification tests.

Appearances of *Salmonella* colonies in various mediums after incubation are as follows.

#### 5.1.3.1 Appearance of typical *Salmonella* colonies in Brillant green agar and Brillant green sulphadiazine agar

It is colorless, pink, semi transparent or opaque. The color of medium which surrounds the colony has become pink or red. Some *Salmonella* colonies make semi-transparent green colonies when lactose or sucrose fermentating organisms are present around them. Lactose or sucrose fermantating colonies make yellow to green colonies (*Figure 4).*

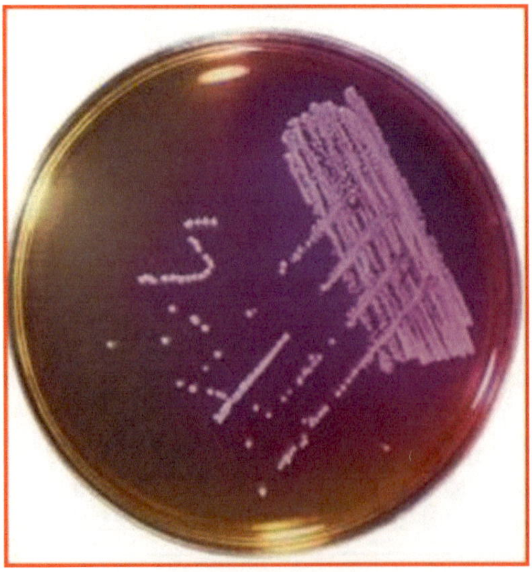

Fig. 4. Appearance of typical *Salmonella* colonies in Brillant green agar

### 5.1.3.2 Appearance of typical *Salmonella* colonies in mac conkey agar

It is colorless and transparent. Coliform organisms precipitate bile salts in the medium. *Salmonella* colonies reproduced near coliforms dissolve precipitated area (*Figure 5*).

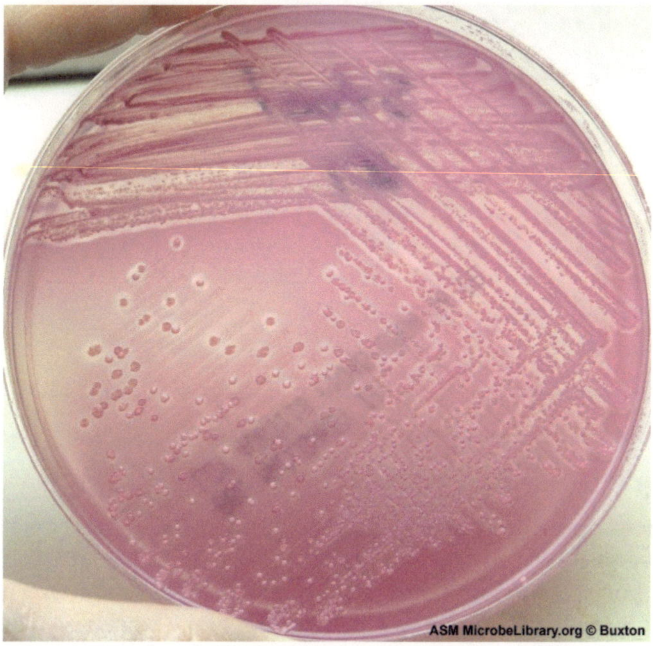


Fig. 5. Appearance of typical *Salmonella* colonies in Mac Conkey agar

### 5.1.3.3 Appearance of *Salmonella* colonies in *Salmonella* - Shigella agar (SS)

Typical *Salmonella* colonies are colorless or very light pink, opaque or semi-transparent. Some of *Salmonellas* make colonies of which the centre is black (*Figure 6*).

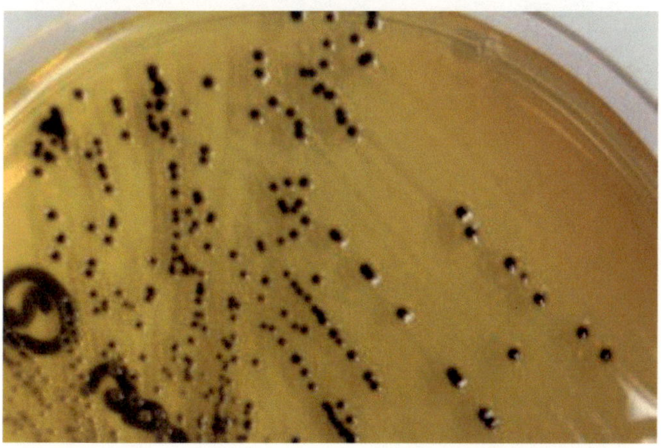

Fig. 6. Appearance of *Salmonella* colonies in *Salmonella* - Shigella agar (SS)

### 5.1.3.4 Appearance of *Salmonella* colonies in desoxyholate citrate agar

*Salmonella* colonies are colorless or very light pink, opaque or semi-transparent. Some of *Salmonellas* reproduce as black or gray in the middle and colorless on the sided (*Figure 7)*.

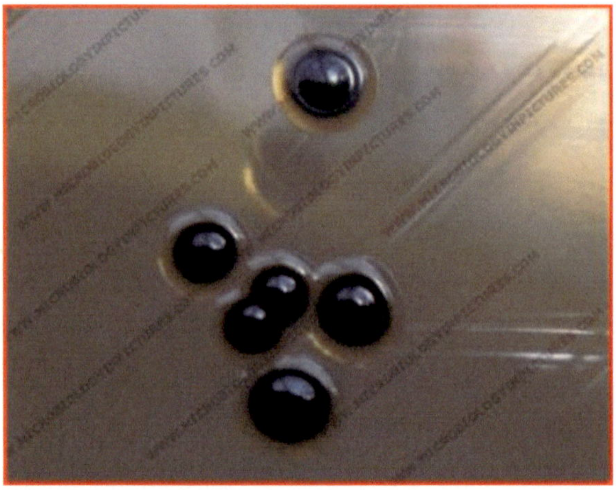

Fig. 7. Appearance of *Salmonella* colonies in desoxyholate citrate agar

### 5.1.3.5 Appearance of *Salmonella* colonies in bismuth sulphite agar

*Salmonella* colonies appear as brown, gray or black. Sometimes they show a metallic brightness. The medium which surrounds the colony is brown at first. It becomes black when incubation period extends. Some strains make green colonies and they make the surrounding medium to black very less or they do not make blackness (*Figure 8)*.

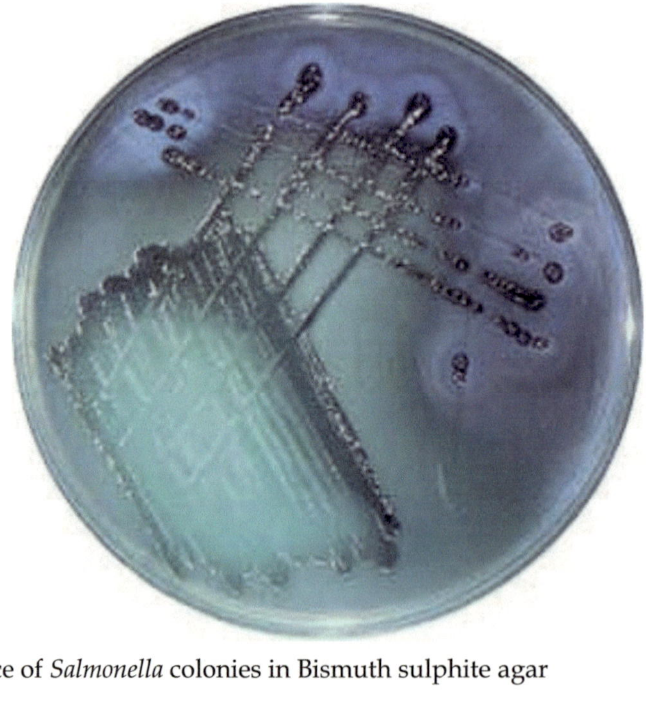

Fig. 8. Appearance of *Salmonella* colonies in Bismuth sulphite agar

#### 5.1.3.6 Appearance of bile-salts-jelatin lactose agar (Tahsin Berkin agar ) (BS) L AGAR)

*Salmonella* colonies make cyclamen colored colonies with a diameter of 1 to 3 mm. These colonies are bright, swollen (s) type colonies.

#### 5.1.3.7 Appearance of *Salmonella* colonies in EMB AGAR

*Salmonella* colonies make transparent, colorless colonies with a diameter of -4 mm (*Figure 9*).

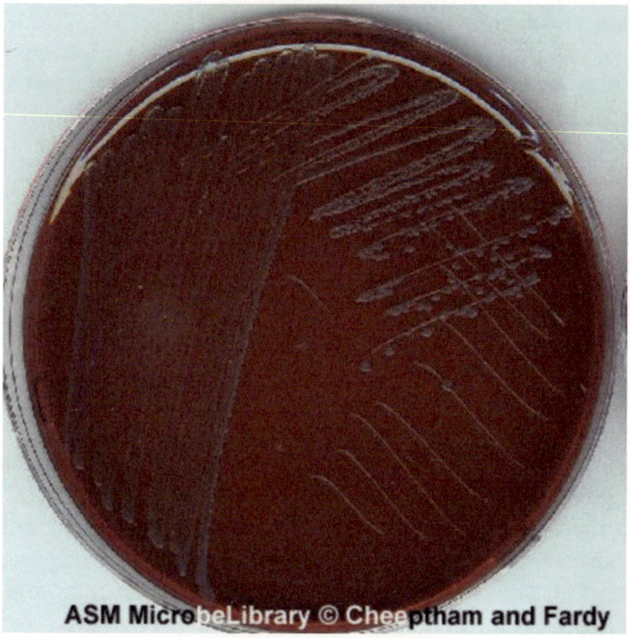


Fig. 9. Apperance of *Salmonella* colonies in *EMB AGAR*

### 5.2 Identification of *Salmonellas*

Identification of suspicious colonies among *Salmonellas* are performed in three steps.

1. Biochemical examination of suspicious colonies,
2. Serological tests (test with polyvalent H and O group antiserums and H pools)
3. Test with bacteriophages

*Salmonellas* uspicious colonies in mediums are examined by staining with gram method. Other detection methods are used for colonies where gram negative bacillus were observed. Although several biochemical tests may be used for identification of *Salmonellas* , sufficient information may be obtained with some of them. Gillen medium 1 and 2 (urea, indole and H2S formation is controlled by fermentation of motility, glucose, mannite, sucrose and salicine ). Triple Sugar Iron Agar (Triple Sugar Iron Agar shows H2S formation by fermentation of Sucrose, Lactose and Glucose). It is used common in laboratories.

Suspicious colonies in terms of *Salmonella* are controlled by polyvalent H and O antiserums following biochemical tests. These antiserums include antibodies collectively against most of *Salmonellas* . Cultures that has given positive reaction with polyvalent antiserums are then examined with 0 group and H pool antiserums. These antiserums include antibodies of *Salmonellas* including the groups in Kauffmann-White sceheme. These groups are classified from A to I alphabetically. Positive agglutination presents the group of the culture. Specific H and 0 antiserums are required for den,itite typing.

## 5.3 Biochemical tests for identification of *Salmonellas*

### 5.3.1 Purificitaion of colonies selected

Colonies selected are purified. If time is restricted, this purifying process may be ignored. The following procedure is applied for purification process.

a. Every colony selected is planted as to allocate single colony to a separate Mac Conkey agar plate.
b. Reversed plates are incubated at 35 to 37 °C for 24 hours.
c. *Salmonella* colonies appear as transparent and colorless in Mac Conkey agar. Sometimes the centre appears as pink. If there are many organisms that fermantates the lactose, the precipitated area around *Salmonella* colonies which are next to them becomes transparent.
d. Planting is performed from typical colonies to normal slant agars. Cultures are incubates at 35 to 37°C for 24 hours.
e. Preparation is prepared from slant agar cultures and stained with gram method. If cultures are pure, the following mediums are used for passages.

A passage specified in the following is performed from 24 hours, purified slant agars to Gillies medium 1 and Gillies medium 2.

### 5.3.2 Planting to Gillies medium 1 and assesment

a. It is immersed to the bottom by a loop and then it is planted into slanted part. It is incubated at 35 to 37°C for 24 hours.
b. Urease reaction, glucose and mannitol fermentation and gas formation are recorded. Cultures with positive urease reaction converts the medium to a dark purple color. Mannitol fermentation is characterized by bottom part turning into yellow; and gas formation is characterized by appearance of gas bubbles in the agar. *Salmonellas* are urease negative. On the other hand, they fermantate glucose and mannitol with or without forming gas.
c. Urease postitive cultures that do not fermentate glucose or mannitol are assessed as negative in terms of *Salmonella*.

### 5.3.3 Planting to Gillies medium II and assessment

a. The tube is hold vertically and planting is performed by immersing to 2 cm depth with a loop.
b. Tubes are incubated at 35 to 37 °C for 24 hours vertically. If reactions are not significant, they are waited for another 24 hours.
c. Sucrose and salicine fermentation, motility, H2S and indole formation are recorded. Color change in the agar, conversion from original blue-green color to yellow shos that sucrose or salicine or both are fermentated. Darkening of the lead acetate paper indicates H2S formation and indol paper becoming red indicates indole formation. Typical *Salmonellas* are motile, indole positive, Sucrose and Salicine negative.

### 5.3.4 Planting to TSI AGAR and assessment

a. Suspicious single colony is taken from purified culture or selective agar medium and inoculation is performed by immersing to the bottom with a loop of triple sugar iron agar (TSI) or by drawing to the slant part.
b. Cultures are incubates at 35 to 37 °C for 18 to 24 hours.
c. Cultures that do not give reactions specific to *Salmonellas* are not taken into the assessment. Typical reaction in TSI agar is red color on the slant part, "alkaline reaction"

and the bottom is yellow. "Acid reaction, glucose fermentation) H2S and gas is positive or negative. H2S reaction manifest itself with blackening of the medium. Typical reactions of *Salmonella* and Arizone species in Lysine-Iron Agar medium are purple colored sloped and red "alkaline reactions", vertical part. They produce H2S and sometimes gas (*Figure 10)*.

Serological tests are continued with positive *Salmonella* cultures.

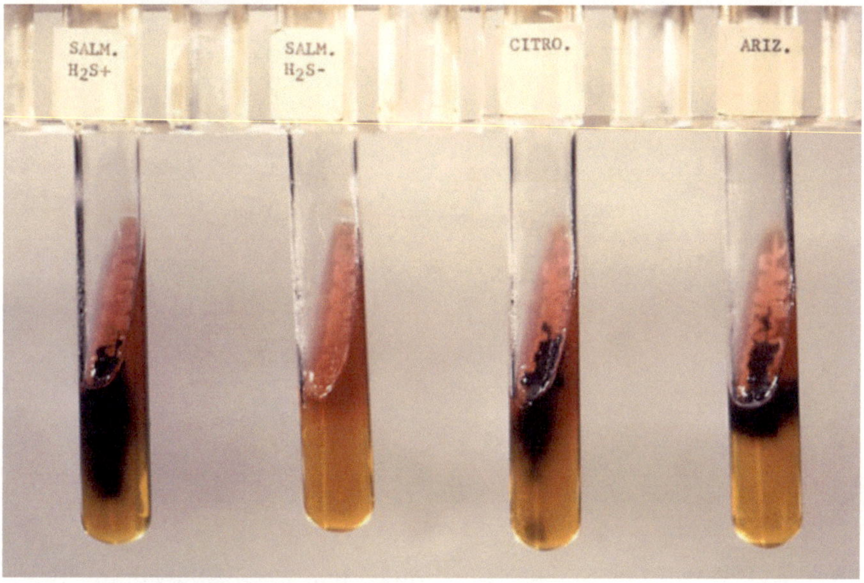


Fig. 10. Appearance of *Salmonella* in TSI Agar

### 5.3.5 Imvic test

(I=indole, M=methyl red, V=voges pros cover, C=citrate)

INDOL= Planting is performed into tryptophan medium. After incubation at 37°C for 24 hours, 0,2 to 0,5 cc of Kovac indicator is dripped into indole medium. Red circle formation is positive (*Figure 11)*.

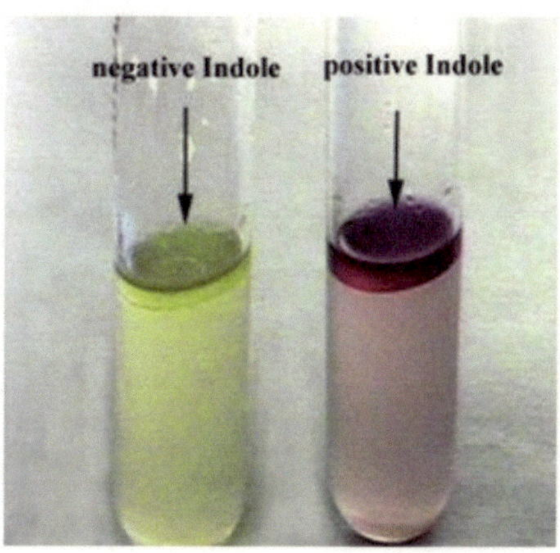


Fig. 11. Indole Test

METHYL RED= Planting is performed into BGB (buffered glucose bouillon) or peptone medium. This test shows pH change in 0,5% buffered glucose medium. 5-6 drops of methyl red indicator is dripped on 1 cc. of medium. If pH drops under 4,2, red color occurs and the result is positive. If there is no color change, it is negative (*Figure 12*).

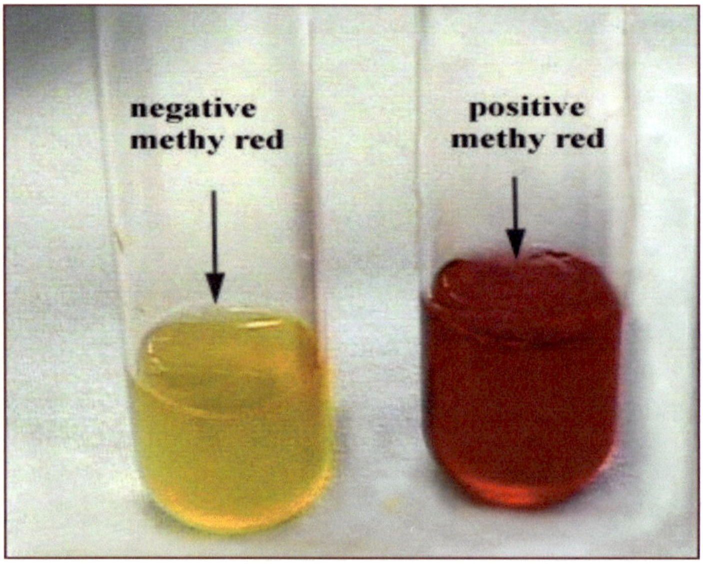


Fig. 12. Methyl RED Test

VOGES PROS COVER= 0,2 cc 40% KOH is dripped into 1 cc BGB medium. Then, 0,6 cc of alpha naphtol indicator is added. Test results 20-30 minutes after.
If red circle appears, the result is positive. In positive cases, acethyl-methyl-carbinol, final catabolism product of glucose occurs. If there is no color change, it is negative (*Figure 13*).

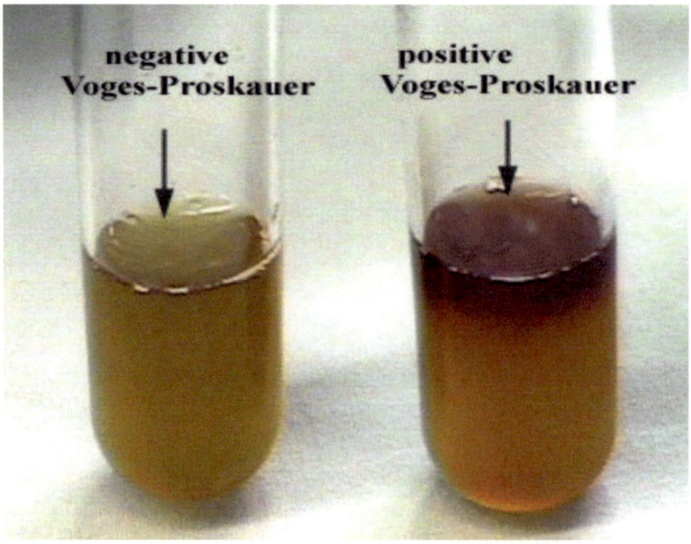


Fig. 13. Voges Pros Cover test

CITRATE=Simmons citrate; line style planting is performed to citrate medium. If the bacteria used citrate as a carbon source, the color of the medium will turn from green into blue. The test is positive (*Figure 14*).

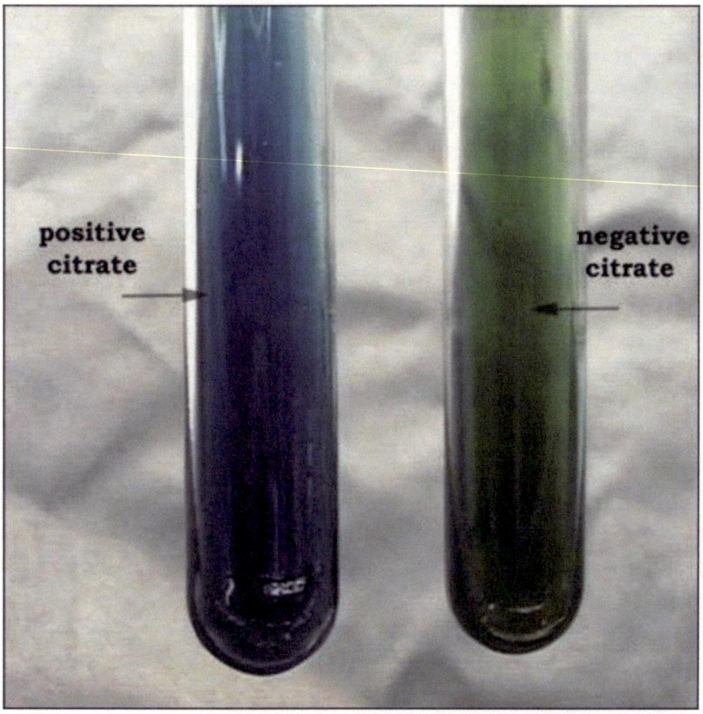


Fig. 14. Citrate test

IMVIC test results for *Salmonella* were given in Table 2.

| Reaction | *Salmonella* |
|---|---|
| Indole | negative |
| Methyl Red | positive |
| Voges Pros Kover | negative |
| Citrate | positive |

Table 2. IMVIC Test Results

#### 5.3.6 Triple tube method

Single colony that identification is desired is made suspension in the bouillon or a 3rd tube. Incubation is performed at 37°C for 3 to 4 hours if required. Plantings are performed to 2nd and 1st tubes. It is left for incubation at 37°C for 18-22 hours.

1. Matters that we may observe in the tube:

a. Glucose fermentation: It is understood by turning of the bottom of the tube to yellow color.
b. Lactose fermentation: The color of sloped surface of the medium turns from orange red into yellow.
c. H2S formation: It is understood by formation of black color in the medium.
d. Lyzine decarboxylase: 4 ml of 4N NaOH and 2 ml of Chloroform are added on the culture. It is kept at room temperature for 15 minutes, 1 ml from chloroform layer is taken by Pasteur pipette. Equal quantities of ninhydrin (from 0,1% solution in chloroform) is added and kept at room temperature for 10 minutes. Formation of violet color at the end of this period shows that the test is positive.
e. Gas formation: It is understood by biodegradation of the medium and occurrence of gas bubbles.
f. ONPG Test: Loop full culture which was taken from the surface of the medium is dispersed with 0,25 ml of physiological saline. 0,25 ml ONPG solution is added on this and it is kept in the drying oven at 37°C for 30 minutes. Formation of fixed yellow color at the end of this period was evaluated as positive.
g. Other tests: Beta galactosidase
   Phennyaline deaminase
   Oxidase

2. Matters that we may observe in the tube:
   a. Mannitol fermentation: It is understood by conversion of the color from red into yellow.
   b. Motility: It is smeared through the middle and it is reproduced to right and left alon the planting line.
   c. Nitrate reduction: 4 drops each from indicators A and B are dripped.
3. Matters that we may observe in the tube:
   a. UREASE formation is observed by conversion o the medium into red color.
   b. Indole: 0,5 ml of Kovacs indicator is added from the side of the tube slowly. Red color indicates that the test is positive.
   c. Tryptophane deaminase: 5 drops of medium is transferred into a sterile agglutination tube via a pipette before addition of Kovacs indicator to the medium. 1 drop of 10% FeCl3 is added on it. If the color turns into red tile color within 3 to 5 minutes, test is positive.

Mediumd used in triple tube method

1. TUBE: klikler I A, or TSI agar are used.

| | |
|---|---|
| Peptone | 20 g |
| Lactose | 10 g |
| Glucose | 1 g |
| Sodyum thiosulphate | 0,2 g |
| Ferroammonium sulphate | 0,3 g |
| NaCl | 6 g |
| Agar | 17 g |
| Phenol red(0,2 %) | 12.5 ml |
| Distilled water | 1,000 ml |
| Ph | 7 |

The mixture is distributed into screw tubes as 7 to 8 ml after boiling. It is sterilized in the autoclave at 121°C for 15 minutes. Tubes are frozen as oblique.

2. TUBE:

| | |
|---|---|
| Peptone (casein) | 5 g |
| Neopeptone | 5 g |
| Mannitol | 2 g |
| Potassium nitrate | 1,7 g |
| Phenol red(0,2 %) | 20 ml |
| Distilled water | 1,000ml |
| Agar | 2,5 g |

The mixture is distributed into screw tubes as 5 to 6 ml after boiling. It is sterilized in the autoclave at 121°C for 15 minutes. Ph is adjusted to 7.

3. TUBE:

| | |
|---|---|
| L-Tryptophane | 0,3 g |
| Potassium dihidrogen phosphate ($KH2PO4$) | 0,1 g |
| Dipotassium hydrogen phosphate ($K2HPO4$) | 0,1 g |
| NaCl | 0,5 g |
| Urea | 2 g |
| Ethanole (95%) | 1ml |
| Phenol red(0,2 %) | 1.25 ml |
| Distilled water | 1,000 ml |
| Ph | 6,5 |

The mixture is sterilized by the filter after dissolving. It is distributed into sterile tubes. If there is no filter, it is sterilized by tyndalisation method (*Table 3*).

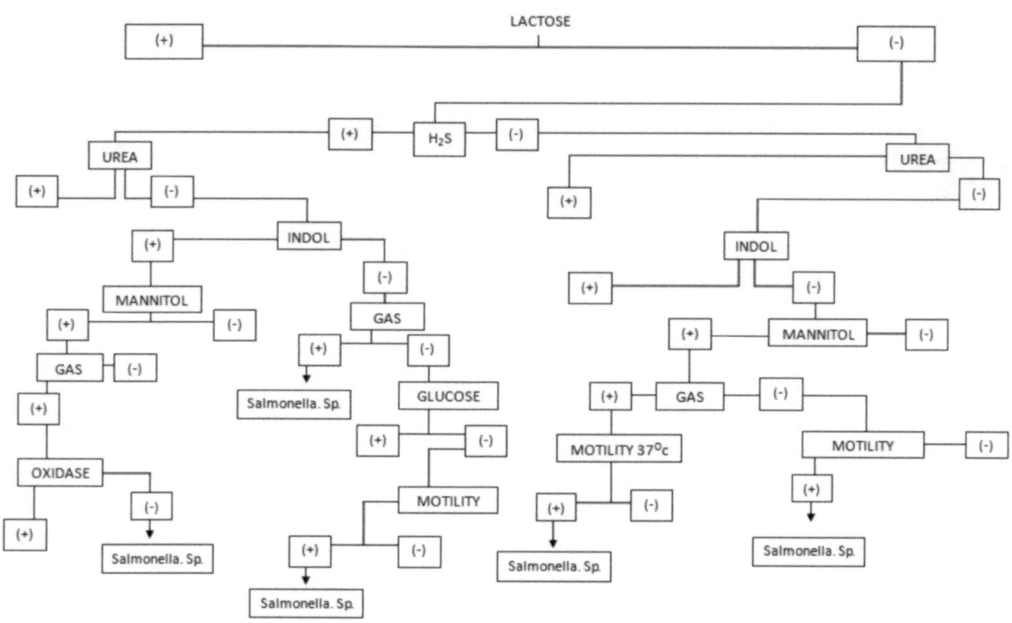


Table 3. Identification Schedule of *Salmonellas* According to triple Tube Method

### 5.3.7 API method

The API-20E test kit for the identification of enteric bacteria (bioMerieux, Inc., Hazelwood, MO) provides an easy way to inoculate and read tests relevant to members of the Family *Enterobacteriaceae* and associated organisms. A plastic strip holding twenty mini-test tubes is inoculated with a saline suspension of a pure culture (as per manufacturer's directions). This process also rehydrates the dessicated medium in each tube. A few tubes are completely filled (CIT, VP and GEL as seen in the photos below), and some tubes are overlaid with mineral oil such that anaerobic reactions can be carried out (ADH, LDC, ODC, $H_2S$, URE).

After incubation in a humidity chamber for 18-24 hours at 37°C, the color reactions are read (some with the aid of added reagents), and the reactions (plus the oxidase reaction done separately) are converted to a seven-digit code which is called the Analytical Profile Index, from which name the initials "API" are derived. The code can be fed into the manufacturer's database via touch-tone telephone, and the computerized voice gives back the identification, usually as genus and species. An on-line database can also be accessed for the identification. The reliability of this system is very high, and one finds systems like these in heavy use in many food and clinical labs.

Note: Discussion and illustration of the API-20E system here does not necessarily constitute any commercial endorsement of this product. It is shown in our laboratory courses as a prime example of a convenient multi-purpose testing method one may encounter out there in the "real world."

In the following photos:

- Note especially the color reactions for **amino acid decarboxylations** (ADH through ODC) and **carbohydrate fermentations** (GLU through ARA).
    - The amino acids tested are (in order) arginine, lysine and ornithine. **Decarboxylation** is shown by an **alkaline** reaction (red color of the particular pH indicator used).
    - The carbohydrates tested are glucose, mannitol, inositol, sorbitol, rhamnose, sucrose, melibiose, amygdalin and arabinose. **Fermentation** is shown by an **acid** reaction (yellow color of indicator).
- Hydrogen sulfide production (H2S) and gelatin hydrolysis (GEL) result in a black color throughout the tube.
- A positive reaction for tryptophan deaminase (TDA) gives a deep brown color with the addition of ferric chloride; positive results for this test correlate with positive phenylalanine and lysine deaminase reactions which are characteristic of *Proteus, Morganella* and *Providencia.*

In the first set of reactions:

- Culture "5B" (isolated from an early stage of sauerkraut fermentation) is identified as *Enterobacter agglomerans* which has been a convenient dumping ground for organisms now being reassigned to better-defined genera and species including the new genus *Pantoea.* This particular isolate produces reddish (lactose +), "pimply" colonies on MacConkey Agar which exude an extremely viscous slime as may be seen here; this appearance is certainly atypical of organisms identified as *E. agglomerans* or *Pantoea* in general.
- Culture "8P44" is identified as *Edwardsiella hoshinae.* The CDC had identified this culture (in 1988) as the ultra-rare Biogroup 1 of *Edwardsiella tarda* which may not be in the API-20E database (*Figure 15).* This system probably would not be able to differentiate between these two organisms. Note that 8P44 shows $H_2S$ production

which is probably typical of *Edwardsiella tarda* Biogroup 1. Clinical laboratories usually run this test in Triple Sugar Iron Agar in which the organism's fermentation of sucrose (with consequent high acid production) tends to negate the $H_2S$ reaction, and - as a result - the organism is mis-characterized throughout the literature as $H_2S$ negative even though it shows a positive reaction in KIA and other $H_2S$-detecting media.

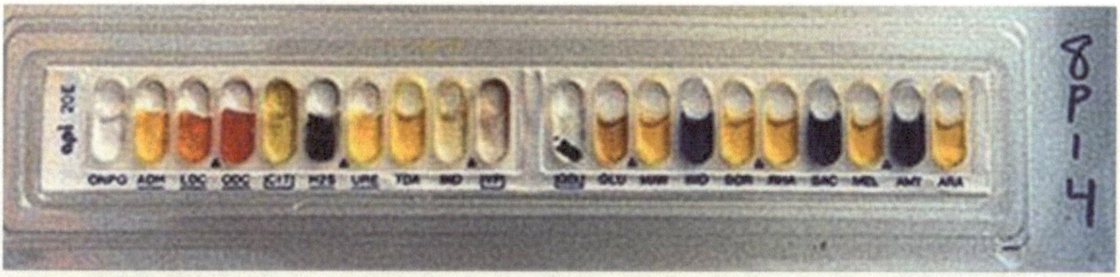

| culture no. | ONPG | ADH | LDC | ODC | CIT | H2S | URE | TDA | IND | VP | GEL | GLU | MAN | INO | SOR | RHA | SAC | MEL | AMY | ARA | identification |
|---|---|---|---|---|---|---|---|---|---|---|---|---|---|---|---|---|---|---|---|---|---|
| 8P14 | – | – | + | + | – | + | – | – | – | – | – | + | + | – | + | + | – | + | – | + | *Salmonella* sp. |

Fig. 15. API Test Result for *Salmonella*

#### 5.3.8 Full automatic bacteria identification device

Some amount of material is taken and transferred into selenite F bouillon (bio-Merieux SA-France). It is incubated at 37°C for 16 to 24 hours in the drying oven. Single colony planting is performed to *Salmonella* -Shigella agar (bio-Merieux SA-France) after the period has passed. It is incubated at 37°C for 16 to 24 hours in the drying oven. Bacteria is made suspension to provide 0,40-0,60 McFarlantd turbidity from reproduced suspicious colonies to Phoenix ID broth.

1 drop of Phoenix AST indicator (Phonex AST Indicator solution, BD Sparks, Benex Limited, Shannon, Ireland) to Phoenix AST broth (Phonex AST borth, BD Sparks, Benex Limited, Shannon, Ireland). 25 µl ID broth is taken and pipetted into AST Broth (BD Phoenix NMIC/ID-82 Sparks- USA). ID and AST broths are transferred to ID and AST pplate. Identification and antibiogram process are performed as full automatically in Phoenix-100 (BD Sparks-USA).

### 5.4 Serologucal tests

Antiserums which are used in serological tests of *Salmonellas* can be classified as follows. Pure *Salmonellas* uspicious culture reproduced in TSI agar, agar agar or bouillon and culture of *Salmonellas* erotypes reproduced in normal or oblique agar can be classified as follows to be used in serological tests:

a. *Salmonella* polyvalent 0 (somatic) antiserum: 1,16,19,22,23,24,25 and vi in the least,
b. *Salmonella* individual (0) somatic group anti-serums: A,B,C1,C2,D E (E1,E2,E3,E4), F,G,H,I, vi,
c. *Salmonella* polyvalent H (flagella) antiserum: It will include agglutinins of a,b,c,d,en,en,enx,fg,tgt,gm,gms,gp,gpu,gq,gst,gt,i,k,lv,lw,lz13,lz28,mt,r,y,z,z4z23,z4z24, z4z32,z6,z10,z29,1,2,1,5,1,6 ve 1,7 antigens.
d. *Salmonellas* picer-Edward's H (flagella) antiserums:

It is consisted of seven antiserums and it gives a reaction as follows:

$d_1$) *Salmonella* H antiserum Spicer –Edwards 3: Gives reaction with a, d, eh, k, z, z4z23, z4z32 ve z29 antigens.

$d_2$) *Salmonella* H antiserum Spicer –Edward 4: Gives reaction with b, d, fg, fgt, gm, gms, gmt, gp, gpu, gq, gst, ms, mt, k, r, z, ve z10 antigens.

$d_3$) *Salmonella* H antiserum e,n complex: It gives reaction with enx and enz 15 antibodies.

$d_4$) *Salmonella* H antiserum L complex: Gives reaction with 1v,1w,1zl3,lz28 antigens.

$d_5$) *Salmonella* H antiserum 1 complex: Gives reaction with 1,2; 1,5 1,6 1,7 ve z6 antigens.

#### 5.4.1 Lame test for polyvalent 0 (somatic) antigen

1. First, reliability of antiserum should be detected. For this, various dilutions of the antiserum should ne prepared and controlled with a certain culture.
2. The lame is divided into two by a glass cutter.
3. A small amount of culture a taken and put on both parts of the lame. (cultures in normal oblique agar and 24 hours cultures of TSI agar should be used.).
4. One drop each from 0,85% sodium chloride solution is put on drops above and it is emulsified well.
5. One drop of *Salmonella* polyvalent (0) antiserum is put into the first section and mixed well.
6. The mixture is mixed by moving to the front and back for one minute and it is examined on a dark base. Positive reaction is rapid and strong reaction.

#### 5.4.2 Polyvalent H (flagella) antigen agglutination test

1. Various dilutions of antiserum is prepared and it is controlled that whether the antiserum is safe with a known culture.
2. 5 ml of 24 hours H bouillon culture is taken, 5 ml of 0,6% formalin physiological saline is added on it. It is kept for one hour. Formalin bouillon is kept for a couple of days at 5 to 8°C if required.
3. A small serological tube (10 X 75 mm or 13X 100 mm) is taken. 0,02 ml (one drop) is put from H (flagella) antiserum which was diluted appropriately and 1 ml of formalin bouillon culture (antigen) is added on it.

4. If formalin culture includes granular particles or thin membrane or sediment, control is performed by adding formalin salty water instead of antiserum (salty water control). For this, 0,02 ml Formalin salty water is put into the tube with the same length and 1 ml of formalin bouillon culture is added on it.
5. Antigen-serum mixture and antigen-salty water mixture are incubated at 50°C warm water bath for one hour. It is controlled by 15 minutes of interval first and the final result is read after one hour.
6. Polyvalent H test is assessed as follows.
   a. If agglutination is present in culture+formalin salty water + serum mixture and agglutination is absent in culture- formalin salty water mixture, reaction is positive.
   b. If there is no agglutination in culture+ formalin salty water + serum mixture, reaction is negative.
   c. If there is agglutination in both mixtures, reaction is non-specific.
7. Immotile *Salmonella* cultures or *Salmonella* polyvalent H (flagella) negative cultures are assessed according to Edwards and Ewing.

### 5.4.3 "0" antiserum groups test

This test is performed to determine the "0" group that the culture belongs to.

1. Various dilutions of antiserums are performed and it is processed with a known culture and reliability of antiserum is controlled.
2. The test is applied as told in section II. But, "0" group antiserums are used in here instead of 0 polyvalent. ( Including Vi).
3. Intense suspensions of cultures which give positive reactions with Vi antiserums in 1 ml physiological saline and it is heated in boiling water for 20-30 minutes and left for cooling. The test is repeated by using D, C and Vi antiserums of 0 group with these heated cultures. Vi positive cultures which react with Soamtic D group antiserums are likely *Salmonella* typhi. Vi positive cultures which react with Somatic C1 group antiserum are probably *Salmonella* paratyphi C. If Vi positive cultures heated which does not react with any of = group antiserum continues to give positive reaction after heating, they are not probably *Salmonella*. They belong to Citrobacter group.
4. The culture is accepted as belonging to the group that the culture reacted positively with which of "0" group antiserums. Cultures that do not react positively with any of 0 group antiserums are accepted as negative.

### 5.4.4 Spicer-Edwards H (flagella) test

These tests may be used instead of polyvalent H test which was specified in 4.4.2. It is used in determination of H antigens.

1. Various dilutions of antiserums are prepared and it is processed with a known culture and reliability of antiserum is detected.
2. Every seven Spiecer-Edwards H antiserum is processed with each of them. This examination is as told in section III. Spiecer-Edwards H antiserums are used instead of polyvalent H antiserum.
3. Positive agglutination shows presence of H antigen. Antigen is detected according to Spiecer-Edwards antiserum agglutinins which was shown in the sollowing table 3.

| H antigen | Positive reaction with Spiecer Edward *Salmonella* H antiserum |
|---|---|
| a | 1, 2, 3 |
| b | 1, 2, 4 |
| c | 1, 2 |
| d | 1, 3, 4 |
| eh | 1, 3 |
| G complex | 1, 4 |
| i | 1 |
| k | 2, 3, 4 |
| r | 2, 4 |
| y | 2 |
| z | 3, 4 |
| $z_4$ complex | 4 |
| $z_{10}$ | 4 |
| $z_9$ | 2, 3 |
| enx, $enz_{15}$ | en complex |
| 1v, 1w, $1z_{13}$, $1z_{28}$ | 1 complex |
| 1,2; 1,5; 1,6; 1,7; $z_6$ | complex |

Table 3.

### 5.5 Gruber-Widal reaction

Gruber Widal reaction is used to reveal infections caused by *Salmonella* group bacteria. *Salmonella* typhi, *Salmonella* paratyphi B bacteria are used in the reaction, because they are most common species in our country. *Salmonella* paratyphi A is added for many times. Bacteria such as *Salmonella* paratyphi C are also important in another countries. Both O and H antigens of bacteria are used separately in the reaction. Because, only O or G agglutinins occur especially in first episode of the disease. O agglutinins appear before H agglutinins generally in typhoid fever. As O antigen fractions of Salmoenalla typhi are present in Salmoenalla paratyphi B, they give common agglutination. H agglutination is more valuable as it is not common.

Gruber Widal reaction is performed quantitatively, because serum titration is important. It is impossible to put definite rules to improve various titrations. Reaction is improved by considering other findings. It should be considered that in which day of the disease serum has been taken, whether an infection appeared previously, whether protective vaccination is performed and normal antibody level in healthy persons in the population.

Agglutinins may exist normally in the serum. H agglutinins of *Salmonella* typhi and *Salmonella* paratyphi B may be 1/40 titration and O agglutinins may be as 1/50 titration. Therefore, reaction is started as final dilution of the serum in the first tube will be as 1/50.

If a non-specific antigen such as fimbria antigen is present in the bacteria suspension, false positive Gruber-Widal reaction occurs with an agglutinin in the human serum.

Specific antibodies occur in serums of those who had typhoid-paratyphoid vaccination and Gruber-Widal reaction is positive in them. If previously vaccinated persons have a pyretic disease, agglutination titration elevates. When vaccinated persons are examined after months, it is seen that they have H agglutinins mainly. Therefore, high H agglutinin titration of those who was vaccinated is meaningless. However, if more than six months has passed from the vaccination date and titration of O agglutination is more than 1/100 and titration elevates in continuous assays, such result is insignificant in the diagnosis.

Presence of both O and H agglutinins in persons who had undergone the infection may last long.

Detection of O antibodies in the serum shows that a new infection was experienced. H agglutinins are 1/400 or higher in those who had new infections and they stay for a long time, sometimes for years. Serum titration elevates during an pyretic disease (anamnestic reaction). O agglutinins decrease rapidly in the blood and it may be shown rarely after one year. High O titration is not seen with anamnestic reaction.

1/100 positive O agglutination and 1/200 positive agglutination are valuable in persons who was not infected and vaccinated. 1/200 O agglutination and 1/400 H agglutination in persons who was infected and vaccinated before is valuable in terms of diagnose of a new infection. Only 1/100-1/200 positive H agglutination shows an undergone infection, new vaccination or anamnestic reaction.

**Making the Assay;**

6 series of tubes are taken, 6 tubes are put in every series as 1/50, 1/100, 1/200, 1/400 serum dilutions, antigen control and serum control. To make serial dilution, 0,5 cm3 salty water except 1st tube and last serum control tube and 0,5 cm3 diluted immunized serum is put into the last tube. Immunized serum which was generally obtained from rabbits as immunized serum is used by diluting 100 or 1000 times and adding 0,5% phenol. First Tube 7.2 cm3 and 0.3 cm3 of saline placed in serum 1 / 25 dilution of each series after the 1st and 2 tube is added 0.5 cm3. Serum was diluted as 1/25 in the 1st tube. Same amount of salty water was diluted as much in the 2nd tube and dilution has become 1/50.

## 6. References


[1] Akman M., Gülmezoglu E. (1976). Tıbbi Mikrobiyoloji, 12. Baskı Ders Kitabı, s: 347-352,Ankara.

[2] Akman, M. (1977). Bakteri Genetiği Test-Pratik, Cumhuriyet Üniversitesi Yayın No:1

[3] Alkış, N. (1982). Gıda Mikrobiyolojisi. Ankara; Yeni İnci Matbaacılık Sanayi

[4] Ang-Küçüker M., Buget E., Dinçer N., Ang Ö. (1992). İstanbul'da izole edilen *Salmonella* enteritidis suslarının özellikleri. İnfeks Derg, 6: 91-93.

[5] Anon, (1988). Salmonellosis Control. The Role of Animal and Product Hygiene. WHO Expert Commitee. Technical Report Series 774.

[6] Anonymous, (1983). Gıd Maddeleri Muayene ve Analiz Yöntemleri Kitabı. Tarım, Orman ve Köy İşleri Bakanlığı Gıda İşleri Genel Müdürlüğü, Genel Yayın No:65, Özel Yayın No:62-105

[7] Anonymous, (2005). Mercek Gıda Mikrobiyolojisi Uygulamaları. Ed: A.K. Halkman. Başak Matbaacılık Ltd. Şti., 358. Sayfa

[8] Arda, M. (1985). Genel Bakteriyoloji Ankara Üniversitesi Veteriner Fakültesi Yayınları:402

[9] Arda, M. (2000). Temel Mikrobiyoloji, Ankara: Medisan Yayınevi.

[10] Arda, M., Minbay, A., Leloğlu, N., Aydin, N., Akay, Ö. (1992). Özel Mikrobiyoloji. Erzurum: Atatürk Üniversitesi Yayınları No: 741

[11] Beşe, M. (1974). Mikrobiyolojide Kullanılan Biyokimyasal Testler ve Besiyerleri. Ankara Üniversitesi Veteriner Fakültesi Yayınları; 298.

[12] Bilgehan, H. (1986). Klinik mikrobiyoloji. İzmir: Bilgehan Basımevi.

[13] Bilgehan, H. (1992). *Salmonella* , Klinik Mikrobiyoloji, Özel Bakteriyoloji ve Bakteriyel İnfeksiyonlar, İzmir: Barış Yayınları, Fakülte Kitabevi,

[14] Bilgehan, H.(1993). Temel Mikrobiyoloji ve Bağışıklık Bilimi, Ankara: Şafak Matbaacılık.

[15] Brenner F.W., Villar R.G., Angulo F.J., Tauxe R., Swaminathan B. (2000). *Salmonella* nomenclature. J Clin Microbiol, 38: 2465–2467.

[16] Chalker, R.B., BLASE, M.J. (1988). A review of human Salmonellosis. III Magnitude of *Salmonella* infection in the United States. Rev. Infect Dis. 10: 111-124

[17] Çarlı K.T., Eyigör A,Goncagül G., Günaydın E (2004). *Salmonellas* tandart ve İleri Tanı Yöntemleri, İstanbul, Türkiye.

[18] Çetin, E.T. (1973). Genel ve Pratik Mikrobiyoloji. İstanbul, Sermet Matbaas

[19] Erganiş, O. (1994). Mikrobiyoloji ve İmmünoloji. Konya Sağlık Eğitim Enstitüsü Yayınları No:11

[20] Kılıçturgay, K.Ed. (1992). Temel Mikrobiyoloji ve Parazitoloji. Bursa Onur Yayıncılık

[21] Lassen J. (1975). Rapid identification of Gram negative rods using A three-tube method combined with a dichotomic key. Acta Pathol Microbiol Scand Sect B, 83: 525–533.

[22] Le Minor, L. (1992). The Genus *Salmonella*. In: A Handbook on the Biology of Bacteria: Ecophysiology, Isolation, Identification, Application 2.th Ed. Vol III , Ed.: A. Balows, H.G. Truper, M. Dworkin, W. Harder, K.H. Schleifer, New York, Berlin, Heidelberg: Springer-Werlag, p.: 2760-2774

[23] Özçelik, S. (2009). Genel Mikrobiyoloji. Süleyman Demirel Üniversitesi Ziraat Fakültesi Yayınları, Yayın No:1

[24] Özçelik, S. (2010). Gıda Mikrobiyolojisi Laboratuar Kılavuzu. Süleyman Demirel Üniversitesi Ziraat Fakültesi Yayınları, Yayın No:7 III. Basım

[25] Özçelik, S. (2010). Gıda Mikrobiyolojisi. Süleyman Demirel Üniversitesi Ziraat Fakültesi Yayınları, Yayın No:6

[26] Özçelik, S. (2011) Genel Mikrobiyoloji Uygulama Kılavuzu. Süleyman Demirel Üniversitesi Ziraat Fakültesi Yayınları, Yayın No:2

[27] Rodrigue, D.C., Tauxe, R.V., Rowe, B. (1990). International Increase in *Salmonella* enteritidis. A New Pandemic. Epidemiol. Infect., 105: 21-27

[28] Tamer, A.Ü. (2000). Genel Mikrobiyoloji, Celal Bayar Üniversitesi Fen Edebiyat Fakültesi Biyoloji Bölümü, Manisa

[29] Temiz, A. (2000). Genel Mikrobiyoloji Uygulama Teknikleri. Ankara; Hatipoğlu Yayınevi

[30] Yund, İ. (1975). Pratik Laboratuar Metotları, İstanbul, Batu Matbaası.

8

# Attachment and Biofilm Formation by *Salmonella* in Food Processing Environments

Efstathios Giaouris[1], Nikos Chorianopoulos[2], Panagiotis Skandamis[3] and George-John Nychas[3]
[1]*Department of Food Science and Nutrition, University of the Aegean*
[2]*Veterinary Research Institute, National Agricultural Research Foundation (NAGREF)*
[3]*Department of Food Science and Technology, Agricultural University of Athens (AUA)*
*Greece*

## 1. Introduction

During the last decades, it has become increasingly clear that bacteria, including foodborne pathogens such as *Salmonella enterica*, grow predominantly as biofilms in most of their natural habitats, rather than in planktonic mode. A biofilm can be broadly defined as a microbially derived sessile community characterized by cells that are irreversibly attached to a substratum or interface or to each other, are embedded in a matrix of extracellular polymeric substances (EPS) that they have produced, and exhibit an altered phenotype with respect to growth rate and gene transcription (Donlan & Costerton, 2002; Kuchma & O'Toole, 2000; Lazazzera, 2005; Shemesh et al., 2007). Interestingly, it has been observed that the resistance of biofilm cells to antimicrobials is significantly increased compared with what is normally seen with the same cells being planktonic (Gilbert et al., 2002; Mah & O'Toole, 2001). Thus, it is believed that biofilm formation enhances the capacity of pathogenic *Salmonella* bacteria to survive stresses that are commonly encountered both within food processing, as well as during host infection.

In food industry, biofilms may create a persistent source of product contamination, leading to serious hygienic problems and also economic losses due to food spoilage (Brooks & Flint, 2008; Carpentier & Cerf, 1993; Ganesh Kumar & Anand, 1998; Lindsay & von Holy, 2006; Zottola & Sasahara, 1994). Improperly cleaned surfaces promote soil build-up, and, in the presence of water, contribute to the development of bacterial biofilms which may contain pathogenic microorganisms, such as *Salmonella*. Cross contamination occurs when cells detach from biofilm structure once food passes over contaminated surfaces or through aerosols originating from contaminated equipment. Till now, there is only limited information on the presence of *Salmonella* in biofilms in real food processing environments. However, numerous studies have shown that *Salmonella* can easily attach to various food-contact surfaces (such as stainless steel, plastic and cement) and form biofilms under laboratory conditions (Chia et al., 2009; Giaouris et al., 2005; Giaouris & Nychas, 2006; Hood & Zottola, 1997a,b; Marin et al., 2009; Oliveira et al., 2006; Rodrigues et al., 2011; Vestby et al., 2009a,b).

The natural environments that most bacteria inhabit are typically complex and dynamic. Unfortunately, this complexity is not fully appreciated when growing microorganisms in monocultures under laboratory conditions. Thus, in real environments, biofilm communities are usually inhabited by numerous different species in close proximity (Wimpenny et al., 2000). Spatial and metabolic interactions between species contribute to the organization of multispecies biofilms, and the production of a dynamic local environment (Goller & Romeo, 2008; Tolker-Nielsen & Molin, 2000). Indeed, cell-to-cell signalling and interspecies interactions have been demonstrated to play a key role in cell attachment and detachment from biofilms, as well as in the resistance of biofilm community members against antimicrobial treatments (Annous et al., 2009; Burmølle et al., 2006; Irie & Parsek, 2008; Nadell et al., 2008; Remis et al., 2010). Mixed-species biofilms are usually more stable than mono-species biofilms, while biofilm formation by *Salmonella* has also been shown to be influenced by either the natural *in situ* presence of other species, or just their metabolic by-products (Chorianopoulos et al., 2010; Girennavar et al., 2008; Habimana et al., 2010b; Jones & Bradshaw, 1997; Prouty et al., 2002; Soni et al., 2008).

In this chapter, we review up-to-date available voluminous literature on the attachment and biofilm formation by *Salmonella* strains on abiotic surfaces, simulating those encountered in food processing areas (section 4). Before this, the advantages of biofilm lifestyle for microorganisms are briefly discussed (section 2), together with the serious negative implications of biofilm formation for the food industry (section 3). Major molecular components building up *Salmonella* biofilm matrix are then reported (section 5). Finally, we review available knowledge on the influence of cell-to-cell communication (quorum sensing) on the establishment of *Salmonella* biofilms (section 6).

## 2. Bacterial attachment to surfaces and advantages of the biofilm lifestyle

For most of the history of microbiology, microorganisms have primarily been characterised as planktonic, freely suspended cells and described on the basis of their growth characteristics in nutritionally rich culture media. Although this traditional way of culturing bacteria in liquid media has been instrumental in the study of microbial pathogenesis and enlightening as to some of the amazing facets of microbial physiology, pure culture planktonic growth is rarely how bacteria exist in nature. On the contrary, direct observation of wide of variety of natural habitats has shown that the majority of microbes persist attached to surfaces within a structured biofilm ecosystem and not as free-floating organisms (Costerton et al., 1987, 1995; Kolter & Greenberg, 2006; Verstraeten et al., 2008).

The data on which this theory is predicated came mostly from natural aquatic ecosystems, in which direct microscopic observations together with direct quantitative recovery techniques showed unequivocally that more than 99.9% of the bacteria grow as biofilms on a wide variety of surfaces. The diversity and distribution of salmonellae in fresh water biofilms has also been recently shown (Sha et al., 2011). Moreover, it is becoming clear that these natural assemblages of bacteria within the biofilm matrix function as a cooperative consortium, in a relatively complex and coordinated manner (James et al., 1995; Moons et al., 2009; Wuertz et al., 2004). Nowadays, besides natural aquatic systems, it is well established that biofilms may form on a wide variety of surfaces, including living tissues, indwelling medical devices and also industrial systems, such as pharmaceutical industries, oil drilling, paper production, waste water treatment and food processing (Hall-Stoodley et al., 2004). Thus, examples of this bacterial lifestyle are abundant in daily life: the slimy material that covers flower vases, pipelines, submerged rocks, and even the surface of teeth (Marsh, 2005; Wimpenny, 2009).

Biofilm formation occurs through sequential steps in which the initial attachment of planktonic bacteria to a solid surface is followed by their subsequent proliferation and accumulation in multilayer cell clusters, and the final formation of the bacterial community enclosed in a self-produced polymeric matrix (Goller & Romeo, 2008; Lasa, 2006; O'Toole et al., 2000; Palmer et al., 2007; Rickard et al., 2003). The initial interaction between solid surface and bacterial cell envelope appears to be mediated by a complex array of chemical and physical interactions, with each affected by the chemical and physical environment to which the bacterial cell and the surface are currently or recently exposed (Palmer et al., 2007). Mature biofilms are highly organized ecosystems in which water channels are dispersed and can provide passages for the exchange of nutrients, metabolites and waste products (Stoodley et al., 2002). Once the biofilm structure has developed, some bacteria are released into the liquid medium, in order to colonize new surfaces, probably when surrounding conditions become less favourable (Gilbert et al., 1993; Hall-Stoodley & Stoodley, 2002, 2005; Klausen et al., 2006).

According to Darwin's theory of evolution, the only true driving force behind the course of action of any organism is reproductive fitness. Outside of the laboratory bacteria rarely, if ever, find themselves in an environment as nutrient rich as culture media, and in these conditions, there are a number of fitness advantages imparted by the biofilm mode of growth (Jefferson, 2004). The process of biofilm formation is believed to begin when bacteria sense certain environmental parameters (extracellular signals) that trigger the transition from planktonic growth to life on a surface (Lopez et al., 2010). Currently, four potential incentives behind the formation of biofilms by bacteria are considered: (i) protection from the harmful environment (as a stress response mechanism), (ii) sequestration to a nutrient rich area, (iii) utilization of cooperative benefits (through metabolic cooperativity), and (iv) acquisition of new genetic traits (Davey & O'Toole, 2000; Molin & Tolker-Nielsen, 2003).

Bacteria experience a certain degree of shelter and homeostasis when residing within a biofilm and one of the key components of this microniche is the surrounding extrapolymeric substance (EPS) matrix (Flemming & Wingender, 2010). This matrix is composed of a mixture of components, such as exopolysaccharides, proteins, nucleic acids, and other substances (Branda et al., 2005). The nature of biofilm matrix and the physiological attributes of biofilm microorganisms confer an inherent resistance to antimicrobial agents, whether these antimicrobial agents are antibiotics, disinfectants or germicides. Thus, established biofilms can tolerate antimicrobial agents at concentrations of 10-1000 times that need to kill genetically equivalent planktonic bacteria, and are also extraordinary resistant to phagocytosis, making rather difficult to eradicate biofilms from living hosts (Cos et al., 2010). Mechanisms responsible for resistance may be one or more of the following: (i) delayed penetration of the antimicrobial agent through the biofilm matrix, (ii) altered growth rate of biofilm microorganisms, and (iii) other physiological changes due to the biofilm mode of growth, e.g. existence of subpopulations of resistant phenotypes in the biofilm, which have been referred to as "persisters" (Donlan & Costerton, 2002; Gilbert et al., 2002; Lewis, 2001; Mah & O'Toole, 2001).

Scientific interest in the process of bacterial biofilm formation has erupted in recent years and studies on the molecular genetics of biofilm formation have begun to shed light on the driving forces behind the transition to the biofilm mode of existence. Evidence is mounting that up- and down-regulation of a number of genes occurs in the attaching cells upon initial interaction with the substratum (Donlan, 2002; Sauer, 2003). Thus, high-throughput DNA microarray studies have been conducted to study biofilm formation in many model microorganisms and have identified a large number of genes showing differential expression under biofilm conditions (Beloin et al., 2004; Hamilton et al., 2009; Lazazzera,

2005; Shemesh et al., 2007; Whiteley et al., 2001). In *S.* Typhimurium, 10% of its genome (i.e. 433 genes) showed a 2-fold or more change in the biofilm, using a silicone rubber tubing as a substratum for growth, compared with planktonic cells (Hamilton et al., 2009). The genes that were significantly up-regulated implicated certain cellular processes in biofilm development, including amino acid metabolism, cell motility, global regulation and tolerance to stress. Obviously, the more we learn about the genetic regulation of biofilm formation, the more we understand about the relative roles of benefits and forces that drive the switch to the biofilm mode of growth.

## 3. Biofilm formation in food processing environments and implications

The ability of bacteria to attach to abiotic surfaces and form biofilms is a cause of concern for many industries, including the food ones (Chmielewski & Frank, 2003). Poor sanitation of food-contact surfaces is believed to be an essential contributing factor in foodborne disease outbreaks, especially those involving *Listeria monocytogenes* and *Salmonella*. This is because the attachment of bacterial cells to such surfaces is the first step of a process which can ultimately lead to the contamination of food products. Thus, biofilms formed in food processing environments are of special importance since they may act as a persistent source of microbial contamination which may lead to food spoilage or/and transmission of diseases (Brooks & Flint, 2008; Zottola & Sasahara, 1994). While food spoilage and deterioration may result in huge economic losses, food safety is a major priority in today's globalizing market with worldwide transportation and consumption of raw, fresh and minimally processed foods (Shi & Zhu, 2009).

Besides food spoilage and safety issues, in the dairy industry, bacterial attachment in heat exchangers (a process commonly known as "biofouling") greatly reduces the heat transfer and operating efficiency of the processing equipment, while it can also causes corrosion problems (Austin & Bergeron, 1995). Additionally, in the various filtration systems, biofilm formation reduces significantly the permeability of the membranes (Tang et al., 2009). However, it should be noted that in the industry of fermented food products (sausages, cheeses etc), biofilm formation by some useful and technological bacteria (e.g. staphylococci, lactococci, lactobacilli) can be desirable, as a mean of the enhancement of food fermentation process, and more importantly as a mean of protection against the establishment of pathogenic biofilms (Chorianopoulos et al., 2008; Zhao et al., 2006).

Adhesion of *Salmonella* to food surfaces was the first published report on foodborne bacterial biofilm (Duguid et al., 1966). Since that time, many documents have described the ability of foodborne pathogens to attach to various surfaces and form biofilms, including *L. monocytogenes* (Blackman & Frank, 1996; Chorianopoulos et al., 2011; di Bonaventura et al., 2008; Poimenidou et al., 2009), *Salmonella enterica* (Chia et al., 2009; Giaouris et al., 2005; Giaouris & Nychas, 2006; Habimana et al., 2010b; Joseph et al., 2001; Kim & Wei, 2007, 2009; Oliveira et al., 2006; Marin et al., 2009; Rodrigues et al., 2011; Solomon et al., 2005; Stepanović et al., 2003, 2004), *Yersinia enterocolitica* (Kim et al., 2008), *Campylobacter jejuni* (Joshua et al., 2006) and *Escherichia coli* O157:H7 (Habimana et al., 2010a; Skandamis et al., 2009).

Modern food processing supports and selects for biofilm forming bacteria on food-contact surfaces due to mass production of products, lengthy production cycles and vast surface areas for biofilm development (Lindsay & von Holy, 2006). *In situ* biofilms have been recognised in various food processing industries, such as processors of cheese and other milk products, raw and cooked/fermented meats, raw and smoked fish etc (Austin & Bergeron, 1995; Bagge-Ravn et al., 2003; Gounadaki et al., 2008; Gunduz & Tuncel, 2006; Sharma & Anand, 2002). Several studies were also focused on the attachment of bacterial pathogens to food surfaces such as *Escherichia coli* to beef muscle and adipose tissue (Rivas et al., 2006) and *S.* Typhimurium, *Yersinia enterocolitica* and *L. monocytogenes* to pork skin (Morild et al., 2011).

Biofilm formation depends on an interaction between three main components: the bacterial cells, the attachment surface and the surrounding medium (Van Houdt & Michiels, 2010). Adhesion of bacterial cells, the first phase of biofilm formation, is influenced by the physicochemical properties of the cells' surface, which in turn are influenced by factors such as microbial growth phase, culture conditions and strain's variability (Briandet et al., 1999; Giaouris et al., 2009). The surfaces of most bacterial cells are negatively charged, and this net negative charge of the cell surface is adverse to bacterial adhesion, due to electrostatic repulsive force. However, the bacterial cell-surface possesses hydrophobicity due to fimbriae, flagella and lipopolysaccharide (LPS) (Ukuku & Fett, 2006). Hydrophobic interactions between the cell surface and the substratum may enable the cell to overcome repulsive forces and attach irreversibly (Donlan, 2002). The properties of the attachment surface (e.g. roughness, cleanability, disinfectability, wettability, vulnerability to wear) are important factors that also affect the biofilm formation potential and thus determine the hygienic status of the material. Stainless steel type 304, commonly used in the food processing industry, is an ideal material for fabricating equipment due to its physico-chemical stability and high resistance to corrosion. Teflon and other plastics are often used for gaskets and accessories of instruments. These surfaces become rough or crevice with continuous reuse and form a harbourage to protect bacteria from shear forces in the food fluid.

Environmental factors such as pH, temperature, osmolarity, $O_2$ levels, nutrient composition and the presence of other bacteria play important roles in the process of biofilm formation (Giaouris et al., 2005; Hood & Zottola, 1997a; Stepanovic et al., 2003). The integration of these influences ultimately determines the pattern of behavior of a given bacterium with respect to biofilm development (Goller & Romeo, 2008). In food processing environments, bacterial attachment is additionally affected by food matrix constituents, which can be adsorbed onto a substratum and create conditioning films (Bernbom et al., 2009). For example, skim milk was found to reduce adhesion of *Staphylococcus aureus*, *L. monocytogenes*, and *Serratia marcescens* to stainless steel coupons (Barnes et al., 1999). Additionally, in real environments, the presence of mixed bacterial communities adds additional complexity to attachment and biofilm formation procedure. For instance, the presence of *Staphylococcus xylosus* and *Pseudomonas fragi* affected the numbers of *L. monocytogenes* biofilm cells on stainless steel (Norwood & Gilmour, 2001), while compounds present in *Hafnia alvei* cell-free culture supernatant inhibited the early stage of *S.* Enteritidis biofilm formation on the same material (Chorianopoulos et al., 2010).

Once biofilms have formed in the factory environment, they are difficult to be removed often resulting in persistent and endemic populations (Vestby et al., 2009b). Interestingly, persistent *L. monocytogenes* strains had the added ability of enhanced adhesion within shorter times to stainless steel surfaces compared to non-persistent strains (Lundén et al., 2000). It has been suggested that such persistence is likely due to physical adaptation of cells in biofilms, particularly resistance to cleaning and sanitizing regimes, since it is generally accepted and well documented that cells within a biofilm are more resistant to biocides than their planktonic counterparts (Carpentier & Cerf, 1993). For example, nine disinfectants commonly used in the feed industry and efficient against planktonic *Salmonella* cells, showed a bactericidal effect that varied considerably for biofilm-grown cells with products containing

70% ethanol being most effective (Møretrø et al., 2009). Other studies similarly indicated that compared to planktonic cells, biofilm cells of *Salmonella* were more resistant to trisodium phosphate (Scher et al., 2005) and to chlorine and iodine (Joseph et al., 2001). In a comparative study of different *S*. Enteritidis phage type 4 isolates it was found that those isolates that survived better on surfaces also survived better in acidic conditions and in the presence of hydrogen peroxide and showed enhanced tolerance towards heat (Humphrey et al., 1995).

The cellular mechanisms underlying microbial biofilm formation and behaviour are beginning to be understood and are targets for novel specific intervention strategies to control problems caused by biofilm formation in fields ranging from industrial processes like food processing, to health-related fields, like medicine and dentistry. In food industry, various preventive and control strategies, like hygienic plant lay-out and design of equipment, choice of materials, correct selection and use of detergents and disinfectants coupled with physical methods can be suitably applied for controlling biofilm formation. Right now, bacterial biofilms have not been specifically addressed in the HACCP system that has been employed in the food processing facilities. However, surveying of biofilms in food environments and developing an effective sanitation plan should be considered in the HACCP system (Sharma & Anand, 2002). An upgraded HACCP with biofilm assessment in food plants will provide clearer information of contamination, and assist the development of biofilm-free processing systems in the food industry.

## 4. Attachment to food-contact surfaces and biofilm forming ability of *Salmonella*

Salmonellae represent a group of Gram-negative bacteria that are recognized worldwide as major zoonotic pathogens for both humans and animals. In the EU, salmonellosis was the second most commonly reported zoonotic infection in 2009, with 108,614 human cases confirmed and a case fatality rate of 0.08%, which approximately corresponds to 90 human deaths (EFSA-ECDC, 2011). That year, *Salmonella* was most often found in fresh broiler, turkey and pig meat where proportions of positive samples, on average 5.4%, 8.7% and 0.7%, were detected respectively. The two most common *Salmonella* serotypes, implicated in the majority of outbreaks, are Typhimurium and Enteritidis (52.3% and 23.3% respectively of all known serovars in human cases). The native habitat of salmonellae is considered to be the intestinal tract of taxonomically diverse group of vertebrates, from which salmonellae can spread to other environments through released faeces (Litrup et al., 2010).

Interestingly, salmonellae have been shown to survive for extended periods of time in non-enteric habitats, including biofilms on abiotic surfaces (White et al., 2006). Thus, several reports have demonstrated the ability of *Salmonella* to form biofilms on abiotic surfaces outside the host, such as stainless steel (Austin et al., 1998; Chorianopoulos et al., 2010; Giaouris et al., 2005; Giaouris & Nychas, 2006; Hood & Zottola, 1997a,b; Joseph et al., 2001; Kim & Wei, 2007, 2009; Møretrø et al., 2009), plastic (Asséré et al., 2008; Iibuchi et al., 2010; Jain & Chen, 2007; Joseph et al., 2001; Ngwai et al., 2006; Stepanović et al., 2003, 2004; Vestby et at., 2009a,b), rubber (Arnold & Yates, 2009), glass (Kim & Wei, 2009; Korber et al., 1997; Prouty & Gunn, 2003; Solano et al., 1998), cement (Joseph et al., 2001), marble and granite (Rodrigues et al., 2011). Taken into account, that all these surfaces are commonly encountered in farms, slaughter houses, food industries and kitchens, it is obvious that the risk for public health is quite serious.

It is strongly believed that the ability of *Salmonella* to form biofilms on inanimate surfaces contributes to its survival and persistence in non-host environments and its transmission to new hosts. To this direction, Vestby et al. (2009b) found a correlation between the biofilm formation capacities of 111 *Salmonella* strains isolated from feed and fish meal factories and their persistence in the factory environment. Another study on colonization and persistence of *Salmonella* on egg conveyor belts indicated that the type of egg belt (i.e. vinyl, nylon, hemp or plastic) was the most important factor in colonization and persistence, while rdar morphotype, a physiological adaptation associated with aggregation and long-term survival which is conserved in *Salmonella* (White & Surette, 2006), surprisingly, was not essential for persistence (Stocki et al., 2007). Interestingly, inoculation onto fresh-cut produce surfaces, as well as onto inert surfaces, such as polyethersufone membranes, was found to significantly increase the survival of salmonellae during otherwise lethal acid challenge (pH 3.0 for 2 hours) (Gawande & Bhagwat, 2002). Similarly, *Salmonella* strains with high biofilm productivity survived longer on polypropylene surfaces under dry conditions than strains with low productivity (Iibuchi et al., 2010).

In the food processing environments, food-contact surfaces come in contact with fluids containing various levels of food components. Under such conditions, one of the first events to occur is the adsorption of food molecules to the surface (conditioning). Both growth media and surface conditioning were found to influence the adherence of *S.* Typhimurium cells to stainless steel (Hood & Zottola, 1997b). A study of 122 *Salmonella* strains indicated that all had the ability to adhere to plastic microwell plates and that, generally, more biofilm was produced in low nutrient conditions, as those found in specific food processing environments, compared to high nutrient conditions (Stepanovic et al., 2004). A study conducted in order to identify the risk factors for *Salmonella* contamination in poultry farms, showed that the most important factors were dust, surfaces and faeces, and nearly 50% of the strains isolated from poultry risk factors were able to produce biofilm, irrespective of the origin of different serotypes (Marin et al., 2009).

There are some studies which have investigated the influence of physicochemical and surface properties (e.g. charge, hydrophobicity, surface free energy, roughness) of *Salmonella* and surface materials on the attachment process. For instance, Sinde & Carballo (2000) found that surface free energies and hydrophobicity do not affect attachment of *Salmonella* to stainless steel, rubber and polytetrafluorethylene, while Ukuku & Fett (2002) found that there was a linear correlation between bacterial cell surface hydrophobicity and charge and the strength of attachment of *Salmonella, E. coli* and *L. monocytogenes* strains to cantaloupe surfaces. Korber et al. (1997) found that surface roughness influences susceptibility of *S.* Enteritidis biofilms, grown in glass flow cells (with or without artificial crevices) to trisodium phosphate. Chia et al. (2009) studied the attachment of 25 *Salmonella* strains to four different materials (Teflon®, stainless steel, rubber and polyurethane) commonly found in poultry industry and found out that materials more positive in interfacial free energies had the highest number of adhering bacteria. However, in that study, authors concluded that *Salmonella* adhesion is strain-dependent, and probably influenced by surface structures, such as cell wall and membrane proteins, fimbriae, flagella and polysaccharides. This was also the conclusion of another similar study which compared the adhesion ability of four *S.* Enteritidis isolates to three different materials (polyethylene, polypropylene and granite) used in kitchens (Oliveira et al., 2006). Ngwai et al. (2006) characterized the biofilm forming ability of eleven antibiotic-resistant *S.* Typhimurium DT104 clinical isolates from human and animal sources and concluded that there was a general lack of correlation between this ability and bacterial physicochemical surface characteristics.

The persistence of *Salmonella* within the food chain has become a major health concern, as biofilms of this pathogen formed in food processing environments can serve as a reservoir for the contamination of food products. The development of materials to be used for food-contact surfaces with improved food safety profiles continues to be a challenge. One approach which has been developed to control microbial attachment is the manufacture of food-contact materials incorporating antimicrobial compounds. Triclosan-impregnated kitchen bench stones (silestones), although prone to bacterial colonization, were found to reduce *S.* Enteritidis biofilm development on them and also the viability of cells within the biofilm (Rodrigues et al., 2011).

## 5. Molecular components of *Salmonella* biofilms formed on abiotic surfaces

Curli fimbriae (formerly designated as thin aggregative fimbriae or Tafi) and cellulose are the two main matrix components (exopolymeric substances, EPS) in *Salmonella* biofilms (Gerstel & Römling, 2003). When co-expressed on Congo Red (CR) agar plates, curli fimbriae and the exopolysaccharide cellulose form the characteristic rdar (red, dry and rough) morphotype (also called rugose or wrinkled) (Römling, 2005). Their syntheses are co-regulated by a complex regulatory system. The LuxR type regulator CsgD protein stimulates the production of curli through transcriptional activation of the *csgBAC* (formerly *agfBAC*) operon, while the activation of cellulose production is indirect through the regulator AdrA which is a member of the GGDEF protein family regulated by *csgD* (Römling et al., 2000). García et al. (2004) demonstrated that most GGDEF proteins of *S.* Typhimurium are functionally related, probably by controlling the levels of the same final product, cyclic di-GMP, a secondary messenger that seems to regulate a variety of cellular functions including cellulose production and biofilm formation. The co-expression of curli fimbriae and cellulose leads to the formation of a highly hydrophobic network with tightly packed cells aligned in parallel in a rigid matrix and enhances biofilm formation on abiotic surfaces (Jain & Chen, 2007). Solomon et al. (2005) showed that 72% of 71 *S. enterica* strains, originating from produce, meat or clinical sources and belonging to 28 different serovars, expressed the rdar morphotype, with curli- and cellulose-deficient isolates being least effective in biofilm formation on polystyrene microtiter plates. White et al. (2006) showed that rdar morphotype significantly enhanced the resistance of *Salmonella* to dessication and sodium hypochlorite, suggesting that this phenotype could play a role in the transmission of *Salmonella* between hosts. However, aggregation via the rdar morphotype does not seem to be a virulence adaptation in *S.* Typhimurium, since competitive infection experiments in mice showed that nonaggregative cells outcompeted rdar-positive wild-type cells in all tissues analyzed (White et al., 2008).

A variety of environmental cues such as nutrients, oxygen tension, temperature, pH, ethanol and osmolarity can influence the expression of the transcriptional regulator CsgD, which regulates the production of both cellulose and curli (Gerstel & Römling, 2003). Transcription of *csgD* is dependent upon the stationary phase-inducible sigma factor RpoS, and is maximal in the late exponential or early stationary phase of growth (Gerstel & Römling, 2001). For an extensive overview on the current understanding of the complex genetic network regulating *Salmonella* biofilm formation, reader is advised to refer to the recently published review of Steenackers et al. (2011). When *csgD* is not expressed the morphotype is a conventional smooth and white (saw) colony, which does not produce any extracellular matrix (Römling et al., 1998b). In wild type *Salmonella* strains, rdar morphotype is restricted to low temperature (below 30°C) and low osmolarity conditions, but biogenesis of curli fimbriae occurs upon iron starvation at 37°C. Römling et al. (2003) showed that the majority (more than 90% of 800 strains) of human disease-associated *S.* Typhimurium and *S.* Enteritidis (isolated from patients, foods and animals) displayed the rdar morphotype at 28°C, but just rarely at 37°C. Interestingly, mutants in the *csgD* promoter have also been found expressing rdar morphotype independently of temperature (Römling et al., 1998b).

Curli fimbriae are amyloid cell-surface proteins, and are involved in adhesion to surfaces, cell aggregation, environmental persistence and biofilm development (Austin et al., 1998; Collinson et al., 1991; White et al., 2006). The *csg* (curli subunit genes) genes (previously called *agf* genes) involved in curli biosynthesis are organized into two adjacent divergently-transcribed operons, *csgBAC* and *csgDEFG* (Collinson et al., 1996; Römling et al., 1998a). Knocking out the gene encoding for the subunit of thin aggregative fimbriae, AgfA, results in pink colony formation, the pdar (pink, dry and rough) morphotype, which is characterised by production of cellulose without curli (Jain & Chen, 2007). Solano et al. (2002) stressed the importance of the applied biofilm system since they noticed that curli were not essential for biofilm mediated glass adherence under adherence test medium (ATM) conditions, while they were indispensable to form a tight pellicle under LB conditions.

In addition to curli, the second component of the extracellular matrix of the *Salmonella* biofilms is cellulose, a *β*-1→4-D-glucose polymer, which is biosynthesized by the *bcsABZC*-*bcsEFG* genes (bacterial cellulose synthesis) (Zogaj et al., 2001). Both operons are responsible for cellulose biosynthesis in both *S.* Enteritidis and *S.* Typhimurium (Jain & Chen, 2007; Solano et al., 2002). Cellulose production impaiment generates a bdar (brown, dry and rough) morphotype on congo red (CR) agar plates, characteristic of the expression of curli. Solano et al. (2002) showed that cellulose is a crucial biofilm determinant for *Salmonella*, under both LB and ATM conditions, without however affecting the virulence of the bacterium. Additionally, cellulose-deficient mutants were more sensitive to chlorine treatments, suggesting that cellulose production and biofilm formation may be an important factor for the survival of *Salmonella* in hostile environments. Prouty & Gunn (2003) identified its crucial importance for biofilm formation on glass coverslips. However, cellulose was not a major constituent of the biofilm matrix of *S.* Agona and *S.* Typhimurium strains isolated from the feed industry, but it contributed to the highly organized matrix structurization (Vestby et al., 2009a). Malcova et al. (2008) found that cellulose was not crucial for *S.* Enteritidis adherence and biofilm formation on polystyrene.

Latasa et al. (2005) also reported another matrix component, BapA, a large cell-surface protein required for biofilm formation of *S.* Enteritidis. This protein was found to be loosely associated with the cell surface, while it is secreted through the BapBCD type I protein secretion system, encoded by the *bapABCD* operon. The expression of *bapA* was demonstrated to be coordinated with the expression of curli and cellulose through the action of *csgD* (Latasa et al., 2005). Also, these authors demonstrated that a *bapA* mutant strain showed a significant lower colonization rate at the intestinal cell barrier and consequently a decreased efficiency for organ invasion compared with the wild-type strain.

Motility was found to be important for *Salmonella* biofilm development on glass (Prouty & Gunn, 2003) and polyvinyl chloride (PVC) (Mireles et al., 2001). On the contrary, Teplitski et al. (2006) noticed that the presence of the flagellum on the surface of the cell, functional or not, is inhibitory to biofilm formation on polystyrene, as mutants lacking intact flagella, showed increased biofilm formation compared to the wild-type. Flagella were not found to be important for *S.* Typhimurium rdar expression on Congo Red (CR) agar plates (Römling & Rohde, 1999). Solano et al. (2002) noticed that flagella affect *S.* Enteritidis biofilm development only under LB but not under ATM conditions. Stafford & Hughes (2007) showed that the conserved flagellar regulon gene *flhE*, while it is not required for flagella production or swimming, appeared to play a role in flagella-dependent swarming and biofilm formation on PVC. Kim & Wei (2009) noticed that flagellar assemply was important during biofilm formation on PVC in different (meat, poultry and produce) broths and on stainless steel and glass in LB broth.

Colanic acid, a capsular extracellular polysaccharide, essential for *S.* Typhimurium biofilm development on epithelial cells was found not to be required for *Salmonella* biofilm formation on abiotic surfaces (Ledeboer & Jones, 2005; Prouty & Gunn, 2003). Solano et al. (2002) showed that colonic acid was important to form a tight pellicle under LB conditions, while it was dispensable under ATM conditions. De Rezende et al. (2005) purified another capsular polysaccharide (CP) from extracellular matrix of multiresistant *S.* Typhimurium DT104 which was found to be important for biofilm formation on polystyrene centrifuge tubes and was detected at both 25°C and 37°C. This was comprised principally of glucose and mannose, with galactose as a minor constituent. Malcova et al. (2008) confirmed the importance of this capsular polysaccharide in the biofilm formation capacity of strains unable to produce either curli fimbriae or cellulose. Due to mucoid and brown appearance on Congo Red agar plates, their morphotype was designated as sbam (smooth, brown and mucoid).

However, other capsular polysaccharides can be present in the extracellular biofilm matrix of *Salmonella* strains (de Rezende et al., 2005; Gibson et al., 2006; White et al., 2003), and the exact composition depends upon the environmental conditions in which the biofilms are formed (Prouty & Gunn, 2003). Another component of the EPS matrix of *Salmonella* bile-induced biofilms, the O-antigen (O-ag) capsule, while it was found to be crucial for *S.* Typhimurium and *S.* Typhi biofilm development on gallstones, this was not necessary for adhesion and biofilm formation on glass and plastic (Crawford et al., 2008). The formation of this O-ag capsule was also found to be important for survival during desiccation stress (Gibson et al., 2006). Anriany et al. (2006) highlighted the importance of an integral lipopolysaccharide (LPS), at both the O-antigen and core polysaccharide levels, in the modulation of curli protein and cellulose production, as well as in biofilm formation, thereby adding another potential component to the complex regulatory system which governs multicellular behavior in *S.* Typhimurium. Mireles et al. (2001) observed that for *S.* Typhimurium LT2, all of the LPS mutants examined were able to form a biofilm on polyvinyl chloride (PVC) but none were able to attach to a hydrophilic surface such as glass. Kim & Wei (2009) noticed that a *rfbA* mutant of *S.* Typhimurium DT104, showing an aberrant LPS profile, was impaired in rdar expression, pellicle formation, biofilm forming capability on PVC in meat, poultry and produce broths and biofilm formation on stainless steel and glass.

## 6. Cell-to-cell communication in *Salmonella* biofilms (quorum sensing)

It has been thoroughly suggested that bacterial cells communicate by releasing and sensing small diffusible signal molecules, in a process commonly known as quorum sensing (QS) (Miller & Bassler, 2001; Smith et al., 2004; Whitehead et al., 2001). Through cell-to-cell signaling mechanisms, bacteria modulate their own behaviour and also respond to signal produced by other species (Ryan & Dow, 2008). QS involves a density-dependent recognition of signaling molecules (autoinducers, AIs), resulting in modulation of gene expression (Bassler, 1999). Gram-negative bacteria primarily use a variety of *N*-acylhomoserine lactones (AHLs) as AI (autoinducer-1, AI-1), while Gram-positive bacteria use a variety of autoinducing polypeptides (AIPs). AHLs are synthesized and recognized by QS circuits composed of LuxI and LuxR homologues, respectively (Whitehead et al., 2001). Both AHLs and AIPs are highly specific to the species that produce them. A third QS system is proposed to be universal, allowing interspecies communication, and is based on the enzyme LuxS which is in part responsible for the production of a furanone-like compound, called autoinducer-2 (AI-2) (Schauder et al., 2001).

Bacteria use QS communication circuits to regulate a diverse array of physiological activities, such as genetic competence, pathogenicity (virulence), motility, sporulation, bioluminescence and production of antimicrobial substances (Miller & Bassler, 2001). Yet, a growing body of evidence demonstrates that QS also contributes to biofilm formation by many different species (Annous et al., 2009; Davies et al., 1998; Irie & Parsek, 2008; Lazar, 2011). As biofilms typically contain high concentration of cells, autoinducer (AI) activity and QS regulation of gene expression have been proposed as essential components of biofilm physiology (Kjelleberg & Molin, 2002; Parsek & Greenberg, 2005).

To date, three QS systems have been identified in *S. enterica* and are thought to be mainly implicated in the regulation of virulence (SdiA, luxS/AI-2 and AI-3/epinephrine/norepinephrine signaling system) (Boyen et al., 2009; Walters & Sperandio, 2006). Firstly, the LuxR homologue SdiA has been characterized in *Salmonella,* but there does not appear to be a corresponding signal-generating enzyme similar to LuxI in this species (Ahmer et al., 1998). Since *Salmonella* does not possess a luxI homologue, it cannot produce its own AHLs (Ahmer, 2004). However, *Salmonella* SdiA can detect AHLs produced by a variety of bacterial species, leading to the suggestion that SdiA can be used in interspecies communication within a mixed-species community (Michael et al., 2001; Smith & Ahmer 2003). Till now, SdiA is known to activate the expression of the *rck* operon and the *srgE* gene (Ahmer et al., 1998; Smith & Ahmer, 2003). In contrast to the function of SdiA in *E. coli* adherence to HEp-2 epithelial cells and also biofilm formation on polystyrene (Lee et al., 2009; Sharma et al., 2010), no direct link between SdiA and *Salmonella* biofilms has been reported. Interestingly, Chorianopoulos et al. (2010) demonstrated that cell-free culture supernatant (CFS) of the psychrotrophic spoilage bacterium *Hafnei alvei,* containing AHLs among other unknown metabolites, negatively influenced the early stage of biofilm formation by *S.* Enteritidis on stainless steel. Similarly, Dheilly et al. (2010) reported the inhibitory activity of CFS from the marine bacterium *Pseudoalteromonas* sp. strain 3J6 against biofilm formation on glass flow cells by *S. enterica* and other Gram-negative bacteria. Taking into account that *Salmonella* possess SdiA, a receptor of AHLs which may be produced by resident flora on food-contact surfaces (Michael et al., 2001; Smith & Ahmer, 2003; Soares & Ahmer, 2011), the effect of AHLs on biofilm formation by this pathogen in multispecies real food processing environments needs to be further studied.

The second QS system of *Salmonella* uses the LuxS enzyme for the synthesis of AI-2 (Schauder et al., 2001; Soni et al., 2008). The Lsr ABC transporter is known to be involved in the detection and transport of AI-2 into the cell (Taga et al., 2001), while the *rbs* transporter has recently been suggested as an alternative AI-2 uptake system (Jesudhasan et al., 2010). A *S.* Typhimurium *luxS* deletion mutant was impaired in biofilm formation on polystyrene (De Keersmaecker et al., 2005; Jesudhasan et al., 2010). However, this phenotype could not be complemented by extracellular addition of QS signal molecules, suggesting that AI-2 is not the actual signal involved in *Salmonella* biofilm formation (De Keersmaecker et al., 2005). To this direction, Kint et al. (2010) analyzed additional *luxS* mutants for their biofilm phenotype. Interestingly, a *luxS* kanamycin insertion mutant and a partial deletion mutant, that only lacked the 3′ part of the *luxS* coding sequence, were found to be able to form mature wild-type biofilms on polystyrene, despite the fact that these strains were unable to produce AI-2. These authors concluded that a small regulatory RNA molecule, MicA, encoded in the *luxS* adjacent genomic region, rather than LuxS itself, infuences *S.* Typhimurium biofilm formation phenotype. On the other hand, Prouty et al. (2002) showed that a *S.* Typhimurium *luxS* insertion mutant formed scattered biofilm on gallstones with little apparent EPS even after 14 days of incubation. Yoon & Sofos (2008) showed that biofilm formation by *S.* Thompson on stainless steel, under monoculture conditions (72 h at 25°C), was similar between AI-2 positive and negative strains. Altogether, these results demonstrate that the relationship between biofilm formation and the presence of an active LuxS system and AI-2 in *S. enterica* is not clear and further research is needed.

The third QS system of *Salmonella* uses the two component system PreA/B (Bearson & Bearson 2008; Merighi et al., 2006). PreA/B is similar to the *luxS*-dependent two component QseB/QseC of enterohemorrhagic *E. coli*, which has been shown to sense the QS signal AI-3, as well the eukaryotic hormones epinephrine and norepinephrine (Sperandio et al., 2002; Walters & Sperandio, 2006). In *S.* Typhimurium, the histidine sensor kinase QseC, which is able to detect norepinephrine, has been implicated in the regulation of virulence traits, such as motility and *in vivo* competitive fitness in pigs (Bearson & Bearson, 2008). Even though the role of AI-3/epinephrine/norepinephrine signaling system in the formation of biofilm by *Salmonella* is still unknown, given that motility is usually an important biofilm determinant in many bacterial species, it is quite possible that this third QS system may also affect *Salmonella* biofilm formation.

## 7. Conclusions

Biofilms are commonly defined as communities of microorganisms attached to a surface and producing an extracellular matrix, in which these microorganisms are embedded. Biofilms are very diverse and unique, not just to the microorganism, but to the particular environment in which they are being formed. This makes *in vitro* characterization of biofilms difficult and requires the establishment of laboratory conditions that mimic the natural setting being studied. Pathogenic biofilms have been of considerable interest in the context of food safety and have provoked interest of many research groups. In particular, biofilm formation by *Salmonella* is a serious concern in food industry, since the persistence of this bacterium in biofilms formed on food-contact surfaces may become a constant source of product contamination.

The discovery of bacterial biofilms in medical and industrial ecosystems has created an urgency to identify and characterize factors that are necessary for biofilm development, which may serve as targets for biofilm prevention and treatment. Thus, researchers in the fields of clinical, food, water, and environmental microbiology have begun to investigate microbiological processes from a biofilm perspective. As the pharmaceutical, health-care and food industries embrace this approach, novel strategies for biofilm formation and control will undoubtedly emerge. Particularly challenging is the attempt to understand the complexity of the interactions within a biofilm community, since these interactions between the different species influence the final outcome of this community. Communication between species may include extracellular compounds whose sole role is to influence gene expression, metabolic cooperativity and competition, physical contact, and the production of antimicrobial exoproducts. One or all of these interactions may be occurring simultaneously. The challenge becomes more intriguing given that microflora on inadequately cleaned and disinfected food processing surfaces is a complex community, contrary to the laboratory studied pure-species biofilms.

Undoubtedly, a clearer understanding of the factors which influence microbial attachment to abiotic surfaces could provide the information necessary to modify processes in food processing environments in order to reduce microbial persistence and therefore reduce the contamination of food products. For instance, the understanding of bacterial attachment to solid surfaces, such as stainless steel, may help in the future development of surfaces with no or reduced attachment, or in developing an effective sanitation programme and thus reducing the potential contamination of processed products by spoilage or/and pathogenic bacteria. Undoubtedly, the ability to recognize how *Salmonella* attach to food-contact surfaces and form biofilms on them is an important area of focus, since a better understanding of this ability may provide valuable ways towards the elimination of this pathogenic bacterium from food processing environments and eventually lead to reduced *Salmonella*-associated human illness.

## 8. Acknowledgement

Authors would like to acknowledge European Union project ProSafeBeef (ref. Food-CT-2006-36241) within the 6th Framework Programme for the financial support of some of the studies on *Salmonella* biofilms performed on our lab.

## 9. References

Ahmer, B.M.M. (2004). Cell-to-cell signalling in *Escherichia coli* and *Salmonella enterica*. *Molecular Microbiology*, Vol.52, No.4, (January 2004), pp. 933-945

Ahmer, B.M.; van Reeuwijk, J.; Timmers, C.D.; Valentine, P.J. & Heffron, F. (1998). *Salmonella typhimurium* encodes an SdiA homolog, a putative quorum sensor of the LuxR family, that regulates genes on the virulence plasmid. *Journal of Bacteriology*, Vol.180, No.5, (March 1998), pp. 1185-1193

Annous, B.A.; Fratamico, P.M & Smith, J.L. (2009). Quorum sensing in biofilms: why bacteria behave the way they do. *Journal of Food Science*, Vol.74, No.1., pp. R24-R37

Anriany, Y.; Sahu, S.N.; Wessels, K.R.; McCann, L.M. & Joseph, S.W. (2006). Alteration of the rugose phenotype in *waaG* and *ddhC* mutants of *Salmonella enterica* serovar Typhimurium DT104 is associated with inverse production of curli and cellulose. *Applied and Environmental Microbiology*, Vol.72, No.7, (July 2006), pp. 5002-5012

Arnold, J.W. & Yates, I.E. (2009). Interventions for control of *Salmonella*: clearance of microbial growth from rubber picker fingers. *Poultry Science*, Vol.88, No.6, (June 2009), pp. 1292-1298

Asséré, A.; Oulahal, N. & Carpentier, B. (2008). Comparative evaluation of methods for counting surviving biofilm cells adhering to a polyvinyl chloride surface exposed to chlorine or drying. *Journal of Applied Microbiology*, Vol.104, No.6, (June 2008), pp. 1692-1702

Austin, J.W. & Bergeron, G. (1995). Development of bacterial biofilms in dairy processing lines. *Journal of Dairy Research*, Vol.62, No.3, (August 1995), pp. 509-519

Austin, J.W.; Sanders, G.; Kay, W.W. & Collinson, S.K. (1998). Thin aggregative fimbriae enhance *Salmonella enteritidis* biofilm formation. *FEMS Microbiology Letters*, Vol.162, No.2, (May 1998), pp. 295-301

Bagge-Ravn, D.; Ng, Y.; Hjelm, M.; Christiansen, J.N.; Johansen, C. & Gram, L. (2003). The microbial ecology of processing equipment in different fish industries - analysis of the microflora during processing and following cleaning and disinfection. *International Journal of Food Microbiology*, Vol.87, No.3, (November 2003), pp. 239-250

Barnes, L.M.; Lo, M.F.; Adams, M.R. & Chamberlain, A.H. (1999). Effect of milk proteins on adhesion of bacteria to stainless steel surfaces. *Applied and Environmental Microbiology*, Vol.65, No.10, (October 1999), pp. 4543-4548

Bassler, B.L. (1999). How bacteria talk to each other: regulation of gene expression by quorum sensing. *Current Opinion in Microbiology*, Vol.2, No.6, (December 1999), pp. 582-587

Bearson, B.L. & Bearson, S.M. (2008). The role of the QseC quorum-sensing sensor kinase in colonization and norepinephrine-enhanced motility of *Salmonella enterica* serovar Typhimurium. *Microbial Pathogenesis*, Vol.44, No.4, (April 2008), pp. 271-278

Beloin, C.; Valle, J.; Latour-Lambert, P.; Faure, P.; Kzreminski, M.; Balestrino, D.; Haagensen, J.A.; Molin, S.; Prensier, G.; Arbeille, B. & Ghigo, J.M. (2004). Global impact of mature biofilm lifestyle on *Escherichia coli* K-12 gene expression. *Molecular Microbiology*, Vol.51, No.3, (February 2004), pp. 659-674

Bernbom, N.; Ng, Y.Y.; Jørgensen, R.L.; Arpanaei, A.; Meyer, R.L.; Kingshott, P.; Vejborg, R.M.; Klemm, P. & Gram, L. (2009). Adhesion of food-borne bacteria to stainless steel is reduced by food conditioning films. *Journal of Applied Microbiology*, Vol.106, No.4, (April 2009), pp. 1268-1279

Blackman, I.C. & Frank, J.F. (1996). Growth of *Listeria monocytogenes* as a biofilm on various food-processing surfaces. *Journal of Food Protection*, Vol.59, No.8, (August 1996), pp. 827-831

Boyen, F.; Eeckhaut, V.; Van Immerseel, F.; Pasmans, F.; Ducatelle, R. & Haesebrouck, F. (2009). Quorum sensing in veterinary pathogens: mechanisms, clinical importance and future perspectives. *Veterinary Microbiology*, Vol.135, No.3-4, (March 2009), pp. 187-195

Branda, S.S.; Vik, S.; Friedman, L. & Kolter, R. (2005). Biofilms: the matrix revisited. *Trends in Microbiology*, Vol.13, No.1, (January 2005), pp. 20-26

Briandet, R.; Meylheuc, T.; Maher, C. & Bellon-Fontaine, M.N. (1999). *Listeria monocytogenes* Scott A: cell surface charge, hydrophobicity, and electron donor and acceptor characteristics under different environmental growth conditions. *Applied and Environmental Microbiology*, Vol.65, No.12, (December 1999), pp. 5328-5333

Brooks, J.D. & Flint, S.H. (2008). Biofilms in the food industry: problems and potential solutions. *International Journal of Food Science and Technology*, Vol.43, (August 2008), pp. 2163-2176

Burmølle, M.; Webb, J.S.; Rao, D.; Hansen, L.H.; Sørensen, S.J. & Kjelleberg, S. (2006). Enhanced biofilm formation and increased resistance to antimicrobial agents and bacterial invasion are caused by synergistic interactions in multispecies biofilms. *Applied and Environmental Microbiology*, Vol.72, No.6, (June 2006), pp. 3916-3923

Carpentier, B. & Cerf, O. (1993). Biofilms and their consequences, with particular reference to hygiene in the food industry. *Journal of Applied Bacteriology*, Vol.75, (June 1993), pp. 499-451

Chia, T.W.R.; Goulter, R.M.; McMeekin, T.; Dykes, G.A. & Fegan, N. (2009). Attachment of different *Salmonella* serovars to materials commonly used in a poultry processing plant. *Food Microbiology*, Vol.26, (May 2009), pp. 853-859

Chmielewski, R.A.N. & Frank, J.F. (2003). Biofilm formation and control in food processing facilities. *Comprehensive Reviews in Food Science and Food Safety*, Vol.2, pp. 22-32

Chorianopoulos, N.G.; Giaouris, E.D.; Kourkoutas, Y. & Nychas, G.-J. (2010). Inhibition of the early stage of *Salmonella enterica* serovar Enteritidis biofilm development on stainless steel by cell-free supernatant of a *Hafnia alvei* culture. *Applied and Environmental Microbiology*, Vol.76, No.6, (January 2010), pp. 2018-2022

Chorianopoulos, N.G.; Giaouris, E.D.; Skandamis, P.N.; Haroutounian, S.A. & Nychas, G.-J. (2008). Disinfectant test against monoculture and mixed-culture biofilms composed of technological, spoilage and pathogenic bacteria: bactericidal effect of essential oil and hydrosol of *Satureja thymbra* and comparison with standard acid-base santitizers. *Journal of Applied Microbiology*, Vol.104, No.6, (November 2007), pp. 1586-1596

Chorianopoulos, N.G.; Tsoukleris, D.S.; Panagou, E.Z.; Falaras, P. & Nychas, G.J. (2011). Use of titanium dioxide ($TiO_2$) photocatalysts as alternative means for *Listeria monocytogenes* biofilm disinfection in food processing. *Food Microbiology*, Vol.28, No.1, (February 2011), pp. 164-170

Collinson, S.K.; Clouthier, S.C.; Doran, J.L.; Banser, P.A. & Kay, W.W. (1996). *Salmonella enteritidis agfBAC* operon encoding thin, aggregative fimbriae. *Journal of Bacteriology*, Vol.178, No.3, (February 1996), pp. 662-667

Collinson, S.K.; Emödy, L.; Müller, K.H.; Trust, T.J. & Kay, W.W. (1991). Purification and characterization of thin, aggregative fimbriae from *Salmonella enteritidis*. *Journal of Bacteriology*, Vol.173, No.15, (August 1991), pp. 4773-4781

Cos, P.; Toté, K.; Horemans, T. & Maes, L. (2010). Biofilms: an extra hurdle for effective antimicrobial therapy. *Current Pharmaceutical Design*, Vol.16, No.20, pp. 2279-2295

Costerton, J.W.; Cheng, K.J.; Geesey, G.G.; Ladd, T.I.; Nickel, J.C.; Dasgupta, M. & Marrie, T.J. (1987). Bacterial biofilms in nature and disease. *Annual Review of Microbiology*, Vol.41, pp. 435-464

Costerton, J.W.; Lewandowski, Z.; Caldwell, D.E.; Korber, D.R. & Lappin-Scott, H.M. (1995). Microbial biofilms. *Annual Review of Microbiology*, Vol.49, pp. 711-745

Crawford, R.W.; Gibson, D.L.; Kay, W.W. & Gunn, J.S. (2008). Identification of a bile-induced exopolysaccharide required for *Salmonella* biofilm formation on gallstone surfaces. *Infection and Immunity*, Vol.76, No.11, (November 2008), pp. 5341-5349

Davey, M.E. & O'Toole, G.A. (2000). Microbial biofilms: from ecology to molecular genetics. *Microbiology and Molecular Biology Reviews*, Vol.64, No.4, pp. 847-867

Davies, D.G.; Parsek, M.R.; Pearson, J.P.; Iglewski, B.H.; Costerton, J.W. & Greenberg, E.P. (1998). The involvement of cell-to-cell signals in the development of a bacterial biofilm. *Science*, Vol.280, No.5361, (April 1998), pp. 295-298

De Keersmaecker, S.C.; Varszegi, C.; van Boxel, N.; Habel, L.W.; Metzger, K.; Daniels, R.; Marchal, K.; De Vos, D. & Vanderleyden, J. (2005). Chemical synthesis of (*S*)-4,5-dihydroxy-2,3-pentanedione, a bacterial signal molecule precursor, and validation of its activity in *Salmonella typhimurium*. *Journal of Biological Chemistry*, Vol.280, No.20, (May 2005), pp. 19563-19568

De Rezende, C.E.; Anriany, Y.; Carr, L.E.; Joseph, S.W. & Weiner, R.M. (2005). Capsular polysaccharide surrounds smooth and rugose types of *Salmonella enterica* serovar Typhimurium DT104. *Applied and Environmental Microbiology*, Vol.71, No.11, (November 2005), pp. 7345-7351

Dheilly, A.; Soum-Soutéra, E.; Klein, G.L.; Bazire, A.; Compère, C.; Haras, D. & Dufour, A. (2010). Antibiofilm activity of the marine bacterium *Pseudoalteromonas* sp. strain 3J6. *Applied and Environmental Microbiology*, Vol.76, No.11, (June 2010), pp. 3452-3461

Di Bonaventura, G.; Piccolomini, R.; Paludi, D.; D'Orio, V.; Vergara, A.; Conter, M. & Ianieri, A. (2008). Influence of temperature on biofilm formation by *Listeria monocytogenes* on various food-contact surfaces: relationship with motility and cell surface hydrophobicity. *Journal of Applied Microbiology*, Vol.104, No.6, (June 2008), pp. 1552-1561

Donlan, R.M. (2002). Biofilms: microbial life on surfaces. *Emerging and Infectious Diseases*, Vol.8, No.9, pp. 881-890

Donlan, R.M. & Costerton, J.W. (2002). Biofilms: survival mechanisms of clinically relevant microorganisms. *Clinical Microbiology Reviews*, Vol.15, No.2, pp. 167-193

Duguid, J.P.; Anderson, E.S. & Campbell, I. (1966). Fimbriae and adhesive properties in Salmonellae. *Journal of Pathology and Bacteriology*, Vol.92, No.1, (July 1966), pp. 107-138

EFSA-ECDC. (2011). The European Union summary report on trends and sources of zoonoses, zoonotic agents and food-borne outbreaks in 2009. *The EFSA Journal*, Vol.9, No.3:2090

Flemming, H.C. & Wingender, J. (2010). The biofilm matrix. *Nature Reviews. Microbiology*, Vol.8, No.9, (August 2010), pp. 623-633.

Ganesh Kumar, S. & Anand, S.K. (1998). Significance of microbial biofilms in food industry: a review. *International Journal of Food Microbiology*, Vol.42, (April 1998), pp. 9-27

García, B.; Latasa, C.; Solano, C.; García-del Portillo, F.; Gamazo, C. & Lasa, I. (2004). Role of the GGDEF protein family in *Salmonella* cellulose biosynthesis and biofilm formation. *Molecular Microbiology*, Vol.54, No.1, (October 2004), pp. 264-277

Gawande, P.V. & Bhagwat, A.A. (2002). Inoculation onto solid surfaces protects *Salmonella* spp. during acid challenge: a model study using polyethersulfone membranes. *Applied and Environmental Microbiology*, Vol.68, No.1, (October 2001), pp. 86-92

Gerstel, U. & Römling, U. (2001). Oxygen tension and nutrient starvation are major signals that regulate *agfD* promoter activity and expression of the multicellular morphotype in *Salmonella typhimurium*. *Environmental Microbiology*, Vol.3, No.10, (October 2001), pp. 638-648

Gerstel, U. & Römling, U. (2003). The *csgD* promoter, a control unit for biofilm formation in *Salmonella typhimurium*. *Research in Microbiology*, Vol.154, No.10, (December 2003), pp. 659-667

Giaouris, E.; Chapot-Chartier, M.P. & Briandet, R. (2009). Surface physicochemical analysis of natural *Lactococcus lactis* strains reveals the existence of hydrophobic and low charged strains with altered adhesive properties. *International Journal of Food Microbiology*, Vol.131, No.1, (April 2009), pp. 2-9

Giaouris, E.; Chorianopoulos, N. & Nychas, G.-J.E. (2005). Effect of temperature, pH, and water activity on biofilm formation by *Salmonella enterica* Enteritidis PT4 on stainless steel surfaces as indicated by the bead vortexing method and conductance measurements. *Journal of Food Protection*, Vol.68, No.10, (May 2005), pp. 2149-2154

Giaouris, E.D. & Nychas, G.-J.E. (2006). The adherence of *Salmonella* Enteritidis PT4 to stainless steel: the importance of the air-liquid interface and nutrient availability. *Food Microbiology*, Vol.23, (February 2006), pp. 747-752

Gibson, D.L.; White, A.P.; Snyder, S.D.; Martin, S.; Heiss, C.; Azadi, P.; Surette, M. & Kay, W.W. (2006). *Salmonella* produces an O-antigen capsule regulated by AgfD and important for environmental persistence. *Journal of Bacteriology*, Vol.188, No.22, (November 2006), pp. 7722-7730

Gilbert, P.; Allison, D.G. & McBain, A.J. (2002). Biofilms *in vitro* and *in vivo*: do singular mechanisms imply cross-resistance? *Journal of Applied Microbiology*, Vol.92, pp. 98S-110S

Gilbert, P.; Evans, D.J. & Brown, M.R. (1993). Formation and dispersal of bacterial biofilms *in vivo* and *in situ*. *Journal of Applied Bacteriology*, Vol.74, Suppl.67S-78S

Girennavar, B.; Cepeda, M.L.; Soni, K.A.; Vikram, A.; Jesudhasan, P.; Jayaprakasha, G.K.; Pillai, S.D. & Patil, B.S. (2008). Grapefruit juice and its furocoumarins inhibits autoinducer signaling and biofilm formation in bacteria. *International Journal of Food Microbiology*, Vol.125, (March 2008), pp. 204-208

Goller, C.C. & Romeo, T. (2008). Environmental influences on biofilm development. *Current Topics in Microbiology and Immunology*, Vol.322, pp. 37-66

Gounadaki, A.S.; Skandamis, P.N.; Drosinos, E.H. & Nychas, G.J. (2008). Microbial ecology of food contact surfaces and products of small-scale facilities producing traditional sausages. *Food Microbiology*, Vol.25, No.2, (April 2008), pp. 313-323

Gunduz, G.T. & Tuncel, G. (2006). Biofilm formation in an ice cream plant. *Antonie van Leeuwenhoek*, Vol.89, pp. 329–336

Habimana, O.; Heir, E.; Langsrud, S.; Asli, A.W. & Møretrø, T. (2010a). Enhanced surface colonization by *Escherichia coli* O157:H7 in biofilms formed by an *Acinetobacter calcoaceticus* isolate from meat-processing environments. *Applied and Environmental Microbiology*, Vol.76, No.13, (July 2010), pp. 4557-4559

Habimana, O.; Møretrø, T.; Langsrud, S.; Vestby, L.K.; Nesse, L.L. & Heir, E. (2010b). Micro ecosystems from feed industry surfaces: a survival and biofilm study of *Salmonella* versus host resident flora strains. *BMC Veterinary Research*, Vol.6, No. 48

Hall-Stoodley, L.; Costerton, J.W. & Stoodley, P. (2004). Bacterial biofilms: from the natural environment to infectious diseases. *Nature Reviews. Microbiology*, Vol.2, (February 2004), pp. 95-108

Hall-Stoodley, L. & Stoodley, P. (2002). Developmental regulation of microbial biofilms. *Current Opinion in Biotechnology*, Vol.13, No.3, (June 2002), pp. 228-233

Hall-Stoodley, L. & Stoodley, P. (2005). Biofilm formation and dispersal and the transmission of human pathogens. *Trends in Microbiology*, Vol.13, No.1, (January 2005), pp. 7-10

Hamilton, S.; Bongaerts, R.J.; Mulholland, F.; Cochrane, B.; Porter, J.; Lucchini, S.; Lappin-Scott, H.M. & Hinton, J.C. (2009). The transcriptional programme of *Salmonella enterica* serovar Typhimurium reveals a key role for tryptophan metabolism in biofilms. *BMC Genomics*, Vol.10, (December 2009), 599

Hood, S.K. & Zottola, E.A. (1997a). Adherence to stainless steel by foodborne microorganisms during growth in model food systems. *International Journal of Food Microbiology*, Vol.37, (June 1997), pp. 145-153

Hood, S.K. & Zottola, E.A. (1997b). Growth media and surface conditioning influence the adherence of *Pseudomonas fragi*, *Salmonella typhimurium*, and *Listeria monocytogenes* cells to stainless steel. *Journal of Food Protection*, Vol.60, No.9, (January 1997), pp. 1034-1037

Humphrey, T.J.; Slater, E.; McAlpine, K.; Rowbury, R.J. & Gilbert, R.J. (1995). *Salmonella* Enteritidis Phage Type 4 isolates more tolerant of heat, acid, or hydrogen peroxide also survive longer on surfaces. *Applied and Environmental Microbiology*, Vol.61, No.8, (May 1995), pp. 3161-3164

Iibuchi, R.; Hara-Kudo, Y.; Hasegawa, A. & Kumagai, S. (2010). Survival of *Salmonella* on a polypropylene surface under dry conditions in relation to biofilm-formation capability. *Journal of Food Protection*, Vol.73, No.8, (December 2009), pp. 1506-1510

Irie, Y. & Parsek, M.R. (2008). Quorum sensing and microbial biofilms. *Current Topics in Microbiology and Immunology*, Vol.322, pp. 67-84

Jain, S. & Chen, J. (2007). Attachment and biofilm formation by various serotypes of *Salmonella* as influenced by cellulose production and thin aggregative fimbriae biosynthesis. *Journal of Food Protection*, Vol.70, No.11, (November 2007), pp. 2473-2479

James, G.A.; Beaudette, L. & Costerton, J.W. (1995). Interspecies bacterial interactions in biofilms. *Journal of Industrial Microbiology*, Vol.15, pp. 257-262

Jefferson, K.K. (2004). What drives bacteria to produce a biofilm? *FEMS Microbiology Letters*, Vol.236, (June 2004), pp. 163-173

Jesudhasan, P.R.; Cepeda, M.L.; Widmer, K.; Dowd, S.E.; Soni, K.A.; Hume, M.E.; Zhu, J. & Pillai, S.D. (2010). Transcriptome analysis of genes controlled by *luxS*/autoinducer-2 in *Salmonella enterica* serovar Typhimurium. *Foodborne Pathogens and Disease*, Vol.7, No.4, (April 2010), pp. 399-410

Jones, K. & Bradshaw, S.B. (1997). Synergism in biofilm formation between *Salmonella enteritidis* and a nitrogen-fixing strain of *Klebsiella pneumoniae*. *Journal of Applied Microbiology*, Vol.82, (October 1996), pp. 663-668

Joseph, B.; Otta, S.K.; Karunasagar, I. & Karunasagar, I. (2001). Biofilm formation by *salmonella* spp. on food contact surfaces and their sensitivity to sanitizers. *International Journal of Food Microbiology*, Vol.64, No.3, (March 2001), pp. 367-372

Joshua, G.W.; Guthrie-Irons, C.; Karlyshev, A.V. & Wren, B.W. (2006). Biofilm formation in *Campylobacter jejuni*. *Microbiology*, Vol.152(Pt2), (February 2006), pp. 387-396

Kim, T.J.; Young, B.M. & Young, G.M. (2008). Effect of flagellar mutations on *Yersinia enterocolitica* biofilm formation. *Applied and Environmental Microbiology*, Vol.74, No.17, (September 2008), pp. 5466-5574

Kim, S.-H. & Wei, C.-I. (2007). Biofilm formation by multidrug-resistant *Salmonella enterica* serotype Typhimurium Phage Type DT104 and other pathogens. *Journal of Food Protection*, Vol.70, No.1, (July 2006), pp. 22-29

Kim, S.-H. & Wei, C.-I. (2009). Molecular characterization of biofilm formation and attachment of *Salmonella enterica* serovar Typhimurium DT104 on food contact surfaces. *Journal of Food Protection*, Vol.72, No.9, (September 2009), pp. 1841-1847

Kint, G.; De Coster, D.; Marchal, K.; Vanderleyden, J. & De Keersmaecker, S.C. (2010). The small regulatory RNA molecule MicA is involved in *Salmonella enterica* serovar Typhimurium biofilm formation. *BMC Microbiology*, Vol.10, (November), 276

Kjelleberg, S. & Molin, S. (2002). Is there a role for quorum sensing signals in bacterial biofilms? *Current Opinion in Microbiology*, Vol.5, No.3, (June 2002), pp. 254-258

Klausen, M.; Gjermansen, M.; Kreft, J.U. & Tolker-Nielsen, T. (2006). Dynamics of development and dispersal in sessile microbial communities: examples from *Pseudomonas aeruginosa* and *Pseudomonas putida* model biofilms. *FEMS Microbiology Letters*, Vol.261, No.1, (August 2006), pp. 1-11

Kolter, R. & Greenberg, E.P. (2006). The superficial life of microbes. *Nature*, Vol.441, No.7091, (May 2006), pp. 300-302

Korber, D.R.; Choi, A.; Wolfaardt, G.M.; Ingham, S.C. & Caldwell, D.E. (1997). Substratum topography influences susceptibility of *Salmonella enteritidis* biofilms to trisodium phosphate. *Applied and Environmental Microbiology*, Vol.63, No.9, (September 1997), pp. 3352-3358

Kuchma, S.L. & O'Toole, G.A. (2000). Surface-induced and biofilm-induced changes in gene expression. *Current Opinion in Biotechnology*, Vol.11, No.5, (October 2000), pp. 429-433

Lasa, I. (2006). Towards the identification of the common features of bacterial biofilm development. *International Microbiology*, Vol.9, (January 2006), pp. 21-28

Latasa, C.; Roux, A.; Toledo-Arana, A.; Ghigo, J.M.; Gamazo, C.; Penadés, J.R. & Lasa, I. (2005). BapA, a large secreted protein required for biofilm formation and host colonization of *Salmonella enterica* serovar Enteritidis. *Molecular Microbiology*, Vol.58, No.5, (December 2005), pp. 1322-1339

Lazar, V. (2011). Quorum sensing in biofilms - How to destroy the bacterial citadels or their cohesion/power? *Anaerobe, in press*

Lazazzera, B.A. (2005). Lessons from DNA microarray analysis: the gene expression profile of biofilms. *Current Opinion in Microbiology*, Vol.8, No.2, (April 2005), pp. 222-227

Ledeboer, N.A. & Jones, B.D. (2005). Exopolysaccharide sugars contribute to biofilm formation by *Salmonella enterica* serovar Typhimurium on HEp-2 cells and chicken intestinal epithelium. *Journal of Bacteriology*, Vol.187, No.9, (May 2005), pp. 3214-3226

Lee, J.; Maeda, T.; Hong, S.H. & Wood, T.K. (2009). Reconfiguring the quorum-sensing regulator SdiA of *Escherichia coli* to control biofilm formation via indole and N-acylhomoserine lactones. *Applied and Environmental Microbiology*, Vol.75, No.6, (March 2009), pp. 1703-1716

Lewis, K. (2001). Riddle of biofilm resistance. *Antimicrobial Agents and Chemotherapy*, Vol.45, No.4, (April 2001), pp. 999-1007

Lindsay, D. & von Holy, A. (2006). What food safety professionals should know about bacterial biofilms. *British Food Journal*, Vol.108, No.1, pp. 27-37

Litrup, E.; Torpdahl, M.; Malorny, B.; Huehn, S.; Christensen, H. & Nielsen, E.M. (2010). Association between phylogeny, virulence potential and serovars of *Salmonella enterica*. *Infection, Genetics and Evolution*, Vol.10, No. 7, (July 2010), pp. 1132-1139

López, D.; Vlamakis, H. & Kolter, R. (2010). Biofilms. *Cold Spring Harbor Perspectives in Biology*, Vol.2, No.7, (June 2010), a000398

Lundén, J.M.; Miettinen, M.K.; Autio, T.J. & Korkeala, H.J. (2000). Persistent *Listeria monocytogenes* strains show enhanced adherence to food contact surface after short contact times. *Journal of Food Protection*, Vol.63, No.9, (September 2000), pp. 1204-1207

Mah, T.-F.C. & O'Toole, G.A. (2001). Mechanisms of biofilm resistance to antimicrobial agents. *Trends in Microbiology*, Vol.9, No.1, (January 2001), pp. 34-39

Malcova, M.; Hradecka, H.; Karpiskova, R. & Rychlik, I. (2008). Biofilm formation in field strains of *Salmonella enterica* serovar Typhimurium: identification of a new colony morphology type and the role of SGI1 in biofilm formation. *Veterinary Microbiology*, Vol.129, No.3-4, (June 2008), pp. 360-366

Marin, C.; Hernandiz, A. & Lainez, M. (2009). Biofilm development capacity of *Salmonella* strains isolated in poultry risk factors and their resistance against disinfectants. *Poultry Science*, Vol.88, (October 2008), pp. 424-431

Marsh, P.D. (2005). Dental plaque: biological significance of a biofilm and community life-style. *Journal of Clinical Periodontology*, Vol.32, Suppl.6, pp. 7-15.

Merighi, M.; Carroll-Portillo, A.; Septer, A.N.; Bhatiya, A. & Gunn, J.S. (2006). Role of *Salmonella enterica* serovar Typhimurium two-component system PreA/PreB in modulating PmrA-regulated gene transcription. *Journal of Bacteriology*, Vol.188, No.1, (January 2006), pp. 141-149

Michael, B.; Smith, J.N.; Swift, S.; Heffron, F. & Ahmer, B.M. (2001). SdiA of *Salmonella enterica* is a LuxR homolog that detects mixed microbial communities. *Journal of Bacteriology*, Vol.183, No.19, (October 2001), pp. 5733-5742

Miller, M.B. & Bassler, B.L. (2001). Quorum sensing in bacteria. *Annual Review of Microbiology*, Vol.55, pp. 165-199

Mireles, J.R. 2$^{nd}$; Toguchi, A. & Harshey, R.M. (2001). *Salmonella enterica* serovar typhimurium swarming mutants with altered biofilm-forming abilities: surfactin inhibits biofilm formation. *Journal of Bacteriology*, Vol.183, No.20, (October 2001), pp. 5848-5854

Molin, S. & Tolker-Nielsen, T. (2003). Gene transfer occurs with enhanced efficiency in biofilms and induces enhanced stabilisation of the biofilm structure. *Current Opinion in Biotechnology*, Vol.14, pp. 255-261

Moons, P.; Michiels, C.W. & Aertsen, A. (2009). Bacterial interactions in biofilms. *Critical Reviews in Microbiology*, Vol.35, No.3, (August 2009), pp. 157-168

Møretrø, T.; Vestby, L.K.; Nesse, L.L.; Storheim, S.E.; Kotlarz, K. & Langsrud, S. (2009). Evaluation of efficacy of disinfectants against *Salmonella* from the feed industry. *Journal of Applied Microbiology*, Vol.106, No.3., (September 2008), pp. 1005-1012

Morild, R.K.; Olsen, J.E. & Aabo, S. (2011). Change in attachment of *Salmonella* Typhimurium, *Yersinia enterocolitica*, and *Listeria monocytogenes* to pork skin and muscle after hot water and lactic acid decontamination. *International Journal of Food Microbiology*, Vol.145, No.1, (January 2011), pp. 353-358

Nadell, C.D.; Xavier, J.B.; Levin, S.A. & Foster, K.R. (2008). The evolution of quorum sensing in bacterial biofilms. *PLoS Biology*, Vol.6, No.1, (January 2008), e14

Norwood, D.E. & Gilmour, A. (2001). The differential adherence capabilities of two *Listeria monocytogenes* strains in monoculture and multispecies biofilms as a function of temperature. *Letters in Applied Microbiology*, Vol.33, No.4, (October 2001), pp. 320-324

Ngwai, Y.B.; Adachi, Y.; Ogawa, Y. & Hara, H. (2006). Characterization of biofilm-forming abilities of antibiotic-resistant *Salmonella typhimurium* DT104 on hydrophobic abiotic surfaces. *Journal of Microbiology, Immunology and Infection*, Vol.39, (December 2005), pp. 278-291

Oliveira, K.; Oliveira, T.; Teixeira, P.; Azeredo, J.; Henriques, M. & Oliveira, R. (2006). Comparison of the adhesion ability of different *Salmonella* Enteritidis serotypes to materials used in kitchens. *Journal of Food Protection*, Vol.69, No.10, (May 2006), pp. 2352-2356

O'Toole, G.; Kaplan, H.B. & Kolter, R. (2000). Biofilm formation as microbial development. *Annual Review of Microbiology*, Vol.54, pp. 49-79

Palmer, J.; Flint, S. & Brooks, J. (2007). Bacterial cell attachment, the beginning of a biofilm. *Journal of Industrial Microbiology and Biotechnology*, Vol.34, (July 2007), pp. 577-578

Parsek, M.R. & Greenberg, E.P. (2005). Sociomicrobiology: the connections between quorum sensing and biofilms. *Trends in Microbiology*, Vol.13, No.1, (January 2005), pp. 27-33

Poimenidou, S.; Belessi, C.A.; Giaouris, E.D.; Gounadaki, A.S.; Nychas, G.J. & Skandamis, P.N. (2009). *Listeria monocytogenes* attachment to and detachment from stainless steel surfaces in a simulated dairy processing environment. *Applied and Environmental Microbiology*, Vol.75, No.22, (November 2009), pp. 7182-7188

Prouty, A.M. & Gunn, J.S. (2003). Comparative analysis of *Salmonella enterica* serovar Typhimurium biofilm formation on gallstones and on glass. *Infection and Immunity*, Vol.71, No.12, (December 2003), pp. 7154-7158

Prouty, A.M.; Schwesinger, W.H. & Gunn, J.S. (2002). Biofilm formation and interaction with the surfaces of gallstones by *Salmonella* spp.. *Infection and Immunity*, Vol.70, No.5, (January 2002), pp. 2640-2649

Remis, J.P.; Costerton, J.W. & Auer, M. (2010). Biofilms: structures that may facilitate cell-cell interactions. *ISME Journal*, Vol.4, No.9, (July 2010), pp. 1085-1087

Rickard, A.H.; Gilbert, P.; High, N.J.; Kolenbrander, P.E. & Handley, P.S. (2003). Bacterial coaggregation: an internal process in the development of multi-species biofilms. *Trends in Microbiology*, Vol.11, No.2, (February 2003), pp. 94-100

Rivas, L.; Dykes, G.A. & Fegan, N. (2006). Attachment of shiga toxigenic *Escherichia coli* to beef muscle and adipose tissue. *Journal of Food Protection*, Vol.69, No.5, (May 2006), pp. 999-1006

Rodrigues, D.; Teixeira, P.; Oliveira, R. & Azeredo, J. (2011). *Salmonella enterica* Enteritidis biofilm formation and viability on regular and triclosan-impregnated bench cover materials. *Journal of Food Protection*, Vol.74, No.1, (July 2010), pp. 32-37

Römling, U. (2005). Characterization of the rdar morphotype, a multicellular behaviour in Enterobacteriaceae. *Cellular and Molecular Life Sciences*, Vol.62, No.11, (June 2005), pp. 1234-1246

Römling, U.; Bian, Z.; Hammar, M.; Sierralta, W.D. & Normark, S. (1998a). Curli fibers are highly conserved between *Salmonella typhimurium* and *Escherichia coli* with respect to operon structure and regulation. *Journal of Bacteriology*, Vol.180, No.3, (February 1998), pp. 722-731

Römling, U.; Bokranz, W.; Rabsch, W.; Zogaj, X.; Nimtz, M. & Tschäpe, H. (2003). Occurrence and regulation of the multicellular morphotype in *Salmonella* serovars important in human disease. *International Journal of Medical Microbiology*, Vol.293, No.4, (August 2003), pp. 273-285

Römling, U. & Rohde, M. (1999). Flagella modulate the multicellular behavior of *Salmonella typhimurium* on the community level. *FEMS Microbiology Letters*, Vol.180, No.1, (November 1999), pp. 91-102

Römling, U.; Rohde, M.; Olsén, A.; Normark, S. & Reinköster, J. (2000). AgfD, the checkpoint of multicellular and aggregative behaviour in *Salmonella typhimurium* regulates at least two independent pathways. *Molecular Microbiology*, Vol.36, No.1, (April 2000), pp. 10-23

Römling, U.; Sierralta, W.D.; Eriksson, K. & Normark, S. (1998b). Multicellular and aggregative behaviour of *Salmonella typhimurium* strains is controlled by mutations in the *agfD* promoter. *Molecular Microbiology*, Vol.28, No.2, (April 1998), pp. 249-264

Ryan, R.P. & Dow, J.M. (2008). Diffusible signals and interspecies communication in bacteria. *Microbiology*, Vol.154(Pt 7), (July 2008), pp. 1845-1858

Sauer, K. (2003). The genomics and proteomics of biofilm formation. *Genome Biology*, Vol.4, No.6, (May 2003), 219

Schauder, S.; Shokat, K.; Surette, M.G. & Bassler, B.L. (2001). The LuxS family of bacterial autoinducers: biosynthesis of a novel quorum-sensing signal molecule. *Molecular Microbiology*, Vol.41, No.2, (July 2001), pp. 463-476

Scher, K., Romling, U. & Yaron, S. (2005). Effect of heat, acidification, and chlorination on *Salmonella enterica* serovar Typhimurium cells in a biofilm formed at the air-liquid interface. *Applied and Environmental Microbiology*, Vol.71, No.3, (September 2004), pp. 1163-1168

Sha, Q.; Gunathilake, A.; Forstner, M.R.J. & Hahn, D. (2011). Temporal analyses of the distribution and diversity of *Salmonella* in natural biofilms. *Systematic and Applied Microbiology*, Vol.34, No.5, (July 2011), pp. 353-359

Sharma, M. & Anand, S.K. (2002). Biofilms evaluation as an essential component of HACCP for food/dairy processing industry - a case. *Food Control*, Vol.13, (July 2001), pp. 469-477

Sharma, V.K.; Bearson, S.M. & Bearson, B.L. (2010). Evaluation of the effects of *sdiA*, a *luxR* homologue, on adherence and motility of *Escherichia coli* O157:H7. *Microbiology*, Vol.156(Pt5), (May 2010), pp. 1303-1312

Shemesh, M.; Tam, A. & Steinberg, D. (2007). Differential gene expression profiling of *Streptococcus mutants* cultured under biofilm and planktonic conditions. *Microbiology*, Vol.153, (May 2007), pp. 1307-1317

Shi, X. & Zhu, X. (2009). Biofilm formation and food safety in food industries. *Trends in Food Science and Technology*, Vol.20, No.9, (September 2009), pp. 407-413

Sinde, E. & Carballo, J. (2000). Attachment of *Salmonella* spp. and *Listeria monocytogenes* to stainless steel, rubber and polytetrafluorethylene: the influence of free energy and the effect of commercial sanitizers. *Food Microbiology*, Vol.17, pp. 439-447

Skandamis, P.N.; Stopforth, J.D.; Ashton, L.V.; Geornaras, I.; Kendall, P.A. & Sofos, J.N. (2009). *Escherichia coli* O157:H7 survival, biofilm formation and acid tolerance under simulated slaughter plant moist and dry conditions. *Food Microbiology*, Vol.26, No.1, (February 2009), pp. 112-119

Smith, J.N. & Ahmer, B.M. (2003). Detection of other microbial species by *Salmonella*: expression of the SdiA regulon. *Journal of Bacteriology*, Vol.185, No.4, (February 2003), pp. 1357-1366

Smith, J.L.; Fratamico, P.M. & Novak, J.S. (2004). Quorum sensing: a primer for food microbiologists. *Journal of Food Protection*, Vol.67, No.5, (May 2004), pp. 1053-1070

Soares, J.A. & Ahmer, B.M. (2011). Detection of acyl-homoserine lactones by *Escherichia* and *Salmonella*. *Current Opinion in Microbiology*, Vol.14, No.2, (April 2011), pp. 188-193

Solano, C.; García, B.; Valle, J.; Berasain, C.; Ghigo, J.M.; Gamazo. C. & Lasa, I. (2002). Genetic analysis of *Salmonella enteritidis* biofilm formation: critical role of cellulose. *Molecular Microbiology*, Vol.43, No.3, (February 2002), pp. 793-808

Solano, C.; Sesma, B.; Alvarez, M.; Humphrey, T.J.; Thorns, C.J. & Gamazo, C. (1998). Discrimination of strains of *Salmonella enteritidis* with differing levels of virulence by an in vitro glass adherence test. *Journal of Clinical Microbiology*, Vol.36, No.3, (March 1998), pp. 674-678

Solomon, E.B.; Niemira, B.A.; Sapers, G.M. & Annous, B.A. (2005). Biofilm formation, cellulose production, and curli biosynthesis by *Salmonella* originating from produce, animal, and clinical sources. *Journal of Food Protection*, Vol.68, No.5, (May 2005), pp. 906-912

Soni, K.A.; Jesudhasan, P.R.; Cepeda, M.; Williams, B.; Hume, M.; Russell, W.K.; Jayaraman, A. & Pillai, S.D. (2008). Autoinducer AI-2 is involved in regulating a variety of cellular processes in *Salmonella* Typhimurium. *Foodborne Pathogens and Disease*, Vol.5, No.2, pp. 147-153

Sperandio, V.; Torres, A.G. & Kaper, J.B. (2002). Quorum sensing *Escherichia coli* regulators B and C (QseBC): a novel two-component regulatory system involved in the regulation of flagella and motility by quorum sensing in *E. coli*. *Molecular Microbiology*, Vol.43, No.3, (February 2002), pp. 809-821

Stafford, G.P. & Hughes, C. (2007). *Salmonella typhimurium flhE*, a conserved flagellar regulon gene required for swarming. *Microbiology*, Vol.153(Pt2), (February 2007), pp. 541-547

Steenackers, H.; Hermans, K.; Vanderleyden, J. & De Keersmaecker, S.C.J. (2011). *Salmonella* biofilms: an overview on occurrence, structure, regulation and eradication. *Food Research International, in press*

Stepanović, S.; Cirković, I; Mijac, V. & Svabić-Vlahović, M. (2003). Influence of the incubation temperature, atmosphere and dynamic conditions on biofilm formation by *Salmonella* spp.. *Food Microbiology*, Vol.20, (September 2002), pp. 339-343

Stepanović, S.; Cirković, I; Ranin, L. & Svabić-Vlahović, M. (2004). Biofilm formation by *Salmonella* spp. and *Listeria monocytogenes* on plastic surface. *Letters in Applied Microbiology*, Vol.38, No.5, pp. 428-432

Stocki, S.L.; Annett, C.B.; Sibley, C.D.; McLaws, M.; Checkley, S.L.; Singh, N.; Surette, M.G. & White, A.P. (2007). Persistence of *Salmonella* on egg conveyor belts is dependent on the belt type but not on the rdar morphotype. *Poultry Science*, Vol.86, (July 2007), pp. 2375-2383

Stoodley, P.; Sauer, K.; Davies, D.G. & Costerton, J.W. (2002). Biofilms as complex differentiated communities. *Annual Review of Microbiology*, Vol.56, (January 2002), pp. 187-209

Taga, M.E.; Semmelhack, J.L. & Bassler, B.L. (2001). The LuxS-dependent autoinducer AI-2 controls the expression of an ABC transporter that functions in AI-2 uptake in *Salmonella typhimurium*. *Molecular Microbiology*, Vol.42, No.3, (November 2001), pp. 777-793

Tang, X.; Flint, S.H.; Bennett, R.J.; Brooks, J.D. & Morton, R.H. (2009). Biofilm growth of individual and dual strains of *Klebsiella oxytoca* from the dairy industry on ultrafiltration membranes. *Journal of Industrial Microbiology and Biotechnology*, Vol.36, No.12, (December 2009), pp. 1491-1497

Teplitski, M.; Al-Agely, A. & Ahmer, B.M. (2006). Contribution of the SirA regulon to biofilm formation in *Salmonella enterica* serovar Typhimurium. *Microbiology*, Vol.152 (Pt 11), (November 2006), pp. 3411-3424

Tolker-Nielsen, T. & Molin, S. (2000). Spatial organization of microbial biofilm communities. *Microbial Ecology*, Vol.40, No.2, (August 2000), pp. 75-84

Ukuku, D.O. & Fett, W.F. (2002). Relationship of cell surface charge and hydrophobicity to strength of attachment of bacteria to cantaloupe rind. *Journal of Food Protection*, Vol.65, No.7, (July 2002), pp. 1093-1099

Ukuku, D.O. & Fett, W.F. (2006). Effects of cell surface charge and hydrophobicity on attachment of 16 *Salmonella* serovars to cantaloupe rind and decontamination with sanitizers. *Journal of Food Protection*, Vol.69, No.8, (August 2006), pp. 1835-1843

Van Houdt, R. & Michiels, S.W. (2010). Biofilm formation and the food industry, a focus on the bacterial outer surface. *Journal of Applied Microbiology*, Vol.109, (April 2010), pp. 1117-1131

Verstraeten, N.; Braeken, K.; Debkumari, B.; Fauvart, M.; Fransaer, J.; Vermant, J. & Michiels, J. (2008). Living on a surface: swarming and biofilm formation. *Trends in Microbiology*, Vol.16, No.10, (October 2008), pp. 496-506

Vestby, L.K.; Møretrø, T.; Balance, S.; Langsrud, S. & Nesse, L.L. (2009a). Survival potential of wild type cellulose deficient *Salmonella* from the feed industry. *BMC Veterinary Research*, Vol.5:43 (November 2009)

Vestby, L.K.; Møretrø, T.; Langsrud, S.; Heir, E. & Nesse, L.L. (2009b). Biofilm forming abilities of *Salmonella* are correlated with persistence in fish meal- and feed factories. *BMC Veterinary Research*, Vol.5:20, (May 2009)

Walters, M. & Sperandio, V. (2006). Quorum sensing in *Escherichia coli* and *Salmonella*. *International Journal of Medical Microbiology*, Vol.296, pp. 125-131

White, A.P.; Gibson, D.L.; Collinson, S.K.; Banser, P.A. & Kay, W.W. (2003). Extracellular polysaccharides associated with thin aggregative fimbriae of *Salmonella enterica* serovar Enteritidis. *Journal of Bacteriology*, Vol.185, No.18, (September 2003), pp. 5398-5407

White, A.P.; Gibson, D.L.; Grassl, G.A.; Kay, W.W.; Finlay, B.B.; Vallance, B.A. & Surette, M,G. (2008). Aggregation via the red, dry, and rough morphotype is not a virulence adaptation in *Salmonella enterica* serovar Typhimurium. *Infection and Immunity*, Vol.76, No.3, (March 2008), pp. 1048-1058

White, A.P.; Gibson, D.L.; Kim, W.; Kay, W.W. & Surette, M.G. (2006). Thin aggregative fimbriae and cellulose enhance long-term survival and persistence of *Salmonella*. *Journal of Bacteriology*, Vol.188, No.9, (May 2006), pp. 3219-3227

White, A.P. & Surette, M.G. (2006). Comparative genetics of the rdar morphotype in *Salmonella*. *Journal of Bacteriology*, Vol.188, No.24, (December 2006), pp. 8395-8406

Whitehead, N.A.; Barnard, A.M.; Slater, H.; Simpson, N.J. & Salmond, G.P. (2001). Quorum-sensing in Gram-negative bacteria. *FEMS Microbiology Reviews*, Vol.25, No.4, (August 2001), pp. 365-404

Whiteley, M.; Bangera, M.G.; Bumgarner, R.E.; Parsek, M.R.; Teitzel, G.M.; Lory, S. & Greenberg, E.P. (2001). Gene expression in *Pseudomonas aeruginosa* biofilms. *Nature*, Vol.413, No.6858, (October 2001), pp. 860-864

Wimpenny, J. (2009). Microbial metropolis. *Advances in Microbial Physiology*, Vol.56, (November 2009), pp. 29-84

Wimpenny, J.; Manz, W. & Szewzyk, U. (2000). Heterogeneity in biofilms. *FEMS Microbiology Reviews*, Vol.24, No.5, (December 2000), pp. 661-671

Wuertz, S.; Okabe, S. & Hausner, M. (2004). Microbial communities and their interactions in biofilm systems: an overview. *Water Science and Technology*, Vol.49, No.11-12, pp. 327-336

Yoon, Y. & Sofos, J.N. (2008). Autoinducer-2 activity of Gram-negative foodborne pathogenic bacteria and its influence on biofilm formation. *Journal of Food Science*, Vol.73, No.3, (January 2008), pp. M140-M147

Zhao, T.; Podtburg, T.C.; Zhao, P.; Schmidt, B.E.; Baker, D.A.; Cords, B. & Doyle, M.P. (2006). Control of *Listeria* spp. by competitive-exclusion bacteria in floor drains of a poultry processing plant. *Applied and Environmental Microbiology*, Vol.72, No.5, (May 2006), pp. 3314-3320

Zogaj, X.; Nimtz, M.; Rohde, M.; Bokranz, W. & Römling, U. (2001). The multicellular morphotypes of *Salmonella typhimurium* and *Escherichia coli* produce cellulose as the second component of the extracellular matrix. *Molecular Microbiology*, Vol.39, No.6, (March 2001), pp. 1452-1463

Zottola, E.A. & Sasahara, K.C. (1994). Microbial biofilms in the food processing industry – Should they be a concern? *International Journal of Food Microbiology*, Vol.23, (February 1994), pp. 125-148

# 9

# Important Aspects of Salmonella in the Poultry Industry and in Public Health

Eliana N. Castiglioni Tessari[1], Ana Maria Iba Kanashiro[1], Greice F. Z. Stoppa[1], Renato L. Luciano[1], Antonio Guilherme M. De Castro[1] and Ana Lucia S. P. Cardoso[1]
[1]*Biological Institute - Advanced Technological Research Center of the Poultry Agribusiness - Agriculture Secretariat of the State of Sao Paulo, Descalvado/SP Brazil*

## 1. Introduction

The objective of this review was to discuss relevant issues related to the pathogeny, epidemiology and antimicrobial resistance of *Salmonella* spp. Due to its economic importance, and because it poses risks to human health, *Salmonella* spp. is one of the most frequently studied enteropathogens. Nowadays, the disease is considered to be a consequence of interrelated factors, such as food, the environment, vectors, men, utensils and equipments, the production line, animal transit and animal reservoirs.

## 2. General aspects

*Salmonellae* are widely distributed in nature. The main reservoir of these bacteria is the intestinal tract of men and warm-and cold-blooded animals (Jakabi et al., 1999), except for fish, mollusks and crustaceans, which may get contaminated after being fished. Among warm-blooded animals, chickens, geese, turkeys and ducks are the most important reservoirs. Domestic animals, such as dogs, cats, turtles and birds may be carriers, and pose great risk, mainly to kids (Franco & Landgraf, 1996).
The natural habitat of *Salmonella* may be divided into three categories based on the specificity of the host and clinical pattern of the disease: highly adapted to men: *Salmonella* Typhi and *Salmonella* Paratyphi A, B and C, agents of typhoid fever; highly adapted to animals: *Salmonella* Dublin (bovines), *Salmonella* Choleraesuis and *Salmonella* Typhisuis (swine), *Salmonella* Pullorum and *Salmonella* Gallinarum (birds), responsible for animal paratyphoid. The third category includes most of the serovars that affect men and animals, called zoonotic *Salmonella*, responsible for worldwide-distributed foodborne diseases, and detected in most species of animals used for human consumption, wild and domestic animals (Gantois et al., 2009).
*Salmonellae* are short bacilli, 0.7-1.5 x 2.5 μm, Gram-negative, aerobic or facultative anaerobic, positive catalase, negative oxidase; they ferment sugars with gas production, produce $H_2S$, are nonsporogenic, and are normally motile with peritricheal flagella, except for *Salmonella* Pullorum and *Salmonella* Gallinarum, which are nonmotile (Forshell & Wierup, 2006).

Optimal pH for multiplication is around 7.0; pH values above 9.0 or below 4.0 are bactericidal. Ideal temperature is between 35 to 37°C, with minimum of 5°C and maximum of 47°C. As for salt concentration, *Salmonellae* do not survive concentrations over 9% (Franco & Landgraf, 1996).

The first bacteria in the genus *Salmonella* were identified towards the end of the 19th century. *Salmonella* Typhy, the first to be recognized as a pathogen, was found in spleen and lymph nodes of humans in 1880. However, isolation and morphological description were only carried out by Gaffky, in 1884.

In 1885, Salmon and Smith isolated a bacillus from diseased pigs, and called it *Bacterium* Suipestifer. They wrongly considered it the agent of swine fever. This bacterium was later on called *Salmonella* Cholerasuis. In 1888, there was a report on *Salmonella* Enteritidis by Gaetner; in 1889, Klein identified fowl typhoid in adult birds in England, and in 1892, Loefer isolated *Salmonella* Typhimurium. In 1899, Rettger described pulorosis and differentiated it from the disease that affected pigs. In 1913, Jones used an agglutination test to identify carriers of *Salmonella* Pullorum (Correa & Correa, 1992).

The genus *Salmonella* started to be classified in 1925, with the use of serological methods. *Salmonella* Typhimurium, created by Loeffler (1892), and *Salmonella* Paratyphi, created by Schottimuller (1899), were included in the genus. Later on, several *Salmonella* serotypes were described, and classified according to White (1829) (Correa & Correa, 1992). Popoff et al. (1996) presented a proposal for the reclassification of the genus *Salmonella*, which would have two species: *Salmonella enterica* and *Salmonella bongori.*

In the current classification of the Bergey's manual, all *Salmonella* serotypes belong to one of two species: *Salmonella bongori*, which has at least 10 extremely rare serotypes; and *Salmonella enterica*, which is phenotypically and genotypically divided into six subspecies *enterica, salamae, arizonae, diarizonae, houtenae* and *indica*, differentiated by their biochemical behavior, mainly in terms of sugar and amino acid metabolism (Forshell & Wierup, 2006).

In the current nomenclature, the name of the serovar begins with an uppercase letter, but it is never written in italics. For example in subspecies enterica: *Salmonella enterica* subespecies *enterica* serovar Typhimurium. The short form would be *Salmonella* ser. Typhimurium or *Salmonella* Typhimurium. Other subspecies are designated by the name of the serovar, followed by its antigenic formula, explained below.

Typification of *Salmonella* spp. serovars is based on the antigens found in bacterial cells, somatic (O), flagellar (H) and capsular (Vi) (Selander et al., 1996). Vi antigen is associated with virulence, and is only expressed by serovars Typhi, Paratyphi C and Dublin (Rycroft, 2000; Grimont et al., 2000). H antigen is thermolabile, whereas O and Vi are thermoresistant, and not destroyed by heating at 100°C for two hours (Franco & Landgraf, 1996). The combination of the antigens O, H1 (flagellar, phase 1) and H2 (flagellar, phase 2) determine the antigenic formula of a serovar. O antigens receive Arabic numerals, whereas H1 antigens are identified by lowercase letters, and H2 antigens by Arabic numerals. For example, *Salmonella* enterica subsp salamae ser. 50: z : e,n,x, or *Salmonella* serotype II 50: z : e,n,x.

Somatic (O) and flagellar (H) antigens, determine different serovars in each subspecies, in a total of 2,610 serovars today, as recognized by Kauffman-White scheme (Grimont & Weill, 2007). Although all of them are considered to be potentially pathogenic to men, only 200 are more frequently related with human disease (Baird-Parker, 1990). Distribution according to species and subspecies is as follows: *Salmonella* enterica subsp. enterica (1,547 serovars); *Salmonella enterica* subsp salamae (513); *Salmonella enterica* subsp arizonae (100); *Salmonella enterica* subsp diarizonae (341); *Salmonella enterica* subsp houtenae (73); *Salmonella* enterica subsp. indica (13); *Salmonella* bongori (23); the newly proposed species *Salmonella* subterranea was not recognized, and is considered a serovar of the bongori species (Rodrigues, 2011).

Serovars may be further subdivided into biotypes and phagotypes. Biotyping uses different sugar fermentation patterns and assimilation of amino acids among strains of the same serovar, whereas phagotyping is based on the difference in strain susceptibility to a series of bacteriophages (Ward et al., 1987; Grimont et al., 2000; Dunkley et al., 2009).

As for their antigenic profile, *Salmonella* has an antigen common to all species in the Enterobacteriaceae family, called Kunin antigen. The presence of this antigen is not routinely analyzed, once it is not a relevant criterion for the differentiation between genus and species.

Some serovars produce a superficial polysaccharide, or capsular antigen, called "Vi". It is found outside the cell wall, and prevents detection of the somatic antigen. It is usually found in strains of *Salmonella* Typhi, *Salmonella* Paratyphi C and *Salmonella* Dublin. Vi antigens are thermolabile, and may be destroyed by heating at 100°C for 10-15 minutes.

The somatic antigen, or "O" (Ohne), on the other hand, is specific. It is a lipopolysaccharide, and is resistant to heat and alcohol. It is made up of three parts: a lipid portion, responsible for toxicity and pyrogenic characteristics; a core portion; and the polysaccharide, which confers stability to smooth (S) variants. The "O" antigen is made up of repetitive chains with a definite spatial arrangement. The specificity of "O" antigen is given by this definite nature and the type of bond. The synthesis of this antigen is encoded by about 20 genes (locus rfb).

Many somatic antigen factors (67) are recognized and used in the serological identification of *Salmonella*. Although these factors are intimately related, they are not always antigenically identical, and can only be characterized when strains are in the smooth phase. In this phase, colonies show homogenous, shiny surfaces, with regular borders, indicative of the complete "O" antigen. Mutations that affect the core portion of the antigen, or the synthesis of its chain, lead to loss of specificity. In this case, strains are called Rough (R), colonies have irregular borders and surfaces, and it is impossible to recover or recognize their original characteristics. They agglutinate in saline solution, are easily phagocyted, and are sensitive to the action of the complement system. Agglutination of bacterial cells (somatic or "O" antigen) using polyclonal (±7) and specific (65) antisera, which is the laboratory procedure for antigen confirmation, is slow and may form fine granules that are not dissociable by stirring. This occurs because the reaction is based on an interrelationship between the walls of the bacterial cells.

Flagellar antigens, or "H" (Hauch) antigens, are made of a protein called flagellin. Antigenic differences are related to variations in the primary structure or amino acid content of different flagellin molecules. The "H" antigen is thermolabile, may be destroyed at 100°C for 10 minutes, and by slow action of alcohol 50%; but it is resistant to formaldehyde 0.5%. Agglutination of flagellar antigen forms large clumps that are quickly dissociated by stirring. Compared with somatic agglutination, it occurs faster due to the large number of flagella in the cell, and because bacterial cells bind to each other.

Spatial arrangement and intrinsic characteristics of the genus lead to the production of two different types of flagella. In a bacterial population of *Salmonella* spp. strains that produce two different types of flagella, the rate of cell variation among those that present one of the two types or phases is about $10^4$. In most *Salmonella* isolates, two genes encode flagellar antigens: fliC (>50 different alleles), with highly conserved terminal sequences in the genus and which encodes phase 1 antigens; and fljB (±30 alleles), also conserved in the genus,

which encodes phase 2 antigens. These genes are expressed by a phase-variation mechanism, with fliC being found in all *Salmonellae,* and having a homologous gene found in *E. coli;* whereas fljB is located in a region exclusive to the *Salmonella* genome, and is found in four of the six subspecies. In some cases, triphasic strains may be isolated. Besides the other two genes, it was described that these strains presented the flagellin gene (flpA) in a plasmid. The genes that encode flagellin in *Salmonella* spp. are generally highly conserved in extremities 5′ and 3′, whereas the central region is highly variable.
In practical conditions, rapid agglutination with polyclonal antisera (12 polivalent and 85 monovalent antisera) may frequently occur in the absence of expression of one of the phases, preventing the identification of the serovar. This may happen in some serovars, when cell subpopulations, each possessing a given antigen or set of antigens associated with their flagella, are able to produce a third or fourth type of flagellum. Identification, in these cases, requires "immobilization" of one of the phases, in order to characterize the unknown phase, a technique called "phase inversion". When the phase is not recognized, the serovar will not be conclusively diagnosed, preventing effective control actions. However, considering the complexity of flagellar antigens, if not all monovalent antisera are used, results on antigenic structure may be incorrect, such as g,m; g,t; g,p; g,q; g,p,s; g,z61; m,t.

## 3. Salmonellosis and public health

Growth in international trade and current facilities for traveling increased not only the dissemination of pathogenic agents and contaminants in foodstuffs, but also our vulnerability. Nowadays, the world is interrelated and interdependent. Thus, local foodborne disease outbreaks have become a potential threat for the whole world. Globalization, commercialization and distribution make it possible for a contaminated foodstuff to affect the health of people in several countries at the same time. The identification of only one contaminated food ingredient may lead to the discard of literally tons of food; to considerable economic losses to the production sector; restrictions to trade; and effects on the tourism industry (Tauxe et al., 2010).
Therefore, there is an ever growing perception of the need and importance for surveillance systems and adoption of measures to ensure food safety, such as the identification of the foods involved in foodborne disease outbreaks. In 1992, the National Surveillance scheme for general Outbreaks of Infectious Intestinal Disease was introduced in England and Wales to provide comprehensive information on causative agents, sources, vehicles of infection and modes of transmission (Oliveira et al., 2010).
*Salmonella* spp. is an intestinal bacterium responsible for severe foodborne intoxications. It is one of the most important agents involved in outbreaks reported in several counties (Tessari et al., 2003). Salmonellosis is an important socioeconomic problem in several counties, mainly in developing countries, where this etiological agent is reported as the main responsible for foodborne disease outbreaks (Alves et al., 2001). There are reports of foodborne salmonellosis in humans since the $19^{th}$ century, caused by the ingestion of contaminated bovine meat (Barrow, 1993). It is one of the most problematic zoonosis in terms of public health all over the world because of the high endemicity, but mainly because of the difficulty in controlling it (Antunes et al., 2003, Santos et al., 2002), and the significant morbidity and mortality rates (Cardoso et al., 2002).

According to the World Health Organization (WHO), *Salmonella* is the bacterial agent most frequently involved in cases of foodborne disease all over the world. The agent is normally transmitted to humans by means of foods of animal origin, such as meat, eggs and milk (Nascimento et al., 2003). In the past, the main motivations for controlling *Salmonella* spp. infections in poultry were the losses caused by clinical (pullorum disease and fowl typhoid) and subclinical diseases (paratyphoid infections) (Calnek, 1997). Nowadays, due to the public health implications, prevention of foodborne transmission of *Salmonella* spp. is a priority for the poultry sector (Oliveira & Silva, 2000).

Historically, *Salmonella* Typhimurium was the most common agent of the foodborne disease in humans, although in the past decades *Salmonella* Enteritidis has been most frequently involved in salmonellosis outbreaks (Berchieri Jr. & Freitas Neto 2009; Kottwitz, et al., 2010). There is a growing concern about human infections caused by other serovars, such as Infantis, Agona, Hadar, Heidelberg and Virchow (Freitas Neto et al., 2010).

Concerns about the presence of *Salmonella* spp. in foodstuffs of poultry origin increased in the 1980s, when *Salmonella* Enteritidis phagotype 4 was responsible for several outbreaks of foodborne disease in England, caused by the ingestion of foods containing poultry ingredients (Colin, 1996; Baxter-Jones, 1996). The vertical transmission of *Salmonella* Enteritidis in commercial poultry was responsible for the increased number of cases of human infection in Europe, North America and other parts of the world (Humphrey et al., 1988; International Commission for Microbiological Safety of Foods (ICMSF), 1998). These species replaced *Salmonella* Typhimurium, which was the most common agent of human foodborne infection until the 1980s (Olsen et al., 2003; Jay, 2000).

The introduction of *Salmonella* Enteritidis in Brazil probably occurred in the end of the 1980s, by means of breeders acquired from European countries. This may have also facilitated the introduction and dissemination of phatogotype PT-4 beginning in 1993 (Irino et al., 1996), the predominant phagotype in Europe at this time (Wall & Ward, 1999).

In the 1990s, there were several reports of foodborne disease outbreaks in humans mainly caused by the ingestion of poultry products (Taunay et al., 1996). Between 1995 and 2011, there were 406 reported outbreaks and 16,304 cases of salmonellosis in Brazil, Chile, Argentina, Peru, Uruguay, Paraguay and Ecuador (Franco et al., 2003).

According to the National Health Surveillance Agency in Brazil [ANVISA; *Agência Nacional de Vigilância Sanitária*], among the etiological agents of foodborne diseases identified between 1999 and 2004, *Salmonella* spp. was the most prevalent in Brazil, with the predominance of *Salmonella* Enteritidis between 2001 and august 2005 (Rodrigues, 2005).

According to the WHO, *Salmonella* is one of the pathogens that causes the greatest impact on population health, and is associated with outbreaks and with sporadic cases of foodborne disease. According to data of the Brazilian Ministry of Health, 6,602 foodborne disease outbreaks were recorded between 1999 and 2008, and *Salmonella* spp. was associated with 43% of the cases in which the etiological agent was identified (Medeiros, 2011).

In the European Union, *Salmonella* Enteritidis, *Salmonella* Typhimurium, *Salmonella* Infantis, *Salmonella* Hadar and *Salmonella* Virchow are considered by the European Food Safety Authority the most important serovars in terms of public health (EFSA, 2007). In Japan, between 1999 and 2002, 32% of the cases of foodborne infection were due to *Salmonella*, with Enteritidis, Typhimurium and Infantis as the predominant serovars. In 2005, in the US, the serovars that were most frequently isolated from human sources were *Salmonella* Typhimurium, *Salmonella* Enteritidis, *Salmonella* Newport, *Salmonella* Heidelberg and *Salmonella* Javiana (Centers For Diseases Control and Prevention - CDC, 2007).

In Denmark, *Salmonella* Infantis was isolated from samples of pork, which was pointed out as the source human infection (Wegener & Baggesen, 1996). In several industrialized countries, cases of human infection caused by this serovar have been described (Raevuori et al., 1978; Pelkonen et al., 1994). In Finland, *Salmonella* Infantis was described as the third most important serovar; it infects humans, and it is the most frequently isolated serovar in poultry (Pelkonen et al., 1994). In Hungary, the rate of occurrence of *Salmonella* Infantis has increased in the past years both in the poultry industry and in humans (Nógrády et al., 2008).

National and international regulations determine the absence of *Salmonella* spp. in 25 grams of sample, including poultry meat and eggs. In spite the technological development in food production and the adoption of better hygiene measures in the food production and handling, the incidence of human salmonellosis has increased in several parts of the world (Anais de Toxiinfecção Alimentar, 1996).

In the US, there are more than 800,000 notified cases of infections caused by *Salmonella* spp., with an average of 500 deaths a year. Worldwide occurrence of salmonellosis is calculated in 1.3 billion cases and 3 million deaths (Thong et al, 1995). In 1988, there were 4 million cases of foodborne disease in the US and Canada, representing an estimated cost of US$ 4.8 billion, including losses in commercialization, productivity and labor (Todd, 1989). In a five-year period (1985-1989), there were 189 outbreaks in the US caused only by *Salmonella* Enteritidis, with 6,604 people involved, and 43 deaths.

Salmonellosis epidemiology and control are highly complex, and hygienic and sanitary standards vary with the region, based on feeding and cooking habits, and animal raising practices. Control of the disease is a challenge to public health because of the emergence/reemergence of serovars in different areas, both in developing and developed countries.

Carriers are the most important epidemiological factors, because of the lack of symptoms, and the technical difficulty in detecting them before or during the inspection of foods of animal origin. Considering that the main route of transmission is in the food chain, the presence of this microorganism in production animals shows that *Salmonella* is the most incident and relevant etiological agent of intestinal infections. It causes million of dollars in losses to the industry, mainly in cattle, swine and poultry production, both in local and international trade. In some countries, rigid food inspection is a constant need to produce foodstuffs of high quality.

Besides the importance of preventive measures against the risk of *Salmonella* infection in humans, control of salmonellosis has a positive economic impact in countries where outbreaks occur. Estimated costs of medical expenses, sick leaves and loss of productivity related to the high incidence of salmonellosis in the US range from US$1.3 to US$4.0 billion a year (Taitt et al., 2004).

As for fowl salmonellosis, paratyphoid *Salmonellae* are the most important ones in terms of animal and public health (Nascimento et al., 1997). These microorganisms remain in the intestinal tract of the birds, making poultry a possible source of foodborne infection for humans (Berchieri Jr., 1991). Transmission of *Salmonella* to men generally occurs by means of contaminated food and water, although person-to-person transmission may take place, mainly in hospitals. Transmission by contact with infected animals, mainly among veterinarians and farm workers (Trabulsi & Landgraf, 2004), is also possible. It should be emphasized that most serotypes in this genus are pathogenic to men; the differences observed in symptoms may be related to variation in the mechanisms of pathogenicity, age and immune response of the host (Trabulsi & Landgraf, 2004; Hofer et al., 1997).

A large number of *Salmonellae* have to be ingested to cause gastroenteritis. Generally, the infective dose depends on the serotype, ranging from $2.0x10^2$ to $1.0x10^6$ CFU/g or mL (Huang, 1999). Variation in the symptoms is also related to the type of food and the species of *Salmonella* involved, once species that are adapted to men require lower infective doses to cause the same characteristics symptoms of the disease (Pinto et al., 2004).

*Salmonella* excretion in human and/or animal feces may contaminate the water, soil, other animals and foodstuffs. Animals are infected by direct contact with feces, contaminated water and food (Argôlo Filho, 2007). Because of the ability to disseminate and survive for a long period of time in the environment, *Salmonella* may be isolated from superficial freshwater bodies, from sea water in coastal areas, and from several raw materials used in food production (Jakabi et al., 1999).

According to Nascimento (1996), contamination of poultry products (meat and eggs) destined for human consumption may occur at the slaughterhouse, during food preparation, or by cross-contamination with material from poultry with intestinal and systemic infections. As for poultry meat, even a small number of infected birds may contaminate the whole slaughter line, multiplying the chances of occurrence of foodborne disease. Because of that, slaughterhouses where carcasses are not correctly processed are a threat to public health (Nascimento, 1996); current practices of broiler slaughtering and processing may spread microorganisms from one carcass to another. When consumed, the product may be responsible for human infection (Santos, 2004). Although broiler carcasses may be contaminated with *Salmonella* Enteritidis, eggs and egg by-products - mainly homemade mayonnaise – are the main products responsible for outbreaks of the disease in humans (Silva, 2000).

Transmission of *Salmonella* in birds may occur vertically, via eggs, with the birth of infected chicks; horizontally, by means of ingestion of water, feed, fecal material, contaminated bedding material or dust; or by oral, nasal, conjunctival, cloacal and umbilical routes (Cox et al., 1996; Navarro, 1995; Nascimento, 1996). Many *Salmonella* serotypes may survive for weeks or months in manure or bedding material, in equipments, in empty sheds, in the dirt around sheds that have been cleaned and disinfected, in feces of wild poultry, in dust particles, and in bird feeders. According to these authors, *Salmonella* may survive in contaminated feed for 26 months, in feces of infected birds for more than 11 days when inside of sheds, or for 9 days in open spaces. Besides, domestic and wild animals may be carriers of *Salmonella*, spreading the microorganism in the environment where they live. These bacteria may cause acute and/or chronic disease in susceptible animals. As stated before, the epidemiological complexity of the disease, which involves vertical transmission, fecal excretion, horizontal transmission, environmental contamination and presence of carriers in different species, make salmonellosis control difficult to be achieved (Soncini & Back, 2001).

*Salmonellae* are distributed all over the world. Multiplication outside the body of the host is facilitated by high temperatures and presence of protein (for example, in residual waters). Therefore, the most important points of transmission of *Salmonella* are tropical and subtropical regions, as well as places where there is a large concentration of animals and people. *Salmonella* may also be found in products refrigerated at 2°C; the microorganism is able to remain viable in frozen products for long periods.

After entering the digestive system together with contaminated food and water, *Salmonellae* reach the intestines, where they attach to intestinal cells and multiply. Depending on the host species and age, and on the pathogenicity of the microorganism and its adaptation to the host, *Salmonellae* may cause severe disease, or go unnoticed and remain in the host for months or years. In this case, the host will be a reservoir of the bacteria for susceptible animals.

The most common symptoms include diarrhea, abdominal pain, vomit and nausea, and may occur together with prostration, muscle pain, drowsiness and fever. Although symptoms generally disappear after 5 days, the microorganisms may be excreted in the feces for many weeks (Jay, 1992). Children, mainly those younger than 1 year of age, elderly and immunocompromised patients are much more susceptible to the disease, and may present more severe infections, such as sepsis, which may lead to death (Gomez & Cleary, 1998; Pinto et al., 2004)

Salmonellosis is not limited to intestinal infection and gastroenterocolitis. The microorganism may infect other organs; as *Salmonellae* are able to reach the circulation, they may cause diffuse extraintestinal infections, such as meningitis, osteomyelitis, arthritis, pneumonia, cholecystitis, peritonitis, pyelonephritis, cystitis, endocarditis, pericarditis, vasculitis and other disorders (Gelli, 1995).

*Salmonellae* cross the intestinal epithelium, and reach the *lamina propria* (the layer where epithelial cells are anchored), where they multiply. They are phagocyted by macrophages and monocytes, causing an inflammatory response as a consequence of the hyperactivity of the reticuloendothelial system. Different from what happens in typhoid fever, penetration of *Salmonella* spp. is limited to the *lamina propria* in cases of enterocolitis. In these cases, sepsis or systemic infection are rarely observed, and infection is restricted to the intestinal mucous membrane. Inflammatory response is also related to the release of prostraglandins, which stimulate adenylate cyclase, leading to increased secretion of water and electrolytes and aqueous diarrhea (Franco & Landgraf, 2004).

From 1980 on, human outbreaks caused by *Salmonella* Enteritidis, showed common sources in the US, Great Britain and other European countries (CDC, 2005). Epidemiological surveys from the CDC identified the consumption of eggs or egg-based foods as responsible for most of the outbreaks involving specific phagotypes (PT) of *Salmonella* Enteritidis; PT-4 in European countries, and PT-8 and PT-13a in the US (Perales & Audicana, 1989). The predominant serotypes involved in foodborne diseases changed, in the past decades, from *Salmonella* Agona, *Salmonella* Hadar and *Salmonella* Typhimurium to *Salmonella* Enteritidis, which is the predominant cause of salmonellosis in several countries (Suresh et al., 2006). Changes in the predominance of serotypes reflect changes in animal raising practices and dissemination of new serotypes due to increased international trade. Nowadays, the main concern is the emergence of *Salmonella* serotypes that are resistant to multiple antibiotics (Huang, 1999).

Cases of disease caused by four serovars of subspecies *enterica* are subject to mandatory reporting, according to regulation number 207 of the Brazilian Agency of Agricultural Defense [SDA; *Secretaria da Defesa Agropecuária*] , reviewed in July 30$^{th}$, 1995. These serovars are part of the list B of the World Organization for Animal Health (OIE), of diseases that cause regional economic losses. Among them, *Salmonella* Pullorum, Gallinarum, Typhimurium and Enteritidis. About 90 serovars of *Salmonella* spp. are more frequent in cases of human and animal infection (Berchieri Jr. & Freitas Neto, 2009).

The typification of serovars is important to track the source of infection. For example, *Salmonella* Agona affected humans in the US, in European countries and in Brazil (Synnott et al., 1998; CDC, 2007). According to Clark et al. (1973), human outbreaks in the US and Europe that occurred around 1970 were caused by poultry meat. Animals were infected by feed containing contaminated fish meal that came from Peru. This case is an example of the epidemiological complexity of this disease.

The intensive breeding system adopted by the poultry industry favors the introduction, establishment, permanence and dissemination of these bacteria (Berchieri Jr. & Freitas Neto, 2009). Therefore, the stage when animals are raised is very important in the dissemination of *Salmonella* spp. among the birds, and consequently, in giving rise to contaminated food products (Bersot, 2006). *Salmonella* may affect all segments of poultry production, such as breeder facilities, incubators, commercial raising operations, feed factories, slaughterhouses, transportation systems and commercialization facilities.

Globalization incorporated the sanitary restrictions imposed by the European Community to international traders of foods of animal origin, mainly poultry. The occurrence of cases of foodborne infection linked to *Salmonella* Enteritidis and *Salmonella* Typhimurium show the sanitary importance of Brazilian poultry production, in social and economic terms. When the World Trade Organization (WTO) was created, the guidelines and Codex Alimentarius regulations were determined for international trade, and for agreements on sanitary and phytosanitary (SPS) measures and technical barriers to trade (TBT). With these agreements, WTO country members should review, establish and implement internal control systems, that is, adopt the Hazard Analysis and Critical Control Points System (HACCP).

## 4. Detection methods

*Salmonellae* are short Gram-negative bacilli, about 0.7-1.5 x 2-5 µm, readily stained, and nonsporulating. Most of them move using peritrichial flagella, although serotypes such as *Salmonella* Pullorum and *Salmonella* Gallinarum are nonmotile. They are either aerobic or facultative anaerobic, and grow between 5 and 45°C. Optimum growth occurs at 37°C. Ideal pH for multiplication is 7, but *Salmonella* survives in pH values between 4 and 9. They grow in culture medium for enterobacteria and in blood agar. Colonies are 2-4 mm in diameter, with smooth and round edges. They are slightly raised in medium containing carbon and nitrogen. Colonies may remain viable for a long time when stored in peptone (Holt et al., 1994; Gast, 1997).

Biochemically, *Salmonella* strains have the ability to metabolize nutrients, and catabolize D-glucose and other carbohydrates, except lactose and sucrose, with production of acid and gas. They are catalase positive and oxidase negative, as are all genera in the *Enterobacteriaceae* family. They do not ferment malonate, do not hydrolyze urea, do not produce indol, use citrate as a sole source of carbon, reduce nitrate to nitrite, and may produce hydrogen sulfide (Quinn et al., 2000).

Conventional culture methods for isolating *Salmonella* spp. in poultry or animal feed or in feed ingredients have been reported in a number of studies, which were summarized by Williams (1981). Although all methods follow the basic strategy of preenrichment followed by selective enrichment, differential plating and biochemical or serological confirmation, there is no single internationally accepted procedure for *Salmonella* spp. detection.

The Food and Drug Administration (FDA), for example, recommends lactose broth for preenrichment (Andrews el al. 1998), while Wyatt et al. (1993) used buffered peptone water. Cox et al. (1982) reported that preenrichment decreased the recovery of *Salmonella* spp. from artificially contaminated poultry feed when compared with direct enrichment. Suggested protocols also vary with the substrate: Kafel (1981) suggested the use of anaerobic lactose broth, followed by selection in tetrathionate brilliant green broth and plating on brilliant green agar, in the analysis of fish meal. Allen et al. (1991) reported that the sensitivity of Rappaport Vassiliadis medium depended on the substrate in the detection of *Salmonella* spp. in high moisture foods, compared with tetrathionate or selenite cystine broth. Eckner et al. (1992) added novobiocin to tetrathionate selective enrichment and increased the incubation temperature to 42°C.

The conventional technique for the detection of the microorganism includes the following steps: preenrichment, selective enrichment, isolation and selection, biochemical characterization, serological characterization and final identification. This technique requires at least four days for a negative result and six to seven days for the identification and confirmation of positive samples (Soumet et al., 1997). The presence of *Salmonella* has to be determined in at least 25g or mL of sample.

New methodologies, such as immunological tests, have been proposed as alternatives for direct detection of this pathogen. For example, ELISA (Enzyme-linked Immunosorbent Assay) was used by Loguercio et al. (2002). Immunoenzymatic technology may be combined with other rapid methods in order to decrease total assay time. Luk et al. (1997) combined a digoxigenin-based ELISA with the polymerase chain reaction (PCR) to detect amplified *rfb*S, a lipopolysaccharide gene of *Salmonella* spp.; in this case, preenrichment was no longer than 16 hours.

Other types of assays have also been used: techniques based on molecular biology, such as nucleic acid hybridization or PCR, which was used by Flôres et al. (2003); and tests based on metabolism measurements (impedance and radiometry) (Franco & Landgraf, 1996). Ribotyping is the most recent addition to the automated identification of bacteria.

The RiboPrinter™ Microbial Characterization System is based on the highly conserved nature of the rRNA operon. Ribotyping provides a reproducible method by which rRNA and polymorphic fragments can be compared with a database for identification of genus, species and strain (Grimont & Grimont, 1986). The system is almost completely automated, requiring only picking up the colonies, suspending them in buffer and submitting them to heat treatment in a special carrier. Once heated, the sample is placed in the device, which automatically lyses the bacteria, releasing DNA; digests it with restriction enzymes; transfers the sample to agarose gel; and separates restricted fragments by electrophoresis. DNA fragments separated by size are then transferred to a nylon membrane, which is hybridized with a chemically-labeled and treated DNA antibody/alkaline phosphatase conjugate.

Resulting stained bands are then photographed, and the image is stored in the computer database and compared with other images in it. The database for this system is less comprehensive than that of other automated systems, but it still adequate for *Salmonella* spp. The system would, however, be invaluable in epidemiological studies related to (HACCP) incidents.

Serotyping is an important epidemiological tool that complements the identification of *Salmonella*, making it possible to determine the prevalence/emergence or to show trends of a given serovar in different geographical regions, as well as to identify outbreaks, and discover sources of infection and routes of transmission. Serotyping is based on the Kauffmann & White classification and involves the identification of somatic and flagellar antigens.

The somatic structure is identified based on the recognition of the serovars, which are represented by uppercase letters. For example, group A (O:2), group B (O:4); group C1 (O:6,7), group C2 (O:6,8,20), group D (O:9), group E1 (O:3,10), group E2 (O:3,15), group E4 (O:1,3,19), etc. Some factors identify the antigenic group, for example, O:4, O:9. Other factors have little or no discriminatory value, and are normally associated because they represent a complex, such as O:12 (121, 122, 123), with O:2, O:4 and O:9. For example, *Salmonella* Paratyphi A (O:1,2,12), *Salmonella* Typhimurium (O:1,4,5,12) and *Salmonella* Enteritidis (O:1,9,12).

Some antigens appear as a consequence of a change in the structure, such as O:1, which is a result of the insertion of galactose in the polysaccharide; O:5 a results of the acetylation of abequose, found in the repetitive units of the polysaccharide responsible for specificity, such as in serovar *Salmonella* Typhimurium O:4,12 and O:1,4,5,12.

As for the characterization of flagellar antigens, it should be taken into account the fact that some *Salmonella* serovars have only one flagellar phase. They are called monophasic: *Salmonella* Enteritidis (9,12: g,m:-), *Salmonella* Typhi (9,12 [Vi]:d:-); however, most serogroups show two flagellar phases, that is, they are diphasic strains, such as *Salmonella* Typhimurium (1,4,5,12: i: 1,2) and *Salmonella* Hadar (6,8: z10: e,n,x), which express phase 1 (antigens i or z10) and phase 2 antigens (respectively, antigens 1,2 or e,n,x). Nonmotile strains, which have no flagella, have also been recognized (Rodrigues, 2011).

## 5. Drug resistance

Microbial resistance is related to strains of microorganisms that are able to multiply in the presence of concentrations of antimicrobial compounds even higher than those given as therapeutic doses to humans. Development of resistance is a natural phenomenon that followed the introduction of antimicrobial agents in clinical practice. The irrational and widespread use of these agents has added to the problem, and resistance rates vary from place to place, depending on the local use of antibiotics.

One of the major concerns of the poultry industry is maintaining the sanitary status of the herds. In the incubators where birds are born, there is an attempt to reduce contamination to minimum levels in all phases of the process. Lack of contact with natural biota soon after birth interferes with the normal development of bird intestines (Silva, 2000). Generally, antimicrobial substances (antibiotic or chemotherapic agents), called growth promoters, are used in the feed from the first day of life to the moment of slaughter of the birds, respecting the recommended withdrawal period (Mota, 1996). These growth promoters improve performance because they "modulate" intestinal microbiota and improve feed efficiency.

Suppliers of growth promoters guarantee that these substances are not absorbed through the intestinal walls and are shed in feces, where they are quickly biodegraded. Thus, they do not leave residues in the animal, and do not pose risks to human health or the environment (Mota, 1996). However, consumers are constantly concerned on the possible risks that antimicrobial resistance poses to human health.

In veterinary medicine, antimicrobial agents are used in therapy, metaphylaxis, prophylaxis, and as growth promoters (Scharwz et al., 2001). The use of subtherapeutic doses of antibiotics as growth promoters is a public health problem, because many resistant microorganisms may transfer resistance to microorganisms found in bird feces. This kind of use may be responsible for selective pressure that generates resistant bacteria, a current, worldwide-spread, public health problem, due to the risk of dissemination of pathogens and transfer of resistance genes, via food chain, to pathogenic and commensal microorganisms of humans, decreasing the treatment options for infections (Medeiros, 2011).

Since antimicrobials started to be widely used by humans at the end of the 1940s, the emergence of resistant strains was observed in most bacterial species, and against all drugs available (Flemming, 2005). The use of antimicrobials, combined with improvements in sanitation, nutrition and immunization, has lead to a dramatic decrease in deaths and a major gain in human life expectancy (WHO, 2002). However, with the increased use of antimicrobials, antimicrobial resistance has emerged as one of the greatest threats to the safety of human health (WHO, 2007), and as a most pressing problem for public health, animal health and food safety authorities (Tenover, 2006; Marchese & Schito, 2007).

The increase in antimicrobial resistance has narrowed the potential uses of antibiotics for the treatment of infections in humans and animals (Angulo et al., 2004). As a striking example, the CDC estimated that the total of methicillin-resistant *Staphylococcus* Infections (MRSI) in US hospitals and communities have increased from 2 % in 1974 to almost 63% in 2004 (CDC, 2010).

In the US, more than 40% of the antibiotics produced are used in animal feed. This non-therapeutic use of antibiotics is a way to promote the selection of a growing number of resistant bacteria (Levy, 1998). As more strains responsible for poultry infections become resistant to therapeutic drugs, these compounds become less available for human treatments. Similarly, with *Salmonella* being an important cause of foodborne diarrheal disease in humans 10/12, the reduction in the number of antibiotics available for effective treatment of *Salmonella*-related infections in humans and animals has become a serious concern (Angulo et al., 2004).

In Europe, besides this concern with resistance, several recent public health episodes were branded on the mind of the consumers. Among them, the connection between eggs and *Salmonella* Enteritidis, BSE/"mad cow disease" and cattle meat and, more recently, avian flu in Asia. Therefore, zoonoses and restricted use of additives and antimicrobials as growth promoters in feeds, together with the occurrence of resistant microorganisms, have become an important challenge in the control of detrimental microorganisms found in the digestive system of birds.

There is a consensus in several countries that the indiscriminate use of antimicrobials in animal production is one of the causes of the increased resistance to antimicrobials. Human infections are more severe when a strain of a given microorganism is resistant to the drug of choice for its treatment. The use of antimicrobials may stimulate the selection of resistant bacteria in this ecosystem. Human pathogens and resistant genes may cross species and ecosystems by contact with, or consumption of contaminated food and water (Kelley et al., 1998). Due to the little knowledge on single, multiple or cross-resistance mechanisms in microorganisms that are highly pathogenic to humans, the WHO has recommended careful use and restrictions to antimicrobials in animal production (WHO, 2001).

Before *Salmonella* Enteritidis outbreaks related to traditional drugs in Europe, different antibiotics - such as nitrofurazone, furazolidone, novobiocine and tetracyclines - were used in drinking water and in feed offered to poultry. In Brazil, tetracyclines, penicillins, chloramphenicol, sulphonamides, furazolidone, nitrofurazone and avoparcin were banned as additives in animal feed in 1998. However, the use of several other drugs is still allowed: 3-nitro acid, arsanilic acid, avilamycin, colistine sulfate, enramycin, flavomycin, lincomycin, spiramycin, tylosin sulfate and zinc bacitracin.

Extensive use of quinolones in birds was made possible by very flexible prescription regulations, use of generic, lower cost drugs in feed and water, and, without a doubt, because of the efficiency of these agents against *Salmonella*. The use of fluoroquinolones, which have a similar mechanism of action, followed quinolones (Rossi, 2005).

Strains of *Salmonella* Enteritidis may become resistant because of the indiscriminate use of drugs in their country of origin, imports of foodstuffs contaminated with bacteria carrying resistance genes, or infected people returning from international trips. Finnish researchers

(Hakanen et al., 2001) observed increased antimicrobial resistance in strains of *Salmonella* Enteritidis isolated from travelers after they came back from Asian countries where quinolones were used indiscriminately. There was an increase from 3.9% to 23.5% in the resistance to fluoroquinolones in samples analyzed between 1995 and 1999 in Finland.

These facts, suggest that drug resistance genes may be associated with virulence, or that humans strains have an improved resistance profile compared with *Salmonella* of animal origin, making the whole situation even more concerning from a public health viewpoint.

The frequency and extent of *Salmonella* resistance to antimicrobials vary based on the use of antibiotics in humans and animals, and on ecological differences in the epidemiology of *Salmonella* infections (McDermott, 2006). Globally, *Salmonella* exhibits extensive resistance profiles which have been associated both with higher rates of morbidity and mortality and the use of antimicrobials in food-producing animals (Angulo et al., 2004). Antibiotics suppress normal intestinal microbiota, breaking its protective effect, increasing the competitive advantage of antibiotic-resistant *Salmonella,* and favoring the occurrence of salmonellosis (Eley, 1994).

Salmonellosis surveillance has been described all over the world, specially after the emergence of strains resistant to multiple antibiotics, making control and treatment even more difficult. The WHO observed an alarming increase in the number of strains of *Salmonella* resistant to antibiotics due to the abusive use in intensive animal raising (Eurosurveillance, 1997). This finding is a concern for surveillance and environmental control organisms, once the use of antibiotics in animal feed as growth promoters contributes for the emergence of resistant and pathogenic strains (Pinto, 2000).

Antibiotics may be either bactericidal or bacteriostatic agents. Bactericidal agents cause changes incompatible with bacterial survival, whereas bacteriostatic agents inhibit bacterial growth and reproduction, without immediately killing microorganisms (Tavares, 2001).

The mechanism of action of antibiotics is essentially related to interference with cell wall synthesis. Cell wall constitution varies in Gram-positive or Gram-negative bacteria, leading to differences in permeability to drugs. Antibiotics that affect the permeability of the cytoplasmic membrane are similar to cationic detergents, due to the presence of basic groups ($NH3$ +) in a lateral chain of the fatty acid.

Insertion of antibiotic molecules disorganizes the membrane, producing leakage of cell components and death. Antibiotics that interfere with DNA replication generate toxic products that get inserted in the DNA molecule, breaking it up and preventing its synthesis. Others compounds loosen the DNA spiral structure, making it larger and breaking the bacterial cell. Agents that affect protein synthesis act on the ribosome, inhibiting protein synthesis by different mechanisms (Tavares, 2001; Trabulsi & Alterthum, 2008).

Some bacterial species are considered naturally resistant to antibacterial compounds (primary resistance), because only concentrations that would be unviable *in vivo* would affect them. Under continuous exposure to antimicrobials, microorganisms show acquired resistance (secondary) caused by the development of new mechanisms of defense (Fuchs & Wannmacher, 1999).

Resistance mechanisms may emerge because of changes in bacterial DNA, or biochemical mechanisms of molecule production, reactions and behaviors, which may be transmissible or not to the daughter cells. Resistance is observed when an antibiotic is administered to patients who are carriers of sensitive, mutant strains. Antimicrobials eliminate microorganisms that are sensitive, "selecting" the ones that are resistant. The rate of emergence of mutant strains is highly variable, and the mutation process may occur quickly in some cases, and slowly and gradually in other cases, taking years to appear. Some cells may present random genetic changes that may lead to resistance to a given antibiotic (Decamp & Moriarty, 2006). The process is called single resistance when the bacterium is resistant to only one drug; multiple resistance, when it is simultaneously resistant to two or more drugs (Tavares, 2001).

According to Claus (1988), mechanisms of antimicrobial resistance may involve chromosomal DNA, by means of mutations; or may be due to the acquisition of extrachromosomal DNA (by means of gene transduction, transformation or conjugation).

Mutations occur by chromosome swapping. These changes may be random, or caused by physical and/or chemical agents, and the process may be caused or not by exposure to antimicrobial agents. Many microorganisms isolated before the use of antibiotics showed mutations, and were not sensitive to antibiotics when these were discovered. Antimicrobials are not necessarily responsible for mutations, but they have an important role in the selection of resistant strains. Commonly, the genetic change that causes the resistance in a microorganism is generated by genes transported in extrachromosomal plasmids (Claus, 1988).

In the transduction process, a bacteriophage transfers, from a resistant to a sensitive bacterium, extrachromosomal bacterial DNA incorporated in its protein. The previously sensitive bacterium, then, will acquire resistance and transfer it to its daughter cells. This mechanism is easily observed in *Staphylococcus aureus* strains that acquired resistance to penicillins.

Transformation occurs when bacteria that are sensitive to one substance incorporate the DNA with genes that encode resistance, that are found in the environment. These bacteria, then, become resistant to one or more antimicrobials. Some bacteria, in certain growth phases, are able to excrete DNA to the environment.

Conjugation is caused by a passage of genes (R factors) from a resistant to a sensitive bacterium by attachment to a sex pilus. The R factor may contain resistance information against several antimicrobials. Conjugation and production of the sex pilus requires intervention of another group of genes, called transference factor. Without them, the process is not carried out. The R determinant complex, plus the resistance transfer factor, are known as R factor. R factor is important to Gram-negative bacteria, specially enterobacteria. *Escherichia coli, Salmonella, Shiguella, Klebsiella* and *Pseudomonas aeruginosa* are among microorganisms capable of transferring this type of resistance to sensitive bacteria. This resistance mechanism has been observed in relation to tetracyclines, chloramphenicol, sulfonamides, penicillins and aminoglycosides.

All these genetic alterations give rise to several biochemical changes in bacterial metabolism. Resistance to antibiotics may be carried out by three basic mechanisms produced by these changes (Strohl et al., 2004): decreased absorption or increase efflux of the antibiotic; change in the target site of the antibiotic, and acquisition of the ability to break or modify the antibiotic.

Acquired resistance to antibiotics is a necessary gain, or temporary or permanent change of bacterial genetic information. Most resistance genes are found in plasmids, which may be swapped with chromosomal elements. Acquired resistance is caused by mutations in the bacterial chromosome (which leads to the emergence of resistance genes in a sensitive bacterium), or by the transfer of resistance genes from one cell to another, with DNA fragments with these genes being inserted in the receptor cell. Both types of resistance, mutation (chromosomal) and transferable (plasmidial) may be found in the same bacterium (Tavares, 2001).

Plasmids are circular, extrachromosomal DNA molecules found in many bacterial species, and in some eukaryotes. They replicate separately or together with the host cell, and are passed on to the daughter cells. Plasmids may removed from the cell by different stress conditions, such as changes in temperature, presence of some stains or lack of certain nutrients. They are not essential to the cell, but may confer some selective advantages: they may have information for the degradation of certain substrates, resistance antibiotics or heavy metals. Plasmids may self-replicate independently of chromosomal replication, and may occur in variable numbers. Sex factors (F factor), antibiotic resistance (R factor), $N_2$-fixation (Trabulsi & Alterthum, 2008) are example of plasmids.

Antimicrobial resistance is one of the most important problems for human and veterinary medicine, and it is recognized by the WHO as an important public health problem (Rossi, 2005).

There was a significant increase in the occurrence of *Salmonella* Enteritidis in poultry carcasses from 2000 to 2005 in the US. Studies in Brazil between 2000 and 2009 show the predominance of this serovar in poultry. More than half of the strains were resistant to multiple antibiotics, and *Salmonella* Enteritidis was the only serovar that showed different degrees of resistance to all antimicrobial compounds. Studies carried out with *Salmonella* Heidelberg demonstrated that all strains showed multiple resistance, including marked resistance to third generation cephalosporins. In the past years in the US, increased resistance to ceftiofur was observed in poultry strains. In 1997, resistance to this antibiotic was 1.6%, and in 2003, 7.4% (Medeiros, 2011).

During decades, ampicillin, chloramphenicol and trimetoprim-sulfametoxazole were the most frequent antimicrobials used in salmonellosis treatment. However, the increase in the number of strains resistant to these drugs reduced their used in medical practice. Consequently, fluoroquinolones became the main antimicrobials used in the treatment of human infections (Souza et al., 2010).

Resistance to *Salmonella* transmitted by contaminated foods of animal origin is undesirable, but it is an inevitable consequence of the use of antimicrobials in animals used in food production (Threlfall et al., 2002). Bacterial resistance is a natural process, but it should and can be prevented with the rational use of antimicrobials in animal production. Therefore, it is very important to follow the evolution of resistance in order to use efficient methods for *Salmonella* control.

## 6. Prevention and control

Prevention and control programs for infections caused by paratyphoid *Salmonellae* aim at protecting the health of the birds, ensure the safety of the consumers, and strengthen the reliability of the poultry production chain. In the case of *Salmonella*, measures recommended for prevention and control are not specific due to the large number of species and their complex epidemiological behavior. Similarly, variability in the implementation of these measures depends on the requisites determined by the international market, or the adaptation of the industry to the chronogram of production.

In the past 10 years, there have been important outbreaks of emerging foodborne diseases all over the world. These outbreaks showed sanitary authorities of the countries affected that there is an increasing need for measures to prevent the risk of transmission. This led the Food and Agriculture Organization (FAO) to create the WTO, which motivated countries to review their innocuousness policies, rules and strategies to ensure that the food consumed by the population had appropriate sanitary conditions for international trade (Pan American Health Organization - PAHO, 2001).

General regulations issued all over the world for *Salmonella* control and prevention are: Proposed Guidelines for the Control *Campylobacter* and *Salmonella* in chicken meat, from the Codex Alimentarius; Prevention, Detection and Control of *Salmonella* in poultry, Chapter 6.5 of the Terrestrial Animal Health Code of 2010, from the World Organization for Animal Health (OIE); Compliance Guideline for Controlling *Salmonella* and *Campylobacter* in Poultry, of May 2010, from the Food Safety Inspection Service and United States Department of Agriculture (FSIS/USDA); and the national programs for eradication control and surveillance of some *Salmonella* serotypes in breeding chickens and broilers, from the Ministry of Environment of Spain.

Together with many other biosafety measures, monitoring of these bacteria, which may be associated with foodborne disease in humans, is one of the great objectives of the poultry industry. Health education actions that emphasize personal hygiene habits, mainly correct hand washing, care in food preparation, handling, storage and distribution, are recommended for food handlers. Main prevention strategies should be: selection of raw materials; carefully cleaning of equipment and utensils; adequate supply of potable water; adequate garbage disposal and sewage treatment; adoption of good manufacturing practices and implementation of the HACCP; removal of asymptomatic carriers from the production area, and adequate methods for transportation and preservation. All these actions are in compliance with the recommendations of public health authorities from all over the world (ICMSF, 2002; Brazil, 2002; Reuben et al., 2003).

Literature information show that one year after the implementation of *Salmonella* control in Finland, prevalence was below 1% in egg and bovine, swine and poultry meat production, decreasing the occurrence of salmonellosis outbreaks (Maijala et al., 2005). Food hygiene, therefore, is based on the adoption of preventive and control measures. The HACCP system is an efficient tool to remove disease-causing agents. The system provides specific protection against foodborne disease, and leads to reduction in costs and warranties of microbiologically safe foods.

The risk of vertical transmission may be minimized by bacteriological and serological monitoring of breeding chicken lots, resulting in *Salmonella*-free birds; by purchasing birds more resistant to *Salmonella* infection (Bumstead, 2000); by culling birds that are carriers of the microorganism; by treatment of eggs that are still in the sheds, and careful incubation of dirty and cracked eggs (Berchieri Jr., 2000).

Biosafety and sanitary management are important to reduce the environmental presence of *Salmonella*. According to Gast (1997), one of the methods employed to achieve this aim is cleaning and disinfection of the sheds with chemical disinfectants. However, not all disinfectants are efficient and depend, for example, on their behavior in the presence of large amounts of organic material (Berchieri Jr. & Barrow, 1996). Together with this, it is important to control rodents found in bird sheds. These animals have an important role in *Salmonella* infection by contaminating the environment and transmitting the microorganism to birds and eggs (Henzler & Opitz, 1992).

Specific procedures that aim at controlling *Salmonella* in bird feed include pelleting and use of organic acids (Silva, 2005). According to Gama (2001), as pelleting is carried out at temperatures over 60°C, the process may eliminate *Salmonella* from poultry feed, provided that the feed is not recontaminated by handling, rats or insects. Iba & Berchieri Jr. (1995), observed that a mixture of formic and propionic acids was efficient in controlling *Salmonella* Typhimurium in artificially contaminated feed.

Another important tool in *Salmonella* prevention and control is the use of quantitative thresholds. These values vary from country to country and correspond to the measures and control systems that are adequate for local production. These limits should be established based on scientific research and special attention should be paid to the use of antibiotics, detergents, disinfectants and process temperature.

Indiscriminate use of antibiotics and addition of growth promoters in animal feed contributed to the emergence of resistance among strains of *Salmonella* and other bacteria (Berchieri Jr. & Barrow, 1998). Besides, according to Barrow (1999), after the therapeutic agent is removed, there may be a period in which birds may become susceptible to *Salmonella* infection, because their normal microbiota - which would inhibit *Salmonella* naturally - is also affected by the use of the antibiotic.

Competitive exclusion is based on oral inoculation of the cecum contents of adult birds in newborn chicks, speeding the establishment of desirable intestinal microbiota (Nurmi & Rantala, 1973). The process attempts to prevent the establishment of pathogenic microorganisms in the intestinal mucous membrane. This is an important method in the control of *Salmonella* infection in birds with immature or debilitated intestinal microbiota (submitted to antibiotic therapy).

Another measure for *Salmonella* control and prevention is vaccination of susceptible birds (Gast, 1997). Nowadays, several studies have been carried out in order to evaluate the efficacy of live (Barrow et al., 1991; Hassan & Curtiss III, 1997) and inactivated vaccines (Timms et al., 1990; Gast et al., 1993; Nakamura et al., 1994; Miyamoto et al., 1999; Woodward et al., 2002). These studies support the use of vaccination, in a safe and efficient manner, as part of the prevention of infection in birds and contamination of eggs by *Salmonella* Enteritidis (Gast et al., 1992).

Notification and epidemiological records are important sources of information for inspection and control agencies, which may estimate which pathogens and foods may possibly be involved in foodborne disease outbreaks. For example, the presence of several *Salmonella* serotypes that did not show high prevalence some years ago, are found now in poultry herds and represent an important public health problem worldwide.

Control of salmonellosis cases will be achieved by the adoption of some measures, such as frequent and systematic surveillance of food production and distribution. An efficient program both provides warranties in the production of safe foods and reduces costs.

## 7. Conclusions

It is concluded that salmonellosis outbreaks still occur daily, even when recommended biosafety measures to ensure the health of poultry herds are in place. This may be due to the lack of awareness on animal health issues and due to the difficult control of this microorganism.

Birds may carry *Salmonella* spp. to inside of the industry by means of utensils, men, rodents, and mainly feces. Therefore, the microorganism may be introduced in all facilities and equipments of a slaughterhouse, negatively affecting the quality of final products and by-products destined for human consumption and animal feed.

Due to the wide distribution and variety of forms of *Salmonella* transmission, and the large number of foodstuffs involved in salmonellosis outbreaks, programs for guiding and

sensitizing the consumers, the trade, food handlers and breeders of animals, mainly of poultry, should be implemented in order to improve health and hygiene conditions of products and processes, and ensure the health of the final consumer.
Resistance of *Salmonella* strains to antimicrobials normally used in poultry raising may serve as a warning against the indiscriminate use of antibiotics in the treatment of infections. Addition of antibiotics in animal feed as growth promoters may contribute for selecting resistant strains, and may affect human health.

## 8. References


Allen, G., Bruce, V.R., Stephenson, P., Satchell, F.B., Andrews, W.H. (1991). Recovery of *Salmonella* from high-moisture foods by abbreviated selective enrichment. *Journal of Food Protection*, v.*54*, p.492-495.

Alves, L.M.C.; Costa, N.F.; Silva, M.S.; Sales, S.S.; Correia, M.R. (2001). Toxinfecção alimentar por *Salmonella* Enteretidis: relato de um surto ocorrido em São Luís-MA. *Higiene Alimentar*, v.15, n.80/81 (jan./fev. 2001), p.57-58.

Anais de Intoxicações Alimentares. UNISUL. Florianóplis. 1996.

Andrews, W.H., June, G.A., Sherrod, P., Hammack, T.S., Amaguana, R.M. (1998). Sulmonella In *Food* und Drug Administration: *Bacteriological Analytical Manual*, 8th ed. (Revision A/1988), AOAC International, Arlington,VA.

Argôlo Filho, R.C.A. (2007). Identificação, sorotipagem e diferenciação pela PCRDGGE de sorotipos de *Salmonella* isolados de teiús criados em cativeiro. 2007. 96f. Dissertação (Mestrado em Genética e Biologia Molecular) - Universidade Estadual de Santa Cruz, Ilhéus-BA, 2007.

Angulo F.J.; Nargund, V.N.; Chiller, T.C. (2004). Evidence of an association between use of antimicrobial agents in food animals and anti-microbial resistance among bacteria isolated from humans and the human health consequences of such resistance. *Journal of Veterinary Medicine. B, Infectious Diseases and Veterinary Public Health*, v.51, p.374-379.

Antunes, P.; Réu, C.; Sousa, J. C.; Peixe, L.; Pestana, N. (2003). Incidence of *Salmonella* from poultry products and their susceptibility to antimicrobial agents. *International Journal of Food Microbiology*, Amsterdam, v.82, n.1, p.97-103.

Baird-Parker, A.C. (1990). Foodborne salmonellosis. *Lancet*, v.336, p.1231-1235.

Barrow, P.A.; Lovell, M.A.; Berchieri JR, A.J. (1991). The use of two live attenuated vaccines to imunize egg-laying hens against *Salmonella* Enteritidis phage type 4. *Avian Pathology*, Huntingdon, v.20, n.4, p.681-692.

Barrow, P.A. (1999). *Salmonella* infections in poultry - problems and new thoughts on the possibilities of control. *Revista Brasileira de Ciência Avícola*, v.1, p.9-16.

Baxter-Jones, C. (1996). Control de la transmisión vertical de *Salmonella*. *Avicultura Professional*, v.14, n.1, p.18-19.

Brazil. Ministério da Saúde. Fundação Nacional da Saúde (FUNASA). (2002). *Guia de Vigilância Epidemiológica*. Brasília: Ministério da Saúde.

Berchieri Jr, A. (1991). Paratifo: Como podemos controlá-lo ou erradicá-lo a nível de produção. In: *Conferência Apinco de Ciência e Tecnologia Avícolas*, 1991, Santos. Anais..., p. 49-62.

Berchieri Jr, A.; Barrow, P.A. (1996). Reduction in incidence of experimental fowl typhoid by incorporation of a commercial formic acid preparation into poultry feed. *Poultry Science,* Champaign, v.75, n.3, p. 339-341.

Berchieri Jr, A.; Barrow, P.A. (1998). O desenvolvimento da microbiota intestinal em pintos de corte: prós e contras. In: Conferencia Apinco de Ciência e Tecnologia Avícolas, 1998, Campinas, Anais..., Campinas, FACTA, 1998, p.183-190.

Berchieri Jr, A. (2000). Salmoneloses Aviárias, In: *Doenças das aves,* Berchieri Jr, A.; Macari, M., cap.4.1, p.185-195. FACTA, Campinas, SP.

Berchieri Jr, A.; Freitas Neto, O.C.S. (2009). Salmoneloses aviárias. In: *Doenças das aves,* Berchieri Jr, A.; Silva, E.N.; Di Fábio, J.; Sesti, L.; Zuanaze, M.A.F. 2 ed. Seção 4, p. 435-454, FACTA, Campinas, SP.

Bersot, L.S. (2006). *Salmonella* no Brasil: Sua importância no abate de aves. In: V Simpósio de sanidade avícola da UFSM, 2006, Santa Maria, RS. Anais..., Santa Maria: UFSM, 2006, p.90-94.

Bumstead, N. (2000). Mecanismos genéticos de resistência a doenças. In: Conferência Apinco de Ciência e Tecnologia Avícolas, Campinas, Anais..., Campinas, FACTA, 2000, p.25-30.

Calnek, B.W. (1997). *Diseases of Poultry***.** Iowa State University Pres. Ames, IA, p.81-121.

Cardoso, A.L.S.P.; Tessari, E.N.C.; Castro, A.G.M.; Kanashiro, A.M.I.; Gama, N.M.S.Q. (2002). Pesquisa de *Salmonella* spp em ovos comerciais, analisados no Laboratório de Patologia avícola de Descalvado, SP. *Revista Higiene Alimentar,* São Paulo, v.16, n.92/93 (jan./fev. 2002), p.76-79.

Centers For Diseases Control and Prevention (CDC). (2005). Outbreaks reported: 1990, 1991; 1992. MMWR 1993. Disponível em: < www.cdc.gov>. Acesso em: 04/07/2011.

Centers For Diseases Control and Prevention (CDC). (2007). Multistate outbreak of human *Salmonella* infections associated with frozen pot pies-United States, 2007, *Morbidity and Mortality Weekly Report,* v.57, n.47, p.1277-1280.

Centers For Diseases Control and Prevention (CDC). (2010). Overview of Healthcare-associated MRSA. Atlantaed.

Clark, G.M.; Kaukmann, A.F.; Gangarosa, E.J. (1973). Epidemiology of an international outbreak of *Salmonella* Agona, *Lancet,* v.2, p.490-493.

Claus, J.W. (1988). Genética molecular e variação genética em bactérias e viroses bacterianas. In: Fundamentos de bacteriologia e micologia veterinária, Carter, G.R, Roca, 1988, p.39-64, São Paulo.

Colin, B.J. (1996). Control de la *Salmonella. Avicultura Professional,* v.14, n.1, p.23.

Correa, W.M, Correa, C.M. (1992). Paratifos em geral. In: Enfermidades infecciosas dos mamíferos domésticos, p.167-174, 2 ed., Rio de Janeiro.

Cox, N.A., Bailey, J.S.; Thomson, J.E. (1982). Effect of various media and incubation conditions on recovery of inoculated *Salmonella* from poultry feed. *Poultry Science,* v.61, p.1314-1321.

Cox, N.A.; Bailey, J.S.; Berrang, M.E. (1996). Extent of Salmonellae contamination in breeder hatcheries, *Poultry Science,* Champaign, v.70, p.416-418.

Decamp, O.; Moriarty, D.J.W.P. (2006). A segurança dos probióticos para a aqüicultura, *Revista da Associação Brasileira de Criadores de Camarão,* v.8, n.2, p.40-41.

Dunkley, K.D.; Callaway, T.R.; Chalova, V.I.; Mcreynolds, J.L.; Hume, M.E.; Dunkley, C.S.; Kubena, L.F.; Nisbet, D.J.; Ricke, S.C. (2009). Foodborne *Salmonella* ecology in the avian gastrointestinal tract, *Anaerobe*, v.15, p. 26-35, London.

Eckner, K.F., Dustman, W.A., Curiale, M.S. (1992). Use of an elevated temperature and novobiocin in modified enzyme-linked immunoabsorbent assay for the improved recovery of *Salmonella* from foods. *Journal Food Protection*, v.55, n.10, p.758-762.

Eley, A.R. (1994). *Microbial food poisoning*. Chapman & Hall, London, 191p.

European Food Safety Authority, EFSA-ECDC report for 2007: *Salmonella* remains most common cause of food-borne outbreaks, 2007.

Eurosurveillance. (1997). *Vigilância da resistência das salmonelas aos antibióticos*. Disponível em: <http://www.ceses.org/eurosurv>. Acesso em: 28/06/2011.

Flemming, J.S. (2005). Utilização de leveduras, probióticos e mananoligossacarídeos (MOS) na avaliação de frangos de corte. 2005. 109f. Tese (Doutorado em Tecnologia de alimentos) - Universidade federal do Paraná, Paraná, 2005.

Flôres, M.L.; Nascimento, V.P.; Kader, I.I.T.A.; Cardoso, M.; Santos, L.R. dos; Lopes, R.F. F.; Wald, V.B.; Barbosa, T.M.C. (2003). Análise da contaminação por *Salmonella* em ovos do tipo colonial através da reação em cadeia da polimerase. *Ciência Rural*, v.33, n.3, p.553-557.

Franco, B.D.G.M.; Landgraf, M. (1996). *Microbiologia dos Alimentos*, Atheneu, São Paulo, 182p.

Franco, B.D.G.M.; Landgraf, M.; Destro, M.T.; Gelli, D.S. (2003). Foodborne diseases in Southern South América. In: *International handbook of foodborn pathogens*, Miliotis, M.D.; Bier, J.W., p.733-743, Marcel Deckker, New York.

Franco, B.D.G.M.; Landgraf, M. (2004). *Microbiologia dos alimentos*. Atheneu, 182p. São Paulo.

Freitas Neto, O.C.; Penha Filho, R.A.C.; Barrow, P.; Berchieri Jr, A. (2010). Sources of human non-typhoid salmonellosis: a review. *Revista Brasileira de Ciencia Avícola*, vol.12, n.1, p.01-11.

Forshell, L.P.; Wierup, M. (2006). *Salmonella* contamination: a significant challenge to the global marketing of animal foods products. *Revue Scientifique Techinique Office International des Epizooties*, Paris, v.25, n.2, p.541-554.

Fuchs, F.D.; Wannmacher, L. (1999). *Farmacologia clínica fundamentos da terapêutica racional*, 2 ed., Editora Guanabara Koogan, Rio de Janeiro, 678p.

Gama, N.M.S.Q. Salmonella spp em aves de postura comercial. (2001). 60f. Dissertação (*Mestrado em Medicina Veterinária)* - Faculdade de Ciências Agrárias e Veterinárias, Universidade Estadual Paulista, Jaboticabal, 2001.

Gantois, I.; Ducatelle, R.; Pasmans, F.; Haesebrouk, F.; Gast, R.; Humphrey, T.J.; Van, I.F. (2009). Mechanisms of egg contamination by *Salmonella* Enteritidis. *FEMS Microbiology Review*, Amsterdam, v.33, n.4, p.718-738.

Gast R. K.; Stone, H.D.; Holt, P.S.; Beard, C.W. (1992). Evaluation of the efficacy of an oil emulsion bacterin for protecting chickens against *Salmonella* Enteritidis. *Avian Diseases*, Kennett Square, v.36, n.4, p.992-999.

Gast, R.K.; Stone, H.D.; Holt, P.S. (1993). Evaluation of the efficacy of oil-emulsion bacterins for reducing fecal shedding of *Salmonella* Enteritidis by laying hens. *Avian Diseases*, Kennett Square, v.37, n.4, p.1085-1091.

Gast, R.K. (1997). Paratyphoid infections. In: *Disease of poultry*, Calnek, B.W.; Barnes, H.J.; Beard, C.W.; Mcdougald, L.R.; Saif, Y.M., p.97-129, 10 ed., Ames: Iowa State University Press.

Gelli, S. D. (1995). Surtos humanos por *Salmonella* em alimentos. *Aves e Ovos*, junho/1995, São Paulo, SP.

Grimont, F.; Grimont, P.A.D. (1986). Ribosomal ribonucleic acid gene restriction patterns as possible taxonomic tools. *Annales de l'Institut Pasteur Microbiology* (Paris), v.137, n.1, Supplement 2, 8 July 1986, p.165-175.

Grimont, P.A.D.; Grimont, F.; Bouvet, P. (2000). Taxonomy of the Genus *Salmonella,* In: *Salmonella* in domestic animals, Wray, C.; Wray, A., p.1-17, cap.1, CABI Publishing, New York.

Grimont, P.A.D.; Weill, F. (2007). *Antigenic Formulae of the Salmonella Serovars.* 9th ed. Paris: WHO Collaborating Center for Reference and Research on *Salmonella* Institute Pasteur, 2007.

Gomez, H.F; Cleary, G.G. (1998). *Salmonella*, 4th ed., v.1, Philadelphia.

Hakanen, A.; Kotilainen, P.; Huovinen, P.; Helenius, H.; Siitonen, A. (2001). Reduced fluoroquinolone susceptibility in *Salmonella enterica* serotypes in travelers returning from Southeast Asia. *Emerging Infectious Diseases*, v.7, p.1-10.

Hassan, J.O.; Curtiss III, R. (1997). Efficacy of a live avirulent *Salmonella* Typhimurium vaccine in preventing colonization and invasion of laying hens by *Salmonella* Typhimurium and *Salmonella* Enteritidis. *Avian Diseases*, Kennett Square, v.41, n.4, p.783-791.

Henzler, D.J.; Opitz, H.M. (1992). The role of mice in the epizootiology of *Salmonella* Enteritidis infection on chicken layer farms. *Avian Diseases,* Kennett Square, v.36, n.3, p.625-631.

Hofer, E.; Silva Filho, S.J.; Reis E.M.F. (1997). Prevalência de sorovares de *Salmonella* isolados de aves no Brasil. *Pesquisa Veterinária Brasileira*, v.17, n.2, p.55-62, Rio de Janeiro.

Holt, J.G. (1994). *Bergey's: Manual of determinative bacteriology*: Williams & Willams, Baltimore, 9 ed., p.186-187.

Huang, H. (1999). Evaluation of culture enrichment for use with *Salmonella* detection in Immunoassay. *International Journal of Food Microbiology*, v.51, n.2-3, p.85-94.

Humphrey, T.J.; Mead, G.C.; Rowe, B. (1988). Poultry meat as a source of human salmonellosis in England and Wales. *Epidemiology Infection*, v.100, p.175-184.

Iba, A.M.; Berchieri JR, A. (1995). Studies on the use of a formic acid-propionic acid mixture (BioaddTM) to control experimental *Salmonella* infection in broiler chickens. *Avian Pathology*, Huntingdon, v.24, n.2, p.303-311.

International Commission for Microbiological Safety of Foods (ICMSF). (1998). Poultry and poultry products. In: *Microorganisms in Foods*, Microbial Ecology of Food Commodities. Blackie Academic and Professional, v.6., p.75-129, London.

International Commission for Microbiological Safety of Food (ICMSF). (2002). *Microorganismos de los alimentos*. Acribia: Zaragoza, 332p.

Irino, K.; Fernandes, S.A.; Tavechio, A.T.; Neves, B.C.; Dias, A.M.G. (1996). Progression of *Salmonella* Enteritidis phage type 4 strains in São Paulo State, Brazil. *Revista do Instituto de Medicina Tropical de São Paulo*, v.38, p.193-196.

Jakabi, M.; Buzzo, A.A.; Ristori, C.A.; Tavechio, A.T.; Sakuma, H.; Paula, A.M.; Gelli, D.S. (1999). Observações laboratoriais sobre surtos alimentares de *Salmonella* spp. ocorridos na Grande São Paulo, no período de 1994 a 1997. *Revista do Instituto Adolfo Lutz*, v.58, n.1, p.47-51.

Jay, J.M. (1992). *Microbiología moderna de los alimentos*. 32th ed. Zaragoza: Acribia, 804p.

Kafel, S. (1981). Effects of preenrichment media and their incubation conditions on isolating Salmonellae from fish meal. *Journal of Food Protection*, v.44, p.268-270.

Kelley, T.R.; Pancorbo, O.C.; Merka, W.C.; Barnhart, H.M. (1998). Antibiotic resistance of bacterial litter isolates. *Poultry Science*, Champaign, v.77, p.243-247.

Kottwitz, L.B.M.; Oliveira, T.C.R.M.; Alcocer, I.; Farah, S.M.S.S.; Abrahão, W.S.M.; Rodrigues, D.P. (2010). Avaliação epidemiológica de surtos de salmoneloses ocorridos no período de 1999 a 2008 no Estado do Paraná, Brasil. *Acta Scientiarum Health Sciences*, v.32, p.9-15.

Levy, S.B. (1998). The challenge of antibiotic resistance. *Scientific American*, v.278, p.32-39.

Loguercio, A.P.; Aleixo, J.A.G.; Vargas, A.C. de; Costa, M.M. da. (2002). ELISA indireto na detecção de *Salmonella* spp. em lingüiça suína. *Ciência Rural*, v.32, n.6, p.1057-1062.

Luk, J.M.; Kongmuang, U.; Tsang, R.W.; Lindberg, A.F. (1997). An enzyme-linked immunosorbent assay to detect PCR products of the *rfbS* gene from serogroup D Salmonellae: a rapid screening prototype. *Journal of Clinical Microbiology*, v.35, p.714-718.

Maijala R, Ranta J, Seuna E. (2005). The efficiency of the Finnish *Salmonella* Control Programme. *Food Control*, v.16, n.8, p.669-675.

Marchese A., Schito G.C. (2007). [Recent results of multinational studies on antibiotic resistance: should we have "Protection" against these resistances?]. *Médecine et Maladies Infectieuses*, 37 Spec, n.1, p.2-5.

McDermott, P.F. (2006). Antimicrobial resistance in nontyphoidal salmonellae. In: Aarestrup FM, ed. *Antimicrobial Resistance in Bacteria of Animal Origin*. Washington, DC: ASM Press, 2006; p.293–314.

Medeiros, M.A.N. (2011). Prevalência de *Salmonella* spp. e resistência antimicrobiana dos isolados em carcaças de frango congelado no varejo. Brasil, 2004 a 2006. In: *Seminário Internacional de Salmoneloses Aviárias*, Rio de Janeiro, RJ, Anais..., CD Room. 2011.

Miyamoto, T.; Kitaoka, D.; Withanage, G.S.; Fukata, T.; Sasai, K.; Baba, E. (1999). Evaluation of the efficacy of *Salmonella* Enteritidis oil-emulsion bacterin in an intravaginal challenge model in hens. *Avian Diseases*, Kennet Square, v.43, n.3, p.497-505.

Mota, E. G. (1996). Restrição e uso de aditivos (promotores de crescimento) em rações de aves. In: *Conferencia Apinco de Ciência e Tecnologia Avícolas*, 1996, Curitiba, PR. Anais..., Campinas: FACTA, 1996. p.57

Nakamura, M.; Nagamine, N.; Takashi, T.; Suzuki, S.; Sato, S. (1994). Evaluation of the efficacy of a bacterin against *Salmonella* Enteritidis infection and the effect of stress after vaccination. *Avian Diseases*, Kennet Square, v.38, n.4, p.717- 724.

Nascimento, V.P. (1996). Salmoneloses paratíficas: uma revisão e situação atual. In: *Simpósio Técnico de Produção de Ovos*, 1996, São Paulo. Anais... São Paulo: APA, 1996. p.93-116.

Nascimento, V.P.; Oliveira, S.D.; Ribeiro, A.R.; Santos, L.R.; Cardoso, M.O.; Pontes, A.P.; Silva, A.B.; Rocha, L.S. (1997). Identificação de sorovares de *Salmonella* em cortes e carcaças de frangos. In *Congresso Brasileiro de Microbiologia*, Rio de Janeiro, RJ, Anais..., 1997. v.1, p.344.

Nascimento, V.P., Salle, C.T.P., Moraes, H.L.S., Fittél,A.P., Kellermann, A., Streck, A.F., Ribeiro, A.R., Santos, L.R. (2003). Prevalência de *Salmonella* spp. em produtos de origem avícola no período de maio de 1995 abril de 1996. In: *Congresso Brasileiro de*

*Microbiologia,* Florianópolis. Anais..., Florianópolis, Brasil: Sociedade Brasileira de Microbiologia, 2003.

Nogrady, N.; Kardos, G.; Bistyak, A.; Turcsanyi, I.; Meszaros, J. Galantai, Z, et al. (2008). Prevalence and characterization of *Salmonella* Infantis isolated originating from different points of the broiler chicken-human food chain in Hungary. *International Journal Food Microbiology,* v.127, p.162-167.

Nurmi, E.; Rantala, M. (1973). New aspects of *Salmonella* infection in broiler production. *Nature,* v.241, p.210-211.

Oliveira, D.D.; Silva, E.N. (2000). Salmonela em ovos comerciais: ocorrência, condições de armazenamento e desinfecção da casca. *Arquivo Brasileiro de Medicina Veterinária e Zootecnia,* Belo Horizonte, v.52, n.6. ISSN 0102-0935

Oliveira, A.B.A.; Paula, C.M.D.; Capalongas, R.; Cardoso, M.R.I.; Tondos, E.C. (2010). Doenças transmitidas por alimentos, principais agentes etiológicos e aspectos gerais: Uma Revisão. *Revista HCPA,* n.30, v.3, p.279-285.

Olsen, J.E.; Brown, D.J.; Madsen, M.; Bisgaard, M. (2003). Cross-contamination with Salmonella on a broiler slaughterhouse line demonstrated by use of epidemiological markets. *Journal of Applied Microbiology,* v.95, n.5, p.826-835.

Organização Pan-Americana da Saúde. (2001). *HACCP: Instrumento essencial para a inocuidade de alimentos.* Buenos Aires: OPAS/INPPAZ. 2001.

Pelkonen, S.; Romppanen, E. L.; Siitonen, A.; Pelkonen, J. (1994). Differentiation of *Salmonella* Serovar Infantis Isolates from Human and Animal Sources by Fingerprinting IS200 and 16S rm Loci. *Journal of Clinical Microbiology,* v.32, n.9, p.2128- 2133.

Perales, I.; Audicana, A. (1989). The role of hens' eggs in outbreaks of salmonellois in north Spain. *International Journal of Food Microbiology,* Amsterdam, v.8, p.175-180.

Pinto, P.S.A. (2000). Aspectos sanitários da salmonelose como uma zoonose. *Revista Higiene Alimentar,* São Paulo, v.14, n.73, p.39-43.

Pinto, U.M.; Cardoso, R.R.; Vanetti, M.C.D. (2004). Detecção de Listeria, Salmonella e Klebsiella em serviço de alimentação hospitalar. *Revista de Nutrição,* v.17, n.3, p.319-326.

Popoff, M.Y.; Bockemuhl, J.; Hickman-Brenner, F.W. (1996). Kauffmann-white seheme. *Research Microbiology,* v.147, n.39, p.756-9, 1996. Supplement.

Quinn, P.J., Carter, M.E., Markey, B., Carter, G.R., (2000). *Clinical Veterinary Microbiology.* Edinburgh: Mosby, 648p.

Raevuori, M.; Seuna, E.; Nurmi, E. (1978). An epidemic of *Salmonella* Infantis infection in Finnish broiler chickens in 1975-76, *Acta Veterinaria Scandinavica,* v.19, p.317-330.

Rodrigues, D.P. Ecologia e prevalência de *Salmonella* spp. em aves e material avícola no Brasil. (2005). In: Conferência Apinco de Ciência e Tecnologia Avícolas, 2005, Santos, SP. Anais..., Campinas: FACTA, v.2, p.223-228, 2005.

Rodrigues, D.P. (2011). Perspectivas atuais e falhas no diagnostico antigênico de *Salmonella* spp: importância no reconhecimento dos sorovares circulantes, emergentes e exóticos In: *Seminário Internacional Sobre Salmoneloses Aviárias,* Rio de Janeiro, RJ. Anais…, CD Room. 2011.

Rossi, A.A. (2005). Biossegurança em frangos de corte e saúde pública: limitações, alternativas e subsídios na prevenção de salmoneloses. 2005. 111f. Dissertação (*Mestrado em Agroecossistemas*) - Centro de Ciências Agrárias, Universidade Federal de Santa Catarina, Florianópolis, 2005.

Rycroft, A.N. (2000). Structure, Function and Synthesis of Surface Polysaccharides in *Salmonella*. In: *Salmonella in domestic animals*, Wray, C.; Wray, A., cap.2, p.19-33, CABI 2000, New York.

Santos, L.R.; Nascimento, V.P.; Flores, M.L.; Rosek H.; D'Andrea A.; Albuquerque M.C.; Rampanelli Y.; Machado N.P.; Rios S.; Fernandes, S.A. (2002). *Salmonella* Enteritidis isoladas de amostras clinicas de humanos e de alimentos envolvidos em episódios de toxinfecções alimentares, ocorridas entre 1995 e 1996, no Estado do Rio Grande do Sul. *Revista Higiene Alimentar*, São Paulo, v.6, n.102/103, p.93-99.

Santos, I. (2004). Desempenho zootécnico e rendimento de carcaça de frangos de corte suplementados com diferentes probióticos e antimicrobianos. *Acta Scientiarum: Animal Sciences*, Maringá, v.26, p.29-33.

Schwarz, S.; Kehrenberg, C.; Walsh, T.R. (2001). Use of antimicrobial agents in veterinary medicine and food animal production. *International Journal of Antimicrobial Agents*, v.17, p.431-437.

Selander, R.K.; Li, J.; Nelson, K. (1996). Evolutionary genetics of *Salmonella enterica*. In: *Escherichia coli and Salmonella - cellular and molecular biology*, Neidhardi, F.C.; Curtiss, R.; Ingraham, J.L.; Lin, E.C.C.; Low, K.B.; Magasanik, B.; Reznikoff, W.S.; Riley, M.; Schaechter, M.; Umbarger, H.E., v.2, p.2691-2707, American Society for Microbiology, Washington.

Silva, E.N. (2000). Probióticos e prebióticos na alimentação de aves. In: Conferencia Apinco de Ciencia e Tecnologia Avicolas, Campinas, SP. Anais..., Campinas: FACTA, 2000. p.242.

Silva, E.N. (2005). Medidas gerais de controle de salmonelas em frangos. In: Conferência Apinco de Ciência e Tecnologia Avícolas, Campinas, SP. Anais..., Campinas: FACTA, 2005, p.229-237.

Soncine, R.A.; Back, A. (2001). *Salmonella* Enteritidis em aves: erradicação ou controle por vacinação. In: Conferência Apinco de Ciência e Tecnologia Avícolas, Campinas. Anais…, São Paulo: FACTA, 2001. v.1, p.21-30.

Soumet, C. Hermel, G., Salvat, G., Collin, P. (1997). Detection of *Salmonella* spp. in food products by polymerase chain reaction and hybridization assay in microplate format. *Letters in Applied Microbiology*, v.24, p.113-116.

Souza, R.B.; Magnani, M.; Oliveira, T.C.R.M. (2010). Mecanismos de resistência às quinolonas em *Salmonella* spp. Revisão. *Semina: Ciências Agrárias*, v.31, n.2, abr./jun., p. 413-428, Londrina.

Suresh, T.; Hatha, A.A.M.; Screenivasa, D. (2006). Prevalence and antimicrobial resistance of *Salmonella* Enteritidis and other salmonella in the eggs and eggstoring trays from retails markets of Coimbatore, south India. *Food Microbiology*, v.23, n.3, p.294-299.

Strohl, W.A.; Rouse, H.; Fisher, B.D. *Microbiologia ilustrada*. (2004). Porto Alegre: Artmed, 531p.

Synnott, M.B.; Brindley, M.; Gray, J.; Dawson, J.K. (1998). An outbreak of *Salmonella* Agona infection associated with precooked turkey meat. *Communicable Disease and Public Health*, v.1, n.3, p.176-179.

Taitt, C.R.; Shubin, Y.S.; Angel, R. (2004). Detection of *Salmonella enterica* Serovar Typhimurium by using a Rapid, Array-Based Immunosensor. *Applied and Environmental Microbiology*, v.70, n.1, p.152-158.

Tavares, W. (2001). *Manual de antibióticos e quimioterápicos antiinfecciosos*. 3 ed. São Paulo: Editora Atheneu, 2001.

Taunay, A.E.; Fernandes, S.A.; Tavechio, A.T.; Neves, B.C.; Dias, A.M.G.; Irino, K. (1996). The role of Public Health Laboratory in the problem of salmonellosis in São Paulo, Brasil. *Revista do Instituto de Medicina Tropical de São Paulo*, v.38, n.2, p.119-127. ISSN 0036-4665

Tauxe, R.V.; Doyle, M.P.; Kuchenmüller, T.; Schlundt, J.; Stein, C.E. (2010). Evolving public health approaches to the global challenge of foodborne infection. *International Journal of Food Microbiology*, v.139, p.16-28.

Tenover, F.C. (2006). Mechanisms of antimicrobial resistance in bacteria. *The American Journal of Medicine*, v.119 (6A), S3-S10.

Tessari, E.N.C.; Cardoso, A.L.S.P.; Castro, A.G.M. (2003). Prevalência de *Salmonella* Enteritidis em carcaças de frango industrialmente processadas. *Revista Higiene Alimentar*, v.17, n.107, p.52-55.

Thong, K.L.; NgeoW, Y.; Altwegg, M.;navaratnam, P.; Pang, T. (1995). Molecular analysis of *Salmonella* Enteritidis by pulsed-field gel electrophoresis and ribotyping. *Journal of Clinical microbiology*, v.33, n.5, p.1070-1074.

Threlfall, E.J. (2002). Antimicrobial drug resistance in *Salmonella*: problems and perspectives in food- and water-borne infections. *FEMS Microbiology Reviews*, v.26, p.141-148.

Timms, L.M.; Marshal, R.N.; Breslin, M.F. (1990). Laboratory assessment of protection given by an experimental *Salmonella Enteritidis* PT4 inactivated, adjuvant vaccine. *The Veterinary Record*, London, v.127, n.25-26, p.611-614.

Todd, E C. (1989). Preliminary estimates of costs of foodborne disease in the United States. *Journal of Food Protection*, v.52, p.595-601.

Trabulsi, L.R, Alterthum, L.F. (2004). *Microbiologia*. 4 ed., p.54-57, Atheneu, São Paulo.

Trabulsi, L. R.; Alterthum, F. (2008). *Microbiologia*. 5 ed.,Atheneu, São Paulo. 760p.

Wall, P.G.; Ward, L.R. (1999). Epidemiology of *Salmonella enterica* serovar Enteritidis phage type 4 in England and Wales. In: *Salmonella enterica* serovar Enteritidis in humans and animals: epidemiology, pathogenesis, and control, Saeed, A.M.; Gast, R.K.; Potter, M.E. Wall, P.G., p.19-25, ed. Ames, Iowa State University Press.

Wegener, H.C.; Baggesen, D.L. (1996). Investigation of an outbreak of human salmonellosis caused by *Salmonella enterica* ssp. enterica serovar Infantis by pulsed field gel electrophoresis. *International Journal of Food Microbiology*, v.32, n.1-2, p.125-131.

Williams, J.E. (1981). *Salmonella* in poultry feeds - a worldwide review. Part I. Introduction. *World's Poultry Science Journal*, v.37, p.6-19.

World Health Organization. WHO consultation on the monitoring of antimicrobial usage in food animals for the protection of human health. Oslo, Norway, 2001. Disponível em: http://www.who.int. Acesso em: 11 fev. 2004.

WHO. Antimicrobial resistance. *Fact Sheet No 194* ed., 2002.

WHO - World Health Report 2007 - A safer future: global public health security in the 21st century. Chapter 2: Threats to public health security. World Health Organizationed, 2007.

Woodward, M.J.; Gettingby, G.; Breslin, M.F.; Corkish, J. D.; Houghton, S. (2002). The efficacy os Salenvac, a *Salmonella enterica* subsp. Enterica serotype Enteritidis iron-restricted bacterin vaccine, in laying chickens. *Avian Patology*, Huntingdon, v.31, n.4, p.383-392.

Wyatt, G.M.; Langley, M.N.; Lee, H.A.; Morgan, M.R. (1993). Further studies on the feasibility of one-day *Salmonella* detection by enzyme-linked immunosorbent assay. Applied and Environmental Microbiology, v.59, n.5, p.1383-1390.

10

# *Salmonella* Saintpaul Outbreak: Export and Trade Economic Impact

Nohelia Castro-del Campo, Cristóbal Chaidez, José A. Medrano-Félix, J. Basilio Heredia, Josefina León-Félix, Gustavo González Aguilar and J. Fernando Ayala Zavala
*Research Center for Food and Development, A.C. Culiacán, Sinaloa México*

## 1. Introduction

Foodborne pathogens cause diarrhea and flulike illnesses. An estimated 1.8 million children death is associated with disease-causing organisms acquired via food consumption with the greatest number of cases occurring in developing countries (WHO 2008). In the United States, the burden of foodborne infections causes an estimated of 48 million cases of sick people, from which 128,000 are hospitalized and 3,000 die anually (CDC, 2011). In addition, around 31 of the acquired pathogens known cause an approximated of 9.4 million episodes of foodborne illnesses while additional episodes are caused by unspecified agents, known agents not yet recognized as causing foodborne illness, and substances known to be in food but unproven pathogenicity (Scallan *et al.*, 2011). According to Allos *et al.* (2004) and Imhoff *et al.* (2004) the economic burden of foodborne illnesses results in an estimated annual cost of $6.9 billion USD because of work absenteeism, cost of medication and hospitalization, being the annual diarrheal burden of 0.72 episodes per person.

According to Buzby *et al.* (1996) and WHO (2008) the most common foodborne pathogens associated with outbreaks are bacteria like *Campylobacter jejunii*, *Escherichia coli* O157:H7, *Listeria monocytogenes* and *Salmonella*. Data from the CDC (2011) indicates the prevalence of *Salmonella* serotypes causing foodborne illnesses, which shows an increasing tendency from 2006 to 2011, involving several food as transmission vehicle, such as tomatoe, cantaloupe, egg, alfalfa sprout, peanut butter, pepper, and papaya. Therefore, the control of foodborne pathogens must be considered as one of the most important goals of authorities and producers. When a pathogen related outbreak is detected, the collaboration among Universities, Research Centers and health authorities from countries involved, is an essential step to source track the origin of the causative agent, and to seek for strategies for problem remediation.

The association of food with pathogens is a critical problem that requires special attention of the Mexican producers, since the presence of disease-causing organisms might provoke the close of borders of the destiny country. Therefore, the Mexican agricultural authorities have established mandatory regulations for fresh produce production and processing, which include Good Agricultural Practices (GAP) and Good Manufacturing Practices (GMP) audit programs that must be implemented in order to avoid the presence of both pesticides and pathogens on the final product (SAGARPA, 2011).

### 1.1 Fresh produce production in the state of Sinaloa

One of the main activities in Sinaloa is the agriculture. Sinaloa state is located at the northwest of Mexico (27° 7´-22° 20´N, 105° 22´-109-109° 30´O) (Figure 1) with a population of 2,767,761 people (INEGI, 2011).

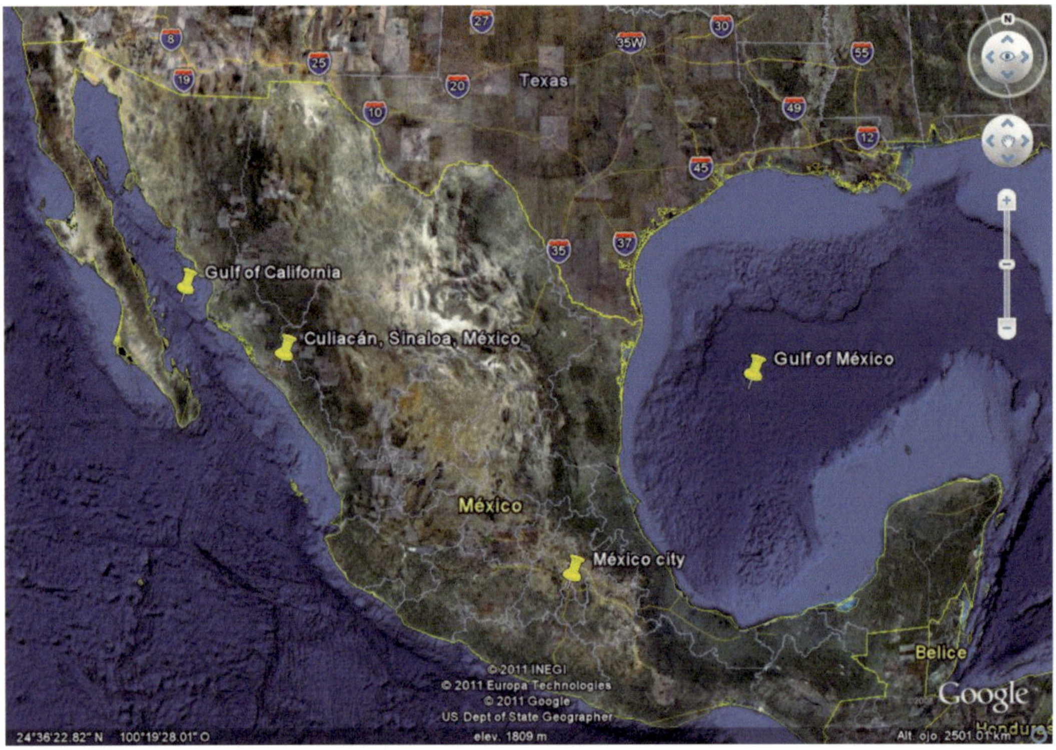


Fig. 1. Location of Sinaloa state.

During the agricultural season of 2006, Confederación de Asociaciones Agrícolas del Estado de Sinaloa (CAADES: Confederation of Agricultural Associations of the State of Sinaloa) reported a total agricultural surface of 1,267,636 ha and a total production worth $1,711,816 USD. Tomato is the most important fresh produce for Sinaloa; from 1980 to 2006, CAADES reported a total of 719,383 ha for red tomato production and profits of $3,098,412 USD, while for green tomato only 130,980 hectares were destined for its production, obtaining profits of $306,662 U.S dollars. In the international trade, the production of tomato favors Mexican economy of America, with a total export of 298,292 t (Figure 2) and profits of $279.7 million USD during the agricultural season of 2008-2009 (Figure 3) (CIDH, 2011).

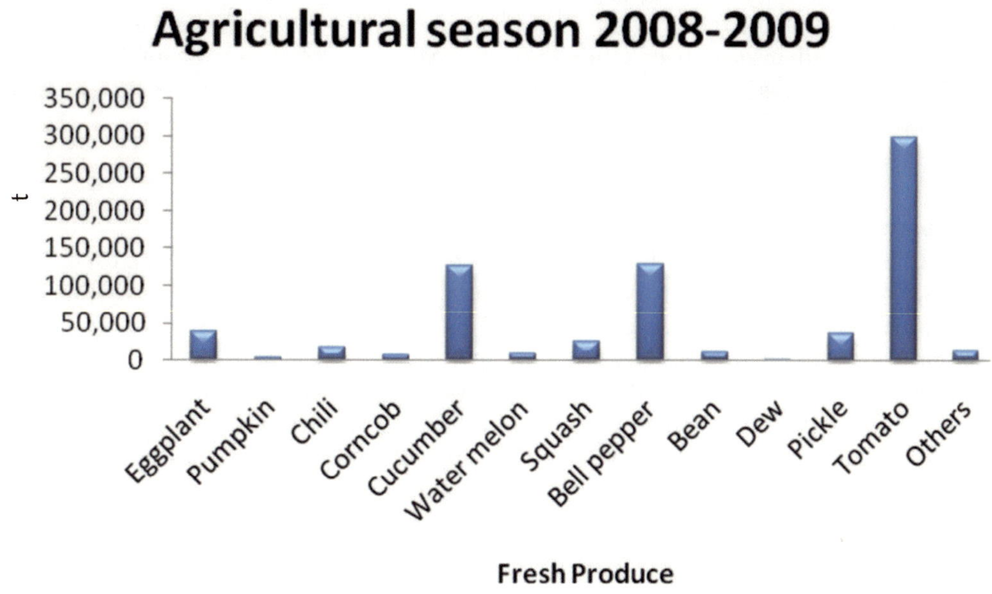


Fig. 2. Total horticultural production expressed in tons from 2008 to 2009 in Sinaloa state. Data from Committee for the Research and Defence of Vegetables, CIDH, 2011.

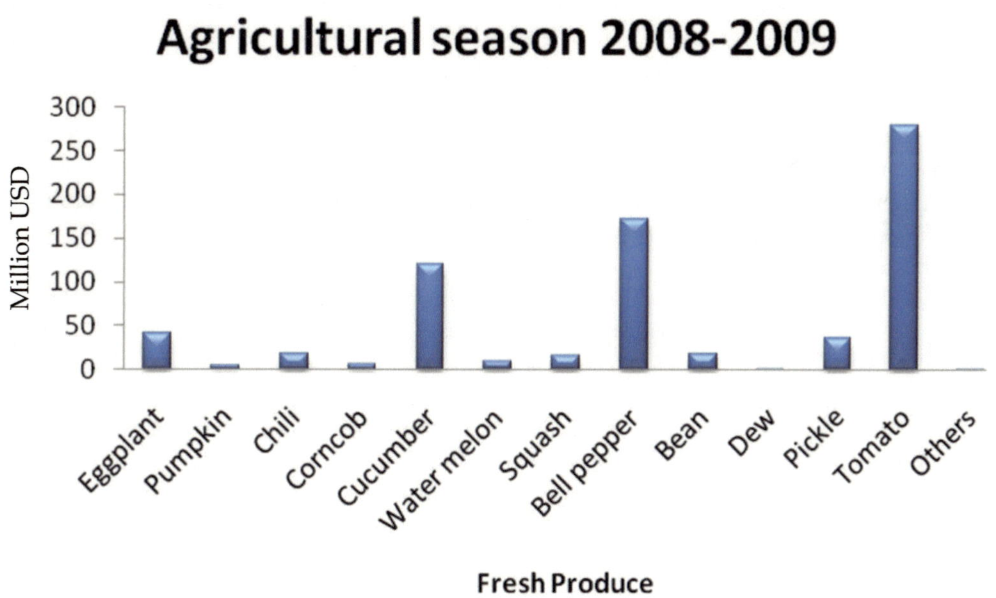


Fig. 3. Global value of horticultural exports from 2008 to 2009 in Sinaloa state expressed in Million USD. Data from CIDH, 2011.

The commercial relationship between Sinaloa state producers and the United States, is given in great majority for the exportation of Mexican fresh produce, which are extensively and carefully produced under strict guidelines of GAP and GMP, to prevent the misuse of pesticides and the presence of pathogens (SENASICA, 2011). As evidence of that, among the different foodborne outbreaks occurred in the United States of America, none of them had been associated to fresh produce grown in fields of Sinaloa.

### 1.2 *Salmonella* Saintpaul outbreak

From April to August of 2008, the US CDC Health Department confirmed the occurrence of a multistate *Salmonella* serotype Saintpaul outbreak affecting 43 US states, Columbia district and Canada (Figure 4). In August of 2008, a total of 1,442 cases and at least 286 hospitalizations and two deaths were reported. The US Health authorities argued high association (85%) of tomato and later jalapeño peppers as the pathogen transmission vehicles and pointed out Sinaloa tomato production as a possible source of the bacterial strain (CDC, 2008). The outbreak and the CDC call alerted both countries, which started to work together to source track the origin of the causative agent.

## 2. Searching the causative agent in Sinaloa fields

### 2.1 Sample collection

In order to confirm or discard the presence of *Salmonella* Saintpaul strain in Sinaloa fields, the U.S Food and Drug Administration (FDA), according to CDC statement, began the traceability of the strain in collaboration with Health and Agricultural Mexican authorities Comisión Federal para la Protección contra Riesgos Sanitarios (COFEPRIS, Federal Commission for Protection against Health Risks) and Servicio Nacional de Sanidad, Inocuidad y Calidad Agroalimentaria (SENASICA, National Health Service, Agri-food Safety and Quality). COFEPRIS and SENASICA are Mexican government institutions responsible to promote the adequate food production and to prevent the microbial risk ensuring food safety. Along with Health and Agricultural authorities of both countries, scientists from the Centro de Investigación en Alimentación y Desarrollo, A.C. (CIAD, Research Center for Food and Development), Culiacán station began collecting samples in Sinaloa fields to search for the *Salmonella enterica* serotype Saintpaul.

The sampling collection was conducted from June 23$^{rd}$ to June 27$^{th}$ of 2008. The sampling areas were divided in agricultural fields and packinghouse´s facilities. From the agricultural fields, canal water, reservoir water, water filtering equipment, soil, and tomato samples were collected; while from packinghouse´s facilities conveyor belts, tomato washing area, drying area and packing lines were sampled.

Sampling procedure was conducted according to the established by the American Public Health Association (APHA, 1998). Water and sediments samples were placed in sterile polypropylene flasks (Nalgene, Miami USA), while hermetic bags and sterile pre-wetted sampling sponges with 15 mL of phosphate-buffered solution (Whirl-Pak, Fort Atkinson, WI, USA) were used for soil and fruit.

### 2.2 *Salmonella* isolation method

*Salmonella* isolation from the collected samples was performed according to the APHA (1998), which consists in the Most Probable Number (MPN) technique by the use of 3x

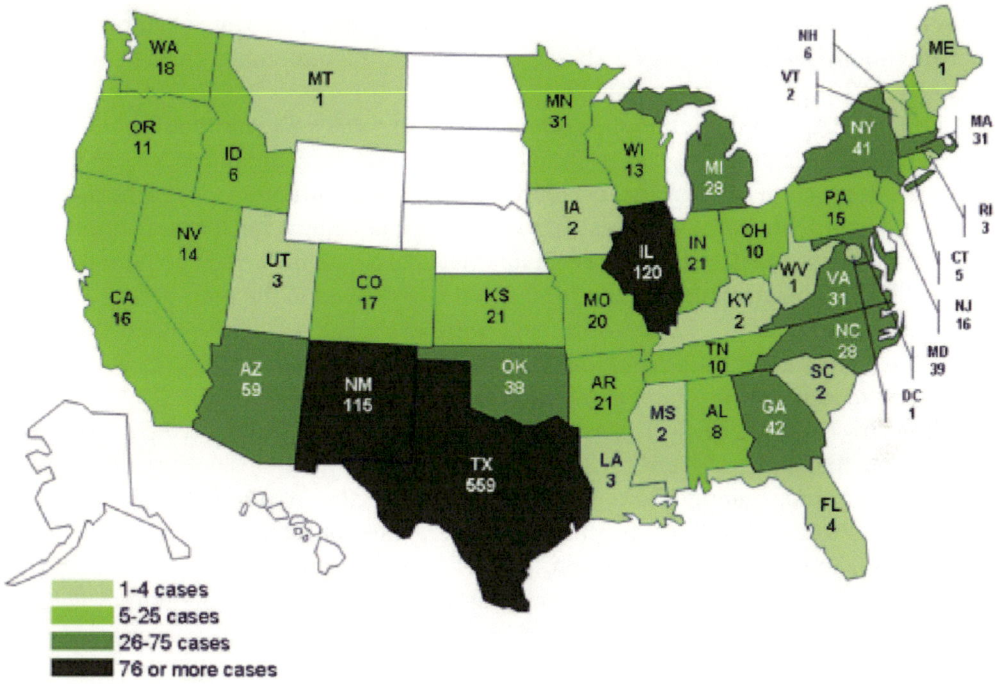


Fig. 4. Distribution and number of infected cases with *Salmonella* Saintpaul, in the United States (CDC, 2008).

Tripticase Soy Broth (3x TSB) (Bioxon, México), modified semi-solid Rappaport Vassiliadis (Difco, USA) and XLD agar (BIoxon, México) as pre enrichment, enrichment and selective isolation, respectively. The homogenized sample was diluted and distributed in 3 sets of 3 tubes each. Once inoculated the tubes were incubated at 37°C during 24 h. After incubation, aliquots were transferred to modified semi-solid Rappaport Vassiliadis (Difco, USA) and incubated at 42°C during 24 h. This process was done by triplicate. Finally a loop of the inoculated semi-solid medium was transferred to the XLD agar (Bioxon, México), which was incubated at 37°C during 24 h to identify presumptive colonies presenting round morphology, black central pigment and a well-defined transparent border. Presumptive colonies were prepared to DNA extraction for confirmation assay by Polymerase Chain Reaction (PCR).

## 3. Results

During the monitoring of packinghouses and agricultural fields, a total of 124 samples were collected and analyzed. According to results, *Salmonella* Saintpaul was absent from any of the samples collected regarding its origin.

It is necessary to remark the absence of *Salmonella* in all the samples analyzed corresponding to packinghouses, which implies a strong evidence of the adherence and following to the GAP and GMP of growers from Sinaloa.

The Ministry of Agriculture announced the absence of *Salmonella* Saintpaul in Sinaloa fields supported by the microbiological traceability conducted by federal and CIAD personnel. During the inspection It was also corroborated the good situation of the horticulture in Sinaloa and that tomatoes from Sinaloa have no responsibility for the unfortunate public health problem occurred in the United States. These actions removed the name of México from the list of countries associated to fresh produce involved in the outbreak.

During this season, only 717,000 t of tomato were exported, a 9.6% less than the previous season due to the *Salmonella* Saintpaul outbreak generating an economic impact for the Sinaloa tomato industry worth $134 million USD losses.

According to United States Department of Agriculture (USDA) 2009, in terms of consumption the tomato is one of the four more consumed fresh produce, as well as potato, lettuce and onion, while in terms of trade, the imports of Mexican tomato represent a strong source of profits. However, this outbreak produced a negative perception for the tomato consumption, not only for Mexican tomato but also to tomato grown in the USA. According to the Center of Agribusiness and Economic Development from The University of Georgia in 2008, the tomato demand decreased significantly during the outbreak, with an average impact of $11,778 USD per acre for tomato not sold and a total of $25.7 million USD only for Georgia State.

The economic impact in México caused by the presumptive responsibility of Mexican tomato as transmission vehicle of *Salmonella* Saintpaul promoted the emergence of the Coordinación Estatal de Inocuidad Hidroagrícola, Pecuaria, Acuícola y Pesquera (CEIHAPAP), which is governed by the Stated of Sinaloa to coordinate efforts among producers and scientific institutions for the development of methods to ensure the safety production of fresh produce, free of biological, chemical and physical agents that can represent risks for the consumer´s health.

Results of the absence of *Salmonella* Saintpaul from Sinaloa tomatoes allowed the re-opening of the international trade for tomatoes, helping the economy and strengthening the commercial relationship between México and the United States of America.

## 4. Conclusions

According to the scientific evidence, it was demonstrated the consistent and effective adherence to the GMP and GAP by the Mexican growers, as well as the proper monitoring of fields to ensure microbiological quality of the fresh produce.

## 5. References

Allos B. M., Moore M. R., Griffin P. M. and Tauxe R. V. 2004. "Surveillance for Sporadic Foodborne Disease in the 21st Century: The foodNet Perspective". *Clinical Infectious Diseases*. 38:S115-S120.

American Public Health Association, 1998. Compendium of Methods for the Microbiological Examination of Foods. 4th ed. ISBN 0-87553-175x.

American Public Health Association, 1998. Standard Methods for the Examination of Water and Wastewater. 20th ed.

Brakstad O., Aasbak K., Maeland J., 1992. "Detection of *Staphylococcus aureus* by Polymerase Chain Reaction Amplification of the nuc Gene". *Journal of Clinical Microbiology* 30:1654-1660.

Buzby J. C., Roberts T., Jordan Lin C-T., MacDonald J. M., 1996. "Bacterial Foodborne Disease: MedicalCosts and Productivity Losses" *Food and Consumer Economics Division, Economic Research Service, U. S.* Department of Agriculture. Agricultural Economic Report No. 741.

Center for Disease control, 2008. "Investigation of outbreak of infections caused by *Salmonella* Saintpaul" www.cdc.gov/salmonella/outbreaks.html

Imhoff B., Morse D, Shiferaw B., Hawkins M., Vugia D., Lance-Parker S., Hadler J., Medus C., Kennedy M., Moore M. R. and Van Gilder T. 2004 "Burden of Self-Reported Acute Diarrheal Illness in FoodNet Surveillance Areas, 1998-1999". *Clinical Infectious Diseases*. 38:S219-S226.

Mead P.S., Slutsker L., Dietz V., McCaig L. F., Bresee J. S., Shapiro C., Griffin P. M. and Tauxe R. V. 1999. "Food-Related Illness and Death in the United States". *Emerging Infectious Diseases* 5:607-625.

Scallan E., 2007. "Activities, Achievements, and Lessons Learned during the First 10 Years of the Foodborne Diseases Active Surveillance Network: 1995-2005". *Clinical Infectious Diseases* 44: 718-25.

Scallan E., Griffin P.M., Angulo F.J., Tauxe R.V., Hoekstra R.M, 2011. "Foodborne Illnesses acquired in the United States-Unspecifies Agents". *Emerging Infectioous Diseases* 17,1: 16-22.

Scott E. 1996. "Foodborne disease and other hygiene issues in the home". *Journal of Applied Bacteriology* 80:5-9.

The University of Georgia, 2008. "Economic Impact of Georgia Tomato Production Value Losses due to the U.S Salmonella Outbreak". Center For Agribusiness and Economic Development. www.caed.uga.edu/publications/2008/pdf/CR-08-17.pdf

Wang R., Cao W., Cerniglia C., 1997. "A universal protocol for PCR detection of 13 species of foodborne pathogens in foods". *Journal of Applied Microbiology* 83:727-736.

World Health Organization (WHO), 2008. "Foodborne disease outbreaks: guidelines for investigation and control". *WHO Library* ISBN 978 924 1547222.

www.cidh.org.mx/publico/plantilla/pl5.aspx?cveseccion=313

www.caades.org.mx

http://www.inegi.org.mx/sistemas/mexicocifras/default.aspx?ent=25

http://www.senasica.gob.mx/?doc=3790

http://www.cdc.gov/salmonella/outbreaks.html
www.cdc.gov/salmonella/saintpaul/jalapeno/map.html
www.ers.usda.gov/briefing/vegetables/tomatoes.htm

# 11

# Antimicrobial Drug Resistance and Molecular Characterization of *Salmonella* Isolated from Domestic Animals, Humans and Meat Products

Margaret. L. Khaitsa and Dawn Doetkott
*North Dakota State University*
*USA*

## 1. Introduction

Infections with nontyphoid *Salmonella enterica* serovars represent an important public health problem worldwide (Zhao et al. 2003) and an economic burden in many parts of the world today (Gomez et al 1997; Vugia et al, 2004). In the United States (US), *Salmonella* is the second most common identifiable cause of illness, and the leading cause of hospitalizations and deaths, due to food-borne bacterial infection (Mead et al, 1999). Each year, 31 major known pathogens acquired in the US caused an estimated 9.4 million episodes of foodborne illness (Scallan et al, 2011), and an estimated 38.4 million episodes of domestically acquired foodborne illness were caused by unspecified agents, resulting in 71,878 hospitalizations and 1,686 deaths (Scallan et al, 2011). The annual economic cost due to foodborne *Salmonella* infections in the US alone is estimated at $2.4 billion (http://www.ers.usda.gov) with an estimated 1.4 million cases of salmonellosis and over 500 deaths annually (Arshad et al. 2007). In 2004 for instance, among 3686 *Salmonella* isolates serotyped, 862 (23%) were serotype Typhimurium, 565 (15%) Enteritidis, 399 (11%) Newport and 248 (7%) Heidelberg (CDC, 2005). Similarly, the same *Salmonella enterica* serovars were reported as major causes of salmonellosis in humans in another study (Oloya et al. 2007). The predominance of *S. Typhimurium* and *S. Newport* in both domestic animals and human case reports further highlights their role in causing cross infections (Arshad et al. 2007; Bacon et al. 2002; Besser et al. 2000).

Although human salmonellosis has been associated with exposure to other vehicles of transmission (e.g. pets, reptiles, and contaminated water), about 95% of human infections have been found to be associated with ingestion of contaminated foods; namely animal products (Gaul et al. 2007; McLaughlin et al. 2006; Padungtod and Kaneene 2006), poultry products (Plym and Wierup 2006; Mead et al. 1999), sea foods (Duran and Marshall 2005; Ozogul et al. 2007; Shabarinath et al. 2007) and fresh produce (Johnston et al. 2006; Puohiniemi et al. 1997). Direct contact with companion and food animals has also been documented as another important route of *Salmonella* transmission to humans (Coburn et al. 2006; Doyle and Erickson 2006; Gorman and Adley 2004; Mead et al. 1999; Padungtod and Kaneene 2006). Consumption of raw or undercooked ground beef and lack of safe food handling practices to prevent cross contamination are considered critical in infections at household levels (Ling et al. 2001). These reports highlight the possibility of increased transmission of these organisms to humans through the food chain (Zhao et al. 2003). Understanding the association between human salmonellosis cases, animal sources and the environment is an important epidemiological factor needed to successfully control the spread of the infection within communities (Ling et al. 2001).

Recently, emergence of resistant and multi-resistant bacteria has become an important worldwide sanitary problem, impacting both veterinary medicine and public health through the potential for therapeutic failures (Lathers, 2001). Antimicrobial resistance among bacterial isolates from animals is also of concern because of the potential for these organisms to be food-borne or zoonotic pathogens or to be donors of resistance genes to human pathogens (Lathers, 2001). For instance, multidrug-resistant Salmonella enterica serovar Typhimurium phage type DT104, resistant to ampicillin, chloramphenicol/florfenicol, streptomycin, sulfonamides, and tetracycline, has disseminated worldwide (Mulvey et al, 2006). The resistance genes reside on the 43-kb Salmonella genomic island 1 (SGI1), which is transferable. Drug-resistant variants of SGI1 have been identified in numerous serotypes. Strains harboring SGI1 may be more virulent and have a tendency to rapidly disseminate (Mulvey et al, 2006).

International agencies, such as the World Health Organization (WHO) have recommended improving resistance surveillance studies in not only human but also animal origin strains (WHO, 2005). Because of its ubiquitous characteristics and zoonotic nature, *Salmonella spp*. can be used as a good indicator microorganism for resistance surveillance studies (Usera, et al, 2002). Yet there is little information available on *Salmonella* isolates from healthy animals on farms across a wide geographic area that uses various production practices (Dargatz, et al, 2002). This chapter will examine the genotypic relatedness of *Salmonella* serovars commonly isolated from domestic animals raised under different production systems, meat products and humans in order to quantify their role in causing human infection. Antimicrobial drug resistance (AMR) and genetic profiles of *Salmonella* will be used to assess their role in transferring drug resistance to humans.

Reliable and powerful typing methods are necessary in order to gain insight into the infection routes of pathogenic microorganisms. Traditionally, *Salmonella* serotyping combined with various molecular techniques such as phage typing, plasmid profiles, pulsed field gel electrophoresis (PFGE) (Gaul et al. 2007; Guerra et al. 2000; Pickard et al. 2008; Rabsch 2007; Trung et al. 2007) have been used to establish this association. The PFGE method particularly has been found to be very discriminatory and reproducible (Guerra et al. 2000; Tsen et al. 2002) and useful in epidemiological analysis of *Salmonella* infections (Refsum et al. 2002) to determine the relatedness of individual cases (Kim et al. 2007), detect and establish outbreaks (Puohiniemi et al. 1997; Xercavins et al. 1997) and determine linkage between human salmonellosis and consumption of foods of animal origin (McLaughlin et al. 2006). PFGE is increasingly being used as well to identify multidrug resistant strains (Bacon et al. 2002; Besser et al. 2000; McLaughlin et al. 2006; Santos et al. 2007). In fact, the method allows for the detection of DNA polymorphisms that were previously undetected by other techniques (Santos et al. 2007). Also, PFGE has been widely used to investigate the ecology of foodborne pathogens at various points along the food chain (Avery et al., 2002; Vali et al., 2005). This technique has also been used to evaluate the genetic diversity in *Salmonella* isolates from humans, animals, and the environment (Refsum et al., 2002; Gaul et al,2007), and from oysters (Brands et al., 2005). PFGE using XbaI restriction was used by Gaul et al (2007) for screening and identifying swine Salmonella serotypes. Additionally, in the US, molecular subtyping network for foodborne bacterial diseases including non-typhoidal *Salmonella* serotypes has been using standardized PFGE technique (Swaminathan, et al., 2001).

Most people who suffer from *Salmonella* infections usually present with temporary gastroenteritis that usually does not require treatment. However, when infection becomes invasive, antimicrobial treatment is mandatory (Winokur et al, 2000). As a result, traditionally ampicillin, chloramphenicol, and trimethoprim-sulfamethoxazole were used to treat such severe cases. However, the increasing number of antimicrobial-resistant *Salmonella* strains has led to a decrease in the efficacy of these treatments (Angulo et al, 2000). Additionally, the frequency of isolation of *Salmonella* strains resistant to one or more antimicrobial agents has risen in the US (Fey et al, 2000), and elsewhere in the world (Al-Tawfiq, 2007). Fluoroquinolones and broad-spectrum cephalosporins have been employed most recently, as the preferred drugs for treatment of adults and children, respectively, due to the low number of *Salmonella* isolates showing resistance to these drugs (Angulo et al, 2000; Chiappini et al, 2002). However, the viability of these drugs may be diminishing as *Salmonella* strains producing β-lactamases conferring resistance to broad-spectrum cephalosporins have been isolated from clinical patients (Dunne et al, 2000; Winokur et al, 2000), some of which have been acquired from cattle (Fey et al, 2000). The situation is reported to be more complex and difficult in developing countries where there is a widespread misuse of antimicrobials both in human and veterinary medicine practices (Okeke et al, 2005). Furthermore, resistance to combinations of several classes of antimicrobials has led to the emergence of multidrug-resistant (MDR) strains that may pass from food animals to humans (Fey et al, 2000).

The spread of antibiotic resistance among bacteria have been associated with mobile genetic elements such as plasmids, transposons (Zhang et al, 2004) and integrons (Miko et al, 2005). Notably, MDR has been frequently linked with microbial genomic elements known as integrons, which have the ability to distribute genes encoding resistance to a number of antimicrobial drugs (Miko et al, 2005). Integrons do have specific structures and can capture genes notably those encoding antimicrobial resistance by a site-specific recombination system and have been located in both chromosomal and extra chromosomal DNA (Bennet, 1999; Hall and Collis 1995). The main classes of integrons are found in the family *Enterobacteriaceae* with class 1 integrons being the most extensively studied. Class 1 integrons are characterized by presence of two conserved segments, the 5′ -conserved segment (5′ -CS) and 3'-conserved segment (3'-CS) (Bennet, 1999), and are defined by an *intI* gene encoding integrase, a recombinant site *attI,* and a strong promoter. Previous studies (Zhang et al, 2004; Zhao et al, 2005) on integrons and associated antimicrobial resistance genes in *Salmonella* revealed a predominance of gene cassettes that confer resistance to aminoglycosides and trimethoprim, with *aadA* genes carried by all the integrons-containing *Salmonella* serovars. The investigation of multi-drug-resistance in foodborne pathogens in general and *Salmonella* in particular is essential for the proper understanding of the epidemiology of emerging multidrug resistance in *Salmonella* serovars (Winokur et al, 2000). The implications of therapeutic failure in public health due to multidrug resistance is particularly important given that *Salmonella* is the leading cause of hospitalizations and deaths, due to food-borne bacterial infection in the US (Mead et al, 1999).

### 1.1 Aim of chapter

This chapter will 1) describe prevalence, antimicrobial drug resistance (AMR) and molecular characterization of *Salmonella* commonly isolated from domestic animals, humans and meat products and 2) assess the relatedness of AMR and genetic profiles of *Salmonella* from various sources and their role in transferring antimicrobial resistance to humans.

## 2. Research methods

### 2.1 *Salmonella* from domestic animals sources

#### 2.1.1 *Salmonella* from feedlot cattle

One hundred and thirty eight (138) 1-year-old steers distributed in 24 pens (6 steers/pen) were used in this study (Tabe et al (2010a, 2010b). Cattle from various private farms were housed at the North Dakota State University feedlot facility in October 2006. From October 2006 to March 26, 2007 cattle were placed on growers diet and then on finishing diet from March 27 to June 2007. Cattle in different pens could not directly contact each other, and there was no sharing of feed or water sources between pens. Fecal samples were collected from cattle every three weeks from March 2007 to June 2007. During the first and second sampling periods (March and April 2007 respectively), one-hundred-thirty eight cattle were available for the study. At the third sampling period (May 2007), two unhealthy cattle were withdrawn from the study while at the last sampling period (June 2007), forty six cattle were available as the rest had been taken for slaughter.

Samples were collected in accordance with the guidelines approved by the Institutional Animal Care and Use Committee (IACUC) following a previously described protocol (Khaitsa et al., 2007a). The feces were put into sterile plastic cups and placed in iced-pack coolers before transport to the laboratory for processing. The sampling procedure was repeated every three weeks for the entire finishing period. For the isolation of *Salmonella*, fecal samples were cultured using conventional culture methods optimized for the detection of *Salmonella* (Khaitsa et al., 2007). Briefly, a sterile swab was loaded with fecal sample and pre-enriched in buffered peptone water (Difco, Becton Dickinson) at 37°C overnight followed by immunomagnetic beads separation specific for *Salmonella* species (Dynabeads anti-*Salmonella*, Dynal Biotech, Inc., Lake Success, N.Y.) according to the **manufacturer's** instructions. After the final wash, the beads were transferred to 10 ml of Rappaport Vassiliadis R10 (RV) broth (Becton Dickinson) and incubated (with constant gentle shaking) at 42$^0$C for 24 h. Following incubation, the RV cultures were streaked onto modified brilliant green agar (Becton Dickinson) and mannitol lysine crystal violet brilliant green agar (Oxoid, Basingstoke, UK). Colonies with typical *Salmonella* characteristics (Fratamico et al., 2000) were stabbed in 10-ml triple sugar iron agar slants (Becton Dickinson), and the biochemical results read after 24-h incubation as described. Presumptive *Salmonella* isolates were stabbed into 2 ml tryptic soy agar (Difco, Becton Dickinson) slants and shipped to the National Veterinary Service Laboratories, Animal and Plant Health Inspection Services, US Department of Agriculture, Ames, Iowa, for serotyping. The detection sensitivity culture post immunomagnetic separation and enrichment using culture media for *Salmonella* was based on growth of bacteria of interest on the culture plates. Fifty eight (58) isolates of *Salmonella* were shipped to the *E. coli* reference center (University Park, PA) for PFGE.

#### 2.1.2 *Salmonella* from ranch cattle

The objective of this study (Theis et al 2005, 2006, 2007) was to determine the prevalence, serotypes, and antimicrobial resistance patterns of *Salmonella* isolates recovered from grass fed cattle in North Dakota. A total of 212 cattle (97 calves and 115 cows) originating from 7 cow-calf farms in the ND counties of Billings, Dunn, Mercer and Stark participated in the study. A random sample of at least 30 cattle (15 calves and 15 adult cows) were selected from each of the 7 herds that participated in the study except where less than 30 animals in each category were available; in that case all of them were sampled. One herd had only calves and 2 herds had only adult cows and so 30 animals of one category were sampled from each of these herds. Approximately 20 grams of feces were obtained from the rectum of individual cattle and shipped by Fedex overnight to the department of Veterinary and Microbiological Sciences, at North Dakota State University. The fecal samples were processed within twenty-four hours of their arrival to the laboratory. The fecal samples were cultured in the laboratory using culture methods optimized for the detection of *Salmonella* (Khaitsa et al., 2007a) in fecal specimens. Presumptive *Salmonella* isolates were sent to NVSL in Ames, IA for serotyping. Antimicrobial susceptibility of *Salmonella* isolates was determined using a custom designed panel according to the manufacturer's instructions (Sensititre, Trek Diagnostics, Westlake, Ohio).

#### 2.1.3 *Salmonella* from dairy cattle

A study (Khaitsa et al, 2004) investigated the prevalence of cattle shedding *Salmonella* in their feces at the NDSU dairy and to test antimicrobial susceptibility of *Salmonella* isolates. In June, 2004, fecal samples from a random sample of thirty cows out of 60 at the NDSU dairy were collected and cultured for *Salmonella* at the Department of Veterinary and Microbiological Sciences. Approximately 20g of fecal matter was obtained from the rectum of each cow and transported on ice to the Department of Veterinary and Microbiology Sciences at NDSU for microbiologic culture. The fecal samples were cultured in the laboratory using culture methods optimized for the detection of *Salmonella* (Khaitsa et al 2007a) in fecal specimens.

#### 2.1.4 *Salmonella* from bison

Twenty bison from one herd in North Dakota, US were run through a chute and approximately 20 grams of feces obtained from the rectum of each animal. Fecal samples were transferred into sterile plastic cups, placed on ice and transported to the laboratory for culturing. *Salmonella* spp were cultured using the procedure described by Khaitsa et al (2007a). All suspect colonies were sent to National Veterinary Services Lab, Ames, IA for serotyping. Antimicrobial susceptibility testing was carried out using Sensititre Trek Diagnostic Systems, Westlake, OH.

### 2.2 *Salmonella* from meats

A study (Khaitsa et al 2007b) investigated the occurrence of *Salmonella* in raw and ready to eat turkey meat products, and factors associated with its occurrence in 959 turkey meat products (raw, n =614; and ready to eat (RTE), n = 345) purchased from four retail outlets in one city in the Midwestern United States. Another study (Kegode et al, 2008) investigated occurrence of *Salmonella* species, in 456 fresh raw meat products (turkey (n=87, 19.1%) chicken (n=123, 27.0%) chicken, pork (n=113, 24.8%) and beef (n=133, 29.2%)) purchased from five retail outlets in the Midwestern United States during a 12-week period (July 11, 2005 to October 3, 2005). Three stores were visited each week until all the stores had been visited a total of five times. The stores were sampled on different days of the week during subsequent sampling times in order to minimize systematic bias associated with a particular day of the week. On each visit to a store, an average of 18 (range 11 to 23) fresh raw samples of all meat types (turkey, chicken, pork, and beef) and different meat products were obtained. Turkey products sampled included: ground breast, breast, breast cutlets, breast tenderloin, drumstick, and thigh. Chicken products comprised whole, quarter, breast, drumstick, thigh, wing, and kebab; pork products included ground, chops, steak, ribs, neck bones, roast, and stew; beef products consisted of ground beef-store brand, steak, stew, chuck, roast, ribs, round, loin, and kebab. Where available, different brands were selected including in-store packaged products. All products were raw and unfrozen. Samples were immediately transported to the laboratory on ice and processed within one hour of purchase.

For *Salmonella* isolation, meat samples were aseptically placed in a plastic WhirlPak bag (Nasco, Fort Atkinson, WI) with 200-400ml buffered peptone water, depending on the size of the meat sample. Approximately 200 ml and 400 ml of buffered peptone water added to any meat sample that was ≤ 1 Ib and > 1Ib, respectively. The bags were shaken manually for 3 minutes and left on ice for 20 minutes. All samples were subjected to an enrichment procedure. The buffered peptone water (BPW) rinse solution (20ml) was mixed with the same volume of double-concentrated lactose broth and enriched overnight at 35°C. To culture *Salmonella,* 1.0 ml of the lactose enrichment broth was transferred into 9.0 ml of tetrathionate broth and incubated (42°C for 24 hr.) The broth culture was then streaked onto XLT4 agar plates and incubated (24h at 37°C). Suspect colonies (yellow with black centers) were stabbed in Triple Sugar Iron (TSI) agar slants and incubated (37°C for 24 hr.) Presumptive *Salmonella* isolates, which formed red slants with black butts, were sent for serotyping to the US National Veterinary Services Laboratories (NVSL, Ames, IA).

Additionally, Tumuhairwe et al (2007) reviewed the temporal and spatial distribution of 1465 human salmonellosis cases associated with consumption of turkey meat in the US during the period 1990 to 2003 involving 49/50 states. Tumuhairwe et al (2007) also described the distribution of salmonellosis cases by vehicle and serotype. Trends in the outbreak numbers over time, and major serotypes across vehicles were tested by Cox-Stuart and chi-square test, respectively. Also, a study (Tumuhairwe et al, 2008) characterized 386 non-typhoidal salmonellosis cases in North Dakota from 2000 to 2005. Salmonellosis cases were extracted from the enteric disease investigation database of the North Dakota Department of Health (NDDoH) for the period 2000 to 2005.

### 2.3 *Salmonella* from clinical cases of humans and animals (cattle, chicken, ducks, swine, turkeys, elk and bison)

A total of 434 frozen presumptive *Salmonella* isolates were included in the study. The isolates were previously obtained from 4 different sources comprising; 1) feces from apparently healthy feedlot, range and dairy cattle in an ongoing surveillance program in ND; 2) Clinical isolates from sick or dead cattle, chicken, ducks, swine, turkeys, elk and bison submitted to North Dakota State University-Veterinary Diagnostic Laboratory (NDSU-VDL) (2000-2005); 3) Frozen isolates from *Salmonella* data bank in the NDSU-Veterinary and Microbiological Services (VMS) Department from previous food surveillance studies involving turkey, chicken and bison meat sold at the grocery stores at ND; and 4) 183 *Salmonella* isolated from stools of human patients in ND (2000-2005) and stored at North Dakota Department of Health (NDDoH) (Table 1).

| Source | Nature/state of the sample | Number | Percent |
|---|---|---|---|
| Humans | sick | 179 | 41.2 |
| Cattle | feedlot (feces) | 112 | 25.8 |
| | dairy (feces) | 5 | 1.2 |
| | range(feces) | 17 | 3.9 |
| | sick or dead cattle | 59 | 13.6 |
| Chicken | retail chicken | 4 | 0.9 |
| Ducks | ill/dead | 1 | 0.2 |
| Swine | ill/dead | 5 | 1.2 |
| Turkeys | ill/dead | 3 | 0.7 |
| | meat | 32 | 7.4 |
| Elk | ill/dead | 1 | 0.2 |
| Bison | fecal samples | 1 | 0.2 |
| | meat | 1 | 0.2 |
| Humans | sick | 179 | 41.2 |
| Others | beddings, linx etc | 14 | 3.2 |
| Total | | 434 | 100 |

Table 1. Sources of *Salmonella* isolates from clinical cases of humans and animals

### 2.4 Antimicrobial resistance (AMR) testing

Antimicrobial susceptibility of *Salmonella* isolates from the various sources was determined using the National Antimicrobial Resistance Monitoring System (NARMS) panel according to Food and Drug Administration and National Committee for Clinical Laboratory Standards (NCCLS) recommendation (Sensititre®, Trek Diagnostics System, Inc, Westlake, Ohio). Each isolate was screened for resistance using full-range minimum inhibitory concentration. The US National Antimicrobial Resistance Monitoring System (NARMS) panels were used to compare AMR levels between domestic animal and human isolates of the same genotype in order to assess a possible role of domestic animals in transfer of AMR of *Salmonella* isolated from human cases. The antimicrobials tested included ampicillin, apramycin, ceftiofur, chlortetracycline, clindamycin, enrofloxacin, erythromycin, florfenicol , gentamicin, neomycin, oxytetracycline, penicillin, spectinomycin, sulphachloropyridazine, sulphadimethoxime, sulphathiazole, tiamulin, tilmicosin, trimethoprim/ sulphamethoxazole and tylosin. Isolates were defined as resistant according to FDA recommended breakpoints. Breakpoints were defined as minimum drug concentration above which growth of the test isolate should not occur (Logue et al. 2003).

### 2.5 *Salmonella* serotyping and genotyping

Frozen (-70°C) presumptive *Salmonella* cultures from the above sources were thawed and stabbed into 2ml tryptic soy agar (Difco, Becton Dickinson) deeps and shipped to the

National Veterinary Service Laboratories, Animal and Plant Health Inspection Services, U.S. Department of Agriculture, Ames, Iowa, for serotyping. PFGE assays on *Salmonella* cultures to investigate their genotypic relatedness were performed at the *E. coli* Reference Centre, Pennsylvania State University, University Park. The sample preparation, restriction digestion, electrophoresis, and gel staining for PFGE were accomplished following the CDC-standardized procedure as described (CDC, 2004) (http://www.cdc.gov/pulsenet/protocols.htm). Restriction endonuclease *XbaI* (Roche Diagnostics Corporation, Indianapolis, IN) was used for restriction digestion of genomic DNA. The size standard used for all gels was *XbaI*-digested DNA from *Salmonella* Braenderup strain H9812 (American Type Culture Collection catalogue no. BAA-664), i.e. the universal size standard used by all PulseNet laboratories. Fingerprints were analyzed using BioNumerics software version 3.5 (Applied Maths, Austin, Texas). Strain relatedness was done based on previously recommended criteria (Gebreyes et al. 2006) using 'different bands' algorithm for clustering and the unweighted pair group for arithmetic means (UPGMA) tree-building approach with optimization of 1 and 0.5% position tolerance. Visual inspection of the patterns was performed as a final step for analysis.

### 2.6 PCR amplification of class 1 and 2 integrons

The bacterial DNA template preparation and the PCR conditions for the detection of class 1 and class 2 integrons were undertaken as previously described (Miko et al, 2005). The screening for the presence of class 1 and class 2 integrons was carried out using PCR with primers specific for the *intI1* ( and *intI2* (Goldstein et al, 2001)). The primer sequences used are shown in Table 2. Amplifications were performed in 10 µL of 5x Taq PCR Master Mix (Qiagen, Valencia, CA, USA), 2 pmol/L each primer, and 2 µg template DNA. Amplification specifications were as follows: 5 min at 94°C followed by 35 cycles of 1 min at 94°C, 1 min at 55°C, and 30 s at 72°C. PCR products were analyzed by gel electrophoresis with 2 % agarose gels. All PCRs included DNA ladder, positive and negative controls.

| Primers | Sequence [a] | Size (bp) | PCR Annealin g Temp (⁰C) | References |
|---|---|---|---|---|
| *intI1* | F: CCTCCCGCACGATGATC | 280 | 55 | *Kraft et al., 1986* |
| | R: TCCACGCATCGTCAGGC | | | |
| *intI2* | F: TATTGCTGGGATTAGGC | 233 | 50 | *Goldstein et al., 2001* |
| | R: ACGGCTACCCTCTGTTATC | | | |

Table 2. PCR primers and conditions used in Screening *Salmonella* isolates for presence of class 1 and class 2 integrons; [a] F, Forward; R, Reverse.

## 3. Key results

### 3.1 *Salmonella* from feedlot cattle

*Salmonella* was isolated from 58 out of 458 (12.7%) fecal samples tested (Tabe et al, 2010a, 2010b). All *Salmonella* belonged to the Typhimurium serotype and the majority 53/58 (91.4%) were Typhimurium *vars* Copenhagen. The rest (3/58, 5%) were reported as

*Salmonella* Typhimurium. AMR testing showed that all isolates were resistant to more than one of the antibiotics (Table 3). All but two of the isolates were resistant to more than two of the antibiotics tested with 96.6% (56 of 58) of the isolates showing MDR antibiogram. All isolates tested were susceptible to amikacin, cefoxitin, cetriaxone, ciprofloxacin, gentamycin, gentamycin, nalidixic acid, and trimethoprim-sulfamethoxazole (Table 3). Almost all the isolates recovered from this study had a similar antimicrobial pattern. Regardless of sampling period (1, 2, or 3), 29 (3 Salmonella serovars Typhimurium and 26 Salmonella serovars Typhimurium var Copenhagen) were positive for class I integron (280 bp product) while only two of the isolates showed a 233-bp PCR product using primers *intI2* thus suggesting the presence of integron 2. These two isolates also had integron 1. Upon PFGE analysis, 9 distinguishable *Salmonella* genotypes were identified. For clarity, the genotypes were numbered I to IX with genotype V (28 of 58; 46.6%) being the most prevalent followed by type VII (15 of 58; 25.9 %) (Figure 1). Genotypes I, II, and III had the least prevalence (1 of 58; 1.7 % each). From the 58 isolates, types IV, V, VII, VIII, and IX (38 of 58; 65.5 %) isolated from the cattle at two sampling periods were observed at a similarity level of 100 %. Type V (28 of 58 isolates; 48.2 %) genotypes comprised of the most common isolates; of the 28 isolates from type V, 8 of 28 (28.6%), 18 of 28 (64.3%), and 2 of 28 (7.1%) were derived from sampling 1, 2 and 3 respectively. (Figure1). The 2 isolates which were positive for both *Int* 1 and 2 belonged to genotypes I and IV, respectively. Sampling time had a significant effect on the recovery of *Salmonella* ($P$ = 0.004) while pen ($P$ = 0.79) did not. All 58 *Salmonella* isolates which were grouped into two clusters (d and e) and five single isolates (a, b, c, f, and g) were observed at a similarity level of 80% (Figure 1).

| Antibiotics | Susceptible Isolates (%) | Intermediate Isolates (%) | Resistant Isolates (%) |
|---|---|---|---|
| Amikacin (0.5–64), | 58(100.0) | - | - |
| Amoxicillin/clavulanic acid (1/0.5–32/16) | 2(3.5) | 1(1.7) | 55(94.8) |
| Ampicillin (2–32) | 2(5.3) | - | 56(94.7) |
| Cefoxitin (0.5–32) | 58(100.0) | - | - |
| Cetriaxone (0.25–64) | 58(100.0) | - | - |
| Chloramphenicol (2–32) | - | 2(5.3) | 56(94.7) |
| Ciprofloxacin (0.015–4) | 58(100.0) | - | - |
| Gentamycin (0.25–16) | 58(100.0) | - | - |
| Kanamycin (6–64) | 58(100.0) | - | - |
| Nalidixic acid (0.5–32) | 58(100.0) | - | - |
| Streptomycin (32–64) | NI | NI | 56(94.7) |
| Sulfizoxazole (16–512) | 2(5.3) | - | 56(94.7) |
| Tetracycline(4–32), | 2(5.3) | - | 56(94.7) |
| Trimethoprim-sulfamethoxazole (4-76) | 58(100.0) | - | - |

Table 3. Number (%) of *Salmonella* isolates resistant/susceptible to various antimicrobials (N = 15)

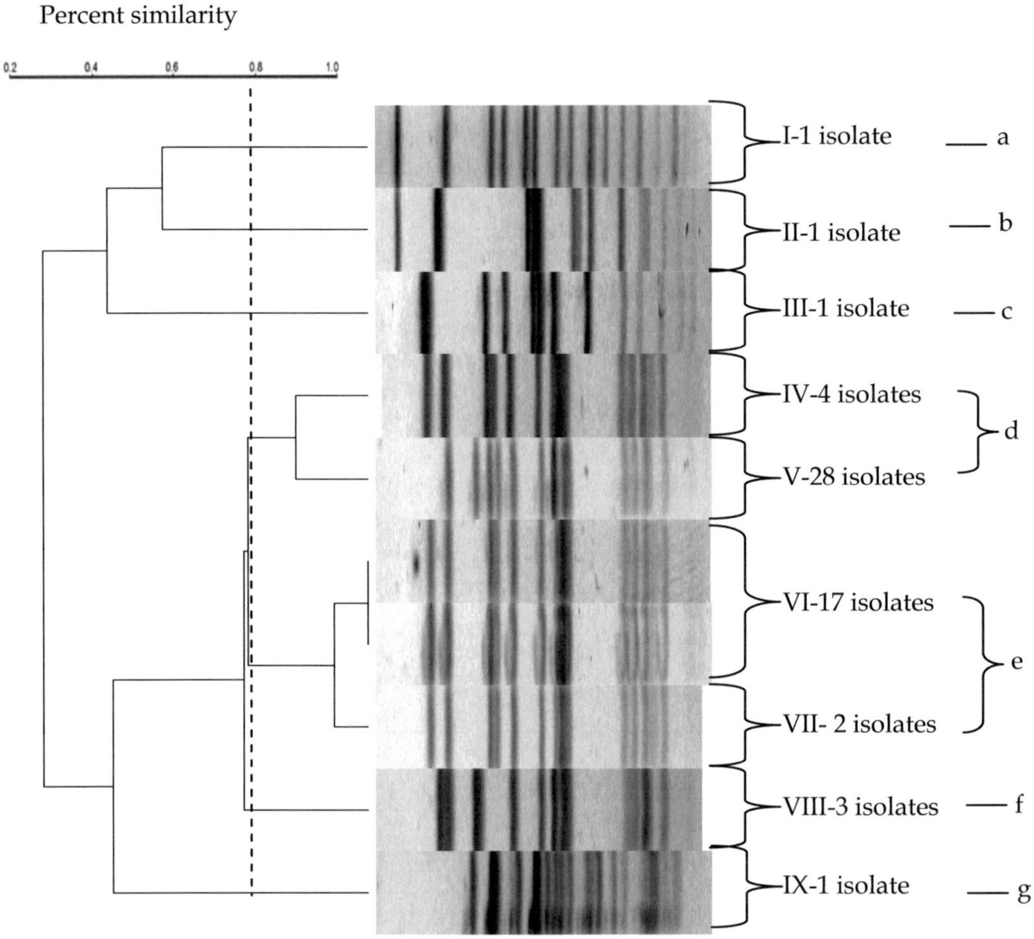


Fig. 1. Dendogram generated from the *XbaI* patterns of the 58 *Salmonella* isolates using UPGMA clustering analysis with the BioNumerics software. A positive tolerance of 1.5 % was chosen.

### 3.1.1 *Salmonella* from ranch cattle

Of the 212 cattle (115 adult cattle, 97 calves) investigated by Theis et al (2007), 15 (7%) tested positive for *Salmonella*. The prevalence of *Salmonella* among adult cattle and calves was 9/115 (7.8%) and 6/97 (6.2%), respectively. The 15 cattle that tested positive to *Salmonella* were distributed in three of the four counties with the majority originating from Billings county and no animal from Mercer county as follows: Stark (7/92, 7.6%), Billings (5/30, 6.6%), Dunn (3/60,5.0%), and Mercer (0/30, 0.0%). Thirteen (87%) of the 15 *Salmonella* isolates recovered were *Salmonella* Typhimurium (Copenhagen) and the rest (2/15, 13%) were *Salmonella* Worthington. All 15 *Salmonella* isolates from healthy cattle were susceptible to Apramycin, Ceftiofur, Entrofloxacin, Gentamicin, and Neomycin. All samples were resistant to Chlortetracycline, Clindamycin, Erythromycin, Florfenicol, Oxytetracycline,

Penicillin, Sulphachlorophridazine, Sulphadimethoxime, Sulphathiazole, Tiamulin, Tilmicosin. Two isolates (both *Salmonella* Worthington), were susceptible to Ampicillin, whereas the other thirteen samples (all *Salmonella* Typhimurium (Copenhagen), were resistant to Ampicillin and to Spectinomycin.

### 3.1.2 *Salmonella* from dairy cattle

In a study of Salmonella occurrence in dairy cattle (Khaitsa et al, 2004), 5 out of 30 cows (17%) tested positive for *Salmonella.* A sensitivity test to 20 antibiotics was performed on the 5 *Salmonella* isolates and the results were similar for all the 5 isolates except for only one isolate that was sensitive to Sulphachloropyridazine and Sulphadimethoxime and gave an intermediate result to Sulphathiazole (Table 4).

| Antimicrobial | All 5 Salmonella Isolates |
|---|---|
| Ampicillin | R |
| Apramycin | S |
| Ceftiofur | S |
| Chlortetracycline | R |
| Clindamycin | R |
| Enrofloxacin | S |
| Erythromycin | R |
| Florfenicol | R |
| Gentamicin | S |
| Neomycin | S |
| Oxytetracycline | R |
| Penicillin | R |
| Spectinomycin | R |
| Sulphachloropyridazine | R (S)* |
| Sulphadimethoxime | R (S)* |
| Sulphathiazole | R *(I)** |
| Tiamulin | R |
| Tilmicosin | R |
| Trimethoprim/Sulphamethoxazole | S |
| Tylosin (Tartrate/Base) | R |

S = Sensitive, I = Intermediate. *These 3 antimicrobials are the only ones that gave a different result (sensitive or intermediate) to 1 of the 5 isolates; the other 4 isolates were all resistant to them).
For all other antimicrobials the results were the same for all 5 Salmonella isolates.

Table 4. Antimicrobial Sensitivity Results to 5 *Salmonella* Isolates from dairy cattle. R = Resistant,

### 3.1.3 *Salmonella* from bison

The prevalence of *Salmonella* in the bison feces was 15% (3/20). The *Salmonella* isolates belonged to the serotypes *Salmonella* Typhimurium (Copenhagen) and *Salmonella* Worthington. In a panel of 20 antimicrobials, *Salmonella* Typhimurium (Copenhagen) was resistant to 13 of 20 antimicrobials (65% resistance), including macrolides (erythromycin, tilmicosin, tylosin), tetracyclines (chlortetracycline, oxytetracycline), chloramphenicol analog – florfenicol, most sulphonamides, and penicillin, and susceptible to 7 antimicrobials including the cephalosporin – ceftiofur, the quinolone – enrofloxacin some aminoglycosides, and ampicillin (Table 5). *Salmonella* Worthington was resistant to 14 of 20 antimicrobials (70% resistance), including macrolides (erythromycin, tilmicosin, tylosin), tetracyclines (chlortetracycline, oxytetracycline), chloramphenicol analog – florfenicol, some sulphonamides, and penicillins (penicillin and ampicillin), and susceptible to 6 antimicrobials including the cephalosporin – ceftiofur, the quinolone - enrofloxacin and some aminoglycosides (Table 5). Except for ampicillin, both *Salmonella* isolates were resistant to similar antimicrobials (Table 5). None of the *Salmonella* isolates were resistant to clinically important antimicrobials.

| | *Salmonella* Isolates | | |
|---|---|---|---|
| **Antibiotics** | **18S** | **24S** | **53S** |
| **Aminoglycosides** | | | |
| Apramycin | S | S | S |
| Gentamycin | S | S | S |
| Neomycin | S | S | S |
| Spectinomycin | R | R | S |
| **Sulphanamides/Potentiated Sulphonamides** | | | |
| Trimethoprim/Sulphamethoxazole | | | |
| Sulphadimethoxime | S | S | S |
| Sulphachloropyridazine | R | R | S |
| Sulphathiazole | R | R | S |
| **Cephalosporins** | R | R | I |
| Ceftiofur | | | |
| **Quinolones/Fluoroquinolones** | S | S | S |
| Enrofloxacin | | | |
| **Pleuromutilins** | S | S | S |
| Tiamulin | | | |
| **Chloramphenicol Analog** | R | R | R |
| Florfenicol | | | |
| **Penicillins** | R | R | R |
| Ampicillin | | | |
| Penicillin | S | R | R |
| **Tetracyclines** | R | R | R |
| Chlortetracycline | | | |
| Oxytetracycline | R | R | S |
| **Macrolides** | R | R | S |
| Erythromycin | | | |
| Tilmicosin | R | R | R |
| Tylosin (Tartrate/Base) | R | R | R |
| **Misc.** | R | R | R |
| Clindamycin | | | |
| | R | R | R |

R = Resistant S = Susceptible I-Intermediate

Table 5. Antibiotic sensitivity and resistance of *Salmonella* isolates from a bison herd

### 3.2 *Salmonella* from meats

In the Khaitsa et al (2007b) study, 2.4% (23/959) of the samples were contaminated with *Salmonella;* with 5% (16/329), and 1% (7/607) of the raw and ready to eat meat samples testing positive for *Salmonella*, respectively. There was a significant difference in recovery of *Salmonella* ($P < 0.05$), between meat type (raw vs RTE; OR =4.2, 95% CI = 1.6, 10.8); and sampling time (OR = 0.4, 95% CI = 0.2, 0.7). Retail store and product brand did not affect *Salmonella* recovery. The twenty three *Salmonella* isolates recovered from meat products were confirmed to belong to 6 different serotypes; the predominant one being *S. hadar* followed by *S. Heidelberg, S.* typhimurium var Copenhagen, *S. newport, S. saintpaul* and *S. agona.* Overall, *Salmonella* isolates from raw turkey products exhibited a higher antimicrobial resistance rate (53%) compared to those from RTE products (33%). Multidrug resistance was exhibited by 54% of the *Salmonella* isolates with the majority (62%) originating from RTE meats compared to 45% from raw ones.

In the Kegode et al (2008) study the distribution of samples that tested positive for *Salmonella* by meat type and meat part is summarized in Table 6. *Salmonella* was recovered from turkey breast (1/8, 13%), ground turkey breast (1/15, 7%), and turkey drumsticks (1/20, 5%) (Table 6). For chicken products *Salmonella* (2/5, 40%) were recovered from whole chicken. Thirteen *Salmonella* isolates recovered from the meat samples were confirmed by NVSL to belong to eight different *Salmonella enterica* serotypes (Table 7). The predominant serotype was *S. enterica* serotype Heidelberg recovered from turkey from which *S.* Typhimurium, *S.* Newport, *S.* Saintpaul and *S.* Senftenberg were also recovered. *S.* Kentucky, *S.* Typhimurium var Copenhagen, *S.* Blockley, and one undetermined serotype were recovered from chicken.

In the study by Tumuhairwe et al, 2007) that investigated the temporal and spatial distribution of 1465 salmonellosis outbreaks involving 49/50 states in the US, turkey meat associated outbreaks (TMAOs) were reported by 24 states, mostly from California and New York. Additionally, turkey meat was implicated in 4.2% of outbreaks, sea-foods (5.8%), pasta (8.3%), milk-products (8.6%), chicken (13.4%), red-meats (15.4%), eggs (21.3%), and fresh-produces (22.9%). Most outbreaks were at restaurants and private-homes for TMAOs (23.2% and 21%). The major serotypes were: S. Enteritidis, S. Heidelberg, S. Reading and S. Newport for TMAOs,

In the study by Tumuhairwe et al (2008), there were 45 different serotypes that were recovered from 71.8% (277/386) of the salmonellosis cases in North Dakota (2000 to 2005). The four major ones contributing over 70% of the cases were: *S.* Typhimurium (93, 33.1%), *S.* Enteritidis (40, 14.2%), *S.* Heidelberg (33, 11.7%) and *S.* Newport (32, 11.4%). The rest of the serotypes were: *S.* Saintpaul and *S.* Montevideo from eight cases each, *S.* Thompson was recovered from five cases, *S.* Hadar from four cases, *S.* Stanley, *S.* Poona, *S.* Mbandaka, *S.* Javiana, *S.* Braenderup, and *S.* Bredeney from three patients each. *S.* Reading, *S.* Oranienburg, *S.* Hillington, *S.* Derby, *S.* Urbana, and *S.* Albany were each recovered from 2 cases. One case each was diagnosed with *S.* Agona, *S.* Berta, *S.* Bleadon, *S.* Blockley, *S.* Chameleon, *S.* Ealing, *S.* Edinburgh, *S.* Havana, *S.* Ibadan, *S.* Indiana, *S.* Infantis, *S.* Istanbul, *S.* Lexington, *S.* Litchfield, *S.* Manhattan, *S.* Marina, *S.* Miami, *S.* Mississippi, *S.* Muenchen, *S.* Newport, *S.* Othmarschen, *S.* Sandiego, *S.* Schwarzengrund, *S.* Senftenberg, *S.* Sepsis, *S.* Syrsis, *S.* Tripoli, *S.* Uppsala, and *S.* Weltevereden.

| Store/Meat Type | *Salmonella* |
|---|---|
| Store A (n=97) | |
| whole chicken | 0 |
| ground turkey | 1 |
| turkey breast | 1 |
| Total | 2 |
| | 2/97 (2%) |
| Store B (n=108) | |
| turkey drumstick | 1 |
| chicken drumstick | 1 |
| chicken thigh | 0 |
| whole chicken | 2 |
| Total | 4 |
| | 4/108 (4%) |
| Store C (n=95) | |
| chicken breast | 0 |
| chicken thigh | 0 |
| chicken wings | 0 |
| whole chicken | 0 |
| ground turkey breast | 1 |
| Total | 1 |
| | 1/95 (1.1%) |
| Store D (n = 93) | |
| ground turkey | 4 |
| chicken thigh | 1 |
| whole chicken | 0 |
| chicken wings | 0 |
| turkey thigh | 0 |
| Total | 5 |
| | 5/93 (5.4%) |
| Store E (n = 63) | |
| chicken breast | 1 |
| Total | 1 |
| | 1/63 (1.6%) |
| Grand Total (n =456) | 13 |
| | 13/456 (2.9%) |

Table 6. Number and percentage of retail meat samples that tested positive for *salmonella* by store and meat type, 2005 (n = 456).

| ***Salmonella* serotypes** | n (%) | Chicken | Turkey |
|---|---|---|---|
| *S.* Heidelberg | 4 (30.8) | 0 | 4 |
| *S.* Kentucky | 2 (15.4) | 2 | 0 |
| *S.* Typhimurium (Copenhagen) | 1 (7.7) | 1 | 0 |
| *S.* Typhimurium | 1 (7.7) | 0 | 1 |
| *S.* Blockley | 1 (7.7) | 1 | 0 |
| *S.* Newport | 1 (7.7) | 0 | 1 |
| *S.* Saintpaul | 1 (7.7) | 0 | 1 |
| *S.* Senftenberg | 1 (7.7) | 0 | 1 |
| Unknown | 1 (7.7) | 1 | 0 |
| Total | 13 (100) | 5 | 8 |

United States metropolitan area, 2005.

Table 7. *Salmonella enterica* serotypes recovered from retail meats in the Midwestern

### 3.3 *Salmonella* from clinical cases of humans and animals (cattle, chicken, ducks, swine, turkeys, elk and bison)

#### 3.3.1 *Salmonella* serotypes

A total of 434 isolates were serotyped, including the 255 (58.8%) isolates from NDSU (from apparently healthy cattle, sick or dead animals and meat products) and 179 (41.2%) isolates from NDDoH (Table 8).

| Serotypes | Cattle | Human | Chicken | Ducks | Swine | Turkey | Bison | Elk | Others | Total |
|---|---|---|---|---|---|---|---|---|---|---|
| Agona | - | 3(0.7) | - | - | - | 1(0.2) | - | - | - | 4(0.9) |
| Anatum | - | 1(0.2) | - | - | - | 2(0.5) | - | - | - | 3(0.7) |
| Arizona | 3 (0.7) | - | - | - | - | - | - | - | - | 3(0.7) |
| Blockley | - | - | 2(0.5) | - | - | - | - | - | - | 2(0.5) |
| Braenderup | - | 1(0.2) | - | - | - | - | - | - | - | 1(0.2) |
| Brandeberg | - | 2(0.5) | - | - | - | - | - | - | - | 2(0.5) |
| Bredeney | - | 2(0.5) | - | - | - | - | - | - | - | 2(0.5) |
| Derby | - | - | - | - | 2(0.5) | - | - | - | - | 2(0.5) |
| Dublin | 2 (0.5) | - | - | - | - | - | - | - | - | 2(0.5) |
| Ealing | - | 1(0.2) | - | - | - | - | - | - | - | 1(0.2) |
| Enteritidis | - | - | - | 1(0.2) | - | - | - | - | - | 1(0.2) |
| Give | 4 (0.9) | - | - | - | - | - | - | - | - | 4(0.9) |
| Hadar | - | - | - | - | - | 10(2.3) | - | - | - | 10(2.3) |
| Havana | - | 1(0.2) | - | - | - | - | - | - | - | 1(0.2) |
| Heidelberg | - | 5(1.2) | - | - | - | 9(2.1) | - | - | - | 14 (3.2) |
| Indiana | - | 2(0.5) | | - | - | - | - | - | - | 2(0.5) |

| Serotypes | Cattle | Human | Chicken | Ducks | Swine | Turkey | Bison | Elk | Others | Total |
|---|---|---|---|---|---|---|---|---|---|---|
| Infantis | 2(0.5) | 2(0.5) | | - | - | - | - | - | - | 4(0.9) |
| Java | - | 1(0.2) | | - | - | - | - | - | - | 1(0.2) |
| Kentucky | - | 1(0.2) | 2(0.5) | - | - | - | - | - | - | 3(0.7) |
| Litchfield | - | 1(0.2) | - | - | - | - | - | - | - | 1(0.2) |
| Mbandaka | 2(0.5) | 2(0.5) | - | - | - | - | - | - | - | 4(0.9) |
| Mississipi | - | 1(0.2) | - | - | - | - | - | - | - | 1(0.2) |
| Montevideo | - | 3(0.7) | - | - | - | - | - | - | - | 3(0.7) |
| Muenchen | - | 3(0.7) | - | - | - | - | - | 1 (0.2) | - | 4(0.9) |
| Muenster | 15 (3.5) | - | - | - | - | - | - | - | - | 15(3.5) |
| Newport | 9(2.1) | 17(3.9) | - | - | - | 2(0.5) | - | - | - | 28(6.5) |
| Oranienburg | - | 2(0.5) | - | - | - | - | - | - | - | 2(0.5) |
| Paratyphi | - | 2(0.5) | - | - | - | - | - | - | - | 2(0.5) |
| Reading | - | 1(0.2) | - | - | - | - | - | - | - | 1(0.2) |
| Reno | - | 1(0.2) | - | - | - | - | - | - | - | 1(0.2) |
| Sandiego | - | 2(0.5) | - | - | - | - | - | - | - | 2(0.5) |
| Senftenberg | - | - | - | - | - | 1(0.2) | - | - | - | 1(0.2) |
| Soesterberg | - | 1(0.2) | - | - | - | - | - | - | - | 1(0.2) |
| Sonnei | - | 3(0.7) | - | - | - | - | - | - | - | 3(0.7) |
| Sovenga | - | 1(0.2) | - | - | - | - | - | - | - | 1(0.2) |
| St paul | - | 7(1.6) | - | - | - | 3(0.7) | - | - | - | 10 (2.3) |
| Stanley | - | 1(0.2) | - | - | - | - | - | - | - | 1(0.2) |
| Thompson | - | 1(0.2) | - | - | - | - | - | - | 11(0.2) (bedding) | 1(0.2) |
| Tripoli | - | 2(0.5) | - | - | - | - | - | - | - | 2(0.5) |
| Typhi | - | 1(0.2) | - | - | - | - | - | - | - | 1(0.2) |
| Typhimurium | 140 (32.3) | 58 (13.4) | - | - | 3(0.7) | 4(0.9) | 1(0.2) | - | 11(0.2) (lynx) | 207 (47.7) |
| Worthingtom | 2 (0.5) | - | - | - | - | - | 1(0.2) | - | - | 3(0.7) |
| unidentified | 14 (3.2) | 47 (10.8) | - | - | - | 3(0.7) | - | - | 12(2.8) | 76 (17.5) |
| Total | 193 (44.5) | 179 (41.2) | 4(0.9) | 1(0.2) | 5(1.2) | 35(8.1) | 2(0.5) | 1 (0.2) | 14(3.2) | 434(100) |

Table 8. *Salmonella* serotypes isolated from different animal species and human cases in North Dakota.

The total number of isolates that were common between domestic animals and humans were 183 (42.2%) and 90 (20.7%) respectively (Table 8). *S. Typhimurium* was the predominant serotype in both humans (13.4%, n=58) and domestic animals (34.3%, n= 159), followed by Newport with 11 (2.6%) and 17(3.9%) isolated in animals and human, respectively. *S. Arizona* (n=3, 0.7%), *S. Give* (n=4, 0.9%) *and S. Muenster* (n=15, 3.5%) were isolated mostly from sick or dead animals submitted to the NDSU-VDL. Of the 42 serotypes involved in animal and human infection, human isolates were highly diverse with 32 serotypes involved compared to cattle (9), turkeys (8), chickens (2), bison (2), swine (2), ducks (1) and elk (1). The detailed distribution of the different serotypes between different host species is provided in Table 8.

### 3.3.2 PFGE Results

The initial 434 *Salmonella* isolates were grouped into 113 distinct PFGE profiles at 85% similarity (Tables 9, 10, 11; Figure 2). The 179 human isolates were distributed within the 98 of the 113 PFGE fingerprint patterns or profiles at the same level of similarity. A detailed examination of the 273 isolates from serotypes commonly isolated from man (n=90) and domestic animals (n=183), revealed that 40 of the human and 55 animal isolates were distributed amongst 8 distinct (i.e. with 100% similarity) PFGE fingerprint profiles. The 40 isolates from the human cases were linked to 2 serotypes - *S. Typhimurium Copenhagen* and *S. Heidelberg* that shared indistinguishable genetic fingerprint patterns (100% homology) with some animal isolates. The biggest clonal group involving *S. Typhimurium Copenhagen* with 100 % similarity in the PFGE fingerprint patterns involved 22 isolates from cattle, 17 Humans and 1 from a sick swine (Figure 2). The second PFGE profile involved 19 isolates of *S. Typhimurium Copenhagen* with indistinguishable fingerprints, isolated from 7 feedlot cattle, 2 range cattle and 10 human cases (Figure 2). The third profile had 10 cattle and 4 humans, fifth profile had 1 human, 1 swine and 1 turkey, sixth profile was identified as *S. Heidelberg* form human (1) and turkey meat (1), seventh profile had *S. Typhimurium Copenhagen* from cattle (4), human (5) and chicken (1) and the eighth profile had S. *Heidelberg,* isolated from human (1) and turkey meat (1). Figure 2 shows details of human and domestic animal serotypes in the eight distinct profiles each with indistinguishable PFGE fingerprint patterns. The isolation of serovars with similar PFGE patterns in cattle preceded those in humans. Most outbreaks were recorded in 2004 (58%), while a few turkey isolates with similar PFGE profile were recorded after (Table 9).

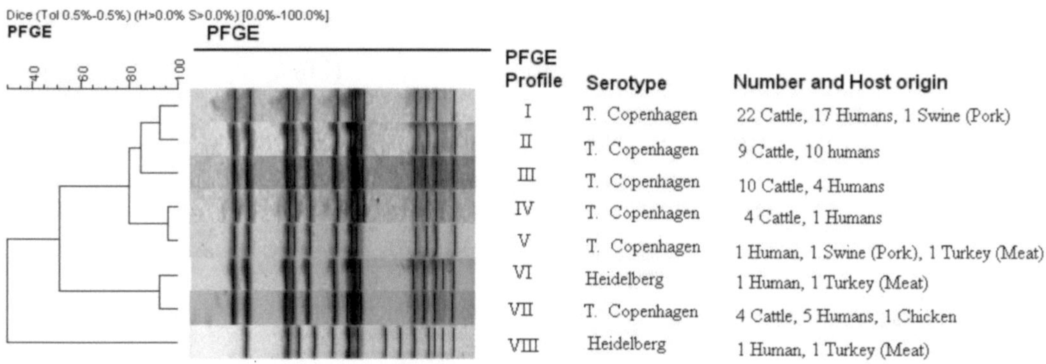


Fig. 2. PGFE profile of the commonly serotypes isolated from domestic animals or their products and humans.

| Xbal profiles with indistinguishable fingerprint | Host | Year of isolation and number isolated (%) | | | | |
|---|---|---|---|---|---|---|
| | | 2003 | 2004 | 2005 | 2006 | Total |
| I | Cattle | - | 19 (19.8) | 2 (2.1) | 1 (1.0) | 22 (22.9) |
| | Human | - | 4 (4.2) | 12 (12.5) | 1 (1.0) | 17(17.7) |
| | Swine | - | - | - | 1(1.0) | (1.0) |
| II | Cattle | 2 (2.1) | 7(7.3) | - | - | 9(9.4) |
| | Human | - | 2 (2.1) | 8(8.3) | - | 10(10.4) |
| III | Cattle | - | 10(10.4) | - | - | 10(10.4) |
| | Human | - | - | 4(4.2) | - | 4(4.2) |
| IV | Cattle | - | 4(4.2) | - | - | 4(4.2) |
| | Human | - | - | 1(1.0) | - | 1(1.0) |
| V | Turkey meat | - | - | 1(1.0) | - | 1(1.0) |
| | Human | - | - | - | 1(1.0) | 1(1.0) |
| | swine | - | - | - | 1(1.0) | 1(1.0) |
| VI | Turkey meat | - | - | - | 1(1.0) | 1(1.0) |
| | Human | - | - | 1(1.0) | - | 1(1.0) |
| VII | Cattle | - | 4(4.2) | - | - | 4(4.2) |
| | Human | - | - | 6(15) | - | 6(12.5) |
| | Chicken | - | - | 1(1.0) | - | 1(1.0) |
| VIII | Turkey meat | - | - | - | 1(1.0) | 1(1.0) |
| | Human | - | 1(1.0) | - | - | 1(1.0) |
| | Total | 2(2.1) | 51(53.1) | 36(37.5) | 7(7.3) | 94(100) |

Table 9. PFGE profiles, host species and year of isolation of the *Salmonella* serotypes.

### 3.3.3 Antimicrobial resistance (AMR) patterns

A comparison of the AMR patterns of isolates with indistinguishable PFGE profiles revealed variations within the groups (Table 11). In profile 1, 2 bovine and 1 human isolates shared similar AMR and PFGE profiles. Second observation was recorded for 1 swine and 20 cattle.

| Xbal patterns with indistinguishable fingerprint | *Salmonella* Serotype | Origin | Antimicrobial resistance profile | Number of matching isolates |
|---|---|---|---|---|
| I | Typhimurium Copenhagen | Cattle | AM,AMP,CL,STR,SU,TET | 20 |
| | | Cattle | AM,AMP,KAN,STR,SU,TET | 2 |
| | | Swine | AM,AMP,CL,STR,SU,TET | 1 |
| | | Human | AM,AMP,KAN,STR,SU,TET | 1 |
| | | Human | CL | 4 |
| | | Human | - | 5 |
| | | Human | AM,AMP | 3 |
| | | Human | GE,STR,SU | 1 |
| | | Human | CL,KAN,TET | 3 |
| II | Typhimurium Copenhagen | Cattle | AM,AMP,CL,STR,SU,TET | 8 |
| | | Cattle | AM,AMP,KAN,STR,SU,TET | 1 |
| | | Human | - | 5 |
| | | Human | CL | 4 |
| | | Human | CL,KAN,TET | 1 |
| III | Typhimurium Copenhagen | Cattle | AM,AMP,CL,STR,SU,TET | 10 |
| | | Human | CL | 2 |
| | | Human | - | 2 |
| IV | Typhimurium Copenhagen | Cattle | AM,AMP,CL,STR,SU,TET | 4 |
| | | Human | - | 1 |
| V | Typhimurium Copenhagen | Human | CL | 1 |
| | | Swine | AM,AMP,CL,STR,SU,TET | 1 |
| | | Turkey meat | AM,AMP,CL,STR,SU,TET | 1 |
| VI | Heidelberg | Human | - | 1 |
| | | Turkey meat | AMP,CL,SU,TET | 1 |
| VII | Typhimurium Copenhagen | Cattle | AM,AMP,CL,STR,SU,TET | 4 |
| | | Chicken | AM,AMP,CL,STR | 1 |
| | | Human | CX | 1 |
| | | Human | CL | 1 |
| | | Human | - | 2 |
| | | Human | AM,AMP | 1 |
| VIII | Heidelberg | Human | CL | 1 |
| | | Turkey meat | SU | 1 |
| | | | *Total* | 95 |

*AM-Amoxacillin/Clavulonic acid, AMP-Ampicillin,CX-Ceftixiaxone, CL-Chloramphenicol, GEN-Gentamicin, KAN-Kanamycin, STR-Streptomycin, SU-Sulfizoxazole,TET-Tetacycline*

Table 10. Relationship of molecular types and antibiotic resistance patterns of *Salmonella enterica* serotype isolated from man, domestic animals and animal products.

The rest shared the PFGE but not the AMR profiles. The AMR profile AM,AMP,CL, STR,SU,TET appeared the most common across many PFGE profiles, recorded in 20 bovines and 1 human (profile 1), 8 bovines (profile II), 10 bovines (profile III), 4 bovine (profile IV), 1 swine and 1 turkey (profile V) and 4 bovines (profile VII). Details of AMR profiles of other PFGE profiles will be provided. For the antibiotic susceptibility tests, a total of 9 antibiotic resistant patterns were found for the 55 animal isolates and 40 human isolates with identical PFGE profiles. Of these, cattle isolates accounted for 7, human 19, swine 2, turkey meat 3 and chicken 1 AMR patterns. A review of susceptibility levels of different isolates was summarized. All human (62), swine (2) and turkey (3) and 97 out of 98 cattle isolates were susceptible to amikacin. Resistance to amoxicillin/clavulanic acid was observed in swine (all 2 isolates) and 75 cattle isolates (76.5%) while turkey (n=2, 100%) and human (n=59, 95.2%) were mostly susceptible. All the 2 swine isolates were susceptible to cefoxitin, ceftriaxone, ciprofloxacin, gentamycin, nalidixic acid and trimethoprim/sulfamethoxazole, while resistant to amoxicillin/clavulanic acid, ampicillin, streptomycin, sulfizoxazole and tetracycline. Detailed antimicrobial susceptibility profiles of the different isolates by origin are shown in Tables 10 and 11.

| | No of susceptibility isolates (%) | | | | No. of intermediate isolates (%) | | | No. of resistant isolates (%) | | | |
|---|---|---|---|---|---|---|---|---|---|---|---|
| | Cattle | Human | Swine | Turkey | Cattle | Human | Turkey | Cattle | Human | Swine | Turkey |
| Amikacin (0.5–64), | 97 (99.0) | 62 (100.0) | 2 (100.0) | 3 (100.0) | - | - | - | 1(1.0) | - | - | - |
| Amoxicillin /clavulanic acid (1/0.5–32/16) | 2 (2.0) | 59 (95.2) | - | 2 (66.7) | 21 (21.4) | 2(3.2) | 1 (33.3) | 75 (76.5) | 1(1.6) | 2 (100.0) | - |
| Ampicillin (2–32) | - | 59 (95.2) | - | 1 (33.3) | - | - | - | 98 (100.0) | 3(4.8) | 2 (100.0) | 2 (66.7) |
| Cefoxitin (0.5–32) | 97 (99.0) | 60 (96.8) | 2 (100.0) | 3 (100.0) | - | 1(1.6) | - | 1(1.0) | 1(1.6) | - | - |
| Ceftriaxone (0.25–64) | 97 (99.0) | 60 (96.8) | 2 (100.0) | 3 (100.0) | - | 1(1.6) | - | 1(1.0) | 1(1.6) | - | - |
| Chlora-mphenicol (2–32) | 1(1.0) | 35 (56.5) | 1 (50.0) | 1 (33.3) | 4(4.1) | 26(41.9) | - | 93 (94.9) | 1(1.6) | 1 (50.0) | 2 (66.7) |
| Ciproflo-xacin (0.015–4) | 97 (99.0) | 62 (100.0) | 2 (100.0) | 3 (100.0) | - | - | - | 1(1.0) | - | - | - |
| Gentamicin (0.25–16) | 97 (99.0) | 60 (96.8) | 2 (100.0) | 3 (100.0) | - | - | - | 1(1.0) | 2(3.2) | - | - |
| Kanamycin (6–64) | 88 (89.8) | 58 (93.5) | 1 (50.0) | 3 (100.0) | - | - | - | 10 (10.2) | 4(6.5) | 1 (50.0) | 0.0 |

| | No of susceptibility isolates (%) | | | | No. of intermediate isolates (%) | | | No. of resistant isolates (%) | | | |
|---|---|---|---|---|---|---|---|---|---|---|---|
| | Cattle | Human | Swine | Turkey | Cattle | Human | Turkey | Cattle | Human | Swine | Turkey |
| Nalidixic acid (0.5–32) | 97 (99.0) | 62 (100.0) | 2 (100.0) | 3 (100.0) | - | - | - | 1(1.0) | - | - | - |
| Streptomycin (32–64) | 2 (2.0) | 58 (93.5) | - | 2 (66.7) | - | - | - | 96 (98.0) | 4(6.5) | 2 (100.0) | 1 (33.3) |
| Sulfizoxazole (16–512) | - | 58 (93.5) | - | - | - | - | - | 98 (100.0) | 4(6.5) | 2 (100.0) | 3 (100.0) |
| Tetracycline (4–32), | - | 57 (91.9) | - | 1 (33.3) | - | - | - | 98 (100) | 5(8.1) | 2 (100) | 2 (66.7) |
| Trimethoprimsulfamethoxazole (4-76) | 97 (99.0) | 62 (100) | 2(100) | 3(100) | - | - | - | 1(1.0) | - | - | - |

Table 11. Drug susceptibility patterns of the common *salmonella* serotypes isolated from domestic animals and human.

## 4. Discussion

### 4.1 *Salmonella* from animals

#### 4.1.1 *Salmonella* in feedlot cattle

The study by Tabe et al (2010a, 2010b) reported *Salmonella* prevalence of 12.7% in fecal samples tested. A larger study (Dargatz et al 2003) that evaluated presence of *Salmonella* in fecal samples from cattle in US feedlots (73 feedlots in 12 states during the period from October 1999 to September 2000) had earlier reported a lower overall *Salmonella* prevalence of 6.3%. However, *Salmonella* prevalence at pen and feedlot level was higher. In that study (Dargatz et al 2003) although overall individual animal prevalence was 6.3% (654/10,417), 22.2% (94/422) of pens and 50.7% (37/73) of feedlots had one or more positive samples. Samples collected during the period of April to June (6.8%, 209/3054) and July to September (11.4%, 286/2500) were more likely to be positive than those collected during October to December (4.0%, 73/1838) and January to March (2.8%, 86/3025). The study by Tabe et al (2010a, 2010b) was conducted from October 2006 to March 26, 2007.

An understanding of the genetic diversity of *Salmonella* isolated from cattle could help determine if contamination at a feedlot is due to bacteria that are transient or resident (Galland et al., 2001) in their gut. Transient bacteria can be introduced into the feedlot by arriving cattle, in ingredients for cattle rations such as legume hay, from contaminated water sources, or by other animals (wild or domestic), motor vehicles, and employees (Galland et al., 2001). In the study by Tabe et al (2010a, 2010b), the isolation of *S.* Typhimurium vars Copenhagen as the major *Salmonella* serovar 95% of the time supported previous reports (Hegde et al., 2005; Khaitsa et al., 2007a) of the existence of common genotypes circulating among the steers. *Salmonella* Typhimurium vars Copenhagen which was primarily reported to be found in pigeons is now frequently isolated from cattle, swine, and other animals (Frech et al., 2003). Another study (NARMS-EB, 2003) reported Typhimurium variant Copenhagen as the most predominant serotype accounting for 16.9% of the total number of isolates examined by U.S. Department of Agriculture's National Animal Health Monitoring System for Enteric Bacteria and reported over a 7-year period (1997 to 2003).

The study by Tabe et al (2010a), reported widespread AMR among the *Salmonella* isolated; all but two of the *Salmonella* isolates were resistant to more than two of the antimicrobials tested with 96.6% of the isolates showing multidrug resistant antibiograms. The widespread AMR of *Salmonella* isolated from cattle in North Dakota had been reported before (Oloya, et al, 2009) with most animal strains showing more multidrug resistance compared to human *Salmonella* isolates possibly due to a difference in antimicrobial selection pressure exerted to the microorganisms in the two populations. Isolation of *S.* Typhimurium vars Copenhagen as the major *Salmonella* serovar 95% of the time supports previous reports of the existence of common genotypes circulating among the steers. This similarity in clonal relationship and antimicrobial resistance of *S.* Typhimurium vars Copenhagen was reported in a study that characterized *Salmonella* isolates from feedlot cattle (Khaitsa et al, 2007a), humans, and ready to eat turkey produce (Oloya et al, 2007, 2009). This could possibly be responsible for the spread of such resistant genes among bacteria, a characteristic typical of gram negative bacteria. Surveillance of antibiotic resistance, especially of integrons distribution among bacteria is therefore critical. The genotypic variation in *Salmonella* isolated in healthy feedlot steers reported in this study plus variation in MDR antibiogram supports previous reports that not all MDR *salmonella* Typhimurium do carry a wide variety of resistance genes (Khaitsa et al, 2007a; White, 2005). Additionally, isolates with the same resistance phenotypes often had different resistance genotypes, a phenomenon that had been observed before by other studies (Frye and Fedorka-Cray, 2007).

In the study by Tabe et al (2010a), although the prevalence of class 1 and 2 integrons were 50% (29/58) and 35% (2/58), respectively, more than 90% of the isolates were multidrug resistant to Amoxicillin/clavulanic acid, Ampicillin, Chloramphenicol, Streptomycin, Sulfizoxazole, and Tetracycline. The lower frequency of class 2 integron relative to class 1 as seen in this study could probably result from lower exposure to selective pressure of antibiotics among the isolates (Zhao et al, 2005). Additionally, two isolates positive for integron 1 had integron 2. These isolates belonged to genotypes I and IV and showed only about 67% genomic similarity (Figure 1). Additionally, these isolates were recovered from different sampling periods (sampling time one and two respectively). It is important to note that, all 29 isolates with integron 1, were susceptible to Amikacin, Cefoxitin, Cetriaxone, Ciprofloxacin, Gentamycin, Kanamycin, Nalidixic acid, and Trimethoprim-sulfamethoxazole possibly due to the presence of defective resistant genes or the presence of quiescent integrons as reported in a previous study (Khaitsa et al, 2008). The fact that integrons 1 and 2 were not detected in some of the isolates (n=29), 93% (27/29) which were resistant to two or more of the antibiotics, with patterns similar to the positive integron isolates, may be an indication that integrons may play a sufficient but not a necessary role in antibiotic resistance in bacteria. This observation is similar to what has been reported in a previous study where class 1 integron was not always involved in the resistance of *E. coli* isolates to antimicrobial agents (Khaitsa et al, 2008). However integrons have been often associated with broad antibiotic resistance, even if they do not encode multiple drug resistant determinants (Zhang et al, 2004). This was also evident in our study as not all integron bearing strains expressed resistance to antibiotics. Additionally, it is possible that our PCR analysis as designed in this study missed some large amplicons and most especially integron 2, which contains some gene cassettes encoding antibiotic resistance (Zhang et al, 2004).

The emergence and dissemination of MDR among *Salmonella* isolates from health cattle may have potential adverse implication in public health. Since the first description of class 1 integron by Stokes and Hall (Stokes, H.W., and R.M. Hall. 1989), integron-mediated resistance has been reported in clinical isolates of various organisms including *K. pneumoniae, K. oxytoka, Pseudomonas aeroginosa, E. coli, C. fruedii* and *V. cholerae* (Orman,et al 2002; Sallen *et al, 1995*). It has been reported (Collis, et al, 2002) that classes 1 and 2 are most common in resistant bacteria, and the mobility of these integrons was undoubtedly important in facilitating their spread into many different bacterial species. A study (Krauland et al, 2009) reported that Salmonella enterica bacteria have become increasingly resistant to antimicrobial agents, partly as a result of genes carried on integrons, and that clonal expansion and horizontal gene transfer may contribute to the spread of antimicrobial drug-resistance integrons in these organisms. Krauland et al (2009) investigated this resistance and integron carriage among 90 isolates with the ACSSuT phenotype (resistance to ampicillin, chloramphenicol, streptomycin, sulfamethoxazole, and tetracycline) in a global collection of S. enterica isolates. Four integrons, dfrA12/orfF/aadA2, dfrA1/aadA1, dfrA7, and arr2/blaOXA30/cmlA5/aadA2, were found in genetically unrelated isolates from 8 countries on 4 continents, which supports a role for horizontal gene transfer in the global dissemination of S. enterica multidrug resistance. Serovar Typhimurium isolates containing identical integrons with the gene cassettes blaPSE1 and aadA2 were found in 4 countries on 3 continents, which supports the role of clonal expansion. The study by Krauland et al (2009) demonstrated that clonal expansion and horizontal gene transfer contribute to the global dissemination of antimicrobial drug resistance in S. enterica.

The 58 isolates of *Salmonella* Typhimurium var. Copenhagen reported by Tabe et al (2010a) belonged to nine PFGE profiles. Multiple genotypes were frequently observed among *Salmonella* isolated within and between pens sampled in one feedlot in this study (Tabe et al, 2010a). A similar result was reported by a previous study (Edrington et al., 2004) which highlighted the genotypic variation in *Salmonella* isolated from cattle within a farm and among four farms. Another study (Alam et al 2009) that investigated antimicrobial susceptibility profiles of 530 Salmonella enterica serotypes recovered from pens of commercial feedlot cattle reported tremendous strain diversity and multidrug resistance (MDR) among *Salmonella* recovered. This study determined antimicrobial susceptibility profiles, serotype, and presence or absence of the integron-encoded intI1 gene for 530 Salmonella isolates recovered using composite rope (n = 335), feces (n = 59), and water (n = 136) samples from 21 pens in 3 feedlots. Most isolates (83.0%) of the 19 Salmonella serotypes identified were susceptible or intermediately susceptible to all the antimicrobials evaluated. Resistance to sulfisoxazole (14.9%), streptomycin (3.8%), and tetracycline (3.6%) were the most common. None of the isolates tested positive for a class 1 integron, and only 2.5% were resistant to multiple antimicrobials. All the MDR isolates, namely, serotypes Uganda (n = 9), Typhimurium (n = 2), and Give (n = 2), were resistant to at least five antimicrobials. Most MDR isolates (n = 11) were from two pens during 1 week within one feedlot. Overall, many Salmonella isolates collected within a pen were similar in terms of serotype and antimicrobial susceptibility regardless of sample type. However, MDR Salmonella and rare serotypes were not recovered frequently enough to suggest a general strategy for appropriate composite sampling of feedlot cattle populations for Salmonella detection and monitoring. This observation offers an insight into the complexity of the population dynamics of foodborne pathogens in food animals preharvest and demonstrates their variability in terms of shedding and environmental contamination (Edrington et al., 2004). In order to reduce the prevalence of foodborne pathogens in food animals at slaughter (which could produce significant reductions in the food supply; Hynes et al., 2000), a thorough understanding of the population dynamics of *Salmonella* at the farm level is crucial before implementation of pathogen reduction strategies can be expected to be successful (Edrington et al., 2004).

#### 4.1.2 *Salmonella* from ranch cattle

The study by Theis et al (2005, 2007) reported a prevalence of *Salmonella* in ranch cattle of 7.1%. Other researchers (Dargatz et al., 2000) have reported a lower prevalence (1.4 to 4.5%) than that observed by Theis et al (2005, 2007) while others (Fegan et al, 2004) have reported *Salmonella* prevalence as high as 16%. It is possible that the lower prevalence reported by Theis et al (2005, 2007) could have been attributed to the smaller sample (N =212) of cattle compared to that of other researchers. It is also possible that the time of sampling may have influenced the prevalence of *Salmonella* reported. Seasonal changes have been reported to affect *Salmonella* prevalence. Samples collected during the period of April to June and July to September were more likely to be positive than those collected during October to December and January to March (Fegan et al, 2004). The study by Theis et al (2005, 2007) was conducted from September to November, 2004.

The *Salmonella* serotypes identified in beef cattle (Theis et al, 2005, 2007) were *Salmonella* Typhimurium (Copenhagen) (87%) and *Salmonella* Worthington (13%). The presence of *S.* Typhimurium in cattle and the consequent cross contamination of beef carcass tissue are of particular concern as this serotype is one of the most common causes of *Salmonella* infection in developed countries (Gomez et al, 1997). Of the twenty most common *Salmonella* serotypes identified by the Centers for Disease Control and Prevention (CDC) eight (*Salmonella* Typhimurium, Heidelberg, Agona, Montevideo, Braenderup, Enteritidis, Saint Paul, and Thompson) are found in both human and non-clinical nonhuman isolates (Chen et al, 2004). All 15 *Salmonella* isolates recovered by Theis et al (2005, 2007) were resistant to more than 10 antimicrobials which is an indication that multiple antimicrobial resistance was widespread. This should be of concern because of the potential for therapeutic failures. Other studies have found various levels of antimicrobial resistance. For example one study of *Salmonella* isolates in food animals found that of the 209 *Salmonella* isolates tested 112 (53.6%) were resistant to more than one antimicrobial (Johnson et al., 2005). AMR has been a topic of interest in many studies and the results of those studies vary widely. For instance one study of AMR patterns of *Salmonella* isolated from beef cattle (Dargatz et al., 2000) showed that all of the 1314 *Salmonella* isolates tested were susceptible to amikacin, cefotaxime, and ciprofloxacin with only 14% susceptible to all antimicrobials tested. The remaining 86% showed resistance to at least one antimicrobial agent. The most common resistance observed was to tetracycline with ampicillin, and co-amoxiclav was the second most common class that the *Salmonella* serotypes were resistant.

#### 4.1.3 *Salmonella* from dairy cattle

In the study by Khaitsa et al (2004) five out of 30 (17%) of the cattle sampled tested positive for *Salmonella*. This result was similar to what had been reported in other dairies (NAHMS, 1996; USDA, 2001) with prevalence values ranging from 5.4% to 75%. This result demonstrated that dairies are a potential source of *Salmonella* for susceptible animals/humans.

The United States National Animal Health Monitoring System's Dairy '96 study reported 5·4% of milk cows shed *Salmonella* and 27·5% of dairy operations had at least one cow shedding *Salmonella* [Wells et al, 1998; NAHMS, 1996]. *Salmonella* has been isolated from all ages of dairy cattle and throughout the production process. Mature dairy cattle typically appear asymptomatic while shedding this pathogen in their faeces (Richardson, 1975; McDonough, 1986; Edrington, 2004; Edrington et al, 2004) and while young calves are more susceptible to salmonellosis, cases in adult cattle have been reported (Gay and Hunsaker, 1993; Anderson, 1997; Sato, 2001). Previous research demonstrated significant variation in the prevalence of faecal *Salmonella* in healthy, lactating dairy cattle, not only among farms across the United States (Edrington et al, 2008) but also in farms within a small geographic area and in individual farms from season to season (Edrington et al, 2004 ) . Additional research examined production parameters (heifers *vs.* mature cows, lactation status, stage of lactation and heat stress) on *Salmonella* prevalence (Edrington, 2004; Fitzgerald et al, 2003). While minor differences were noted in *Salmonella* shedding, results were generally inconsistent with no significant trends noted.

As part of a national study of US dairy operations, another study (Blau et al 2005) conducted between March and September 2002, in 97 dairy herds in 21 states reported an overall prevalence of 7.3% of fecal samples that were culture positive for *Salmonella*. In another study of dairy cattle (Warnick et al. 2003) , *Salmonella* was isolated from 9.3% of 4049 fecal samples collected from a 2 months study of 12 dairy herds originating from Michigan, Minnesota, New York and Wisconsin(Warnick et al, 2003). Also, Fossler et al (2004) sampled dairy cattle to describe the occurrence of fecal shedding, persistence of shedding over time, and serogroup classification of *Salmonella* spp on a large number of dairy farms of various sizes. The design was that of a longitudinal study and the sample population comprised 22,417 fecal samples from cattle and 4,570 samples from the farm environment on 110 organic and conventional dairy farms in Minnesota, Wisconsin, Michigan, and NewYork. Five visits were made to each farm at 2-month intervals from August 2000 to October 2001. Fecal samples from healthy cows, calves, and other targeted cattle groups and samples from bulk tank milk, milk line filters, water, feed sources, and pen floors were collected at each visit. *Salmonella* spp were isolated from 4.8% of fecal samples and 5.9% of environmental samples; 92.7% of farms had at least 1 *Salmonella*-positive sample.

Results from the various studies conducted indicated some variability in the prevalence of fecal shedding of *Salmonella* among the different cattle and production systems sampled possibly due to several factors such as state of origin, treatment with antimicrobials, herd size and season that have previously been reported (Fossler et al, 2005). The study by Fossler et al (2005) that investigated environmental sample-level factors associated with the presence of *Salmonella* in a multi-state study of conventional and organic dairy farms reported that State of origin was associated with the presence of *Salmonella* in samples from cattle and the farm environment; Midwestern states were more likely to have *Salmonella*-positive samples compared to New York. Cattle treated with antimicrobials within 14 days of sampling were more likely to be *Salmonella*-negative compared with nontreated cattle (OR=2.0, 95% CI: 1.1, 3.4). Farms with at least 100 cows were more likely to have *Salmonella*-positive cattle compared with smaller farms (OR=2.6, 95% CI: 1.4, 4.6). Season was associated with *Salmonella* shedding in cattle, and compared to the winter period, summer had the highest odds for shedding (OR=2.4, 95% CI: 1.5, 3.7), followed by fall (OR=1.9, 95% CI: 1.2, 3.1) and spring (OR=1.8, 95% CI: 1.2, 2.6). Environmental samples significantly more likely to be *Salmonella*-positive (compared to bulk tank milk) included, in descending order,

were; samples from sick pens (OR=7.4, 95% CI: 3.4, 15.8), manure storage areas (OR=6.4, 95% CI: 3.5, 11.7), maternity pens (OR=4.2, 95% CI: 2.2, 8.1), hair coats of cows due to be culled (OR=3.9, 95% CI: 2.2, 7.7), milk filters (OR=3.3, 95% CI: 1.8, 6.0), cow waterers (OR=2.8, 95% CI: 1.4, 5.7), calf pens (OR=2.7, 95% CI: 1.3, 5.3), and bird droppings from cow housing (OR=2.4, 95% CI: 1.3, 4.4). Parity, stage of lactation, and calf age were not associated with *Salmonella* shedding. Another study (Fitzgerald et al, 2003)
that examined factors affecting fecal shedding of *Salmonella* in dairy cattle reported that multiparous lactating cows tended to shed more ($P = 0.06$) *Salmonella* than primiparous lactating cows (39% vs 27%, respectively), and that parity did not influence ($P > 0.10$) *Salmonella* shedding in non lactating cows. Unfortunately, information on parity of the cows in Khaitsa et al (2004) was not obtained so comparisons of *Salmonella* prevalence by parity could not be made.
The fact that *Salmonella* isolates recovered by Khaitsa et al (2004) were resistant to more than 10 out of the 20 antimicrobials tested was a concern. Dairy cattle serve as an important reservoir for *Salmonella* and have been implicated in cases of human salmonellosis [CDC, 2003]. In the study by Edrington et al (2008), seven and nine different *Salmonella* serotypes were identified in the healthy and sick dairy cattle, respectively. The serotypes Senftenberg and Kentucky were not detected in any of the healthy cattle and accounted for 34% of the sick isolates. No differences in antimicrobial susceptibility patterns were observed in any the *Salmonella* isolates from sick and healthy cattle. Isolates were susceptible to all antimicrobials examined with the exception of spectinomycin, with three and five isolates resistant in the healthy and diarrhoeic groups, respectively. PFGE was used to compare the genetic relatedness of isolates cultured from the faecal samples of healthy and sick cattle. Seventeen serotypes representing 84 isolates were examined. No genotypic differences were noted when comparing sick *vs.* healthy isolates However, multiple genotypes within serotype were observed for a number of the isolates examined.

#### 4.1.4 *Salmonella* from bison

*Salmonella* prevalence of 15% reported in the bison herd was comparable to that reported in cattle herds (Beach et al, 2002; Huston et al, 2002; Warnick et al, 2003) and other livestock (Branham et al, 2005) from the US. This is an indication that *Salmonella* prevalence in bison may be more widespread than is currently known. Unfortunately, not many studies of Salmonella occurrence in bison have been reported; it is possible, Khaitsa et al (2008) was the first of such studies reported. A cross-sectional study of 212 cattle from 7 cow-calf operations in North Dakota reported *Salmonella* spp. shedding point prevalence of 7% (15 of 212) of cattle sampled (Theis, 2006). This prevalence was similar to that reported for bison given the limitation of number of animals sampled in both studies. It is also possible that the time of sampling may have influenced the prevalence of *Salmonella* reported. Seasonal changes have been reported to affect prevalence of *Salmonella* fecal shedding in cattle (Dargatz et al, 2003). Samples collected during the period of April to June and July to September were more likely to be positive than those collected during October to December and January to March (Dargatz et al, 2003). In this study we sampled bison in June 2005 while Theis (2006) sampled cattle from September to November, 2004. Another longitudinal study (Branham et al, 2005) that assessed *Salmonella* spp. presence in white-tailed deer (*Odocoileus virginianus*) and livestock simultaneously grazing the same rangeland, reported *Salmonella* prevalence of 2/26 (7.69%) and 6/82 (7.32%) in deer and sheep, respectively, and a lower prevalence of (3/81 (3.70%), and 1/80 (1.25%) in goats and cattle, respectively, all from samples taken in September.

The *Salmonella* isolated from bison feces (Khaitsa et al, 2008) belonged to the serotypes *Salmonella* Typhimurium (Copenhagen) and *Salmonella* Worthington. This was not a total surprise since bovine are a common source of *Salmonella* Typhimurium (Cray et al, 2006). It is interesting to note that the same serotypes, *Salmonella* Typhimurium (Copenhagen) and *Salmonella* Worthington, were recovered from cattle on cow-calf operations in North Dakota during the same year[35] (Theis, 2006). However, a larger study of beef cattle (Beach et al 2002), reported that the five serotypes most commonly associated with feedlot cattle and their environment were Salmonella Anatum (18.3% of the isolates), Salmonella Kentucky (17.5%), Salmonella Montevideo (9.2%), Salmonella Senftenberg (8.3%), and Salmonella Mbandaka (7.5%). The five serotypes most commonly associated with nonfeedlot cattle and their environment were Salmonella Kentucky (35.4%), Salmonella Montevideo (21.7%). Salmonella Cerro (7.5%), Salmonella Anatum (6.8%), and Salmonella Mbandaka (5.0%) (Beach et al 2002).

Other studies[9], (Edrington et al 2004) have reported different *Salmonella* serotypes recovered from cattle originating from other states, possibly due to regional differences. In one study (Edrington et al 2004)[9] mature dairy cattle were sampled over a 2-year period (2001-2002) on six farms in New Mexico and Texas. Fecal samples (n = 1560) were collected via rectal palpation and cultured for *Salmonella*, and one isolate from each positive sample was serotyped. Twenty-two different serotypes were identified from a total of 393 Salmonella isolates. Montevideo was the predominant serotype (27%) followed by Mbandaka (15%), Senftenberg (11.4%), Newport (6.4%), Anatum (4.8%), and Give (4.8%). Salmonella Typhimurium and Dublin, two frequently reported serotypes, accounted for only 1% of the observed serotypes in this study. A national *Salmonella* study of 97 dairy herds in 21 states in the US reported *Salmonella* Meleagridis (24.1%), Salmonella Montevideo (11.9%), and *Salmonella* Typhimurium (9.9%) as the three most frequently recovered serotypes (Blau et al 2005). It is noteworthy that *Salmonella enterica* serovar Hadar was the major *Salmonella* serotype isolated from processed bison carcasses originating in the same region as our sampled animals[25] (Li et al, 2006). In the absence of studies that correlate recovery of *Salmonella* from the same bison pre and post-harvest, it is difficult to ascertain the sources of contamination of bison carcasses post-harvest.

In the study Khaitsa et al (2008) both *Salmonella* isolates were susceptible to at least 6 antimicrobials on the panel including the cephalosporin - ceftiofur and the quinolone/fluoroquinolone - enrofloxacin that are clinically important. However, both isolates (100%) demonstrated widespread multi-drug resistance (resitance to ≥ 13 antimicrobials) in a panel of 20.antimicrobials with resistance most frequently to tetracycline, streptomycin, and/or ampicillin). In a larger study (Dargatz et al 2003) of 73 feedlots in 12 states the antimicrobial resistance patterns of *Salmonella* spp recovered were determined. The susceptibilities of all isolates were determined using a panel of 17 antimicrobials. The majority of isolates (62.8%, 441/702) were sensitive to all of the antimicrobials tested. Resistance was most frequently observed to tetracycline (35.9%, 252/702) followed by streptomycin (11.1%, 78/702), ampicillin (10.4%, 73/702) and chloramphenicol (10.4%, 73/702). Multiple resistance (resistance to > or =2 antimicrobials) was observed for 11.7% (82/702) of the isolates. However, overall, most of the *Salmonella* isolates were sensitive to all the antimicrobials tested. Interestingly, antimicrobial testing of *Salmonella enterica* serovar

Hadar recovered from bison carcasses originating from the same region as our sample bison also demonstrated resistance to tetracycline, gentamicin, sulfamethoxazole, and streptomycin[25], results that were quite similar to what we reported for isolates from apparently healthy bison. Additionally, both isolates recovered in our study were susceptible to apramycin. In comparison with human isolates, of the 2613 isolates tested in 1999-2000 at the 17 public health laboratories participating in NARMS, 26% (679) were resistant to >1 agent; 21% (546) were multidrug resistant (resistant to >2 agents)[1] (Angulo et al, 2001). Three multidrug resistant strains accounted for 10% (263/2613) of all Salmonella isolates, 38% (263/679) of the resistant isolates and 48% (263/546) of the multidrug resistant isolates. In particular, 30% (162/546) of multidrug resistant *Salmonella* were *S*. Typhimurium R-type ACSSuT, 12% (63/546) were S. Typhimurium R-type AKSSuT, and 7% (38/546) were S. Newport R-type ACSSuT; no other multidrug resistant patterns accounted for more than 5% of multidrug resistant Salmonellae.

It was interesting to note that in spite of the reports that antibiotics were not routinely used in the study herd, and that no other animals were raised on the farm together with the bison, antimicrobial resistance was detected in the *Salmonella* isolates recovered. It is possible that since the animals were not housed, and the pasture was not completely fenced, wild life, birds and other domestic livestock had access to the animals. It is possible therefore that even when antibiotics were not used in the bison, *Salmonella* isolated from the bison could have acquired resistance through horizontal transfer from other multidrug resistant organisms originating from wild life, birds or other domestic livestock that had access to the bison. Hoyle et al., 2005 discuss the problem of possible transfer of resistance, which may occur horizontally or vertically from enteric organisms such as *Salmonella* to other organisms. Many pathogenic and commensal organisms are multidrug resistant due to exposure to various antibiotics. Often, this antimicrobial resistance is encoded by integrons that occur on plasmids or that are integrated into the bacterial chromosome. Integrons are commonly associated with bacterial genera in the family *Enterobacteriaceae* (Goldstein et al 2001). Most of the resistance integrons found to date in clinical isolates of *Enterobacteriaceae* are class 1 integrons, which are highly associated with resistance to antimicrobial agents (Norrby 2005). Multi-drug resistant phenotypes have been associated with large, transferable plasmids such as integrons (Schoeder et al 2003). These plasmids are stable, transfer readily to other microorganisms in the same environment, and often contain cassettes encoding resistance to one or more classes of antimicrobials (Schoeder et al 2003) thus, resistance to an antimicrobial not routinely used in clinical medicine can mean resistance to one that is (Schoeder et al 2003). This finding has implications for animal and public health due to the potential for failure to treat some infections in animals and humans with the drugs that are currently on the market.

### 4.2 *Salmonella* from meats

In the study by Khaitsa et al (2007b) that investigated the occurrence of *Salmonella* in raw and ready to eat turkey meat products, in 959 turkey meat products (raw, n =614; and ready to eat (RTE), n = 345) purchased from four retail outlets in the Midwestern United States, overall, *Salmonella* was detected in 2.4% (23 of 959) of the retail meat samples with most 5% (16/329), recovered from raw meats and only 1% (7/607) from ready to eat meat samples. This finding was significant as it demonstrated that control strategies for this pathogen post-production are meeting with some success. However, recovery of *Salmonella* from the ready to eat meat products was a concern as it indicated that control strategies for this pathogen post-processing in these ready to eat turkey products was not completely successful. This may be attributed to the way the meats are handled after processing (CDC, 1998).

Other researchers have reported similar low recovery of *Salmonella* in retail meats (Ono, 1999; , Mayrhofer et al, 2004, Whyte et al, 2004, Zhao et al, 2001). It was also reported that among raw turkey meat products, ground turkey had higher *Salmonella* contamination rates than whole turkey or other turkey parts (drumsticks, thighs, breast, breast cutlets, wings, breakfast link, bratwurst, sausage and bacon). This was not a total surprise as ground turkey samples have traditionally had higher food borne pathogens compared to whole turkey or turkey parts (Cloak et al, 2001). This is possibly due to the fact that ground turkey is an amalgamation of large numbers of meat parts from different sources that are eventually ground together. *Salmonella* contamination of poultry meat has been reported to be seasonal with higher prevalence in summer than other seasons (Wallace et al, 1997). Although *Salmonella* recovery was reported to be higher in spring than winter, the study was limited in that it spanned over a period of only 6 months so could not possibly provide us with the best estimates of seasonal occurrence of *Salmonella.*

While some previous researchers (Zhao et al, 2001) reported similar *Salmonella* prevalence (4.2%) to ours, others (Soultos et al, 2003) reported lower levels. Low *Salmonella* incidence rates in chicken of 1.5% were reported by Soultos et al *(2003)*. Another study (Zhao et al, 2006) of *Salmonella* from retail foods of animal origin reported a higher prevalence (6%) than what we observed. However, the *Salmonella* distribution within the meat products was similar to ours, with ground turkey and chicken having the highest *Salmonella* contamination rates; overall, six percent of 6,046 retail meat samples (n = 365) were contaminated with *Salmonella,* the bulk recovered from either ground turkey (52%) or chicken breast (39%). There are other studies that have reported higher *Salmonella* prevalence (16.4% to 35.8%) than reported here (Domínguez et al, 2002; Duffy et al, 199; Mayrhofer et al, 2004, White et al, 2001). In one study (White et al, 2001), 200 meat samples were processed and 41 (20 percent) contained *Salmonella,* with a total of 13 serotypes. The majority of *Salmonella* isolates (61.5%) in the Khaitsa et al (2007b) study were recovered from ground turkey. In the study by Kegode et al (2008), *Salmonella* prevalence was 3% (13/ 456) of all retail meat samples. The *Salmonella* contamination rate for chicken was 4.1% (5/123), which is strikingly similar to what Zhao et al (2001) reported for grocery stores in the Washington, DC metropolitan area. In that study, *Salmonella* was isolated from 3.0% of the 825 meat samples, and chicken had a *Salmonella* contamination rate of 4.2%. Furthermore, the percentage of *Salmonella* recovered in the assorted turkey and chicken parts was similar to findings of the larger FoodNet study conducted in 2002 to 2003 (Zhao et al, 2006). Kegode et al (2008) did not report any *Salmonella* from beef and pork products tested.

Recovery of *Salmonella* from the retail meat products was not influenced by the store type (Khaitsa et al, 2007b). The possible explanations for this finding include; similar product batches within stores, the location of stores within one city, low number of stores sampled, short sampling time and the relatively smaller number of samples tested. It is possible that the relatively low prevalence of *Salmonella* recovered from our study hindered our ability to detect a significant difference among the stores. Also, the relatively smaller number of stores in our study (5 compared to 58 in that study (Zhao et al, 2001) may have explained the difference in results.

Khaitsa et al (2007b) reported the predominant *Salmonella* serotype in retail meats as *S. heidelberg* (30.8%) followed by *S. kentucky* (15.4%). Studies have reported different serotypes and proportions recovered from meat products. One study found that *S. heidelberg* was predominant in chicken, *S. Montevideo* in beef, *S. hadar* in turkey and *S. derby* in pork (Schlosser et al, 2000). The three major *Salmonella* serotypes (Heidelberg, Typhimurium and Kentucky) reported by Kegode et al (2008) were similar to major serotypes reported by the larger studies conducted by FoodNet and others (Zhao et al, 2001; CDC, 2005; CDC, 2006). For example, in 2005, the *Salmonella* serotypes accounting for 56% of human infections included Typhimurium (20%), Enteritidis (15%), Newport (10%), Javiana (7%), and Heidelberg (5%) (CDC, 2006). Another study found the predominant serotype to be *S. typhimurium* var Copenhagen (Sorensen et al, 2002). Other studies have reported the predominant serotype to be *S. enteritidis* (Domínguezet al, 2002; Mayrhofer et, 2004), *S. bredeney* (Duffy et al, 1999) and *S. anatum* (Mrema et al, 2006). The different results may reflect the different meat types examined (meat cuts vs ground meat) or different geographic locations of sampling. Regional variation in predominant serotypes of bacterial foodborne pathogens has previously been reported (CDC, 1998).

In the study by Tumuhairwe et al, 2007) that investigated the temporal and spatial distribution of 1465 salmonellosis outbreaks involving 49/50 states in the US , overall, when the incidence rates were computed, the states with higher rates were not necessarily those with higher outbreak occurrences, an indication that these states probably had better reporting systems. Membership in FoodNet (US federal agency that actively monitors seven foodborne disease trends including *Salmonella*) may have explained the comparatively large number of reports originating from California, Maryland, and New York. The four major *Salmonella* serotypes commonly isolated in humans in the US are: S. Enteritidis, S. Typhimurium, S. Heidelberg and S. Newport; Three of these serotypes (S. Enteritidis, S. Heidelberg and S. Newport) were the most implicated in both TMAOs and SOOVs compared to the other serotypes. Additionally, S. Reading was frequently isolated in TMAOs in this study. This observation was in agreement with other studies (CDC, 2005; CDC, 2006) that have cited S. Reading as a common serotype in turkey meats. Also, it is interesting to note that S. Reading and S. Heidelberg were among the serotypes recovered from turkey farms and their environment, where S. Heidelberg was relatively more common in both humans and turkeys than S. Reading.

The Centers for Disease Control Foodborne Diseases Active Surveillance Network (FoodNet) data indicate that outbreaks and clusters of food-borne infections peak during the warmest months of the year (CDC, 2006). Additionally, some studies have shown that the rate of microbial contamination of food products follows the same trend (CDC, 2003; CDC, 2006). Since our study was conducted during the warmest months of the year, the prevalence estimates of the food-borne pathogens obtained should be fairly representative of their true estimate. One limitation of the study was that we could not evaluate the seasonality of microbial contamination of retail meats due to the short sampling period; the study was conducted only during one season (summer). It has been suggested that future food safety studies focusing on seasonality components of microbial contamination of retail meats may require larger sample sizes and longer analysis periods (Zhao et al, 2006. Also, the location of sampling, the relatively smaller number of samples tested and low number of stores sampled may have influenced the results of this study. S. Heidelberg was the predominant serotype identified (23%), followed by S. Saintpaul (12%), S. Typhimurium (11%), and S. Kentucky (10%). Overall, resistance was most often observed to tetracycline (40%), streptomycin (37%), ampicillin (26%), and sulfamethoxazole (25%). Twelve percent of isolates were resistant to cefoxitin and ceftiofur, though only one isolate was resistant to ceftriaxone. All isolates were susceptible to amikacin and ciprofloxacin; however, 3% of isolates were resistant to nalidixic acid and were almost exclusive to ground turkey samples (n = 11/12). All Salmonella isolates were analyzed for genetic relatedness using pulsed-field gel electrophoresis (PFGE) patterns generated by digestion with Xba1 or Xba1 plus Bln1. PFGE fingerprinting profiles showed that Salmonella, in general, were genetically diverse with a total of 175 Xba1 PFGE profiles generated from the 365 isolates. PFGE profiles showed good correlation with serotypes and in some instances, antimicrobial resistance profiles. Results demonstrated a varied spectrum of antimicrobial resistance and PFGE patterns, including several multidrug resistant clonal groups among Salmonella isolates, and signify the importance of sustained surveillance of foodborne pathogens in retail meats. (Zhao et al, 2006).

### 4.3 *Salmonella* from clinical cases of animals and humans

In the study by Oloya et al (2007), more *Salmonella* isolates were recovered from feces of apparently healthy feedlot cattle (25.8%) than range or beef cattle (3.9%) or dairy (1.2%) cattle. A similar *Salmonella* prevalence in feedlot cattle had been reported before and been attributed to low hygiene in feedlots (Vanselow et al. 2007; Khaitsa et al. 2007a). Also, previous reports of *Salmonella* prevalence in range cattle (Ranta et al. 2005) and dairy cattle (Sorensen et al. 2003; Huston et al. 2002) have been comparable to what is reported by this study, and have been consistently lower than in feedlot cattle. However, the isolation of *Salmonella* in sick or dead cattle (13.6%) and sick humans (41.2%) was indicative of its increasing role in causing disease in both groups of hosts (Besser et al. 2000; Padungtod and Kaneene 2006). Previous studies have reported lower prevalence of salmonellosis in both humans and cattle in ND (Tumuhairwe et al. 2008) and the US (Tumuhairwe et al. 2007).

Human isolates were more diverse (32 different serotypes) than cattle (9 serotypes) or other domestic animal species with the following predominant serotypes; *S. Typhimurium* (cattle and man), S. *Newport* (cattle, man and turkey) and *S. Heidelberg* (man and turkey) (Oloya et al, 2007). The occurrence of *Salmonella* serovars; Agona, Anatum, Heidelberg, Newport, St. Paul and Typhimurium in turkey and man, Infantis, Mbandaka, Newport and Typhimurium in cattle and man and many other less frequently recovered serotypes in both domestic animals and man, highlights the scope and magnitude of risk of *Salmonella* infection from individual species of domestic animals to man (Besser et al. 2000; Gorman and Adley 2004; Oloya et al. 2007; Padungtod and Kaneene 2006). Previous studies had reported clonal relationships of *Salmonella* serovars from humans and non-animal and animal sources and products (Gorman and Adley 2004; Padungtod and Kaneene 2006; Zhao et al. 2003).

The PFGE results showed occurrence of similar genotypes of *Salmonella* isolates in both domestic animals and humans (Oloya et al, 2007). However, it was not possible to ascertain whether the transmission was from domestic animals to humans or either way. Previous studies (Besser et al. 2000; Gorman and Adley 2004) have provided incriminating evidence against food animals or their products as being responsible for transmission of *Salmonella* to humans. The most common PFGE fingerprint profiles I, II, III and IV had strong cattle and human involvement (Figure 2). Since *Salmonella* serovar Typhimurium was a major infection in both domestic animals and humans the isolation of *Salmonella* serotypes with similar PFGE fingerprints profiles in both groups confirms existence of common clones or genotypes between human and animal sources and suggests occurrence of an epidemic strain circulating between the two groups (Tsen et al. 2002). Interestingly, the isolation of serovars with the exact similar PFGE fingerprint patterns in cattle preceded those in humans, suggesting a difference in timing of outbreak and possibly, the direction of infection from domestic animals to humans. Recent evidence of clustering of *S. Typhimurium* infection in domestic animals and correspondingly high case reports of the same serovars in humans in the same counties of ND (Oloya et al. 2007), concurs with an earlier observation that region and infection of domestic animals influence *Salmonella* occurrence in humans (Torpdahl et al. 2006).

AMR profiles showed that most domestic animal strains were multidrug resistant (Oloya et al, 2007). Cattle isolates were resistant (>76.5%) to Amoxicillin/clavulanic acid, ampicillin, chloramphenicol, streptomycin and tetracycline, while human isolates were of comparatively lower resistance to the similar individual drugs (1.6-8.1%) or drug combinations. Only 1 human isolate with similar PFGE profile as the main group of cattle isolates, had similar range of multidrug resistance, providing a single evidence of a possible AMR transmission from cattle to humans. Whereas parallel development of resistance in humans as result of using antibiotics that are identical to those used in animals (Phillips et al. 2004; Tumuhairwe et al. 2007) could not be ruled out, this scenario is less likely. Various epidemiological studies (Besser et al. 2000; Padungtod and Kaneene 2006; Zhao et al. 2003) have provided insights into the roles of domestic animals or their products in the transmission of *Salmonella* and associated antimicrobial drug resistance to humans. Occurrence of serovars with similar PFGE profile may suggest that some cases of human salmonellosis are the results of the circulation of certain strains between animal and human hosts (Phillips et al. 2004). However, the occurrence of different AMR profiles within the similar PFGE patterns suggests fairly established strains in which the domestic animal isolates are more subjected to antimicrobial pressure in the production systems (Zhao et al. 2003), hence the higher resistance compared to the human isolates. If the widespread use of antimicrobial agents in animal husbandry is selecting for antimicrobial-resistant serotypes and there is transmission to humans, then these ought to be reflected in the resistance profiles of salmonella isolates from humans in the same period.

The presence of resistance to chloramphenicol or drug patterns; amoxicillin-ampicillin and chloramphenicol-kanamycin-tetracycline combinations in humans but not in domestic animals could have equally resulted from use of these antibiotic drugs in humans (Phillips et al. 2004). The fact that most isolates with multi-drug resistance were from cattle and only a single human case had the similar resistance profile suggests that *Salmonella* in cattle or predominantly food animals may not play a significant role in transmitting AMR to *Salmonella* in humans. This observation may also support the argument that adequate cooking destroys bacteria in the food (Phillips et al. 2004) and could be that one important barrier to both human infection and AMR transfer. Evidence linking antimicrobial use in food animals to human health risk points to but does not prove a human health threat (Barza and Travers 2002). Attempts could also be made to explain this difference in light of the time lag between time of outbreaks in cattle and humans. Reduction in the antibiotic selection pressure from cattle to humans could result in loss of expression of specific resistance genes (Dowd et al. 2008) as well as loss of the mobile genetic elements responsible for resistance (Kang et al. 2006), but this is beyond the scope of this study.

The diverse *Salmonella* serotypes observed infecting man, suggests other possible sources of infection in human environment. Differences could also arise from the fact that not all infections arise directly from farm animals in contact with the farmers, but also from other sources such as pets and contaminated produce (Johnston et al. 2006) or water sources (Phillips et al. 2004) that may not have been captured in this study. In conclusion, this study demonstrated that although there were similarities in *Salmonella* genotypes responsible for infection in both domestic animals and humans in the 2000-2005 period, both the AMR and multidrug resistance levels in animals were higher than in humans suggesting that resistance acquired in domestic animals did not translate directly into the burden of resistance in humans.

Greene et al (2008) conducted a nationwide study in the US to test for regional differences in risk factors for human infection with salmonellosis. The study analyzed distributions of the two most prevalent MDR Salmonella phenotypes in the United States, 2003-2005: (i) MDR-ACSSuT (resistant to at least ampicillin, chloramphenicol, streptomycin, sulfonamides, and tetracycline) Typhimurium; (ii) MDR-AmpC (resistant to at least ampicillin, chloramphenicol, streptomycin, sulfonamides, tetracycline, amoxicillin/clavulanic acid, and ceftiofur, and with decreased susceptibility to ceftriaxone) Newport. Participating public health laboratories in all states forwarded every 20th Salmonella isolate from humans to the National Antimicrobial Resistance Monitoring System for Enteric Bacteria for antimicrobial susceptibility testing. Among the serotypes Typhimurium and Newport isolates submitted 2003-2005, pansusceptible, MDR-ACSSuT Typhimurium, and MDR-AmpC Newport were identified. Patterns of resistance, demographic factors, and cattle density were compared across regions. Of 1195 serotype Typhimurium isolates, 289 (24%) were MDR-ACSSuT. There were no significant differences in region, age, or sex distribution for pansusceptible versus MDR-ACSSuT Typhimurium. Of 612 serotype Newport isolates, 97 (16%) were MDR-AmpC, but the percentage of MDR-AmpC isolates varied significantly across regions: South 3%, Midwest 28%, West 32%, and Northeast 38% ($p < 0.0001$). The South had the lowest percentage of MDR-AmpC Newport isolates and also the lowest density of milk cows. More Newport isolates were MDR-AmpC in the 10 states with the highest milk cow density compared with the remaining states. Overall, 22% of pansusceptible Newport isolates but only 7% of MDR-AmpC Newport isolates were from patients <2 years of age. For both serotypes, MDR phenotypes had less seasonal variation than pansusceptible phenotypes. This was the first analysis of the distribution of clinically important MDR Salmonella isolates in the United States. MDR-ACSSuT Typhimurium was evenly distributed across regions. However, MDR-AmpC Newport was less common in the South and in children <2 years of age. Information on individuals' exposures was needed to fully explain the observed patterns. Moreover, another study (Nielsen, 2009) reported variation in antimicrobial resistance in sporadic and outbreak-related Salmonella enterica serovar Typhimurium from patients in Denmark. Variation in antimicrobial resistance and corresponding changes of SGI1 were shown among isolates from a foodborne outbreak (Nielsen, 2009).

## 5. Conclusion

The study on *Salmonella* occurrence from naturally infected feedlot cattle housed at the North Dakota State University cattle feedlot research facility highlighted the genotypic variation in *Salmonella* isolated in healthy feedlot steers and also supported previous reports that not all MDR *salmonella* Typhimurium do carry a wide variety of resistance genes, and also that isolates with the same resistance phenotype often have different resistance genotypes. Also the widespread AMR observed in the majority of *Salmonella* isolates was not matched with presence of integrons, an indication that besides integrons, AMR in *Salmonella* may be explained by other mechanisms that warrant further research. Prevalence of *Salmonella* in grass fed cattle in ND was 7.1%, relatively higher than some studies have reported. *Salmonella* Typhimurium was the most common cause of salmonellosis in animals in North Dakota. *Salmonella* Typhimurium (Copenhagen) serotype was identified as the major serotype that was being shed by ranch beef cattle. The data show that multi-drug resistance was widespread among the *Salmonella* recovered from apparently healthy grass fed cattle. The emergence of multi-drug resistant *Salmonella* reduces the therapeutic options in cases of invasive infections and has been shown to be associated with an increased burden of illness.

The study of salmonella occurrence in dairy cattle demonstrated that a substantial percentage of cattle in this dairy was shedding *Salmonella* in the feces, and antimicrobial resistance among the five *Salmonella* isolates was widespread. It is possible that some management practices of dairies related to antimicrobial use may contribute to developing *Salmonella* serotypes that are resistant to antimicrobials. The study on *Salmonella* occurrence in a bison herd indicated that Salmonellae were shed in feces of bison at a comparable prevalence to that of cattle herds in the US, and that the isolates were multidrug resistant. The data contribute to risk assessment of *Salmonella* in bison and highlight the possible existence of antimicrobial resistance in bison. The multi-drug resistance reported among the *Salmonella* isolates warrants further study considering that the serotype *S.* Typhimurium is widely distributed and has the potential of greatly impacting human and animal health. The study on retail meats indicate that turkey meat products from retail stores may occasionally be contaminated with *Salmonella* possessing a varied spectrum of antimicrobial resistance. The contamination was dependent on the type of meat and the time of sampling. These data confirm that both raw and ready to eat retail turkey meat products may be vehicles for transmitting salmonellosis, some of which is resistant to antimicrobials justifying the need for sustained surveillance of foodborne pathogens in retail meats.

The study that compared *Salmonella* isolates from clinical cases of humans and animals reported that human isolates were more diverse than cattle or other domestic animal species. PFGE results confirmed occurrence of similar *Salmonella* genotypes in both domestic animals and humans, with the isolation in cattle preceding those in humans. This suggests a spread of infection from domestic animals to humans. AMR profiles showed that domestic animal strains were multidrug resistant. Only 1 human isolate had similar PFGE profile as cattle isolates with a similar range of multidrug resistance, providing a single evidence of a possible AMR transmission from cattle to humans. This study demonstrated that although there were similar *Salmonella* genotypes from domestic animals and humans, the AMR levels observed in domestic animal isolates was higher than in humans, implying that cattle or food animals may not play a significant role in transmitting AMR to S*almonella* in humans and that the occurrence of resistance in animal isolates may not translate directly into resistance in human isolates in this area.

## 6. Acknowledgements

The authors would like to thank the US National Veterinary Service Laboratories, Animal and Plant Health Inspection Services, US Department of Agriculture, Ames, Iowa, for serotyping. We also thank the *E. coli* reference center (University Park, PA) for the genomic subtyping of the isolates. The authors thank North Dakota State University-Veterinary Diagnostic Laboratory, North Dakota producers, graduate students and postdoctoral researchers for participating in the studies. Funding for these studies was provided by

USDA-APHIS (Agrosecurity: Disease Surveillance and Public Health) and USDA-CSREES (Food Safety Risk Assessment) grants.

## 7. References

Alam M.J., Renter D., Taylor E., Mina D., Moxley R., Smith D. 2009. Antimicrobial susceptibility profiles of Salmonella enterica serotypes recovered from pens of commercial feedlot cattle using different types of composite samples. Curr Microbiol. 2009 Apr;58(4):354-9. Epub 2009 Feb 14.

Al-Tawfiq, J.A. 2007.Antimicrobial susceptibility of *Salmonella* typhi and non-typhi in a hospital in eastern Saudi Arabia. *J Chemother* 19, 62–65.

Anderson, R. J. 1997. Case-control study of an outbreak of clinical disease attributable to *Salmonella* menhaden infection in eight dairy herds. *Journal of the American Veterinary Medical Association*. 210:528–530.

Angulo, F. J., K. R. Johnson, R. V. Tauxe, and M. L. Cohen. 2000. Origins and consequences of antimicrobial-resistant nontyphoidal *Salmonella*: implications for the use of fluoroquinolones in food animals. *Microb. Drug Resist.* 6:77–83.

Arshad, M. M., M. J. Wilkins, F. P. Downes, M. H. Rahbar, R. J. Erskine, M. L. Boulton, and A. M. Saeed. 2007. A registry-based study on the association between human salmonellosis and routinely collected parameters in Michigan, 1995-2001. *Foodborne Pathog Dis* 4 (1):16-25.

Avery, S.M. A. Small, C.A. Reid and S. Buncic. 2002. Pulsed-field gel electrophoresis characterization of Shiga toxin-producing *Escherichia coli* O157 from hides of cattle at slaughter, *J. Food Prot.* 65 (2002), pp. 1172–1176

Bacon, R. T., J. N. Sofos, K. E. Belk, D. R. Hyatt, and G. C. Smith. 2002. Prevalence and antibiotic susceptibility of Salmonella isolated from beef animal hides and carcasses. *J Food Prot* 65 (2):284-290.

Barza, M., and K. Travers. 2002. Excess infections due to antimicrobial resistance: the "Attributable Fraction". *Clin Infect Dis* 34 Suppl 3:S126-130.

Beach, J. C., Murano E. A, Acuff G. R. 2002. Serotyping and antibiotic resistance profiling of Salmonella in feedlot and nonfeedlot beef cattle. *J Food Prot* 65:1694-1699.

Besser, T. E., M. Goldoft, L. C. Pritchett, R. Khakhria, D. D. Hancock, D. H. Rice, J. M. Gay, W. Johnson, and C. C. Gay. 2000. Multiresistant Salmonella Typhimurium DT104 infections of humans and domestic animals in the Pacific Northwest of the United States. *Epidemiol Infect* 124 (2):193-200.

Blau, D. M, McCluskey B. J, Ladely S. R, Dargatz D. A, Fedorka-Cray P. J, Ferris K. E, Headrick M. L: Salmonella in dairy operations in the United States: prevalence and antimicrobial drug susceptibility. J Food Prot 68:696-702, 2005.

Brands, D.A., S.J. Billington, J.F. Levine, L.A. Joens. 2005. Genotypes and antibiotic resistance of *Salmonella* Newport isolates from U. S. market oysters. *Foodborne Patho Dis.* 2:111–114.

Branham L.A., Carr M.A., Scott C.B., Callaway T.R.: *E. coli* O157 and *Salmonella* spp. in white-tailed deer and livestock. Curr Issues Intest Microbiol 6:25-29, 2005.

Centers for Disease Control and Prevention (CDC). 2005. Preliminary FoodNet Data on the Incidence of Infection with Pathogens Transmitted Commonly Through Food - 10 Sites, United States, 2004. *MMWR.* 54:352-356.

Centers for Disease Control and Prevention (CDC). 2006. Preliminary FoodNet Data on the Incidence of Infection with Pathogens Transmitted Commonly Through Food -10 States, United States, 2005. *MMWR.* 55:392-395.

Centers for Disease Control and Prevention (CDC). 2003. *Salmonellosis.* http://www.cdc.gov/icidod/dbmd/diseaseinfo/salmonellosis_t.htm

Chen, S., S. Zhao, D. G. White, C. M. Schroeder, R. Lu, H. Yang, P. F. McDermott, S. Ayers, and J. Meng. 2004.

Characterization of multiple-antimicrobial-resistant *Salmonella* serovars isolated from retail Meats. *Appl. Environ. Microbiol.* 70:1-7.

Chiappini, E., L. Galli, P. Pecile, A. Vierucci, and M. de Martino. 2002. Results of a five year prospective surveillance study of antibiotic resistance among *Salmonella* enterica isolates and ceftriaxone therapy among children hospitalized for acute diarrhea. *Clin. Ther.* 24:1585–1594.

Cloak, O. M., G. Duffy, J. J. Sheridan, I. S. Blair, and D. A. McDowell. 2001. A survey on the incidence of *Campylobacter* spp. and the development of a surface adhesion polymerase chain reaction (SA-PCR) assay for the detection of *Campylobacter jejuni* in retail meat products. *Food Microbiol.* 18:287-298.

Coburn, B., G. A. Grassl, and B. B. Finlay. 2006. Salmonella, the host and disease: a brief review. *Immunol Cell Biol.*

Cray P. J, Bailey J. S, Frye J. G, Jackson C. R, Englen M. D, Berrang M. E, Meinersmann R. J, Wineland N. E, Dargatz D.A,

Anandarama N. 2006. Update: The National Antimicrobial Resistance Monitoring System Enteric Bacteria (NARMS): Animal Arm. *United States Animal Health Association Proceedings.*

Dargatz D.A., Fedorka-Cray P.J., Ladely S.R., Koprai C.A., Ferris K.E., Headrick M.L.: Prevalence and antimicrobial susceptibility of *Salmonella* spp. isolates from US cattle in feedlot in 1999 and 2000. 2003. *J Appl Microbiol* 95:753-761.

Dargatz, D. A., P. J. Fedorka-Cray, S. R. Ladely, K. E. Ferris, A. L. Green, and M. L. Headrick. 2002. Antimicrobial susceptibility patterns of *Salmonella* isolates from cattle in feedlots. *JAVMA.* 221:268-272.

Domínguez, C., I. Gómez, and J. Zumalacárregui. 2002. Prevalence of *Salmonella* and *Campylobacter* in retail chicken in Spain. *Int. J. Food Microbiol.* 72:165-168.

Dowd, S. E., K. Killinger-Mann, M. Brashears, and J. Fralick. 2008. Evaluation of gene expression in a single antibiotic exposure-derived isolate of Salmonella enterica typhimurium 14028 possessing resistance to multiple antibiotics. *Foodborne Pathog Dis* 5 (2):205-221.

Doyle, M. P., and M. C. Erickson. 2006. Reducing the carriage of foodborne pathogens in livestock and poultry. *Poult Sci* 85 (6):960-973.

Duffy, G., O. M. Cloak, M. G. O'Sullivan, A. Guillet, J. J. Sheridan, I. S. Blair, and D. A McDowell. 1999. The incidence and antibiotic resistance profiles of *Salmonella* spp. on Irish retail meat products. *Food Microbiol.* 16:623-631.

Dunne, E. F., P. D. Fey, P. Kludt, R. Reporter, F. Mostashari, P. Shillam, J. Wicklund, C. Miller, B. Holland, K. Stamey, T. J Barrett, J. K. Rasheed, F. C. Tenover, E. M. Ribot, and F. J. Angulo. 2000. Emergence of domestically acquired ceftriaxone-resistant *Salmonella* infections associated with AmpC beta-lactamase. *JAMA* 284:3151–3156.

Duran, G. M., and D. L. Marshall. 2005. Ready-to-eat shrimp as an international vehicle of antibiotic-resistant bacteria. *J Food Prot* 68 (11):2395-2401.

Edrington, T. S., T. Ross, R. Callaway, H. Martinez, E. Hume, J. Genovese, L. Poole, C. Anderson, and J. Nisbet. 2008. Investigation into the seasonal salmonellosis in lactating dairy cattle. *Epidemiol Infect.* 2008 March; 136(3): 381–390.

Edrington T. S., M. E. Hume, Looper M. L. Looper, 2004. Variation in the Fecal shedding of *Salmonella* and *E. coli* O157:H7 in lactating dairy cattle and examination of *Salmonella* genotypes using pulsed-field gel electrophoresis. Lett in Applied Microbiol 2004; 366 - 372. 366-372.

Edrington T.S. 2004. Examination of heat stress and stage of lactation (early versus late) on fecal shedding of *E. coli* O157:H7 and *Salmonella* in dairy cattle. Foodborne Pathogens and Disease. 2004;**1**:114–119.

Fegan N. P., Vanderlinde, G. Higgs, P. Desmarchelier. 2004. Quantification and prevalence of *Salmonella* in beef cattle presenting at slaughter. J Appl Microbiol. 97(5):892-8.

Fey, P. D., T. J. Safranek, M. E. Rupp, E. F. Dunne, E. Ribot, P. C. Iwen, P. A. Bradford, F. J. Angulo, and S. H. Hinrichs. 2000. Ceftriaxone-resistant *Salmonella* infection acquired by a child from cattle. *N. Engl. J. Med.* 342:1242–1249.

Fitzgerald, A. C, Edrington T. S, Looper M. L, Callaway T. R, Genovese K. J, Bischoff K. M, McReynolds J. L, Thomas J. D, Anderson R. C, Nisbet D. J. 2003. Antimicrobial susceptibility and factors affecting the shedding of *E. coli* O157:H7 and Salmonella in dairy cattle. Lett Appl Microbiol 37:392-8.

Fossler, C. P, Wells S. J, Kaneene J. B, Ruegg P. L, Warnick L. D, Eberly L. E, Godden S. M, Halbert L. W, Campbell A. M,

Bolin C. A, Zwald A. M. 2005. Cattle and environmental sample-level factors associated with the presence of Salmonella in a multi-state study of conventional and organic dairy farms. Prev Vet Med 67:39-53.

Fossler C. P. Wells S. J, Kaneene J.B., Ruegg P.L., Warnick L.D., Bender J.B., Godden S.M., Halbert L.W., Campbell A.M., Zwald A.M. 2004. Prevalence of Salmonella spp on conventional and organic dairy farms. *J Am Vet Med Assoc* 225(4):567-73.

Fratamico, P. M., L. K. Bagi, and T. Pepe. 2000. A multiplex polymerase chain reaction assay for rapid detection and identification of *Escherichia coli* O157:H7 in foods and bovine feces. *J. Food Prot.* 63:1032–1037.

Frech G, Kehrenberg C, and Schwarz S**.** Resistance phenotypes and genotypes of multiresistant *Salmonella enterica* subsp. *enterica* serovar Typhimurium var. Copenhagen isolates from animal sources. J. Antimicrob. Chemother. 2003.51:180.

Frye, J.G. and Fedorka-Cray, P.J. 2007. Prevalence, distribution and characterization of ceftiofur resistance in *Salmonella enterica* isolated from animals in the USA from 1999 to 2003. *Int J Antimicrob Agents* 30, 134–142.

Galland J.C. et al. Diversity of *Salmonella* serotypes in cull (market) dairy cows at slaughter. Journal of the American Veterinary Medical Association. 2001;**219**:1216–1220. [PubMed]

Gaul, S. B., S. Wedel, M. M. Erdman, D. L. Harris, I. T. Harris, K. E. Ferris, and L. Hoffman. 2007. Use of pulsed-field gel electrophoresis of conserved XbaI fragments for identification of swine Salmonella serotypes. *J Clin Microbiol* 45 (2):472-476.

Gay, J. M, Hunsaker M. E. 1993. Isolation of multiple *Salmonella* serovars from a dairy two years after a clinical salmonellosis outbreak. *Journal of the American Veterinary Medical Association*. 203:1314–1320.

Gebreyes, W. A., C. Altier, and S. Thakur. 2006. Molecular epidemiology and diversity of Salmonella serovar Typhimurium in pigs using phenotypic and genotypic approaches. *Epidemiol Infect* 134 (1):187-198.

Gold stein, C., M. D. Lee, S. Sanchez, C. Hudson, B. Phillips, B. Register, M. Grady, C. Liebert, A. O. Summers, D. G. White, and J. J. Maurer. 2001. Incidence of class 1 and 2 integrases in clinical and commensal bacteria from livestock, companion animals, and exotics. *Antimicrob Agents Chemother* 45:723–6.

Gomez, T. M., Y. Motarjemi, and S. Miyagawa . 1997. Foodborne salmonellosis. *World Health Stat Q*; 50: 81–9.

Gorman, R., and C. C. Adley. 2004. Characterization of Salmonella enterica serotype Typhimurium isolates from human, food, and animal sources in the Republic of Ireland. *J Clin Microbiol* 42 (5):2314-2316.

Greene S.K., Stuart A.M., Medalla F.M., Whichard J.M., Hoekstra R.M., Chiller T.M. Distribution of multidrug-resistant human isolates of MDR-ACSSuT Salmonella Typhimurium and MDR-AmpC Salmonella Newport in the United States, 2003-2005. Foodborne Pathog Dis. 2008 Oct;5(5):669-80.

Guerra, B., P. Schrors, and M. C. Mendoza. 2000. Application of PFGE performed with XbaI to an epidemiological and phylogenetic study of Salmonella serotype typhimurium. Relations between genetic types and phage types. *New Microbiol* 23 (1):11-20.

Hegde N.V., Cook M.L., Wolfgang, D.R., et al. 2005. Dissemination of *Salmonella enterica* subsp. *enterica* Serovar Typhimurium var. Copenhagen clonal types through a contract heifer-raising operation. J. Clin. Microbiol. 2005.43:4208–4211.

Huston, C. L., T. E. Wittum, B. C. Love, and J. E. Keen. 2002. Prevalence of fecal shedding of Salmonella spp in dairy herds. *J Am Vet Med Assoc* 220 (5):645-649.

Hynes N. A, and I. K Wachsmuth. *Escherichia coli* O157:H7 risk assessment in ground beef: a public health tool. Proceedings of the 4th International Symposium on Shiga Toxin-Producing *Escherichia coli* infections. Kyoto, Japan. 2000. p. 46. Abstract T3-4

Johnston, L. M., L. A. Jaykus, D. Moll, J. Anciso, B. Mora, and C. L. Moe. 2006. A field study of the microbiological quality of fresh produce of domestic and Mexican origin. *Int J Food Microbiol* 112 (2):83-95.

Kang, M. S., T. E. Besser, D. D. Hancock, S. Porwollik, M. McClelland, and D. R. Call. 2006. Identification of specific gene sequences conserved in contemporary epidemic strains of Salmonella enterica. *Appl Environ Microbiol* 72 (11):6938-6947.

Kegode, R. B., D. K. Doetkott, I.V. Wesley, M. L. Khaitsa. 2008. Occurrence of *Campylobacter* species, *Salmonella* species, and generic *Escherichia coli* in meat products from retail outlets in the Midwestern United States. *Journal of Food Safety* 28:111–125.

Khaitsa, M. L., R.B. Kegode, D. K. Doetkott. 2008. Occurrence of Antimicrobial-resistant *Salmonella* serotypes shed in feces of bison in North Dakota. *The Bovine Practitioner, 2008,* 42(2) 148-154.

Khaitsa, M. L., R. B. Kegode, M. L. Bauer, P. S. Gibbs, G. P. Lardy, and D. K. Doetkott. 2007a. A longitudinal study of Salmonella shedding and antimicrobial resistance patterns in North Dakota feedlot cattle. *J Food Prot* 70 (2):476-481.

Khaitsa, M. L., R. B. Kegode, and D. K. Doetkott. 2007b. Occurrence of antimicrobial-resistant salmonella species in raw and ready to eat turkey meat products from retail outlets in the midwestern United States. *Foodborne Pathog Dis* 4 (4):517-525.

Khaitsa M.L., Mantz A. and Doetkott, D. 2004. Prevalence of *Escherichia coli* 0157:H7 and *Salmonella* in North Dakota State University (NDSU) Dairy Cattle and antimicrobial susceptibility patterns of the Salmonella isolates. In: Proceedings of the 38th Annual North Dakota Dairy Convention. Mandan, ND. Nov.18-19, 2004. pp 32-35.

Kim, A., Y. J. Lee, M. S. Kang, S. I. Kwag, and J. K. Cho. 2007. Dissemination and tracking of Salmonella spp. in integrated broiler operation. *J Vet Sci* 8 (2):155-161.

Krauland M.G., Marsh J.W., Paterson D.L., Harrison L.H. 2009. Integron-mediated multidrug resistance in a global collection of nontyphoidal Salmonella enterica isolates. Emerg Infect Dis. 2009 Mar;15(3):388-96

Lathers, C. M. 2001. Role of Veterinary Medicine in Public Health: Antibiotic Use in Food Animals and Humans and the effect on Evolution of Antibacterial Resistance. *J. Clin Pharmacol.* 41:595-599.

Ling, J. M., E. W. Chan, and A. F. Cheng. 2001. Molecular epidemiological analysis of Salmonella enterica serotype Derby infections in Hong Kong. *J Infect* 42 (2):145-153.

Logue, C. M., J. S. Sherwood, P. A. Olah, L. M. Elijah, and M. R. Dockter. 2003. The incidence of antimicrobial-resistant Salmonella spp on freshly processed poultry from US Midwestern processing plants. *J Appl Microbiol* 94 (1):16-24.

Mayrhofer, S., P. Paulsen, J. M. S. Smulders, and F. Hilbert. 2004. Antimicrobial resistance profile of five major food-borne pathogens isolated from beef, pork and poultry. *Int. J. Food Microbiol.* 97:23-29.

McDonough P.I. Epidemiology of bovine salmonellosis. *Proceedings of the American Association of Bovine Practitioners Annual Meeting*1986 ; pp. 169–173.173.

McLaughlin, J. B., L. J. Castrodale, M. J. Gardner, R. Ahmed, and B. D. Gessner. 2006. Outbreak of multidrug-resistant Salmonella typhimurium associated with ground beef served at a school potluck. *J Food Prot* 69 (3):666-670.

Mead, P. S., L. Slutsker, V. Dietz, L. F. McCaig, J. S. Bresee, C. Shapiro, P. M. Griffin, and R. V. Tauxe. 1999. Food-related illness and death in the United States. *Emerg Infect Dis* 5 (5):607-625.

Miko, A., K. Pries, A. Schroeter and R. Helmuth.2005. Molecular mechanisms of resistance in multidrug-resistant serovars of *Salmonella enterica* isolated from foods in Germany. *J. Antimicrob. Chemother*. December. 56: 1025 – 1033.

Mrema, N., S. Mpuchane, and B. A. Gashe. 2006. Prevalence of *Salmonella* in raw minced meat, raw fresh sausages and raw burger patties from retail outlets in Gaborone, Botswana. *Food Control.* 17:207-212.

Mulvey M.R., Boyd D.A., Olson A.B., Doublet B., Cloeckaert A. 2006. The genetics of Salmonella genomic island 1. Microbes Infect. 2006 Jun;8(7):1915-22. Epub 2006 Mar 27.

National Antimicrobial Resistance Monitoring System-Enteric Bacteria (NARMS-EB). 2003. Report. [Online.]http://www.cdc.gov/narms

National Animal Health Monitoring System (NAHMS) 1996. NAHMS Dairy '96: Salmonella Status on U.S. Dairy Operations. www.cvmbs.colostate.edu/ilm/cdn/98articles/July/Salmonella.htm

Nielsen, E. M, Torpdahl M, Ethelberg S, Hammerum AM. 2009. Variation in Antimicrobial resistance in sporadic and outbreak-related Salmonella enterica serovar Typhimurium. Emerg Infect Dis. 2009 Jan;15(1):101-3.

Norrby, S. R. 2005. Integrons: adding another threat to the use of antibiotic therapy. *Clin Infect Dis* 41:10–1.

Okeke, I.N., K. P. Klugman, Z. A. Bhutta, A. G. Duse, P. Jenkins, T. F. O'Brien, A. Pablos-Mendez, R. Laxminarayan. 2005. Antimicrobial resistance in developing countries. Part II: Strategies for containment. *Lancet Infect. Dis*. 5:568–580.

Oloya, D. Doetkott, M.L. Khaitsa. 2009. Antimicrobial drug resistance and molecular characterization of *Salmonella* isolated from domestic animals, humans and meat products. *J. Foodborne Pathogens & Disease*, 2009, 6(3) 273-284.

Oloya, J., M. Theis, D. Doetkott, N. Dyer, P. Gibbs, and M. L. Khaitsa. 2007. Evaluation of salmonella occurrence in domestic animals and humans in north dakota (2000-2005). *Foodborne Pathog Dis* 4 (4):551-563.

Ono, K., and K. Yamamoto. 1999. Contamination of meat with *Campylobacter jejuni* in Saitama, Japan. *Int. J. Food Microbiol.* 47:211-219.

Orman, B. E., Pineiro, S. A., Arduino, S., Galas, M., Melano, R., Caffer, M., Sordelli, D. O., and Centrón, D. 2002. Evolution of multiresistance in nontyphoid *Salmonella* serovars from 1984-1988 in Argentina. *Antimicrob. Agents Chemother*. 46: 3963–3970.

Ozogul, Y., F. Ozogul, I. A. Olgunoglu, and E. Kuley. 2007. Bacteriological and biochemical assessment of marinating cephalopods, crustaceans and gastropoda during 24 weeks of storage. *Int J Food Sci Nutr*:1-12.

Padungtod, P., and J. B. Kaneene. 2006. Salmonella in food animals and humans in northern Thailand. *Int J Food Microbiol* 108 (3):346-354.

Phillips, I., M. Casewell, T. Cox, B. De Groot, C. Friis, R. Jones, C. Nightingale, R. Preston, and J. Waddell. 2004. Does the use of antibiotics in food animals pose a risk to human health? A critical review of published data. *J Antimicrob Chemother* 53 (1):28-52.

Pickard, D., N. R. Thomson, S. Baker, J. Wain, M. Pardo, D. Goulding, N. Hamlin, J. Choudhary, J. Threfall, and G. Dougan. 2008. Molecular characterization of the Salmonella enterica serovar Typhi Vi-typing bacteriophage E1. *J Bacteriol* 190 (7):2580-2587.

Plym, F. L., and M. Wierup. 2006. Salmonella contamination: a significant challenge to the global marketing of animal food products. *Rev Sci Tech* 25 (2):541-554.

Puohiniemi, R., T. Heiskanen, and A. Siitonen. 1997. Molecular epidemiology of two international sprout-borne Salmonella outbreaks. *J Clin Microbiol* 35 (10):2487-2491.

Rabsch, W. 2007. Salmonella typhimurium phage typing for pathogens. *Methods Mol Biol* 394:177-211.

Ranta, J., P. Tuominen, and R. Maijala. 2005. Estimation of true Salmonella prevalence jointly in cattle herd and animal populations using Bayesian hierarchical modeling. *Risk Anal* 25 (1):23-37.

Refsum, T., E. Heir, G. Kapperud, T. Vardund, and G. Holstad. 2002. Molecular epidemiology of Salmonella enterica serovar typhimurium isolates determined by pulsed-field gel electrophoresis: comparison of isolates from avian wildlife, domestic animals, and the environment in Norway. *Appl Environ Microbiol* 68 (11):5600-5606.

Richardson A. Salmonellosis in cattle. Veterinary Record. 1975;96:329–331.

Sallen, B., Rajoharison, A., Desvarenne, S., and Mabilat, C. 1995. Molecular epidemiology of integron-associated antibiotic resistance genes in clinical isolates of *Enterobacteriaceae. Microb. Drug Resist.* 1: 195–202.

Santos, F. B., D. H. Dsouza, L. Jaykus, P. R. Ferket, and B. W. Sheldon. 2007. Genotypes, serotypes, and antibiotic resistance profiles of Salmonella isolated from commercial North Carolina turkey farms. *J Food Prot* 70 (6):1328-1333.

Sato, K. 2001. Spatial and temporal clustering of *Salmonella* serotypes isolated from adult diarrhetic dairy cattle in California. Journal of Veterinary Diagnostic Investigation. 13:206–212. Scallan E, Griffin PM, Angulo FJ, Tauxe RV, Hoekstra RM. 2011. Foodborne illness acquired in the United States--unspecified agents. Emerg Infect Dis. 2011 Jan;17(1):16-22.

Shabarinath, S., H. Sanath Kumar, R. Khushiramani, I. Karunasagar, and I. Karunasagar. 2007. Detection and characterization of Salmonella associated with tropical seafood. *Int J Food Microbiol* 114 (2):227-233.

Schlosser, W., A. Hogue, E. Ebel, B. Rose, R. Umholtz, K. Ferris, and W. James. 2000. Analysis of *Salmonella* serotypes from selected carcasses and raw ground products sampled prior to implementation of the pathogen reduction; hazard analysis and critical control point final rule in the US. *Int. J. Food Microbiol.* 58:107-111.

Schroeder C.M., White D.G., Ge B., Zhang Y., McDermott P.F., Ayers S., Zhao S., and Meng J.: Isolation of antimicrobial-resistant *Escherichia coli* from retail meats purchased in greater Washington, DC, USA. *Int J Food Microbiol* 85:197-202, 2003.

Sorensen, O., M. McFall, and K. Manninen. 2003. Prevalence of Salmonella in dairy herds in Alberta. *Can Vet J* 44 (3):230-231.

Sorensen, O., J. van Donkersgoed, M. McFall, K. Manninen, G. Gensler, and G. Ollis. 2002. *Salmonella* spp. shedding by

Alberta beef cattle and the detection of *Salmonella* spp. in ground beef. *J. Food Prot.* 65:484-491.

Soultos, N., P. Koidis, and R. H. Madden. 2003. Presence of *Listeria* and *Salmenella* spp. in retail chicken in Northern Ireland. *Lett. Applied Microbiol.* 37:421-423.

Stokes, H.W., and R.M. Hall. 1989. A novel family of potentially mobile DNA elements encoding site-specific gene-integration functions: integrons. *Mol Microbiol* 3:1669–1683.

Swaminathan, B., T. J. Barrett, S. B. Hunter, and R. V. Tauxe. 2001. PulseNet: the molecular subtyping network for foodborne bacterial disease surveillance, United States. *Emerg. Infect. Dis.* 7:382–389.

Tabe, E. S., J. Oloya, D. K. Doetkott, M. L. Khaitsa. 2010a. Characterization of multidrug-resistant *Salmonella* Typhimurium serovar Copenhagen isolated from feedlot cattle. *Journal of Food Protection Trends, Journal of Food Protection Trends,* Vol. 30, No. 5, Pages 273–279.

Tabe, E. S., J. Oloya, D. K. Doetkott, M. L. Khaitsa. 2010b. Genotypic diversity of *Escherichia coli* O157:H7 and *Salmonella enterica typhimurium* var Copenhagen isolated from feedlot cattle during finishing. *Africa Journal of Animal and Biomedical Sciences* 5 (3), 2010.ISSN: 1819-4214. http://www.ajabs.net/journals/article%202%20AJABS%202010%205.pdf

Theis, M., J. Oloya, D. Doetkott, N.W. Dyer, P.S. Gibbs, M.L. Khaitsa, 2007. *Salmonella* Occurrence in North Dakota forage-fed beef cattle: Prevalence, Characterization and comparison with reports from the Veterinary Diagnostic Laboratory. *Unified Beef Cattle and Range Research Report:* Agricultural Experiment Station, Department. Animal and Range Sciences, North Dakota State University.

Theis, M. J. 2006. *Salmonella* Occurrence in Beef Cattle: Characterization and Comparison with Clinical Salmonellosis; *Thesis* submitted to North Dakota State University, Fargo, ND.

Theis, M., M.L. Khaitsa, D. Doetkott, N. Dyer, P. Gibbs. 2005. *Salmonella* Occurrence in North Dakota Grass Fed Beef Cattle: Prevalence and Characterization. *Proceedings of the 3rd International Rushmore Conference on Enteric Diseases,* Rapid City, South Dakota, USA, September 29-October 1, 2005.

Torpdahl, M., G. Sorensen, S. Ethelberg, G. Sando, K. Gammelgard, and L. J. Porsbo. 2006. A regional outbreak of S. Typhimurium in Denmark and identification of the source using MLVA typing. *Euro Surveill* 11 (5):134-136.

Trung, N. D., U. Suthisarnsuntorn, T. Kalambaheti, W. Wonglumsom, and W. Tunyong. 2007. Antimicrobial susceptibility patterns and phage types of Salmonella typhi from Vietnam. *Southeast Asian J Trop Med Public Health* 38 (3):487-492.

Tsen, H. Y., J. S. Lin, and H. Y. Hsih. 2002. Pulsed field gel electrophoresis for animal Salmonella enterica serovar Typhimurium isolates in Taiwan. *Vet Microbiol* 87 (1):73-80.

Tumuhairwe, E., R. Magel, M. Bhandary, and M. L. Khaitsa. 2007. Salmonellosis outbreaks in humans in the United States 1990-2003: The contribution of turkey as a vehicle. *Food Protection Trends* 27 (5):300-306.

Tumuhairwe, E., T. Murase, M. Bhandary, and M. L. Khaitsa. 2008. Characterization of 386 Non-typhoidal Salmonellosis cases in North Dakota from 2000 to 2005. *Food Protection Trends* 28 (5):304-313.

USDA, 2001. Preventing Biological Hazards from Cull Dairy Cattle. http://www.fsis.usda.gov/ofo/hrds/internat/seminar/slideshows/10 tamu5/index.htm

Usera, M. A., A. Aladuena, R. Gonzalez, M. De la Fuente, J. Garcia-Pena, N. Frias, and M. A. Echeita, 2002. Antibiotic resistance of *Salmonella* spp. from animal sources in Spain in 1996 and 2000. *J Food Prot.* 65:768-73.

Vali, L., M.C. Pearce, K.A. Wisely, A. Hamouda, H.I. Knight, A.W. Smith and S.G. Amyes. 2005. Comparison of diversities of *Escherichia coli* O157 shed from a cohort of spring-born beef calves at pasture and in housing, *Appl. Environ. Microbiol.* 71 : 1648–1652.

Vanselow, B. A., M. A. Hornitzky, K. H. Walker, G. J. Eamens, G. D. Bailey, P. A. Gill, K. Coates, B. Corney, J. P. Cronin, and S. Renilson. 2007. Salmonella and on-farm risk factors in healthy slaughter-age cattle and sheep in eastern Australia. *Aust Vet J* 85 (12):498-502.

Vugia, D. J., M. Samuel, M. M. Farley, R. Marcus, B. Shiferaw, S. Shallow, K. Smith, and F. J. Angulo. 2004. Invasive *Salmonella* infections in the United States, FoodNet, 1996-1999: incidence, serotype distribution, and outcome. *Clin. Infect. Dis.* 38:S149–S156.

Wallace, J., K. Stanley, J. Currie, P. Diggle, and J. Jones. 1997. Seasonality of thermophilic *Campylobacter* populations in chickens. *J. Appl. Microbiol.* 82:224-230.

Warnick, L. D, Kaneene J. B, Ruegg P. L, Wells S. J, Fossler C, Halbert L, Campbell A. 2003. Evaluation of herd sampling for Salmonella isolation on midwest and northeast US dairy farms. Prev Vet Med 60:195-206.

Wells S. et al. *E. coli* O157:H7 and Salmonella - Status on U.S. Dairy Operations. USDA/APHIS/VS. Fort Collins, CO: Centers for Epidemiology and Animal Health; 1998.

White, D.G., 2005. Characterization of *Salmonella* Typhimurium of animal origin obtained from the national antimicrobial resistance monitoring system. *Foodborne Pathog.Dis.* 2, 169–181.

White, D. G., S. Zhao, R. Sugler, S. Ayers, S. Friedman, S. Chen, P. F. McDermott, S. McDermott, D. D. Wagner, and J. Meng. 2001. The isolation of antibiotic-resistant *Salmonella* from retail ground meats. *New Eng. J. Med.* 345:1147-1154.

Whyte, P., K. McGill, D. Cowley, R. H. Madden, L. Moran, P. Scates, C. Carroll, A. O'Leary, S. Fanning, J. D. Collins, E.

McNamara, J. E. Moore, and M Cormican. 2004. Occurrence of *Campylobacter* in retail foods in Ireland. *Int. J. Food Microbiol.* 95:111-118.

Winokur, P. L., A. Brueggemann, D. L. DeSalvo, L. Hoffmann, M. D. Apley, E. K. Uhlenhopp, M. A. Pfaller, and G. V. Doern.

2000. Animal and human multidrug-resistant, cephalosporin-resistant *Salmonella* isolates expressing a plasmid-mediated CMY-2 AmpC beta-lactamase. Antimicrob. Agents Chemother. 44:2777–2783.

World Health Organization (2005). Drug resistant *Salmonella* fact sheet. Available at URL: http://www.who.int/mediacentre/factsheets/fs139/en/

Xercavins, M., T. Llovet, F. Navarro, M. A. Morera, J. More, F. Bella, N. Freixas, M. Simo, A. Echeita, P. Coll, J. Garau, and G. Prats. 1997. Epidemiology of an unusually prolonged outbreak of typhoid fever in Terrassa, Spain. *Clin Infect Dis* 24 (3):506-510.

Zhang, H., Shi, L., Li, L., Guo, S., Zhang, X., Yamasaki, S., Mioyoshi, S., Shinoda, S., 2004. Identification and characterisation of Class 1 integron resistance gene cassettes among *Salmonella* strains isolated from humans in China. *Microbiol. Immunol.* 48, 639- 645.

Zhao, C., B. Ge, J. Villena, R.Sudler, E. Yeh, S. Zhao, D. White, D. Wagner, and J. Meng. 2001. Prevalence of *Campylobacter* spp., *Escherichia coli*, and *Salmonella* serovars in retail chicken, turkey, pork, and beef from the greater Washington, D.C. area. *Appl. Environ Microbiol.* 67:5431-5436.

Zhao, S., S. Qaiyumi, S. Friedman, R. Singh, S. L. Foley, D. G. White, P. F. McDermott, T. Donkar, C. Bolin, S. Munro, E. J. Baron, and R. D. Walker. 2003. Characterization of Salmonella enterica serotype newport isolated from humans and food animals. *J Clin Microbiol* 41 (12):5366-5371.

Zhao S, Fedorka-Cray PJ, Friedman S, McDermott PF, Walker RD, Qaiyumi S, Foley SL, Hubert SK, Ayers S, English L, Dargatz DA, Salamone B, White DG. 2005. Characterization of Salmonella Typhimurium of animal origin obtained from the National Antimicrobial Resistance Monitoring System. Foodborne Pathog Dis. 2005 Summer;2(2):169-81.

Zhao, S., P. F. McDermott , S. Friedman, J. Abbott, S. Ayers, A. Glenn, E. Hall-Robinson, S. K. Hubert, H. Harbottle, R. D. Walker, T. M. Chiller, D. G. White. 2006. Antimicrobial resistance and genetic relatedness among *Salmonella* from retail foods of animal origin: NARMS retail meat surveillance. Foodborne Pathog. Dis. 3:106-17.

# 12

# Alternative Strategies for *Salmonella* Control in Poultry

G. Tellez, Lisa R. Bielke and B. M. Hargis
*Department of Poultry Science, University of Arkansas, Fayetteville*
*USA*

## 1. Introduction

*Salmonella enterica* serovars continue to be among the most important foodborne pathogens worldwide due to the considerable human rates of illness reported and the wide range of hosts that are colonized by members of this genus, which serve as vectors and reservoirs for spreading these agents to animal and human populations. Furthermore, public concern for the appearance of resistant strains to many antibiotics, particularly among zoonotic pathogens such as common *Salmonella* isolates, is also challenging the poultry industry to find alternative means of control (Boyle, Bishop, Grassl, & Finlay, 2007). For example, in January 2006 Europe implemented a complete ban on growth promoting antibiotics in animal feed (Anadon, Martinez-Larranaga, & Aranzazu Martinez, 2006). Thus, while attempting to control human foodborne pathogens poultry producers are simultaneously challenged to improve production in the face of increasing feed costs while using fewer antibiotics due to increased restriction of antimicrobial usage. These regulations were implemented because of export market restrictions and consumer or customer preferences in local markets. For these reasons continued research on sustainable alternatives to antibiotic growth promoters for animal production such as probiotics or direct fed microbials (DFM) consisting of live or dead organisms and spores (Patterson & Burkholder, 2003), non-traditional chemicals (Ko, Mendoncam, Ismail, & Ahn, 2009), bacteriophages (Andreatti Filho et al., 2007; Bielke, Higgins, Donoghue, Donoghue, & Hargis, 2007; J. P. Higgins et al., 2005; J. P. Higgins, Andreatti Filho et al., 2008), organic acids and other plant extracts and essential oils (Aengwanich & Suttajit, 2010; Allen-Hall, Arnason, Cano, & Lafrenie, 2010; Bagchi et al., 2000; Kubena, Byrd, Young, & Corrier, 2001; Over, Hettiarachchy, Johnson, & Davis, 2009; Van Immerseel et al., 2006), and vaccines (Kremer et al., 2011; O'Meara et al., 2010; Wolfenden et al., 2010; Van Immerseel et al., 2005; Dueger et al., 2001, 2003) are increasingly more important. These potential solutions have emerged in the last decade as tools that could be potentially useful in the near future for pathogen control and poultry performance improvement.

Probiosis, although not a new concept, has only recently begun to receive an increasing level of scientific interest. In agriculture, probiotics and DFMs used in animal feed are becoming accepted as potential alternatives to antibiotics for use as growth promoters, and in select cases, for control of specific enteric pathogens (Anadón, Rosa Martínez-Larrañaga, & Aranzazu Martínez, 2006; Boyle et al., 2007; Cartman, La Ragione, & Woodward, 2008; Vila et al., 2009; L. D. Williams, Burdock, Jimenez, & Castillo, 2009). For these reasons the development of new and more effective probiotic products that can be licensed for animal use continues to receive considerable interest (Hong, Duc le, & Cutting, 2005; Hong, Huang, Khaneja, Hiep, Urdaci, & Cutting, 2008a; Jadamus, Vahjen, & Simon, 2001; Osipova, Makhailova, Sorokulova, Vasil'eva, & Gaiderov, 2003; P. Williams, 2007b; Wolken, Tramper, & van der Werf, 2003).

Currently, there is no universal class of probiotic bacterium. However, the most common types that have been indisputably effective involve LAB. These bacteria are found normally in the gastrointestinal tract (GIT) of vertebrates and invertebrates, and the use of some LAB cultures are able to restore the natural microflora within the gut (Shahani & Ayebo, 1980). Lactic acid bacteria include the genera *Lactobacillus*, *Pediococcus*, and others that have long been associated with health benefits and which have been used for fermentation of certain foods. While speciation of members of these genera is difficult and inconsistent, these organisms are considered uniformly safe and are not associated with disease in healthy animals or humans (Tellez et al., 2006).

A second classification of probiotic cultures are those microorganisms that are not normally found in the GIT (such as allochthonous flora). For example, *Saccharomyces boulardii*, a strain of yeast found on some tropical fruits, has been shown to be effective in preventing the recurrence of *Clostridium difficile* infections (Czerucka, Piche, & Rampal, 2007) and some colibacillosis in humans (Czerucka& Rampal, 2002). Otherallochthonous probiotic microbes are the spore-forming bacteria, normally members of the genus *Bacillus*.

## 2. Lactic acid bacteria-based probiotic for *Salmonella* control and performance in poultry

The selection of individual enteric bacteria capable of inhibiting *Salmonella* growth *in vitro* and the ability of selected oxygen-tolerant bacteria to also protect neonatal poults and broilers from *Salmonella* infection following challenge has been a goal of multiple research laboratories (Menconi et al., 2011; Vicente et al., 2008; Bielke et al., 2003; Hollister et al., 1999; Corrier et al., 1998; Hume et al., 1998). Tellez and co-workers (2006) evaluated a simple method to select for individual enteric bacteria capable of inhibiting *Salmonella* growth *in vitro* and the ability of selected oxygen tolerant bacteria, in combination, to protect neonatal poults from *Salmonella* infection following challenge. Concurrently, they also worked toward the isolation, selection, further evaluation and combination of LAB to control additional foodborne pathogens. Extensive laboratory and field research conducted with this defined LAB culture has demonstrated accelerated development of normal microflora in chickens and turkeys, providing increased resistance to *Salmonella spp.* infections (Farnell et al., 2006; J. P. Higgins et al., 2007; J. P. Higgins et al., 2008; J. P. Higgins et al., 2010; S. E. Higgins et al., 2008; Vicente et al., 2008). Published experimental and commercial studies have shown that these selected probiotic organisms are able to reduce idiopathic diarrhea in commercial turkey brooding houses (S. E. Higgins et al., 2005). Large scale commercial trials indicated that appropriate administration of this probiotic mixture to turkeys and chickens increased performance and reduced costs of production (Torres-Rodriguez et al., 2007a; Torres-Rodriguez et al., 2007b; Vicente et al., 2007a; Vicente et al., 2007b; Vicente et al., 2007c).

These data have clearly demonstrated that selection of therapeutically efficacious probiotic cultures with marked performance benefits in poultry is possible, and that defined cultures can sometimes provide an attractive alternative to conventional antimicrobial therapy (seehttp://www.pacificvetgroup.com/ for more information).

## 3. Mechanism of action of probiotics against *Salmonella*

Probiotics are defined as live microorganisms that, when administered in adequate amounts, confer a health benefit on the host. Amongst the many benefits associated with the consumption of probiotics, modulation of the immune system has received considerable attention (Borchers, Keen, & Gershwin, 2002; Borchers, Selmi, Meyers, Keen, & Gershwin, 2009).

Previously, it was thought that administration of bacteria such as probiotics to neonates directly reduced infection by pathogens due to competition amongst the bacteria for attachment sites and nutrients and, that beneficial bacteria would out-compete pathogens within the GIT. This competition, coined as "competitive exclusion" was first described in 1973 by Nurmi and Rantala (Nurmi& Rantala, 1973). Their data indicated that early administration of beneficial bacteria to chicks prevented infection by pathogens. Since Nurmi and Rantala proposed competitive exclusion could be used as a method to prevent *Salmonella* infection, numerous researchers have reported the ability of live bacterial cultures to also reduce colonization of opportunistic microorganisms in the gastrointestinal tract (Callaway et al., 2008; Wagner et al., 2003; Hollister et al., 1999; Corrier et al., 1998; Hume et al., 1998; Nisbet et al., 1998) and probiotic organisms (J. P. Higgins et al., 2010; S. E. Higgins et al., 2008; Vicente et al., 2008; J. P. Higgins et al., 2007; Bielke et al., 2003; Patterson & Burkholder, 2003). Yet, understanding of how probiotics mediate these health benefits, specifically reduction of *Salmonella* infection, is very limited.

Balanced gastrointestinal microflora and immune-stimulation are major functional effects attributed to the consumption of probiotics (Amit-Romach, Uni, & Reifen, 2010; Boirivant & Strober, 2007; Boirivant, Amendola, & Butera, 2008; Flint, O'Toole, & Walker, 2010; Flore, Francois, & Felicite, 2010; Ibrahim et al., 2010; Klein, Sanders, Duong, & Young, 2010; Nayak, 2010). Many probiotic effects are mediated through immune regulation, particularly through balance control of pro-inflammatory and anti-inflammatory cytokines (Di Giacinto, Marinaro, Sanchez, Strober, & Boirivant, 2005; Foligne et al., 2010; Hacini-Rachinel et al., 2009; Jobin, 2010; Li, Xia, & Li, 2009). However, several animal and human studies have provided unequivocal evidence that specific strains of probiotics are able to stimulate multiple aspects of innate immunity (Amit-Romach et al., 2010; Boirivant & Strober, 2007; Boirivant et al., 2008; Farnell et al., 2006; Romanin et al., 2010; Weiss et al., 2010) as well as to increase humoral immunity (Fang, Elina, Heikki, & Seppo, 2000; Galdeano, de Leblanc Ade, Carmuega, Weill, & Perdigon, 2009; Leblanc, Fliss, & Matar, 2004; Nermes, Kantele, Atosuo, Salminen, & Isolauri, 2011).

Using a *Salmonella* challenge model, an effective LAB probiotic, administered 2 hours after *Salmonella* challenge, had no effect during the first 12 hours on increasing cecal colonization by this pathogen, although marked and rapid decreases were observed between 12 and 24 hours post-challenge (J. P. Higgins et al., 2007; J. P. Higgins et al., 2010). Later, using the same model and microarray analysis of gut mRNA expression, gene expression differences in birds treated with a *Lactobacillus*-based probiotic were compared to saline treated birds. At 12h post-probiotic treatment, 170 genes were significantly different ($P<0.05$), but by 24h post treatment, the number of differentially regulated genes were 201. Pathway analysis revealed that at both time points, genes associated with the NFκB complex were significantly regulated, as well as genes involved in apoptosis. Probiotic-induced differential regulation of the genes *GAS2* and *CYR61* may result in increased apoptosis in the ceca of chicks. Because *Salmonella* is an intracellular pathogen, it was suggested that increased apoptosis may be a mechanism by which B11 reduces *Salmonella* infection (S. E. Higgins et al., 2011).

## 4. Comparisons between genotypic 16S rRNA, MIDI, and biolog identifications of FloraMax™ lactic acid bacteria

A well-characterized LAB-based probiotic has been investigated in numerous studies (Tellez et al., 2006; Torres-Rodriguez et al., 2007a; Torres-Rodriguez et al., 2007b; Vicente et al., 2007a; Vicente et al., 2007b; Vicente et al., 2007c) and has now been commercialized (Pacific Vet Group USA Inc., Fayetteville AR 72703). Struggles with speciation of the LAB isolates during development of this product illustrate the well recognized problem for speciation of LAB. The identification techniques of choice for many facultative anaerobes are biochemical analyses, but the standard identification system for lactic acid bacteria is cellular fatty acid profiling. Nevertheless, these phenotypic methods can yield variable results. Genotypic methods that rely on comparisons of 16S rRNA sequences from unknown bacteria are proving to be valuable for use in a wide range of genera and are not sensitive to variable culture conditions. Genotypic 16S rRNA identification of organisms from probiotic cultures may be more consistent than the current standard microbial techniques applied separately to different microbial groups. However, this approach comes with its own limitations and issues. As identification is based on specific sequence homology as compared with a known database of microflora previously identified through conventional methodologies, the speciation is dependent upon the closest match with what was previously identified, correctly or incorrectly, in the database. As databases constantly expand and change, the same sequence submission over time may match other names with greater homology. Thus, at this moment, it is nearly impossible to really know the speciation of LAB except under specific examples with very highly characterized isolates. In fact, 16S rRNA sequencing of isolates from internationally-known name brands of commercially-produced yogurt with live cultures has consistently resulted in database matches with LAB species that are labeled as other species on the yogurt labels (unpublished). Thus, while 16s RNA sequencing can positively identify one LAB isolate as unique among several, true accuracy of homology comparisons is a somewhat subjective exercise.

Even though there are many new experimental molecular identification techniques, such as microarray hybridization, sequence analysis of 16S rRNA is the predominant molecular technology presently available for microbial identification of these commensal microorganisms (Wagner et al., 2003), even with the known problem of database accuracy and consistency over time. The detailed information needed to identify each species represented in a commercial probiotic product can only be fully obtained from the 16S rRNA at the level of the nucleotide sequence. As an example, an identification scheme was designed using the MIDI System ID from two different private laboratories (Micro Test Lab Inc., Agawam, MA 01001, USA; and Microbial ID Inc., Newark, DE 19713, USA) the Biolog ID System (Biolog, Inc., Hayward, CA 94545, USA) and compared those results with the 16S rRNA Sequence Analyses (Microbial ID Inc., Newark, DE 19713, USA) for identification of the individual component bacteria present in the commercial probiotic FloraMax™ (Table 1). The results of that study showed that the complex populations of bacteria present in FloraMax™ are not easy to accurately identify, especially with phenotypic techniques. Conventional technologies can detect human pathogens, because they are well-established in comparative databases, but emerging and opportunistic pathogens are not. Despite the fact that uncertainty exists between different methods of identification of non-pathogenic probiotic bacteria, identification of known pathogens is much more consistent. Therefore, the use of fully defined cultures for competitive exclusion or probiotic use are still inherently safer than undefined cultures or those where organisms are identified after the culture has been produced.

| LAB ID | 16S RNA Sequencing (FIRST 500 bp) Microbial ID Inc. | Midi system ID Micro Test Lab Inc. | Midi system ID Microbial ID Inc. | Biolog ID Dept. of Poultry Sc. U. of Arkansas |
|---|---|---|---|---|
| 18 | *Pediococcus parvulus* | *Enterococcus cecorum* | *Lactobacillus gasseri* | *Unable to identify* |
| 24 | *Weissella confusa* | *Lactobacillus casei* | *Lactobacillus casei* | *Clostridium clostridiiforme* |
| 27 | *Weissella confusa* | *Lactobacillus casei* | *Lactobacillus casei* | *Weissella confusa* |
| 29 | *Pediococcus parvulus* | *Lactobacillus delbreuckii-bulgaricus* | *Lactobacillus delbreuckii-bulgaricus* | *Lactobacillus hamsteri* |
| 36 | *Lactobacillus salivaruis* | *Lactobacillus cellobiosus* | *Lactobacillus casei* | *Weissella confusa* |
| 37B | *Weissella confusa* | *Pediococcus acidilactici* | *Pediococcus ruminis* | *Unable to identify* |
| 40 | *Weissella confusa* | *Lactobacillus casei* | *Lactobacillus cellobiosus* | *Weissella paramesenteroides* |
| 44 | *Weissella paramesenteroides* | *Lactobacillus fermentum* | *Lactobacillus fermentum* | *Unable to identify* |
| 46 | *Lactobacillus salivaruis* | *Lactobacillus helveticus* | *Lactobacillus sanfranciscensis* | *Lactobacillus salivaruis* |
| 48 | *Lactobacillus salivarius* | *Lactobacillus helveticus* | *Lactobacillus gasseri* | *Lactobacillus salivarius* |
| 52 | *Pediococcus parvulus* | *Unable to identify* | *Lactobacillus cellobiosus* | *Unable to identify* |

Table 1. Comparisons between MicroSeq , MIDI, and Biolog identifications of FloraMax™ lactic acid bacteria[1]

## 5. *Bacillus* spore-based probiotic for *Salmonella* control and performance enhancement in poultry

In spite of the success showed by the development of the LAB probiotic for use in commercial poultry as described above, there is still an urgent need for commercial probiotics that are shelf-stable, cost-effective and feed-stable (tolerance to heat pelletization process) to increase compliance and widespread utilization. Among the large number of probiotic products in use today some are bacterial spore formers, mostly of the genus

[1]Adapted from Tellez et al., 2006

*Bacillus*. Used primarily in their spore form, some (though not all) have been shown to prevent selected gastrointestinal disorders and the diversity of species used and their applications are astonishing. While not all *Bacillus* spores are highly heat tolerant, some specific isolates are the toughest life form known on earth (Vreeland, Rosenzweig, & Powers, 2000) and can be used under extreme heat conditions. Several studies have shown that either live vegetative cells or endospores of some isolates can prevent colon carcinogenesis (Parket al., 2007) or discharge antimicrobial substances against Gram-positive bacteria, such as *Staphylococcus aureus*, *Enterococcus faecium*, and *Clostridium difficile* (O'Mahony et al., 2001). These results provided evidence of colonization and antimicrobial activity of probiotic bacteria, thus, products containing *Bacillus* spores are used commercially as probiotics, and they offer potential advantages over the more common LAB products since they can be used as direct feed microbials (Anadón et al., 2006; Barbosa et al., 2005; Duc le et al., 2004; Hong et al., 2005; Hong et al., 2008a; Hong et al., 2008b; McNulty et al., 2007; Osipova et al., 2003; P. Williams, 2007a; Wolken et al., 2003). There is scientific evidence suggesting that some but not all isolates of ingested *B. subtilis* spores can, in fact, germinate in the small intestine (Casula & Cutting, 2002; Casula & Cutting, 2002; Duc le & Cutting, 2003; Hoa et al., 2001). Together, these studies not only show that spores are not transient passengers in the gut, but they have an intimate interaction with the host cells or microflora that can enhance their potential probiotic effect. Several commercial spore-forming *Bacillus* cultures have been shown to reduce food borne pathogens (Aureli et al., 2010). However, cost issues associated with achieving necessary concentrations of spores in feed have greatly limited commercial acceptance in the animal industry (Hong et al., 2005).

While the majority of clear-cut research with regard to beneficial probiotic cultures has focused on LAB, as discussed above, a major question in several laboratories is whether or not selected spore-former bacteria (genus *Bacillus* or related) can be as effective as the best known LAB cultures. Recently, one *Bacillus subtilis* spore isolate was as effective as a well-established LAB-based probiotic for *Salmonella* reduction in poultry (Wolfenden R.E. et al., 2010; Shivaramaiah et al., 2011), and was equal to bacitracin for prevention of experimental necrotic enteritis, and was able to markedly reduce necrotic enteritis issues in large scale feed trials (unpublished from the author's laboratory).

Other isolates or combinations of isolates with increased potency and efficacy may be identified with continued research. Some of these environmental *Bacillus* isolates have been evaluated *in vitro* for antimicrobial activity against selected bacterial pathogens, heat stability, and the ability to grow to high numbers. Unpublished experimental evaluations have confirmed improved body weight gain as well as *Salmonella sp.* or *Clostridium perfringens* reduction in commercial turkey and broiler operations when compared with medicated (nitarsone) or control nonmedicated diets respectively. Indeed, preliminary data suggests that these isolates could be an effective alternative to antibiotic growth promoters for commercial poultry.

Importantly, improved efficiency of amplification and sporulation is absolutely essential to gain widespread industry acceptance of a feed-based probiotic for ante mortem foodborne pathogen intervention, as well as cost effectiveness. Recently, both vegetative growth and sporulation rates have been optimized, which may lead to new efficiencies for commercial amplification and manufacture of a cost-effective product at very high spore counts (Wolfenden R.E. et al., 2010). In order to select even more effective isolates, current research is focused on the mechanistic action of new *Bacillus* candidates. Preliminary studies indicate a potential mechanistic action of these new *Bacillus* candidates at least partially involve rapid activation of innate host immune mechanisms (system or responses) in chickens and turkeys (unpublished data). This data provides an exciting possibility for identification of vastly superior and more potent probiotics in the near future.

## 6. Prospects of bacteriophage therapy to control gastrointestinal disease

### 6.1 Overview

During the last approximately 60 years, there have been sporadic published reports of efficacy in treating Enterobacteriaceae infections systemically and within the gastrointestinal tract. While a number of reports have rather consistently indicated that systemic or tissue-associated infections were treatable by parenteral administration of appropriate bacteriophage cocktails, reports of successful treatment of enteric Enterobacteriaceae are much more sporadic, and are interspersed with a number of reports of failed attempts for enteric treatment. The following sections will discuss selected successes and failures and describe the possible differences in these studies and the potential for development of more effective strategies.

### 6.2 Successes

The bacteriocidal effects of bacteriophages have long been studied for their usefulness in treating gastrointestinal infections. Early studies originating from the former Soviet Union, Eastern Europe, and Eastern Asia suggested bacteriophages could prevent and treat *Vibrio cholera* infections (Dubos et al, 1943; Dutta, 1963; Sayamov, 1963; and Marčuk et al, 1971). In the 1980s Slopek and co-workers (1983a-b, 1984, 1985a-c, 1987) published numerous papers showing the promising results of treating septic patients with bacteriophages. While the validity of these studies has been questioned, in part due to relaxed scientific rigor in these regions during the time when these studies were completed (Merril et al, 2003; Alisky et al, 1998) and are not often cited by bacteriophage researchers in recent years, they have served as an inspiration for continued research into the possibility that bacteriophages can cure gastrointestinal diseases in humans and animals.

Smith and Huggins (1982) compared the efficacy of phages with that of antibiotics in treating both generalized and cerebral infections in mice. They isolated anti-K1 bacteriophages that were able to lyse K1-positive *E. coli*. These bacteriophages were able to cure infection caused by K1-positive, even when used at a low titer. The bacteriophages were more effective than several antibiotics for curing mice. Smith and Huggins (1983) also successfully used bacteriophage therapy to treat calves, pigs, and lambs that had been infected with *E. coli*. Perhaps key to their success, they selected a bacteriophage that would lyse *E. coli* and also selected a second bacteriophage that would lyse the target *E. coli* that had become resistant to the first bacteriophage. In 1987, Smith and Huggins used bacteriophages to treat calves with *E. coli*-caused diarrhea. They selected their bacteriophages by administering *E. coli* to a calf followed by a bacteriophage cocktail. Bacteriophages able to survive the gastrointestinal tract were collected in the feces 24 hours post-administration. These bacteriophages were used to treat subsequent calves. Calves given bacteriophages within 24 hours of the onset of diarrhea recovered within 20 hours. Also, sick calves placed on litter that had been sprayed with bacteriophages recovered from diarrhea. Smith and Huggins noted that during the period of disease, bacteriophages continued to persist in the feces, but after recovery, bacteriophage numbers dropped dramatically.

Biswas et al. (2002) successfully cured *Enterococcus faecium*-infected mice with bacteriophage therapy. Mice were treated with bacteriophages just 45 minutes after infection with bacteria. Treatment at a multiplicity of infection (MOI) level of 0.3 to 3.0 was able to cure all of the infected mice. However, lower MOIs of 0.03 to 0.003 resulted in just 60% and 40% survival of mice, respectively. They also noted that bacteriophage treatment could be delayed for up to five hours after infection. However, if treatment was delayed for 18 or 24 hours, only 50% recovery was seen.

Berchieri et al. (1991) treated broiler chickens infected with *Salmonella typhimurium* (ST) with bacteriophages and found that the levels of ST could be reduced by several logs, and mortality associated with ST was reduced significantly. However, ST was not eliminated and it returned to its original levels within six hours of treatment. Also, the bacteriophages did not persist in the gastrointestinal tract for as long as the *Salmonella* was present. In fact, bacteriophages persisted only as long as they were added to the feed. In order to be effective, bacteriophages had to be administered in large numbers, and soon after infection with ST.

In 1998 Barrow et al. prevented morbidity and mortality in chickens using bacteriophages lytic for *E. coli*. When chickens were challenged intramuscularly with *E. coli* and simultaneously treated with $10^6$ - $10^8$ pfu of bacteriophages the mortality was reduced by 100%. This study also demonstrated that bacteriophages can cross the blood brain barrier, and furthermore that they can amplify in both the brain and the blood. Similarly, a number of other researchers have shown that bacteriophages can be useful for treating non-enteric *E. coli* infections. Extensive research about the effects of bacteriophages on colibacillosis in broiler chickens has shown that bacteriophages can treat respiratory infections (Huff et al, 2002a-b; Huff et al, 2003a-b). Treatment was most successful when bacteriophages were directly applied to the infected area or injected into the bloodstream. This observation is consistent with previous research discussed above.

However, such successes do not necessarily translate into effective enteric treatments. Host-associated pressure against pathogen infections may predispose systemic bacteriophage therapy toward success. In these cases, where bacteriophage(s) are used to treat systemic or tissue-associated infections, an acute efficacy of merely reducing the infection load by 90% or more, could greatly reduce mortality and reduce the duration and magnitude of disease. In the intestinal lumen, host pressures against the infection may not be as severe and many Enterobacteriaceae are capable of free living status within the gut without eliciting robust acquired immune responses from the infected animal. In these cases, a temporary reduction in enteric colonization may not be as likely to be curative, as discussed below.

### 6.3 Failures

As the history of published successful bacteriophage treatments of enteric disease is reviewed, it is readily evident that such reports, while often dramatic in effect, are relatively sporadic during the last approximately 60 years. Given that experimental failures frequently are not published, as the cause of failure can often not be ascertained, the authors suspect that history is replete with unpublished examples of failures to treat enteric Enterobacteriaceae infections.

Our laboratory, and others, have demonstrated that resistance to bacteriophages selected against *Salmonella* isolates quickly occurs, often in a single passage (Bastias et al, 2010). When bacteriophage cocktails of 71 different bacteriophages selected for treatment of experimental *Salmonella enteritidis* infections in chickens, a brief reduction in enteric colonization was noted during the first 24 hours, but rebound levels were similar to controls within 48 hours, even with repeated or continuous dosage of the bacteriophage cocktail (Higgins et al, 2007). Because of the demonstrated temporary reduction in enteric colonization in these studies, effective bacteriophages were demonstrably able to pass to the lower gastrointestinal tract. As continued treatments failed to maintain this reduction, development of resistance by the enteric *Salmonella enteritidis* is the most likely explanation.

In order to potentially deliver higher levels of bacteriophage, several attempts to protect the bacteriophage cocktail through the upper gastrointestinal tract were made in our laboratory. Pre-treatment of infected poultry with antacid preparations designed to reduce the acidity of the proventriculus (true stomach) were successful in increasing the number of administered bacteriophage that successfully passed into the intestinal tract, but this treatment did not improve the outcome of bacteriophage treatment of *Salmonella enteritidis* infection (Higgins et al, 2007).

An alternative approach is to select for alternative non-pathogenic bacteriophage hosts which could potentially "carry" bacteriophage through the gastrointestinal tract and, with continuous dietary administration of the non-infected alternative host bacterium, provide a means of amplification within the gut of the host (Bielke et al., 2007a). Bielke and co-workers demonstrated that non-pathogenic alternative hosts can be selected for some bacteriophages that were originally isolated using a *Salmonella enteritidis* target (2007b). This approach, which has potential utility for amplification of large numbers of phage without the necessity to thoroughly separate bacteriophage from a pathogenic target host, was also used to create a potential "Trojan Horse" model for protecting the bacteriophages through the upper gastrointestinal tract, thus potentially providing a vehicle for enteric amplification of those surviving bacteriophages. In these studies, neither the Trojan Horse approach, nor the continuous feeding of the alternative host bacteria as a source of enteric amplification, were effective in producing even more than a transient reduction in enteric *Salmonella* infections.

Through these failures, many investigators have concluded that the escape of even a minority of target bacteria within the enteric ecosystem allows for almost immediate selection of resistant target bacteria and rebound to pre-treatment levels of infection may even exceed the levels of non-treated controls in some cases.

### 6.4 Potential strategies to overcome failures

Bacteriophage resistance is an important component of therapy to overcome before bacteriophages can really be a viable antimicrobial for infection. The generation time for bacteria is typically short enough that mutants with bacteriophage resistance can emerge within hours (Higgins et al, 2007; Lowbury and Hood, 1953). One possibly strategy to overcome this problem is administration of multiple bacteriophage isolates for treatment, but resistance is difficult, if not impossible, to predict and combining the correct cocktail of bacteriophages to overcome resistance would be a blind guess in most cases.

The most success is likely to come from treating points in the system that are continually bombarded with bacteria that have not been previously subjected to the bacteriophages being used for treatment. Also important for this system is keeping exposure of the bacteria to bacteriophages to a minimal amount of time. If the bacteriophages interact with the bacteria for long periods of time, the bacteria will become resistant. Food and meat processing facilities are an excellent example. As live animals enter a processing facility, the bacteria have not likely been exposed to the bacteriophages used to treat the infection. This greatly increases the chances of success.

Higgins and co-workers (2005) successfully treated turkey carcasses at a processing facility with bacteriophages specific to the *Salmonella* to which they were infected. This process was effective when either an autogenous bacteriophage treatment targeted to the specific *Salmonella* strain infecting the turkeys was used, or a cocktail of nine wide host-range *Salmonella*-targeting bacteriophage were used. Similarly, a bacteriophage treatment for cattle carcass contamination has been effective at reducing the *E. coli* 0157:H7 load at processing has been developed and commercially licensed in the United States. These successes avoid development of bacteriophage resistance by applying treatment at a single point during production, in an environment where proliferation of the target organism is extremely limited. In this way, since the target organism is never intentionally exposed twice to the same treatment, resistance is unlikely to ever increase beyond the naturally-occurring resistance to the bacteriophage (or cocktail) used.

One of the most well documented successes of published treatment of enteric Enterobacteriaceae infections with bacteriophages was the study of Smith and Huggins (1983) as described above. It is notable that in this successful study, the bacteriophage cocktail used was a combination of two bacteriophages, but the second was isolated using the target organism which was resistant to the first bacteriophage. This approach of selecting for bacteriophage isolates using target bacteria that are resistant to sequential bacteriophage treatments was not used in the work of Higgins et al (2007), or in several other published studies. Higgins and co-workers (2007) used a collection bacteriophages, independently isolated from different sources and with several different plaque morphologies, suggesting that a number of different bacteriophages were employed - and failed to persistently reduce enteric colonization.

It is possible that one of the most notable exceptions to the many failures to treat enteric Enterobacteraceae infections during recent years, that of Smith and Huggins (1983), provides a singular clue as to the potential for enhancing the likelihood of enteric Enterobacteriaceae efficacy. It is possible that selection of multiple bacteriophages for the same target cell phenotype results in selection of bacteriophages that are effective through identical mechanisms of adhesion, penetration, replication, and release. When new bacteriophages are isolated for efficacy against sequentially resistant isolates of the target bacteria, and these are combined for administration as a cocktail, the ability of the target cell to shift phenotype may be severely limited, resulting in a much larger proportion of target cell reduction, thereby increasing the probability of elimination or cure.

Clearly, widespread bacteriophage treatments with Enterobacteriaceae have not been adopted for any animal species during the last 60 years and successful research in this area has been modest and sporadic. Nevertheless, the occasional reports by reputable scientists in solid journals must indicate that there is potential for improved therapeutic efficacy of bacteriophages for this purpose. With the diminution of new antimicrobial pharmaceuticals and the widespread resistance among many pathogenic enteric Enterobacteriaceaes, a breakthrough in this area is sorely needed.

## 7. Vaccination for control of *Salmonella* in poultry

Killed whole-cell bacterins and live attenuated vaccines are the most common types of vaccines currently used in the poultry industry. Vaccination programs depend on the recognition of specific antigens, called epitopes, by the immune system of the host to prevent or reduce the spread of pathogenic viruses and bacteria. Because there are a large number of *Salmonella* serovars, each with individual epitopes that do not elicit cross-protection against other serovars, there has been little traditional emphasis on development of generic *Salmonella* vaccines. Primarily, killed vaccines, which generally must be administered parenterally (through injection), have been applied to protect against systemic infections, and although they have been shown to reduce colonization and shedding, the protection provided by these vaccines has limited ability to stop intestinal colonization. They predominantly stimulate both humoral (circulating IgM and IgG) and cell-mediated responses, but are quite ineffective at generating mucosal immunity as secretory IgA antibody stimulation is very low through this type of vaccination. This is important because, whereas both systemic (humoral and cell-mediated) and mucosal immunity can reduce the chances of disease and mortality, only the mucosal portion of this adaptive immune response is capable of protecting animals from infection. The key to inducing both an adaptive systemic and mucosal response has traditionally been through the use of the mucosa as a "portal of entry" for live but weakened (attenuated) vaccines. However, the use of such vaccines for protection against *Salmonella* infection have been tremendously limited due to the very large number of different antigens presented by the more than 200 serotypes that can infect domestic animals and man, with more than 38 of these commonly infecting poultry within the United States, as discussed below (Hargis et al., 2010).

One approach to solving the problem of serotype variation among the common paratyphoid strains of *Salmonella*, which are often not a disease-causing problem for poultry but rather create a source of foodborne illness for consumers, is the identification of "universal epitopes" that are shared among all *Salmonella* isolates. This concept has been established for a number of pathogens and is based on the identification of a minor surface structure (antigen or epitope) which does not cause robust immune reaction during infection, but which can be targeted for protection if the antigen is presented in a way that tricks the animal into responding robustly. Some of these are relatively minor antigens which are highly conserved among related organisms - usually because they involve biological function. Since small peptide sequences that are biologically functional cannot vary in sequence, organisms that carry a mutation for such sequences are often either lethal or sufficiently detrimental to cause these to not be successful over time (Neirynck et al., 1999).

A well-described example of this phenomenon is a small 23 amino acid peptide on the surface of Type A Influenza viruses named M2e. This peptide is part of an ion transport channel which is necessary for viral activation. Mutations in this sequence undoubtedly occur frequently, but since the 1918 Spanish Influenza outbreak, all Type A Influenza isolates share a highly conserved core sequence for this peptide (Layton et al., 2009). Although natural influenza infection does not result in a robust immune response to this peptide sequence, tricking the animal into producing a robust response has resulted in protective immunity in several animal species (Neirynck et al., 1999; Mozdzanowska et al., 2003; Fiers et al., 2004; Zou et al., 2004). In recent years, the rapid increase in molecular biological techniques has led to the development of more sophisticated vaccines, of which live recombinant bacterial vectored vaccines are one of the most promising (Ashby et al., 2005; Zhang et al., 2006; Duc et al., 2007; Kajikawa et al., 2007; Uyen et al., 2007; Yang et al., 2007; Huang et al., 2008; Liu et al., 2008; Ceragioli et al., 2009; Deguchi et al., 2009).

This type of vaccine uses a genetically modified bacterium to express a heterologous antigen. Oral live attenuated *Salmonella* vaccine vectors expressing recombinant foreign antigens have previously been shown to stimulate systemic, mucosal, humoral, and cell-mediated immune responses against *Salmonella* (Mollenkopf et al., 2001; Koton and

Hohmann, 2004; Ashby et al., 2005). *Salmonella* vectors have the potential advantage of being extremely inexpensive to manufacture and, because they do not have to be injected and can be administered by spray or drinking water, they are much more acceptable for widespread administration to commercial poultry.

Currently, some laboratories are exploiting this concept by identifying candidate antigens/epitopes that are evolutionarily conserved between the many different serotypes of *Salmonella* and which do not elicit a robust response when animals are infected with wild type *Salmonella* (or vaccinated with conventional vaccines), but which may protect against infection when delivered in an appropriate way using a recombinant vaccine platform (Wolfenden, RE et al., 2010; Kremer et al., 2011). Recently, bacterial carriers of antigens (vectors), including *Salmonella* Enteritidis and *Bacillus subtilis*, have been manipulated to express protein antigens to protect against bacterial, viral, and protozoal pathogens (Layton et al., 2009; O'Meara et al., 2010; Kremer et al., 2011; Layton et al., 2011). These vaccines have an advantage over many other types of vaccines in that they are able to be delivered directly to a mucosal surface via nasal, ocular, or oral administration. Because most pathogens invade the host through a mucosal surface, an enhanced mucosal immune response is the only portion of acquired immunity that can markedly reduce the probability of an animal or flock to become infected, as discussed above. While prevention of morbidity and mortality alone are useful traits of conventional vaccines for most poultry disease-causing agents, in the case of the common *Salmonella* serotypes which cause foodborne illness, these isolates generally cause little or no disease in the animals. Thus, recombinant vaccines that are able to provide wide-range protection against common *Salmonella* serotypes of poultry, by mucosal presentation, may be a critical component for controlling this problem in the next few years.

Along with presentation of conserved antigens through mucosally-administered recombinant vaccines, there is a need to trick the immune system of the animal to respond robustly to these recombinant bacteria that are not capable of infecting or causing disease. Co-expression of molecules that may enhance the immune response or may be recognized by receptors located on the mucosal surface of the gastrointestinal tract is a promising area of work. Several such molecules may enhance the response to these recombinant vaccines (Layton et al., 2009; O'Meara et al., 2010; Wolfenden et al., 2010).

Presently, there are no broad-spectrum recombinant vaccines approved for use in agricultural animals to protect against the wide range of serotypes which plague poultry producers worldwide. Specific serotype vaccines, such as *S.* Enteritidis or *S.* Gallinarum, have gained considerable acceptance in countries with endemic problems with these more devastating serovars, particularly in breeders and table egg production chickens (see Shivaprasad, 1997, for a review). These vaccines generally do not provide robust protection against infection with even the identical serotype, and even less protection against heterologous serotypes (Hargis et al., 2010). However, there is a general consensus that some protection is provided and for valuable birds, these vaccines may offer a much-needed modicum of protection, though often through reduced persistence and shedding of the organism, thus limiting spread. For example, studies have shown that oil emulsion *Salmonella* Enteritidis bacterins administered to breeders caused a three $\log_{10}$ cfu/g cecal content reduction in recovery from progeny chicks (Inoue et al., 2008), and a two $\log_{10}$ cfu/g cecal content reduction in breeders after molting (Nakamura et al., 2004). Thus, these vaccines have value at the present time, especially for breeders and at-risk laying hens.

Live-type vaccines with gene deletions assuring avirulence while allowing immunogenicity have been reported (Curtiss and Kelly, 1987; Dueger et al., 2003), and other specific deletion mutants have been proposed (Zhang-Barber et al., 1999; Sydenham et al., 2000). Day-of-hatch chicks vaccinated with this type of attenuated *Salmonella* vaccine have been shown to have serological protection to homologous and heterologous *Salmonella* serotypes, possibly through a mechanism similar to competitive exclusion (Hassan and Curtiss, 1994; Hassan and Curtiss, 1997; Dueger et al., 2003; Holt et al., 2003; Bohez et al., 2008). Furthermore, maternal antibodies can be demonstrated in eggs and chicks from breeders vaccinated with this vaccine. These antibodies were reported to reduce *Salmonella*e colonization and to provide protection to laying hens up to 11 months post-inoculation (Hassan and Curtiss, 1997). However, susceptibility to antimicrobial agents commonly used in poultry production can reduce or eliminate the efficacy of live vaccines, and these vaccines are subject to the serotype limitations as discussed above.

Autogenous vaccines provide for yet another mechanism for vaccinating poultry. In many (but not all) countries, there are regulatory provisions under certain circumstances for production of specific killed vaccines using the specific isolate plaguing a given poultry flock or complex. These "autogenous" *Salmonella* isolates are typically grown, killed and mixed with an adjuvant (a chemical that potentiates the immune response) for parenteral administration. Some veterinarians associated with valuable breeder flocks believe that these vaccines are highly preferred for vaccination against endemic and common serotypes for which no commercial vaccine exists.

Taken together, there are tremendous future opportunities for manipulating the acquired immune response, particularly the mucosal secretory IgA response, for reduceing *Salmonella* infections in poultry. However, current vaccine availability is limited and progress is greatly needed on two fronts: 1) improving mucosal immune responses for *Salmonella* vaccines; and 2) targeting shared protective epitopes for broad-spectrum serotype coverage for the paratyphoid *Salmonella*e that currently plague poultry producers world-wide. Currently-available commercial vaccines are enjoying significant popularity due to the intense regulatory pressures facing meat and egg producing poultry, although applications are generally limited to breeder or layer flocks except under intense regulatory pressure.

## 8. Conclusions

The interest in digestive physiology and the role of microorganisms has generated data whereby human and animal well-being can be enhanced and the risk of disease reduced. New molecular techniques that allow an accurate assessment of the flora composition, resulting in improved strategies for elucidating mechanisms. Given the recent international legislation and domestic consumer pressures to withdraw growth-promoting antibiotics and limit antibiotics available for treatment of bacterial infections, probiotics can offer alternative options. New advances in the application of probiotics, are directed to produce significant changes in gut physiology and provide even higher levels of health as well as increase performance parameters in poultry.

Metchnikoff founded the research field of probiotics, aimed at modulating the intestinal microflora (Dobrogosz, Peacock, & Hassan, 2010; Schmalstieg & Goldman, 2010; Weissmann, 2010). However, other parts of the body containing endogenous microflora or problems relating to the immune system may also be candidates for probiotic therapy. Research has shown that probiotics have potential for human health issues such as: vaginal candidiasis (Ehrstrom et al., 2010; Ya, Reifer, & Miller, 2010); dental caries (Chen & Wang, 2010; Stamatova & Meurman, 2009); allergies (Gourbeyre, Denery, & Bodinier, 2011; Schiavi, Barletta, Butteroni,

Corinti, Boirivant, & Di Felice, 2010b); autoimmune diseases (Lavasani et al., 2010; Tlaskalova-Hogenova et al., 2011); urogenital infections (Pascual, Ruiz, Giordano, & Barberis, 2010; Ruiz et al., 2009); atopic diseases (Hoang, Shaw, Pham, & Levine, 2010; Nermes et al., 2011); rheumatoid arthritis (Lee et al., 2010; Mandel, Eichas, & Holmes, 2010); and respiratory infections (Harikrishnan, Balasundaram, & Heo, 2010; Silvestri et al., 2010). Current research is still heavily biased toward gastrointestinal applications for probiotics, such as: chronic constipation (Bu, Chang, Ni, Chen, & Cheng, 2007; Coccorullo et al., 2010); chronic diarrhea (Preidis et al., 2011; Swidsinski, Loening-Baucke, Verstraelen, Osowska, & Doerffel, 2008); inflammatory bowel disease (Ng, Chan, & Sung, 2011; Vanderpool, Yan, & Polk, 2008); irritable bowel syndrome (Camilleri & Tack, 2010; Enck, Klosterhalfen, & Martens, 2011); and food allergy (Gourbeyre et al., 2011; Schiavi, Barletta, Butteroni, Corinti, Boirivant, & Di Felice, 2010a), but the possibilities for impacting many areas of health are numerous. Much research has been completed in efforts to understand and apply the natural benefits of non-pathogenic bacteria, but there is much still to do.

New approaches to vaccination-based prophylaxis for *Salmonella* infection in poultry offer tremendous hope that highly effective vaccines may be on the horizion for commercial poultry. However, currently available and autogenous vaccines for *Salmonella* offer a modicum of protection that is generally only useful for breeders and laying hens at this time.

Although there are occasional successes with treatment of enteric *Salmonella* infections in live birds with bacteriophage cocktails, as described above, resistance to bacteriophage lysis generally develops very quickly, leading most scientist to conclude that these offer little promise for treating *Salmonella* infections in live poultry. However, when broadly-effective bacteriophage cocktails have been applied to poultry carcasses at processing, these cocktails have been highly efficacious and potentially cost-effective for inducing marked reductions in *Salmonella* contamination (Higgins et al., 2005). This latter approach has the probability of avoiding the resistance issues associated with treatment of live animals in that *Salmonella* contaminants would only be exposed to the bacteriophage cocktail at a single point in the vertical production scheme, thereby avoiding re-introduction of resistant *Salmonella* isolates into the integrated poultry production operation.

The scientific progress outlined in this chapter show highly encouraging progress toward intervention methods for *Salmonella* infections of poultry, and opportunities that are just becoming available to potentially impact poultry as a source of *Salmonella*-related food borne illness. *Salmonella* infections of poultry continue to be hugely problematic in both developed and developing countries. To date, no single "silver bullet" has been identified which can be applied commercially to eliminate this risk for this important and healthy human food source. Nevertheless, several tools, as described above, have been shown to be highly effective in reducing *Salmonella* levels in poultry production operations worldwide, particularly when used in combination. New probiotic/DFM products, with isolate selection based on better understanding of the mechanisms of efficacy, along with eventual regulatory approval and commercialization of exciting new vaccine technologies may make a tremendous impact in the very near future.

## 9. References

Aengwanich, W., & Suttajit, M. (2010). Effect of polyphenols extracted from tamarind (tamarindus indica L.) seed coat on physiological changes, heterophil/lymphocyte ratio, oxidative stress and body weight of broilers (gallus domesticus) under chronic heat stress. Animal Science Journal. 81(2), 264-270. doi:10.1111/j.1740-0929.2009.00736.x

Allen-Hall, L., Arnason, J. T., Cano, P., & Lafrenie, R. M. (2010). Uncaria tomentosa acts as a potent TNF-alpha inhibitor through NF-kappaB. Journal of Ethnopharmacology, 127(3), 685-693. doi:10.1016/j.jep.2009.12.004

Alisky, J., K. Iczkowski, A. Rapoport, and N. Troitsky, 1998. Bacteriophage show promise as antimicrobial agents.J Infect 36: 5-15

Amit-Romach, E., Uni, Z., & Reifen, R. (2010). Multistep mechanism of probiotic bacterium, the effect on innate immune system. Molecular Nutrition & Food Research, 54(2), 277-284. doi:10.1002/mnfr.200800591

Anadon, A., Martinez-Larranaga, M. R., & Aranzazu Martinez, M. (2006). Probiotics for animal nutrition in the european union. regulation and safety assessment. Regulatory Toxicology and Pharmacology: RTP, 45(1), 91-95. doi:10.1016/j.yrtph.2006.02.004

Anadón, A., Rosa Martínez-Larrañaga, M., & Aranzazu Martínez, M. (2006). Probiotics for animal nutrition in the european union regulation and safety assessment. Regulatory Toxicology and Pharmacology, 45(1), 91-95. doi:DOI: 10.1016/j.yrtph.2006.02.004

Andreatti Filho, R. L., Higgins, J. P., Higgins, S. E., Gaona, G., Wolfenden, A. D., Tellez, G., & Hargis, B. M. (2007). Ability of bacteriophages isolated from different sources to reduce Salmonella enterica serovar enteritidis in vitro and in vivo. Poultry Science, 86(9), 1904-1909.

Ashby, D., I. Leduc, W. Lauzon, B.C. Lee, N. Singhal, and D.W. Cameron, 2005. Attenuated Salmonella Typhimurium SL3261 asa vaccine vector for recombinant antigen in rabbits.J ImmunolMethods 299:153–164.

Aureli, P., Fiore, A., Scalfaro, C., Casale, M., & Franciosa, G. (2010). National survey outcomes on commercial probiotic food supplements in italy. International Journal of Food Microbiology, 137(2-3), 265-273. doi:10.1016/j.ijfoodmicro.2009.12.016

Bagchi, D., Bagchi, M., Stohs, S. J., Das, D. K., Ray, S. D., Kuszynski, C. A., Pruess, H. G. (2000). Free radicals and grape seed proanthocyanidin extract: Importance in human health and disease prevention. Toxicology, 148(2-3), 187-197.

Barbosa, T. M., Serra, C. R., La Ragione, R. M., Woodward, M. J., & Henriques, A. O. (2005). Screening for bacillus isolates in the broiler gastrointestinal tract. Applied and Environmental Microbiology, 71(2), 968-978. doi:10.1128/AEM.71.2.968-978.2005

Barrow, P., M. Lovell and A. Berchieri, Jr., 1998. Use of Lytic Bacteriophages for Control of Experimental Escherichia coli Septicemia and Meningitis in chickens and calves.ClinDiag Lab Immun 5: 294-298

Bastias, R., G. Higuera, W. Sierralta, and R.T. Espejo, 2010. A new group of cosmopolitan bacteriophages induce a carier state in the pandemic strain of Vibrio parahaemolyticus. EnivironMicrobiol 12: 990-1000

Berchieri, A., M.A. Lovell, and P.A. Barrow, 1991. The activity in the chicken alimentary tract of bacteriophages lytic for Salmonella typhimurium.Res Microbiol 142: 541-549

Bielke L.R.,Elwood A.L.,Donoghue D.J.,Donoghue A.M.,Newberry L.A.,Neighbor N.K., and Hargis BM, 2003.Approach for selection of individual enteric bacteria for competitive exclusion in turkey poults. Poultry Science 82: 1378-82.

Bielke, L., S. Higgins, A. Donoghue, D. Donoghue, and B.M. Hargis, 2007b. Salmonella host range of bacteriophages that infect multiple genera. PoultSci 86: 2536–2540

Bielke, L., Higgins, S., Donoghue, A., Donoghue, D., & Hargis, B. M. (2007). Salmonella host range of bacteriophages that infect multiple genera. Poultry Science, 86(12), 2536-2540. doi:10.3382/ps.2007-00250

Bielke, L.R., S.E. Higgins, A.M. Donoghue, T. Kral, D.J. Donoghue, B.M. Hargis, and G.I. Tellez, 2007a. Evaluation of alternative host bacteria as vehicles for oral administration of bacteriophages.Int J PoultSci 6: 758-761

Biswas, B., S. Adhya, P. Washart, B. Paul, A.N. Trostel, B. Powell, R. Carlton, and C.R. Merril, 2002. Bacteriophage therapy rescues mice bacteremic from a clinical isolate of vancomycin-resistant Enterococcus faecium. Infect Immunol 70: 204-210

Bohez, L., J. Dewulf, R. Ducatelle, F. Pasmans, F. Haesebrouk, and F. Van Immerseel, 2008. The effect or oral administration of a homologous hilA mutant strain of Salmonella enteritidis in broiler chickens.Vaccine 26: 372.

Boirivant, M., & Strober, W. (2007). The mechanism of action of probiotics. Current Opinion in Gastroenterology, 23(6), 679-692. doi:10.1097/MOG.0b013e3282f0cffc

Boirivant, M., Amendola, A., & Butera, A. (2008). Intestinal microflora and immunoregulation. Mucosal Immunology, 1 Suppl 1, S47-9. doi:10.1038/mi.2008.52

Borchers, A. T., Keen, C. L., & Gershwin, M. E. (2002). The influence of yogurt/Lactobacillus on the innate and acquired immune response. Clinical Reviews in Allergy & Immunology, 22(3), 207-230. doi:10.1007/s12016-002-0009-7

Borchers, A. T., Selmi, C., Meyers, F. J., Keen, C. L., & Gershwin, M. E. (2009). Probiotics and immunity. Journal of Gastroenterology, 44(1), 26-46. doi:10.1007/s00535-008-2296-0

Boyle, E. C., Bishop, J. L., Grassl, G. A., & Finlay, B. B. (2007). Salmonella: From pathogenesis to therapeutics. Journal of Bacteriology, 189(5), 1489-1495. doi:10.1128/JB.01730-06

Bu, L. N., Chang, M. H., Ni, Y. H., Chen, H. L., & Cheng, C. C. (2007). Lactobacillus casei rhamnosus Lcr35 in children with chronic constipation. Pediatrics International : Official Journal of the Japan Pediatric Society, 49(4), 485-490. doi:10.1111/j.1442-200X.2007.02397.x

Callaway, T. R., Edrington, T. S., Anderson, R. C., Harvey, R. B., Genovese, K. J., Kennedy, C. N., Nisbet, D. J. (2008). Probiotics, prebiotics and competitive exclusion for prophylaxis against bacterial disease. Animal Health Research Reviews / Conference of Research Workers in Animal Diseases, 9(2), 217-225. doi:10.1017/S1466252308001540

Camilleri, M., & Tack, J. F. (2010). Current medical treatments of dyspepsia and irritable bowel syndrome. Gastroenterology Clinics of North America, 39(3), 481-493. doi:10.1016/j.gtc.2010.08.005

Cartman, S. T., La Ragione, R. M., & Woodward, M. J. (2008). Bacillus subtilis spores germinate in the chicken gastrointestinal tract. Applied and Environmental Microbiology, 74(16), 5254-5258. doi:10.1128/AEM.00580-08

Casula, G., & Cutting, S. M. (2002). Bacillus probiotics: Spore germination in the gastrointestinal tract. Applied and Environmental Microbiology, 68(5), 2344-2352.

Ceragioli, M., G. Cangiano, S. Esin, E. Ghelardi, E. Ricca, and S. Senesi, 2009. Phagocytosis, germination and killing of Bacillussubtilisspores presenting heterologous antigens in human macrophages.Microbiology 155:338–346.

Chen, F., & Wang, D. (2010). Novel technologies for the prevention and treatment of dental caries: A patent survey. Expert Opinion on Therapeutic Patents, 20(5), 681-694. doi:10.1517/13543771003720491

Coccorullo, P., Strisciuglio, C., Martinelli, M., Miele, E., Greco, L., & Staiano, A. (2010). Lactobacillus reuteri (DSM 17938) in infants with functional chronic constipation: A double-blind, randomized, placebo-controlled study. The Journal of Pediatrics, 157(4), 598-602. doi:10.1016/j.jpeds.2010.04.066

Corrier, D. E., Nisbet, D. J., Byrd, J. A., 2nd, Hargis, B. M., Keith, N. K., Peterson, M., & Deloach, J. R. (1998). Dosage titration of a characterized competitive exclusion culture to inhibit Salmonella colonization in broiler chickens during growout. Journal of Food Protection, 61(7), 796-801.

Curtiss, R.S. and M. Kelly, 1987. Salmonella typhimurium deletion mutants lacking adenylatecyclase and cyclic AMP receptor protein are avirulent and immunogenic. Infect Immun 55: 3035.

Czerucka, D., & Rampal, P. (2002). Experimental effects of saccharomyces boulardii on diarrheal pathogens. Microbes and Infection / Institut Pasteur, 4(7), 733-739.

Czerucka, D., Piche, T., & Rampal, P. (2007). Review article: Yeast as probiotics -- saccharomyces boulardii. Alimentary Pharmacology & Therapeutics, 26(6), 767-778. doi:10.1111/j.1365-2036.2007.03442.x

Deguchi, K., E. Yokoyama, T. Honda, and K. Mizuno, 2009. Efficacyof a novel trivalent inactivated vaccine against the sheddingof Salmonella in a chicken challenge model.Avian Dis53:281–286.

Di Giacinto, C., Marinaro, M., Sanchez, M., Strober, W., & Boirivant, M. (2005). Probiotics ameliorate recurrent Th1-mediated murine colitis by inducing IL-10 and IL-10-dependent TGF-beta-bearing regulatory cells. Journal of Immunology (Baltimore, Md.: 1950), 174(6), 3237-3246.

Dobrogosz, W. J., Peacock, T. J., & Hassan, H. M. (2010). Evolution of the probiotic concept from conception to validation and acceptance in medical science. Advances in Applied Microbiology, 72, 1-41. doi:10.1016/S0065-2164(10)72001-3

Dubos, R.J., J.H. Straus, and C. Pierce (1943). The multiplication of bacteriophage in vivo and its protective effect against an experimental infection with Shigelladysenteriae.J Exp Med78: 161–168

Duc le, H., & Cutting, S. M. (2003). Bacterial spores as heat stable vaccine vehicles. Expert Opinion on Biological Therapy, 3(8), 1263-1270. doi:10.1517/14712598.3.8.1263

Duc le, H., Hong, H. A., Barbosa, T. M., Henriques, A. O., & Cutting, S. M. (2004). Characterization of bacillus probiotics available for human use. Applied and Environmental Microbiology, 70(4), 2161-2171.

Duc, H., H.A. Hong, H.S. Atkins, H.C. Flick-Smith, Z. Durrani, S. Rijpkema, R.W. Titball, and S. M. Cutting, 2007. Immunizationagainst anthrax using Bacillus subtilisspores expressing theanthrax protective antigen.Vaccine 25:346–355.

Dueger, E. L., J. K. House, D. M. Heithoff, and M. J. Mahan (2001). Salmonella DNA adenine methylase mutants elicit protectiveimmune responses to homologous and heterologous serovars inchickens. Infect. Immun. 69:7950:t. Imm

Dueger, E. L., J. K. House, D. M. Heithoff, and M. J. Mahan (2003). Salmonella DNA adenine methylase mutants prevent colonizationof newly hatched chickens by homologous and heterologousserovars. Int. J. Food Microbiol. 80:1530:J.

Dueger, E.L., J.K. House, D.M. Heithoff, and M.J. Mahan (2003). Salmonella DNA adenine methylase mutants prevent colonization of newly hatched chickens by homologous and heterologous serovars. Int J Food Microbiol 80: 153.

Dutta, N.K. (1963). An experimental study on the usefulness of bacteriophage in the prophylaxis and treatment of cholera.Bull Org mond Santé Bull WldHlth Org 28: 357-360

Ehrstrom, S., Daroczy, K., Rylander, E., Samuelsson, C., Johannesson, U., Anzen, B., & Pahlson, C. (2010). Lactic acid bacteria colonization and clinical outcome after probiotic supplementation in conventionally treated bacterial vaginosis and vulvovaginal candidiasis. Microbes and Infection / Institut Pasteur, 12(10), 691-699. doi:10.1016/j.micinf.2010.04.010

Enck, P., Klosterhalfen, S., & Martens, U. (2011). Probiotic therapy of the irritable bowel syndrome. [Probiotische Behandlung des Reizdarmsyndroms] Deutsche Medizinische Wochenschrift (1946), 136(8), 371-375. doi:10.1055/s-0031-1272538

Fang, H., Elina, T., Heikki, A., & Seppo, S. (2000). Modulation of humoral immune response through probiotic intake. FEMS Immunology and Medical Microbiology, 29(1), 47-52.

Farnell, M. B., Donoghue, A. M., de los Santos, F. S., Blore, P. J., Hargis, B. M., Tellez, G., & Donoghue, D. J. (2006). Upregulation of oxidative burst and degranulation in chicken heterophils stimulated with probiotic bacteria. Poultry Science, 85(11), 1900-1906.

Fiers, W., M. De Filette, A. Birkett, S. Neirynck, and W. MinJou (2004). A universal human influenza A vaccine. Virus Res103:173–176.

Flint, H. J., O'Toole, P. W., & Walker, A. W. (2010). Special issue: The human intestinal microbiota. Microbiology (Reading, England), 156(Pt 11), 3203-3204. doi:10.1099/mic.0.045443-0

Flore, T. N., Francois, Z. N., & Felicite, T. M. (2010). Immune system stimulation in rats by lactobacillus sp. isolates from raffia wine (raphia vinifera). Cellular Immunology, 260(2), 63-65. doi:10.1016/j.cellimm.2009.09.002

Foligne, B., Dewulf, J., Breton, J., Claisse, O., Lonvaud-Funel, A., & Pot, B. (2010). Probiotic properties of non-conventional lactic acid bacteria: Immunomodulation by oenococcus oeni. International Journal of Food Microbiology, 140(2-3), 136-145. doi:10.1016/j.ijfoodmicro.2010.04.007

Galdeano, C. M., de Leblanc Ade, M., Carmuega, E., Weill, R., & Perdigon, G. (2009). Mechanisms involved in the immunostimulation by probiotic fermented milk. The Journal of Dairy Research, 76(4), 446-454. doi:10.1017/S0022029909990021

Gourbeyre, P., Denery, S., & Bodinier, M. (2011). Probiotics, prebiotics, and synbiotics: Impact on the gut immune system and allergic reactions. Journal of Leukocyte Biology, doi:10.1189/jlb.1109753

Hacini-Rachinel, F., Nancey, S., Boschetti, G., Sardi, F., Doucet-Ladeveze, R., Durand, P. Y., Kaiserlian, D. (2009). CD4+ T cells and lactobacillus casei control relapsing colitis mediated by CD8+ T cells. Journal of Immunology (Baltimore, Md.: 1950), 183(9), 5477-5486. doi:10.4049/jimmunol.0804267

Hargis, B.M., D.J. Caldwell, and J.A. Byrd (2010). Microbial pathogens: Live poultry considerations. In: Owens, CM, CZ Alvarado, and AR Sams, Poultry Meat Processing. CRC Press, Boca Raton, FL.

Harikrishnan, R., Balasundaram, C., & Heo, M. S. (2010). Lactobacillus sakei BK19 enriched diet enhances the immunity status and disease resistance to streptococcosis infection in kelp grouper, epinephelus bruneus. Fish & Shellfish Immunology, 29(6), 1037-1043. doi:10.1016/j.fsi.2010.08.017

Hassan, J.O. and R. Curtiss (1997). Efficacy of live avirulentSalmonella typhimurium vaccine in preventing colonization and invasion of laying hens by Salmonella typhimurium and Salmonella enteritidis.Avian Diseases 41: 783.

Higgins S. E., A. Torres-Rodriguez, J. L. Vicente, C. D. Sartor, C. M. Pixley, G. M. Nava, G. Tellez, J. T. Barton, & Hargis (2005). Evaluation of Intervention Strategies for Idiopathic Diarrhea in Commercial Turkey Brooding Houses. J. Appl. Poult. Res. 14(1), 345-348.

Higgins, J. P., Andreatti Filho, R. L., Higgins, S. E., Wolfenden, A. D., Tellez, G., & Hargis, B. M. (2008). Evaluation of Salmonella-lytic properties of bacteriophages isolated from commercial broiler houses. Avian Diseases, 52(1), 139-142. doi:10.1637/8017-050807-ResNote

Higgins, J. P., Andreatti Filho, R. L., Higgins, S. E., Wolfenden, A. D., Tellez, G., & Hargis, B. M. (2008). Evaluation of Salmonella-lytic properties of bacteriophages isolated from commercial broiler houses. Avian Diseases, 52(1), 139-142.

Higgins, J. P., Higgins, S. E., Guenther, K. L., Huff, W., Donoghue, A. M., Donoghue, D. J., & Hargis, B. M. (2005). Use of a specific bacteriophage treatment to reduce Salmonella in poultry products. Poultry Science, 84(7), 1141-1145.

Higgins, J. P., Higgins, S. E., Vicente, J. L., Wolfenden, A. D., Tellez, G., & Hargis, B. M. (2007). Temporal effects of lactic acid bacteria probiotic culture on Salmonella in neonatal broilers. Poultry Science, 86(8), 1662-1666.

Higgins, J. P., Higgins, S. E., Wolfenden, A. D., Henderson, S. N., Torres-Rodriguez, A., Vicente, J. L., Tellez, G. (2010). Effect of lactic acid bacteria probiotic culture treatment timing on Salmonella enteritidis in neonatal broilers. Poultry Science, 89(2), 243-247. doi:10.3382/ps.2009-00436

Higgins, JP, SE Higgins, KL Guenther, LA Newberry, WE Huff, and BM Hargis, 2005. Use of a specific bacteriophage treatment to reduce Salmonella in poultry.PoultSci 84:1141-1145

Higgins, S. E., Higgins, J. P., Wolfenden, A. D., Henderson, S. N., Torres-Rodriguez, A., Tellez, G., & Hargis, B. (2008). Evaluation of a lactobacillus-based probiotic culture for the reduction of Salmonella enteritidis in neonatal broiler chicks. Poultry Science, 87(1), 27-31. doi:10.3382/ps.2007-00210

Higgins, S.E., J.P. Higgins, L.R. Bielke, and B.M. Hargis (2007). Selection and application of bacteriophages for treating Salmonella enteritidis infections in poultry.Int J PoultSci 6: 163-168

Higgins, S. E., Wolfenden, A. D., Tellez,G., Hargis, B. M., & Porter T. (2011). Transcriptional profiling of cecal gene expression in probioticandSalmonella-challenged neonatal chicks. Poultry Science"in press".

Hoa, T. T., Duc, L. H., Isticato, R., Baccigalupi, L., Ricca, E., Van, P. H., & Cutting, S. M. (2001). Fate and dissemination of bacillus subtilis spores in a murine model. Applied and Environmental Microbiology, 67(9), 3819-3823.

Hoang, B. X., Shaw, G., Pham, P., & Levine, S. A. (2010). Lactobacillus rhamnosus cell lysate in the management of resistant childhood atopic eczema. Inflammation & Allergy Drug Targets, 9(3), 192-196.

Hollister, A. G., Corrier, D. E., Nisbet, D. J., & DeLoach, J. R. (1999). Effects of chicken-derived cecal microorganisms maintained in continuous culture on cecal colonization by Salmonella typhimurium in turkey poults. Poultry Science, 78(4), 546-549.

Holt, P.S., R.K. Gast, and S. Kelly-Aehle (2003). Use of a live attenuated Salmonella typhimurium vaccine to protect against Salmonella enteritidis infection while undergoing molt.Avian Diseases 47: 656.

Hong, H. A., Duc le, H., & Cutting, S. M. (2005). The use of bacterial spore formers as probiotics. FEMS Microbiology Reviews, 29(4), 813-835. doi:10.1016/j.femsre. 2004.12.001

Hong, H. A., Huang, J. M., Khaneja, R., Hiep, L. V., Urdaci, M. C., & Cutting, S. M. (2008a). The safety of bacillus subtilis and bacillus indicus as food probiotics. Journal of Applied Microbiology, 105(2), 510-520. doi:10.1111/j.1365-2672.2008.03773.x

Hong, H. A., Huang, J. M., Khaneja, R., Hiep, L. V., Urdaci, M. C., & Cutting, S. M. (2008b). The safety of bacillus subtilis and bacillus indicus as food probiotics. Journal of Applied Microbiology, 105(2), 510-520. doi:10.1111/j.1365-2672.2008.03773.x

Huang, J.M., R.M. La Ragione, A. Nunez, and S.M. Cutting (2008). Immunostimulatory activity of Bacillus spores. FEMS ImmunolMed Microbiol 53:195–203.

Huff, W.E., G.R. Huff, N.C. Rath, J.M. Balog, H. Xie, P.A. Moore, Jr., and A.M. Donoghue, 2002b. Prevention of Escherichia coli respiratory infection in broiler chickens with bacteriophage (SPR02).PoultSci 81: 437-441

Huff, W.E., G.R. Huff, N.C. Rath, J.M. Balog, and A.M. Donoghue (2002a). Prevention of Escherichia coli infection in broiler chickens with a bacteriophage aerosol spray.PoultSci 81: 1486-1491

Huff, W.E., G.R. Huff, N.C. Rath, J.M. Balog, and A.M. Donoghue (2003a). Evaluation of aerosol spray and intramuscular injection of bacteriophage to treat an Escherichia coli respiratory infection.PoultSci 82: 1108-1112

Huff, W.E., G.R. Huff, N.C. Rath, J.M. Balog, and A.M. Donoghue (2003b). Bacteriophage treatment of severe Escherichia coli respiratory infection in broiler chickens.Avian Dis 47: 1399-1405

Hume, M. E., Corrier, D. E., Nisbet, D. J., & DeLoach, J. R. (1998). Early Salmonella challenge time and reduction in chick cecal colonization following treatment with a characterized competitive exclusion culture. Journal of Food Protection, 61(6), 673-676.

Ibrahim, F., Ruvio, S., Granlund, L., Salminen, S., Viitanen, M., & Ouwehand, A. C. (2010). Probiotics and immunosenescence: Cheese as a carrier. FEMS Immunology and Medical Microbiology, 59(1), 53-59. doi:10.1111/j.1574-695X.2010.00658.x

Inoue, A.Y., A. Berchieri, Jr., A. Bernardino, A., J.B. Paiva, and E.V. Sterzo (2008). Passive immunity of progeny from broiler breeders vaccinated with oil-emulsion bacterin against Salmonella enteritidis. Avian Diseases 48: 567-571.

Jadamus, A., Vahjen, W., & Simon, O. (2001). Growth behaviour of a spore forming probiotic strain in the gastrointestinal tract of broiler chicken and piglets. Archiv Fur Tierernahrung, 54(1), 1-17.

Jobin, C. (2010). Probiotics and ileitis: Could augmentation of TNF/NFkappaB activity be the answer? Gut Microbes, 1(3), 196-199. doi:10.4161/gmic.1.3.12485

Kajikawa, A., E. Satoh, R.J. Leer, S. Yamamoto, and S. Igimi (2007). Intragastric immunization with recombinant Lactobacilluscaseiexpressing flagellar antigen confers antibody-independentprotective immunity against Salmonella entericaserovar Enteritidis.Vaccine 25:3599–3605.

Klein, M., Sanders, M. E., Duong, T., & Young, H. A. (2010). Probiotics: From bench to market. Annals of the New York Academy of Sciences, 1212 Suppl 1, E1-14. doi:10.1111/j.1749-6632.2010.05839.x; 10.1111/j.1749-6632.2010.05839.x

Ko, K. Y., Mendoncam, A. F., Ismail, H., & Ahn, D. U. (2009). Ethylenediaminetetraacetate and lysozyme improves antimicrobial activities of ovotransferrin against escherichia coli O157:H7. Poultry Science, 88(2), 406-414. doi:10.3382/ps.2008-00218

Kotton, C.N., and E.L. Hohmann (2004). Enteric pathogens asvaccine vectors for foreign antigen delivery. Infect Immun72:5535–5547.

Kremer, C.H., KM O' Meara, S.L. Layton, B.M. Hargis, and K. Cole (2011). Evaluatin of recombinant Salmonella expressing the flagellar protein fliC for persistence and enhanced antibody response in commercial turkeys.Poultry Science 90: 752-758.

Kremer, C.H., K.M. O'Meara, S.L. Layton, B.M. Hargis, and K. Cole (2011). Evaluation of recominant Salmonella expressing the flagellar protein fliC for persistence and enhanced antibody response in commercial turkeys.Poultry Science 90: 752-758.

Kubena, L. F., Byrd, J. A., Young, C. R., & Corrier, D. E. (2001). Effects of tannic acid on cecal volatile fatty acids and susceptibility to Salmonella typhimurium colonization in broiler chicks. Poultry Science, 80(9), 1293-1298.

Lavasani, S., Dzhambazov, B., Nouri, M., Fak, F., Buske, S., Molin, G.,. Westrom, B. (2010). A novel probiotic mixture exerts a therapeutic effect on experimental autoimmune encephalomyelitis mediated by IL-10 producing regulatory T cells. PloS One, 5(2), e9009. doi:10.1371/journal.pone.0009009

Layton, S.L., D.R. Kapzcynski, S. Higgins, J. Higgins, A.D. Wolfenden, K.A. Liljebjelke, W.G. Bottje, D. Swayne, L.R. Berghman, Y.M. Kwon, B.M. Hargis, and K. Cole (2009). Vaccination of chickens with recombinant Salmonella expressing M2e and CD154 epitopes increases protection and decreases viral shedding after low pathogenic avian influenza challenge. Poultry Science 88: 2244-2252.

Layton, S.L., M.J. Morgan, K. Cole, Y.M. Kwon, D.J. Donoghue, B.M. Hargis, and N.R. Pumford (2011). Evaluation of Salmonella-vectored Campylobacter peptide epitopes for reduction of Campylobacter jejuni in broiler chickens.Clinical Vaccine Immunol 18: 449-454.

Leblanc, J., Fliss, I., & Matar, C. (2004). Induction of a humoral immune response following an escherichia coli O157:H7 infection with an immunomodulatory peptidic fraction derived from lactobacillus helveticus-fermented milk. Clinical and Diagnostic Laboratory Immunology, 11(6), 1171-1181. doi:10.1128/CDLI.11.6.1171-1181.2004

Lee, H. J., Waller, R. D., Stebbings, S., Highton, J., Orlovich, D. A., Schmierer, D., & Fawcett, J. P. (2010). The effects of an orally administered probiotic on sulfasalazine metabolism in individuals with rheumatoid arthritis: A preliminary study. International Journal of Rheumatic Diseases, 13(1), 48-54. doi:10.1111/j.1756-185X.2009.01449.x

Li, X., Xia, C., & Li, Y. (2009). Induced expression of alpha-toxin gene of clostridium perfringens in recombinant lactobacillus casei and their immunoprotective in mice.Wei Sheng Wu Xue Bao = Acta Microbiologica Sinica, 49(8), 1115-1120.

Liu, M., S. Li, S. Hu, C. Zhao, D. Bi, and M. Sun (2008). Display ofavian influenza virus nucleoprotein on Bacillus thuringiensiscellsurface using CTC as a fusion partner.ApplMicrobiolBiotechnol78:669–676.

Mandel, D. R., Eichas, K., & Holmes, J. (2010). Bacillus coagulans: A viable adjunct therapy for relieving symptoms of rheumatoid arthritis according to a randomized, controlled trial. BMC Complementary and Alternative Medicine, 10, 1. doi:10.1186/1472-6882-10-1

Marčuk, L.M., V.N. Nikiforov, JaFŠčerbak, T.A. Levitov, R.I. Kotljanova, M.S. Nanmŝina, S.U. Davydov, K.A. Monsur, M.A. Rahman, M.A. Latif, R.S. Northrup, R.A. Cash, I. Huq, C.R. Dey, and R.A. Phillips (1971). Clinical studies in the use of bacteriophage in the treatment of Cholera. Bull Org mond Santé Bull WldHlth Org 45: 77-83

McNulty, C. A., Boyle, P., Nichols, T., Clappison, P., & Davey, P. (2007). The public's attitudes to and compliance with antibiotics. The Journal of Antimicrobial Chemotherapy, 60 Suppl 1, i63-8. doi:10.1093/jac/dkm161

Menconi A., Wolfenden A.D., Shivaramaiah S., Terraes J.C., Urbano T., Kuttel J., Kremer C., Hargis B.M., and Tellez G. (2011). Effect of lactic acid bacteria probiotic culture for the treatment of Salmonella enterica serovar Heidelberg in neonatal broiler chickens and turkey poults. Poultry Science 90: 561-565.

Merril, C.R., D. Scholl, and S.L. Adhya (2003). The prospect for bacteriophage therapy in Western medicine.Nat Rev 2: 489-497

Mollenkopf, H., G. Dietrich, and S.H.E. Kaufmann (2001). Intracellularbacteria as targets and carriers for vaccination. BiolChem382:521–532.

Mozdzanowska, K., J. Feng, M. Eid, G. Kragol, M. Cudic, L. Otvos,and W. Gerhard (2003). Induction of influenza type A virus-specificresistance by immunization of mice with a synthetic multipleantigenic peptide vaccine that contains ectodomains of matrixprotein 2. Vaccine 21:2616–2626.

Nakamura, M., T. Nagata, S. Okamura, K. Takehara, and P.S. Holt (2004). The effect of killed Salmonella enteritidisvaccine prior toinduced molting on the shedding of S. enteritidisin laying hens.Avian Dis 48:183–188.

Nayak, S. K. (2010). Probiotics and immunity: A fish perspective. Fish & Shellfish Immunology, 29(1), 2-14. doi:10.1016/j.fsi.2010.02.017

Neirynck, S., T. Deroo, X. Saelens, P. Vanlandschoot, W. Min Jou and W. Fiers (1999). Universal vaccine based on the extracellulardomain of the M2 protein. Nature 5:1157–1163.

Nermes, M., Kantele, J. M., Atosuo, T. J., Salminen, S., & Isolauri, E. (2011). Interaction of orally administered lactobacillus rhamnosus GG with skin and gut microbiota and humoral immunity in infants with atopic dermatitis. Clinical and Experimental Allergy : Journal of the British Society for Allergy and Clinical Immunology, 41(3), 370-377. doi:10.1111/j.1365-2222.2010.03657.x; 10.1111/j.1365-2222.2010.03657.x

Ng, S. C., Chan, F. K., & Sung, J. J. (2011). Review article: The role of non-biological drugs in refractory inflammatory bowel disease. Alimentary Pharmacology & Therapeutics, 33(4), 417-427. doi:10.1111/j.1365-2036.2010.04541.x; 10.1111/j.1365-2036.2010.04541.x

Nisbet, D. J., Tellez, G. I., Lowry, V. K., Anderson, R. C., Garcia, G., Nava, G., Stanker, L. H. (1998). Effect of a commercial competitive exclusion culture (preempt) on mortality and horizontal transmission of Salmonella gallinarum in broiler chickens. Avian Diseases, 42(4), 651-656.

Nurmi, E. and Rantalla M. 1973. New aspects in Salmonella infection in broiler production. Nature, 241: 210-211.

O'Meara, K.M., C.J. Kremer, S.L. Layton, L.R. Berghman, B.M. Hargis, and K. Cole (2010). Evaluation of recombinant Salmonellaexpressing CD154 for persistence and enhanced antibodyresponse in commercial turkeys. Poultry Science 89:1399–1405.

O'Murphy, L., Kiely, B.M. Hargis, and K. Cole (2010). Evaluation of recombinant Salmonellaexpressing CD154 for persistence and enhanced antibodyresponse in commercial turkeys. Poult. Sci. 89:1399t. Sci

O'Mahony, L., Feeney, M., O'Halloran, S., Murphy, L., Kiely, B., Fitzgibbon, J., Collins, J. K. (2001). Probiotic impact on microbial flora, inflammation and tumour development in IL-10 knockout mice. Alimentary Pharmacology & Therapeutics, 15(8), 1219-1225.

Osipova, I. G., Makhailova, N. A., Sorokulova, I. B., Vasil'eva, E. A., & Gaiderov, A. A. (2003). Spore probiotics. [Sporovye probiotiki] Zhurnal Mikrobiologii, Epidemiologii, i Immunobiologii, (3)(3), 113-119.

Over, K. F., Hettiarachchy, N., Johnson, M. G., & Davis, B. (2009). Effect of organic acids and plant extracts on escherichia coli O157:H7, listeria monocytogenes, and Salmonella typhimurium in broth culture model and chicken meat systems. Journal of Food Science, 74(9), M515-21. doi:10.1111/j.1750-3841.2009.01375.x

Park, E., Jeon, G. I., Park, J. S., & Paik, H. D. (2007). A probiotic strain of bacillus polyfermenticus reduces DMH induced precancerous lesions in F344 male rat. Biological & Pharmaceutical Bulletin, 30(3), 569-574.

Pascual, L., Ruiz, F., Giordano, W., & Barberis, I. L. (2010). Vaginal colonization and activity of the probiotic bacterium lactobacillus fermentum L23 in a murine model of vaginal tract infection. Journal of Medical Microbiology, 59(Pt 3), 360-364. doi:10.1099/jmm.0.012583-0

Patterson, J. A., & Burkholder, K. M. (2003). Application of prebiotics and probiotics in poultry production. Poultry Science, 82(4), 627-631.

Preidis, G. A., Hill, C., Guerrant, R. L., Ramakrishna, B. S., Tannock, G. W., & Versalovic, J. (2011). Probiotics, enteric and diarrheal diseases, and global health. Gastroenterology, 140(1), 8-14. doi:10.1053/j.gastro.2010.11.010

Romanin, D., Serradell, M., Gonzalez Maciel, D., Lausada, N., Garrote, G. L., & Rumbo, M. (2010). Down-regulation of intestinal epithelial innate response by probiotic yeasts isolated from kefir. International Journal of Food Microbiology, 140(2-3), 102-108. doi:10.1016/j.ijfoodmicro.2010.04.014

Ruiz, F. O., Gerbaldo, G., Asurmendi, P., Pascual, L. M., Giordano, W., & Barberis, I. L. (2009). Antimicrobial activity, inhibition of urogenital pathogens, and synergistic interactions between lactobacillus strains. Current Microbiology, 59(5), 497-501. doi:10.1007/s00284-009-9465-0

Sayamov, R.M., 1963. Treatment and prophylaxis of Cholera with bacteriophage.Bull Org mond Santé Bull WldHlth Org 28: 361-367

Schiavi, E., Barletta, B., Butteroni, C., Corinti, S., Boirivant, M., & Di Felice, G. (2010a). Oral therapeutic administration of a probiotic mixture suppresses established Th2 responses and systemic anaphylaxis in a murine model of food allergy. Allergy, doi:10.1111/j.1398-9995.2010.02501.x; 10.1111/j.1398-9995.2010.02501.x

Schiavi, E., Barletta, B., Butteroni, C., Corinti, S., Boirivant, M., & Di Felice, G. (2010b). Oral therapeutic administration of a probiotic mixture suppresses established Th2 responses and systemic anaphylaxis in a murine model of food allergy. Allergy, doi:10.1111/j.1398-9995.2010.02501.x; 10.1111/j.1398-9995.2010.02501.x

Schmalstieg, F. C.,Jr, & Goldman, A. S. (2010). Birth of the science of immunology. Journal of Medical Biography, 18(2), 88-98. doi:10.1258/jmb.2010.010009

Shahani, K., & Ayebo, A. (1980). Role of dietary lactobacilli in gastrointestinal microecology. American Journal of Clinical Nutrition, 33(11), 2448-2457.

Shivaprasad H.L. Pullorum disease and fowl typhoid. In: Calnek BW, John Barnes H, Beard CW, McDougald LR, Saif YM, eds. Diseases of poultry.London: Mosby-Wolfe, 1997: 82-121.

Shivaramaiah, S., N. R. Pumford, M. J. Morgan, R. E. Wolfenden, A. D. Wolfenden, A. Torres-Rodríguez, B. M. Hargis, & Téllez, G. (2011). Evaluation of Bacillus Species as Potential Candidates for Direct Fed Microbials in Commercial Poultry.Poultry Science,"in press".

Silvestri, L., van Saene, H. K., Gregori, D., Agostini, S., Francescon, M., & Taylor, N. (2010). Probiotics to prevent ventilator-associated pneumonia: No robust evidence from randomized controlled trials. Critical Care Medicine, 38(7), 1616-7; author reply 1617. doi:10.1097/CCM.0b013e3181dd0a67

Slopek, S., I. Durlakowa, B. Weber-Dabrowska, A. Kucharewicz-Krukowska, M. Dabrowski, and R. Bisikiewicz (1983a). Results of bacteriophage treatment of supperative bacterial infections. I. General evaluation of the results. Arch ImmunolTherExp31: 267-91

Slopek, S., I. Durlakowa, B. Weber-Dabrowska, A. Kucharewicz-Krukowska, M. Dabrowski, and R. Bisikiewicz (1983b). Results of bacteriophage treatment of supperative bacterial infections. II. Detailed evaluation of the results. Arch ImmunolTherExp31: 293-327

Slopek, S., I. Durlakowa, B. Weber-Dabrowska, A. Kucharewicz-Krukowska, M. Dabrowski, and R. Bisikiewicz (1984). Results of bacteriophage treatment of supparative bacterial infections. III. Detailed evaluation of the results obtained in further 150 cases. Arch ImmunolTherExp 32: 317-35

Slopek, S., I. Durlakowa, B. Weber-Dabrowska, A. Kucharewicz-Krukowska, M. Dabrowski, and R. Bisikiewicz (1985a). Results of bacteriophage treatment of supparative bacterial infections. IV. Evaluation of the results obtained in 370 cases. Arch ImmunolTherExp 33: 219-40

Slopek, S., I. Durlakowa, B. Weber-Dabrowska, A. Kucharewicz-Krukowska, M. Dabrowski, and R. Bisikiewicz (1985b). Results of bacteriophage treatment of supparative bacterial infections. V. Evaluation of the results obtained in children. Arch ImmunolTherExp 33: 241-59

Slopek, S., I. Durlakowa, B. Weber-Dabrowska, A. Kucharewicz-Krukowska, M. Dabrowski, and R. Bisikiewicz (1985c). Results of bacteriophage treatment of supparative bacterial infections. VI. Analysis of treatment of suppurative staphylococcal infections. Arch ImmunolTherExp 33: 261-73

Smith, H.W. and M.B. Huggins (1982). Successful treatment of experimental Escherichia coli infection in mice using phage: its general superiority over antibiotics. J Gen Microbiol 128: 307-318

Smith, H.W. and M.B. Huggins (1983). Effectiveness of phages in treating experimental Escherichia coli diarrhea in calves, piglets, and lambs.J Gen Microbiol 129: 2659-2675

Smith, H.W., M.B. Huggins, and K.M. Shaw (1987).The control of experimental Escherichia coli diarrhea in calves by means of bacteriophages.J Gen Microbiol 133: 1111-1126

Stamatova, I., & Meurman, J. H. (2009). Probiotics: Health benefits in the mouth. American Journal of Dentistry, 22(6), 329-338.

Swidsinski, A., Loening-Baucke, V., Verstraelen, H., Osowska, S., & Doerffel, Y. (2008). Biostructure of fecal microbiota in healthy subjects and patients with chronic idiopathic diarrhea. Gastroenterology, 135(2), 568-579. doi:10.1053/j.gastro.2008.04.017

Sydenham, M., D. Gillian, F. Bowe, S. Ahmed, S. Chatfield, and G. Dougan (2000). Salmonella entericaserovartyphimuriumsurA mutants are attenuated and effective live oral vaccines. Infect Immun 68: 1109.

Tellez G., S. E. Higgins, A. M. Donoghue, & Hargis, B.. (2006). Digestive Physiology and the Role of Microorganisms,J. Appl. Poult. Res., 15(1),136-144.

Tlaskalova-Hogenova, H., Stepankova, R., Kozakova, H., Hudcovic, T., Vannucci, L., Tuckova, L., Funda, D. P. (2011). The role of gut microbiota (commensal bacteria) and the mucosal barrier in the pathogenesis of inflammatory and autoimmune diseases and cancer: Contribution of germ-free and gnotobiotic animal models of human diseases. Cellular & Molecular Immunology, doi:10.1038/cmi.2010.67

Torres-Rodriguez A., A. M. Donoghue, D. J. Donoghue, J. T. Barton, G. Tellez, & Hargis,B. (2007a). Performance and Condemnation Rate Analysis of Commercial Turkey Flocks Treated with a Lactobacillus spp.-Based Probiotic.Poultry Science, 86(1),444–446.

Torres-Rodriguez A., Higgins, S., J. Vicente, Wolfenden, A., Gaona-Ramirez, G., Barton, J., A. M. Donoghue, G. Tellez, & Hargis, B. (2007b). Effect of Lactose as a Prebiotic on Turkey Body Weight Under Commercial Conditions. J. Appl. Poult. Res., 16(1), 635–641.

Uyen, N.Q., H.A. Hong, and S.M. Cutting (2007). Enhanced immunization and expression strategies using bacterial spores asheat-stable vaccine delivery vehicles. Vaccine 25:356–365.

Van Immerseel, F., Russell, J. B., Flythe, M. D., Gantois, I., Timbermont, L., Pasmans, F., Ducatelle, R. (2006). The use of organic acids to combat Salmonella in poultry: A mechanistic explanation of the efficacy. Avian Pathology : Journal of the W.V.P.A, 35(3), 182-188. doi:10.1080/03079450600711045

Van Immerseel, F., U. Methner, I. Rychlik, B. Nagy, P. Velge, G.Martin, N. Foster, R. Ducatelle, and P. A. Barrow. 2005. Vaccinationand early protection against non host-specific Salmonellaserotypes in poultry: Exploitation of innate immunity and microbialactivity. Epidemiol. Infect. 133:95933:io

Vanderpool, C., Yan, F., & Polk, D. B. (2008). Mechanisms of probiotic action: Implications for therapeutic applications in inflammatory bowel diseases. Inflammatory Bowel Diseases, 14(11), 1585-1596. doi:10.1002/ibd.20525

Vicente, J., A. Wolfenden, A. Torres-Rodriguez, S. Higgins, G. Tellez & B. M. Hargis. (2007c). Effect of a Lactobacillus-based Probiotic and Dietary Lactose Prebiotic on Turkey Poult Performance With or Without Salmonella enteritidis challenge. J. Appl. Poult. Res. 16(1), 361–364.

Vicente, J., S. Higgins, L. Bilke, G. Tellez, D. Donoghue, A. Donoghue, & Hargis, B. (2007a). Effect of Probiotic Culture Candidates on Salmonella Prevalence in Commercial Turkey Houses.J. Appl. Poult. Res., 16(1), 471-476.

Vicente, J.L., L. Aviña, A. Torres-Rodriguez, B. M. Hargis & G. Tellez. (2007b). Effect of a Lactobacillus spp-based Probiotic Culture Product on Broiler Chicks Performance under Commercial Conditions. International Journal of Poultry Science, 6(3), 154-156.

Vicente, J., A. Torres-Rodriguez, S. Higgins, C. Pixley, G. Tellez, A. M. Donoghue, & B. M. Hargis. (2008). Effect of a selected Lactobacillus spp-based probiotic on Salmonella enteritidis-infected broiler chicks. Avian Diseases, 52(1),143–146.

Vila, B., Fontgibell, A., Badiola, I., Esteve-Garcia, E., Jimenez, G., Castillo, M., & Brufau, J. (2009). Reduction of Salmonella enterica var. enteritidis colonization and invasion by bacillus cereus var. toyoi inclusion in poultry feeds. Poultry Science, 88(5), 975-979. doi:10.3382/ps.2008-00483

Vreeland, R. H., Rosenzweig, W. D., & Powers, D. W. (2000). Isolation of a 250 million-year-old halotolerant bacterium from a primary salt crystal. Nature, 407(6806), 897-900. doi:10.1038/35038060

Wagner, R. D., Paine, D. D., & Cerniglia, C. E. (2003). Phenotypic and genotypic characterization of competitive exclusion products for use in poultry. Journal of Applied Microbiology, 94(6), 1098-1107.

Weiss, G., Rasmussen, S., Zeuthen, L. H., Nielsen, B. N., Jarmer, H., Jespersen, L., & Frokiaer, H. (2010). Lactobacillus acidophilus induces virus immune defence genes in murine dendritic cells by a toll-like receptor-2-dependent mechanism. Immunology, 131(2), 268-281. doi:10.1111/j.1365-2567.2010.03301.x; 10.1111/j.1365-2567.2010.03301.x

Weissmann, G. (2010). It's complicated: Inflammation from metchnikoff to meryl streep. The FASEB Journal: Official Publication of the Federation of American Societies for Experimental Biology, 24(11), 4129-4132. doi:10.1096/fj.10-1101ufm

Williams, L. D., Burdock, G. A., Jimenez, G., & Castillo, M. (2009). Literature review on the safety of toyocerin, a non-toxigenic and non-pathogenic bacillus cereus var. toyoi preparation. Regulatory Toxicology and Pharmacology : RTP, 55(2), 236-246. doi:10.1016/j.yrtph.2009.07.009

Williams, P. (2007a). Bacillus subtilis: A shocking message from a probiotic. Cell Host & Microbe, 1(4), 248-249. doi:10.1016/j.chom.2007.05.010

Williams, P. (2007b). Bacillus subtilis: A shocking message from a probiotic. Cell Host & Microbe, 1(4), 248-249. doi:10.1016/j.chom.2007.05.010

Wolfenden, A.D., C.M. Pixley, J.P. Higgins, S.E. Higgins, A. Torres, J.L. Vicente, B.M. Hargis, & G. Tellez. (2007a). Evaluation of spray application of a Lactobacillus-based probiotic on Salmonella enteritidis colonization in broiler chickens. International Journal of Poultry Science, 6(7), 493-496.

Wolfenden, A.D., J.L. Vicente, L.R. Bielke, C.M. Pixley, S.E. Higgins, D.J. Donoghue, A.M. Donoghue, B.M. Hargis & G. Tellez. (2007b). Effect of a define competitive exclusion culture for prophylaxis and reduction of horizontal transmission of Salmonella enteritidis in broiler chickens. International Journal of Poultry Science, 6(7), 489-492.

Wolfenden, A.D., J.L. Vicente, J.P. Higgins, R. Andreatti, S.E. Higgins, B.M. Hargis, &G. Tellez. (2007c). Effect of organic acids and probiotics on Salmonella enteritidis infection in broiler chickens. International Journal of Poultry Science, 6(6), 403-405.

Wolfenden, R.E., S.E. Layton, A.D. Wolfenden, A. Khatiwara, G. Gaono-Ramirez, N.R. Pumford, K. Cole, Y.M. Kwon, G. Tellez, L.R. Bergman, and B.M. Hargis (2010). Development and evaluation of candidate recombinant Salmonella-vectored Salmonella vaccines.Poultry Science 89: 2370-2379.

Yang, X., B.J. Hinnebusch, T. Trunkle, C.M. Bosio, Z. Suo, M. Tighe, A. Harmsen, T. Becker, K. Crist, N. Walters, R. Avci, and D.W. Pascual (2007). Oral vaccination with Salmonella simultaneously expressing Yersinia pestisF1 and V antigens protects against bubonic and pneumonic plague. JImmunol 178:1059–1067.

Zhang, Q.J., J.C. Meitzler, S.X. Huang, and T. Morishita (2000). Sequence polymorphism, predicted secondary structures, and surface-exposed conformationalepitopes of Campylobacter major outer membrane protein.InfectImmun68:5679–5689.

Zhang-Barber, L., A.K. Turner, P.A. Barrow (1999). Vaccination for control of Salmonella in poultry.Vaccine 17: 2538.

Zou, P., W. Liu, and Y. Chen (2004). The epitope recognized by amonoclonal antibody in influenza A virus M2 protein is immunogenicand confers immune protection. IntImmunopharmacol5:631–635.

Wolfenden, A.D., Pixley, C., Vicente, J. L, L. Aviña, B.M. Hargis,& G. Tellez. (2007d). Effect of organic acids during feed withdrawal on mortality, shrinkage and carcass condemnation during transportation to the processing plant. International Journal of Poultry Science,6(7), 497-500.

Wolfenden, R.E., N.R. Pumford, M.J. Morgan, S. Shivaramaiah, A.D. Wolfenden, G. Tellez & B.M. Hargis. (2010). Evaluation of a Screening and Selection Method for Bacillus Isolates for Use as Effective Direct-fed Microbials in Commercial Poultry. International Journal of Poultry Science, 9(4), 317-323.

Wolfenden, R.E., S.L. Layton, A.D. Wolfenden, A. Khatiwara, G. Gaona-Ramirez, N.R. Pumford, K. Cole, Y.M. Kwon, G. Tellez, L.R. Bergman, and B.M. Hargis (2010). Development and evaluation of candidate recombinant Salmoenlla-vectored Salmonella vaccines.Poultry Science89:2370try S.

Wolken, W. A., Tramper, J., & van der Werf, M. J. (2003). What can spores do for us? Trends in Biotechnology, 21(8), 338-345.

Ya, W., Reifer, C., & Miller, L. E. (2010). Efficacy of vaginal probiotic capsules for recurrent bacterial vaginosis: A double-blind, randomized, placebo-controlled study. American Journal of Obstetrics and Gynecology, 203(2), 120.e1-120.e6. doi:10.1016/j.ajog.2010.05.023

# 13

# Recent Advances in the Application of Non Thermal Methods for the Prevention of *Salmonella* in Foods

Shilpi Gupta and Nissreen Abu-Ghannam
*School of Food Science and Environmental Health*
*College of Sciences and Health*
*Dublin Institute of Technology, Dublin*
*Ireland*

## 1. Introduction

Food-borne illness as a result of consumption of foods contaminated with pathogenic bacteria is a world-wide concern. The presence and subsequent growth of micro-organisms in food in addition to improper storage not only results in spoilage but also in a reduction of food quality. The microbiological safety in ready to eat products is a cause of big concern not only for the consumers and food industries but also for the regulatory agencies. The number of documented outbreaks of foodborne diseases has increased in the last decade with *Salmonella* spp., *Listeria monocytogenes* and *Escherichia coli* being responsible for the largest number of outbreaks and deaths.

The European Food Safety Authority (EFSA) reported *Salmonella* to be the most common cause of food-borne outbreaks in the EU (EFSA, 2009). As high as 50,000 and 35,000 people were reported to be suffering from salmonellosis in the Netherlands during 1999-2000 and 2002, respectively (Bouwknegt et al., 2003). The symptoms include diarrhoea, vomiting, nausea, abdominal pain and fever. *Salmonella enterica* Typhimurium and *Salmonella enterica* Enteritidis are the most frequently isolated serovars in the EU which are responsible for diarrhoea and fever (EFSA-ECDC, 2007). Some strains of *Salmonella* such as *S*. Senftenberg are more heat resistant than other strains. Even in the United States, *Salmonella* is considered to be one of the most prevalent bacteria amongst the foodborne pathogens, causing an estimated 1.6 million foodborne illnesses with annual cost of ~$14 billion. *Salmonella* Typhimurium has been implicated in the US as the major causative agent for food borne salmonellosis.

## 2. *Salmonella*

*Salmonella* is a gram negative, non-spore forming bacilli belonging to the family Enterobacteriaceae and is one of the most prominent food pathogenic bacteria. This pathogen has the ability to grow at a wide range of temperatures (8-45 °C), pH (4 to 9) and foods with high moisture content (thus high water activity). Since the organism is heat sensitive, it is more prevalent in raw and under-cooked foods. In general, consumption of contaminated foods such as raw or under-cooked eggs, meat, poultry or even dairy products can act as vehicles for salmonellosis in humans. Because of the ability of *Salmonella* cells to exist under dormant conditions and regain active growth phase when favourable conditions return, it also has the ability to survive in dry products. As fresh cut fruits lack any skin barrier they are also likely to be contaminated by *Salmonella*. Storage of raw or pasteurized foods under refrigerated conditions or with treatments that reduce pH can help to increase the shelf life by retarding or avoiding the growth but certain strains of *Salmonella* have been reported to survive even under chilling conditions. It is now evident that these conditions cannot stop the chromosomal replication and are only bacteriostatic in nature (Tahergorabi et al., 2011). Risco (2009) reported survival of *Salmonella* inoculated into chicken nuggets during 16 weeks at -20ºC. This further adds to the problems that can arise by the consumption of ready to eat frozen products that are just pre-warmed in a microwave prior to consumption.

Although any person can contract food poisoning due to *Salmonella*, the disease can be more serious in infants, elderly and people with weak immune system. Treatment with antibiotics becomes essential for the eradication of this bacterial species. However, excessive use of antibiotics has made several strains to develop resistance against such drugs resulting in increased prevalence of these resistant strains in humans and animals. In order to minimize its presence in foods, synthetic antimicrobial agents such as sodium benzoate and sodium nitrite were used. However, these are also losing popularity due to consumer demand for food products with natural preservatives. Thermal processing is the most efficient way for eliminating *Salmonella* from foods. However, consumer's demand for minimally processed foods in addition to the negative effect of heat on nutritional properties of foods is making this technology less popular in the food industry. Novel remedies for safe and efficient removal of this bacterium from foods are becoming vital. Nowadays, non thermal techniques such as the addition of naturally occurring compounds having antibacterial activity, the use of high pressure carbon dioxide (HPCD), use of electrolysed water, high intensity pulsed electric field (PEF) or irraditation are increasingly gaining attention as a means of food preservation. In addition, it is imperative for the non thermal applications to have similar or higher inactivation as compared to the traditional heat treatments. According to US-FDA guidelines, the main requirement is to reduce the pathogen load by 5 logs (FDA, 2001). The major advantage of these non-thermal technologies (table 1) is that they are environmentally friendly and act at ambient or sub-lethal temperatures resulting in minimal impact on color, flavor and nutritional quality of foods. These techniques help in retaining the "fresh-like" characteristics of food and may also help to preserve functionalities.

However, the use of essential oils and other plant extracts is often limited by organoleptical criteria. Moreover, high pressures can cause cell wall breakdown and result in loss of cell turgidity. Thus, under these conditions, it might be necessary to combine two or more technologies in order to achieve the desired preservative effect. The technique of combination or "hurdle technology" is slowly becoming eminent. Thus, the use of natural antimicrobials along with pulsed electric field, ozone or super critical carbon dioxide can be used to curtail the growth of *Salmonella* with a minimal effect on the sensory characteristics such as flavor.

| | **Advantages** | **Limitations** |
|---|---|---|
| Irradiation | Effective for several foods<br>Many different sources available (Gamma rays, electron beam) | Limited public acceptance<br>Lipid oxidation of meat products |
| UV radiation | No chemicals are used<br>Non-heat related method<br>Lesser changes in quality attributes of food | Long term exposure can be harmful to the industry workers |
| HPP | Independent of the shape of food<br>Can be used for both solid and liquid samples. | Changes in quality of food has been observed |
| HPCD | Can be used in a batch or continuous process<br>$CO_2$ is GRAS, nonflammable and non-toxic | Not very successful for solid foods<br>Commercial application is still not a success |
| PEF | Pulse applied for a short period so no generation of heat<br>Less usage of energy | Cannot be applied to foods which cannot withstand high fields<br>Cannot be applied to foods that form bubbles |
| Natural antimicrobials | Natural "green" preservatives<br>Have "GRAS" status | Can have a negative effect on the sensory properties of foods |

Table 1. Limitations and advantages of non thermal processing techniques

## 3. Thermal processing

Heating of food is the most common and effective method for eliminating pathogens. Thermal pasteurization, involving the reduction or inactivation of micro-organisms, was traditionally the most common method for the production of microbiologically safe food products. The method involves generation of heat outside the food which gets transferred into the food through conduction or convection. Although the method is inexpensive, preservative free and environmental friendly, it does result in undesirable changes related to the nutritional and organoleptical properties of foods. At the same time, the content or bioavailability of some bioactive compounds such as ascorbic acid, phenolic compounds or carotenoids may be severely diminished. The case becomes even worse if the food product is heat sensitive. Nonetheless the extent of destruction depends on the temperature used for processing in addition to the time for which it is applied. In order to circumvent the shortcomings of thermal processing, several non-thermal methods such as the use of radiation, high pressure processing and natural antimicrobials are receiving considerable attention (table 2).

| Food Product | Strain | Condition | Reduction | Reference | Technique |
|---|---|---|---|---|---|
| Chicken meat | *S.* Typhimurium | 13.7 MPa, 35 °C , 2 h | 94-98% | Wei et al., 1991 | *hpcd* |
| Beef Trimmings | *Salmonella spp.* | 10.3 MPa, 36 °C , 15 min | 0.83 log | Meurehg, 2006 | *hpcd* |
| Ground beef | *Salmonella spp.* | 10.3 MPa, 36 °C , 15 min | 1.23 log | Meurehg, 2006 | *hpcd* |
| Physiological saline | *S.* Typhimurium | 6 MPa, 35 °C , 15 min | 7 log | Erkmen and Karaman 2001 | *hpcd* |
| Orange juice | *S.* Typhimurium | 38 MPa, 25 °C , 10 min | 6 log | Kincal et al., 2005 | *hpcd* |
| Melon juice | *S.* Enteritidis | 2000 μs and 100 Hz | 4.27 log | Mosqueda-Melgar et al., 2007 | PEF |
| Watermelon juice | *S.* Enteritidis | 1250 μs and 175 Hz | 3.75 log | Mosqueda-Melgar et al., 2007 | PEF |
| Orange juice | *S.* Typhimurium | 90 kV/cm and 55 °C | 5.0 log | Liang et al., (2002) | PEF |
| UHT Milk | *Salmonella spp.* | 600 MPa for 10 min and 21.5 °C | 6.5-8.2 log | Chen et al., 2006 | HPP |
| Orange juice | *Salmonella spp.* | 600 MPa and 20 °C | 7 log | Bull et al., 2004 | HPP |
| Sliced Ham | *S.* Typhimurium | 2 kGy | 3.78 | Song et al., 2011 | Electron beam |
| Sliced Ham | *S.* Typhimurium | 8000 J/ $m^2$ | 2.02 logs | Chun et al., 2009 | UV-C |

Table 2. Inactivation of *Salmonella* spp. achieved by application of non-thermal techniques in foods

## 4. Non thermal approaches

### 4.1 Application of radiation

#### 4.1.1 Irradiation

The use of ionizing radiation as a means of food preservation is being extensively researched and is approved in many countries such as the United States, France, Netherlands and Canada. The use of radiation dose up to 7 kiloGray (kGy) has been sanctioned by WHO as safe. The critical target of ionizing radiation is the bacterial DNA. Gamma rays, X-rays and electron beam are the most common types of ionizing radiation. Gamma radiation is generated using radioactive isotopes such as cobalt-60 or Cesium-137 (FDA approved) whereas for electron beam high speed electrons are generated using electricity. Generation of X-rays involves interposition of a metal target between the food and the electron beam. The choice of use between e-beam and X-ray is typically made as an exchange between efficiency and product penetration depth. Unlike gamma radiation, the processing time using electron beam is very short and the technique does not produce radioactive waste. The effect of both techniques on the quality is minimal as no heat is generated during the process. However, electron beam can penetrate only up to 8 cm in foods which is its major limitation. Nonetheless both these techniques are being studied for eliminating *Salmonella*. Irradiation in the range of 2-3 kGy has been used for the elimination of *Salmonella* in meat products. Park et al. (2010) reported lower total aerobic counts in gamma rays treated beef sausage patties as compared to electron beam treated samples. Reduction of 3.78 and 2.04 logs has been reported using electron beam irradiation (2 kGy) for *S.* Typhimurium inoculated in sliced ham (Song et al., 2011) and powdered weaning foods (Hong et al., 2008), respectively whereas Martins et al., (2004) reported a 4 log reduction in a cocktail of *Salmonella* strains using 1.7 kGy in watercress thereby showing the applicability of gamma radiation in salad vegetables. Application of 3 kGy electron beam resulted in a reduction of 6.75 and 4.85 logs of *S.* Tennessee and *S.* Typhimurium inoculated in Peanut butter (Hvizdzak et al., 2010). In contrast, irradiation by electron beam was found to be an unacceptable method for destroying *Salmonella* on raw almonds (Prakash et al., 2010). A dose of 5 kGy was reported to be required for achieving a 4 log reduction whereas radiation intensity higher than 2.98 kGy induced significant sensory changes in raw almonds (Prakash et al., 2010). Mahmoud (2010) reported 3.7 logs reduction in *S.* enterica per tomato upon the application of 0.75 kGy X-rays. Increasing the dose to more than 1 kGy resulted in more than 5 logs reduction. X-ray has shown to result in more than 6 logs reduction in ready to eat shrimps (Mahmoud, 2009) and spinach leaves and shredded iceberg lettuce (Mahmoud et al., 2010). However, several adverse effects (lipid oxidation, textural degradation) caused by ionizing radiation have prevented this technology from being extended. Especially, lipid oxidation of meat products by irradiation is the most important factor for quality decline. An increase in the off-odors of irradiated ground pork and pork chops upon refrigerated storage were observed (Ohene-Adjei et al., 2004). The negative effects of gamma radiation on the appearance and color of chicken breasts, pork loin and beef loin, has also been reported (Kim et al., 2002). Additionally just like other inactivation techniques, *S.* Typhimurium has been reported to develop resistance against the radiation if the cells are repeatedly processed with electron beam at sub-lethal doses (Tesfai et al., 2011). Although irradiation has a high potential to be used for food preservation, its use is limited by an uncorroborated view that irradiated foods are not well accepted by the public as safe and desirable.

#### 4.1.2 Ultravoilet radiation

Irradiation using non-ionizing rays, especially ultraviolet (UV)-C (wavelengths of 220–300 nm with 90% emission at 253.7 nm) has been approved as a non thermal method by the U.S. Food and Drug Administration (FDA) for surface sterilization (US Food and Drug Administration (2007)). This technique has been used extensively to decontaminate food surfaces directly or other materials which come in contact with food surfaces. The main industrial application of UV is its use in disinfection of drinking water. The mechanism of action of UV light involves the interruption of bacterial replication due to the formation of thymine dimers in the bacterial chromosome either killing them or making them unable to reproduce.

Chun et al., (2009) reported a reduction of 2.02 logs of *S.* Typhimurium in sliced ham upon the application of 8000 $J/m^2$ of UV-C whereas in the case of chicken breasts a reduction of only 1.19 logs were observed upon the application of 5 $kJ/m^2$ UV-C radiation (Chun et al.,

2010). At the same time, storage of UV-C treated chicken breasts resulted in an increase in the TBARS values and a negligible change in the Hunter L, a and b values for the product. The effects of UV-C on the quality attributes and decontamination efficiency against *Salmonella* Enteritidis were evaluated in different egg fractions (de Souza and Fernández, 2011). In terms of quality attributes, UV-C did not affect the viscosity and the pH however, browning due to maillard reaction was detectable in egg yolk and whole egg at low UV-C doses. The TBARS value was not significantly different to untreated samples. At the same time, a reduction of 5.3, 3.3 and 3.8 log was achieved under dynamic conditions (9.22 J/cm$^2$, 39 min) in egg white, egg yolk and whole egg, respectively.

The main drawback of UV irradiation is that it is a surface sterilization method. The efficiency of the treatment will strongly depend on the actual location of the bacterial contaminant as well as the composition, surface topography and transmissivity of the food (Allende et al., 2006). Moreover, the penetration of UV in liquid foods will strongly depend on the characteristics of the liquid product. The presence of solid particles and other components can seriously hinder the penetration. In addition the actual physical arrangement, power and wavelength of the UV source will also play a significant role. Besides, care has to be taken while using short wave UV regarding the damage that it can cause to human eyes in addition to being a cause of skin cancers and burns in humans upon excessive exposure.

### 4.2 Application of pressure

#### 4.2.1 High pressure processing (HPP)

High pressure processing (HPP) is a food processing method involving the application of pressure throughout the food. The technique is independent of the shape of food and can be used for both solid and liquid samples. Pressures in the range of 100-800 MPa are generally applied with temperatures ranging from 0-100 °C. The main target for HPP is the bacterial cytoplasmic membrane. In addition to the loss of solute, enzyme inactivation and protein coagulation might also occur as a result of excess pressure. HPP technique has been used for reducing or eliminating *Salmonella* in foods or culture media. Reduction of 6.5-8.2 logs in *Salmonella* inoculated in UHT whole milk was achieved at a pressure of 600 MPa for 10 min and 21.5 °C (Chen et al., 2006). Several instances regarding the growth of *Salmonella* spp. on the surface of tomatoes have been reported. HPP has been applied for the removal of this bacterium from the tomatoes surface. Application of pressures in the range of 350-550 MPa has been reported to result in 0.46-3.67 log reduction in *S. enterica* serovar Braenderup inoculated on diced and whole tomatoes (Maitland et al., 2011). Exposure to a pressure of 550 MPa for 2 min resulted in a reduction of several *S. enterica* serovars (Baildon, Gaminara, Michigan and Typhimurium) in the range of 4 log cfu/ml or greater for broth, water and apple juice (Whitney et al., 2007). Time did not seem to be an important factor when HPP was applied in a chicken meat model system. Treatment at 400 MPa for 2 min and 20 °C resulted in an inactivation between 3.26 and 4.35 log in a chicken meat model system (Escriu and Mor-Mur, 2009). The applicability of HPP as a preservation method against *Salmonella* has also been evaluated for products with lower water activity such as raw almonds. Goodridge et al. (2006) studied the effect of continuous and oscillatory HPP treatment on the viability of two *Salmonella* Enteriditis strains (FDA and PT30) inoculated onto raw almonds. Continuous pressurization of raw almonds resulted in less than one log reduction whereas the oscillatory process provided 1.27 and 1.16 log reduction for FDA and PT30 strains, respectively. However, a reduction of 3.37 logs was achieved when the almonds were directly suspended in water and then given the treatment. The effect was attributed to the fact that low water activity provided a protective effect to the bacterial cells. Application of HPP to orange juice resulted in 7-log inactivation of *Salmonella* at 600 MPa and 20 °C (Bull et al., 2004) and 615MPa and 15 °C (Teo et al., 2001) for 60 s. At the same time, HPP was reported not to have any significant effect on the quality parameters of orange juice such as titratable acid content, °Brix, viscosity, alcohol insoluble acids, color, ascorbic acid and β-carotene concentrations (Bull et al., 2004).

However, the application of high pressure at high temperatures may result in undesirable changes in the quality of many foods. Moreover, in the case of meat products, high pressure can increase the susceptibility of meat products to attack by oxygen thus resulting in increased lipid oxidation. For instance, Ma et al. (2007) reported almost 5-fold increase in TBARS values after 7 days storage at 4 °C in beef exposed to a pressure ≥400MPa. In other studies, pressures higher than 300 or 400 MPa (at ambient temperatures) caused increased rate of oxidation in pork (Cheah and Ledward, 1996) and cod muscles (Angsupanich and Ledward, 1998), respectively. McArdle et al. (2011) reported detrimental effect of HPP at 600MPa on texture, oxidation and water binding properties of beef. However lower TBARS and cook loss for beef processed by HPP were obtained as compared to raw or conventional heat processed samples. Besides, HPP carried out at high temperatures can cause cell wall breakdown and result in loss of cell turgidity. In addition, large-scale industrial application will only be possible if the technique becomes economical. The treatment time and the pressures applied are the major factors involved in deciding the cost and in achieving the desirable microbial inactivation. Hence, it is important to optimize conditions wherein minimal pressure is applied for the shortest time so that a food product with a reasonable cost is obtained.

### 4.2.2 High pressure carbon dioxide (HPCD)

High pressure carbon dioxide (HPCD) is another upcoming treatment that is being extensively used as a non-thermal technique for food pasteurization. The process is not only environmentally friendly due to the non-toxic nature of carbon dioxide but also involves application of lower $CO_2$ pressure as compared to those employed for HPP. The use of lower pressures makes this technique an energy-saving process. The major factor involved in the destruction is $CO_2$ although pressure helps in greater penetration of $CO_2$ in the cells. Lethality imparted by pressurized $CO_2$ is a result of disassociation of $CO_2$ (in foods with high water content) into reactive ions such as carbonates ($CO_3^{2-}$), bicarbonates ($HCO_3^-$) and hydrogen ($H^+$). These reactive ionic species can then have an effect on the permeability of the cell membrane and properties of cell constituents. In addition, generation of carbonic acid ($H_2CO_3$) in the water present in food products further results in a reduction in the pH of the food products enhancing the penetration of $CO_2$ (Wei et al., 1991).

Studies involving the use of HPCD for the inactivation of *S.* Typhimurium (Kim et al., 2007; Erkmen and Karaman, 2001; Erkmen 2000; Wei et al., 1991) have clearly reported the microbial strain, pressure applied, pH of the medium, type of medium and temperature to be important factors for the inactivation. *S.* Typhimurium in orange juice was effectively reduced by 5-6 logs when subjected to continuous dense phase carbon dioxide (DPCD) for 10 min at 21–107 MPa and 25 °C (Kincal et al., 2005) whereas in another study reduction as high as 8 logs was achieved when the growth media was changed to physiological saline (PS) or phosphate buffer solution (Kim et al., 2007). Kim et al. (2007) also analyzed the structural changes in *S.* Typhimurium cells upon the application of super-critical $CO_2$. A complete loss of colony forming activity was observed for the treated cells with a formation of veins and small vesicles on the surface. TEM images showed the inner areas to be highly disrupted accompanied by a membrane deformation. In addition, shrinking and uneven dispersion of cytoplasmic materials was also observed (Figure 1). Liao et al. (2010) obtained a remarkable reduction of 5 logs for *S.* Typhimurium when carrot juice was subjected to DPCD treatment. Both temperature and pressure had a noticeable effect as the inactivation was enhanced with increasing pressure at a constant temperature or increasing temperature at a constant pressure. In contrast, inactivation of *S.* Typhimurium in PS or PS containing 10% brain–heart infusion (PS-BHI) broth was completed in 35 min in PS whereas it took 140 min in the case of PS-BHI (Erkmen, 2000). Besides, the previous study reported the presence of two phases during the destruction characterized by a slow rate of reduction in the cell number which increased sharply at the later stage. Erkmen and Karaman (2001) observed that the exposure time required to achieve the same level of *Salmonella* inactivation was drastically reduced as the pressure during the inactivation increased. Complete inactivation of *Salmonella* was reported in egg yolk, 94-98% in chicken meat strips and limited inactivation in whole egg at a pressure of 13.7 MPa at 35 °C for 2 h (Wei et al., 1991). The variation in the results clearly indicates the complex nature of food systems. A treatment of 14 MPa at 45 °C for 40 min resulted in a 34.48% and 32.74% reduction for *S.* Typhimurium in soy sauce and hot-pepper paste marinated pork products, respectively (Choi et al., 2009a). However, the technique is more suitable for liquid foods as the diffusion of $CO_2$ into solid samples becomes a limitation due to the absence of agitation in solid foods. Also, high concentrations of $CO_2$ can cause darkening of color of certain animal products due to the formation of metmyoglobin. Due to the complex nature of foods conflicting results are available on the effect of HPCD on sensory, chemical and physical properties of foods. In spite of the potential advantages of HPCD more research is needed to monitor and quantify sensory and chemical characteristics of foods undergoing this preservation technique.

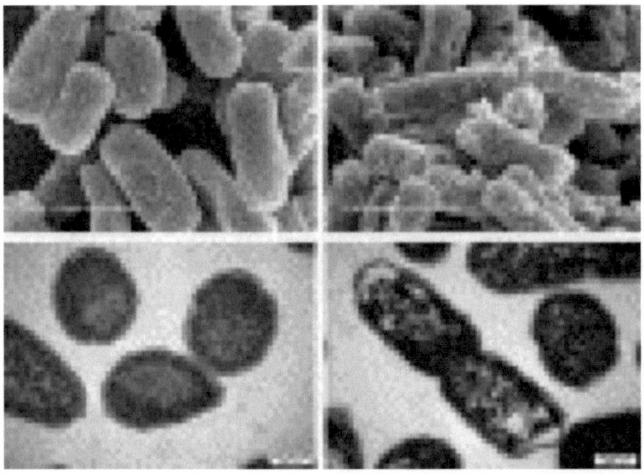

Fig. 1. Scanning electron micrograph (upper; magnification: 20,000) and Transmission electron micrograph (lower; magnification: 50,000) images of *S.* Typhimurium cells (left: untreated; right: treated) upon application of super critical carbon dioxide at 35°C and 100 bar for 30 min (Kim et al., 2007)

### 4.3 Pulsed electric field (PEF)

Pulsed electric field (PEF) is another non-thermal technology that can be used to inactivate bacterial cells at ambient temperatures. The process involves placing the food material between two electrodes and passing pulses of high electric field (1-50 kV/cm) strengths. Since the pulses are applied for short durations (2µs to 1 ms) the negative impact on food quality due to heat processing is highly diminished (Barbosa-Cánovas et al., 2001). The technique is more suitable for liquid or semi-liquid foods which can be easily pumped. It can be used to increase the shelf life of soups, milk, whole liquid eggs and fruit juices. PEF as a non-thermal preservation method has been implemented by Genesis Juices, Oregon, USA. The application of electric field results in cellular death due to generation of pores (electroporation) in the bacterial cell membrane without having an effect on enzymes or proteins present in foods (Wouters et al., 2001). The effectiveness of the technique will strongly depend on the treatment time, electric field strength and specific energy of the pulses. For instance, Monfort et al., (2010) achieved an inactivation of 4 log for *Salmonella* Typhimurium when 45 kV/cm of electric field was applied for 30 µs. Higher number of pulses and electric field was reported to be a stronger factor for reducing the number of *S.* Typhimurium population in orange juice (Liang et al., 2002) whereas in another study on melon and water melon juices, treatment time was found be a more important factor (Mosqueda-Melgar et al., 2007). Treatment of watermelon and melon juice with PEF resulted in a reduction of 4.27 log (at 2000 µs and 100 Hz) and 3.75 log (at 1250 µs and 175 Hz) of *S.* Enteritidis, respectively (Mosqueda-Melgar et al., 2007). In contrast, Liang et al. (2002) reported a 5 log reduction of *S.* Typhimurium in orange juice exposed to a PEF of 90 kV/cm at a temperature of 55 °C. However, the higher reduction could be a result of combination of higher acidity of orange juice in addition to relatively higher temperature and high intensity of the PEF applied. Although the technique is useful, inactivation has only been achieved in the range of 3-4 logs.

### 4.4 Natural antimicrobials

Since ancient times, spices and herbs have been used for preventing food spoilage and deterioration, and also for extending food shelf life. The antimicrobial effect of these components is a result of an increase in the permeability of the cytoplasmic membrane which leads to the loss of cellular constituents. At the same time, plant secondary metabolites such as essential oils and natural plant extracts have also been reported to have antibacterial, antifungal and anti-insecticidal properties. Extracts from capsicum, seaweeds and green tea have been found to inhibit the growth of *Salmonella* spp. in-vitro. Studies are also available wherein inhibitory effect of plant extracts was evaluated against *Salmonella* inoculated in minced beef, salad vegetables, fresh cut apples and minced sheep meat.

#### 4.4.1 Extracts from vegetables

Vegetable extracts have shown a good potential when applied under laboratory conditions in culture media. For instance, application of 6% seaweed extract was shown to result in complete inhibition of *S. abony* whereas 3% extract resulted in 93% inhibition (Gupta et al., 2011). In contrast, 2.8% methanolic extract from Irish York cabbage was shown to result in only 64% inhibition of *S. abony* (Jaiswal et al., 2011). Xu et al. (2007) reported a minimal inhibitory concentration (MIC) of 15µl of grapefruit seed extract to inhibit *Salmonella*. Careaga et al. (2003) reported that a minimum concentration of 1.5 ml of capsicum extract per 100g of meat was needed in order to prevent the growth of *S.* Typhimurium inoculated in minced beef. Karapinar and Sengun (2007) evaluated the antimicrobial activity of koruk (unripe grape— *Vitis vinifera*) juice against *S.* Typhimurium on cucumber and parsley samples which resulted in 1-1.5 log reduction upon immediate contact with korak juice and the reduction increased as the time of exposure of the vegetables to the juice increased.

The antimicrobial efficacy of plant extracts has been attributed to the presence of phenolic compounds, quinones, alkaloids, flavanols/flavonoids and lectins. Solubility of the extract in the food systems and the pH of the extract are important factors determining their efficacy in foods. Mechanism of action of these phenolic compounds involves alteration in the cell morphology which results in a disruption of the cytoplasmic membrane and leakage of cell constituents. Although the use of vegetable extracts for controlling the growth of *Salmonella* is promising the actual application in foods is in its budding stage.

#### 4.4.2 Extracts of herbs and spices

In addition to providing flavor and fragrance, spices and herbs have also antimicrobial potential and thus can be used for preventing food deterioration and shelf life extension. Sumac, rosemary, sage, basil and ginger are some of the spices commonly being used for imparting antimicrobial effects on food. The flower, buds, leaf, stem or bark of these plants contains aromatic oily liquid which is the essential oil (EO). These EO are rich in phytochemicals such as terpenoids, polyphenols, flavonoids, antocyanin and organic acids which are responsible for the antimicrobial activity. Compounds such as carvacrol, citral, thymol, eugenol and citric acid have been shown to inhibit the growth of *Salmonella*. Eugenol has been reported to strongly inhibit the growth of *Listeria monocytogenes, Salmonella Enteritidis, Escherichia coli* and *Staphylococcus aureus*. Carvacrol and thymol are reported to be the principal constituents of EO of certain herbs. Burt et al. (2007) evaluated the antimicrobial activity of carvacrol vapour against *S.* Enteritidis on pieces of raw chicken. UV sterilized chicken pieces treated with carvacrol vapour (2 µl) showed reduced viable numbers of salmonellae at 4, 20 and 37 °C and a concentration of 4 µl resulted in a complete elimination of all viable cells in a minimum of 3 h at 37 °C. Govaris et al. (2010) studied the antimicrobial effect of oregano EO, nisin and their combination against *S.* Enteritidis in minced sheep meat during refrigerated storage (4 or 10 °C) for 12 days. Addition of nisin, at 500 or 1000 IU/g, proved insufficient to inhibit *S.* Enteritidis. The addition of oregano EO at 0.9% caused the population of *S.* Enteritidis to be maintained below 1 log cfu/g whereas a combination of 0.9% oregano EO and nisin at 500 or 1000 IU/g showed a bactericidal effect. The addition of 0.6% or 0.9% EO was found to be organoleptically acceptable also. EOs have also been applied for the elimination of *Salmonella* on fresh tomatoes. Gündüz et al. (2010) tested the antimicrobial potential of essential oil extracts on tomatoes. The tomatoes were inoculated with the nalidixic acid resistant strain of *Salmonella* Typhimurium ATCC 13311 and treated for 5-20 min with water extracts of sumac or oregano oil. Tomatoes treated with 100 ppm oregano or 4% sumac extract resulted in 2.78 and 2.38 log reduction, respectively. Hayouni et al. (2008) studied the antimicrobial effect of extracts from *Salvia officinalis* L. and berries of *Schinus molle* L against *S. anatum* or *S.* Enteritidis inoculated on minced beef meat. Concentrations in the range of 0.02-0.1% showed bacteriostatic effect against both the bacteria by the extracts from *S. officinalis* and *S. molle* for over 15 days. In case of *S. molle,* the bacteriostatic effect was seen up to a concentration of 1%. At concentrations higher than 1.5% for *S. officinalis* and 2% for *S. molle,* immediate bactericidal effect was observed with a 2.6 log cfu /g reduction at 1.5% *S. officinalis* and 1 log cfu/g at 2% *S. molle.* However, sensory analysis of meat containing more than 2% of *S. molle* and 1.5% of *S. officinalis* showed a distinguished effect on the flavour and taste. In order to reduce the amount of EO being used, combinations of EO with NaCl were studied. The use of 0.1% or 1.5% *S. officinalis* with 6% or 4% NaCl or 0.1% or 1.5% *S. molle* with 4 or 8% Nacl could effectively eliminate *S. anatum* from refrigerated raw beef (Hayouni et al., 2008). The positive effect of spices on the inactivation of *S.* Typhimurium DT104 was observed when in direct contact, however, the activity reduced when added to food system such as ground beef (Uhart et al., 2006). Utilization of packaging materials containing these antimicrobial compounds is also becoming an attractive option in the food industry. However, a major limitation in using the EO in foods is the effect they have on the sensory properties of foods. At times, the concentration required to show the antimicrobial effect can surpass the organoleptically levels resulting in alteration in the flavor of foods.

## 5. Hurdle technology or synergism

Hurdle approach or the process of using multiple technologies is an effective approach to improve microbial decontamination in comparison to that of a single technology alone. Deliberate and intelligent combination of preservative treatments can help in maintaining the quality of food and delivering almost similar levels of microbial destruction as conventional methods alone. At the same time it warranties to counteract the negative effect of individual technologies on food quality. The choice of hurdles will strongly depend on the type of food it is being applied to in addition to the mode of inactivation. Potential synergistic effects among different technologies have been reported to be more effective than individual technologies applied alone. The outer membrane of gram negative cells prevents the entry of hydrophobic compounds. A combined treatment of heat and irradiation can result in sub-lethal injury to the cells. The sublethally injured cells can be more vulnerable to attack by antimicrobial compounds thereby reducing the dose of each individual technique.

For instance, combined effect of UV-C (0.5 J/cm$^2$) and potassium lactate, lauric arginate ester and sodium diacetate (FDA approved) resulted in a 3.6-4.1 log reduction of *Salmonella, L. monocytogenes* and *Staphylococcus aureus* on the surface of frankfurters (12 weeks storage at 10 °C). In addition, UV-C and antimicrobials had no significant impact on frankfurter color or texture (Sommers et al., 2010). Amiali et al. (2007) studied the synergistic effects of temperature, treatment time and electric field strength on inactivation of *S.* Enteritidis and *Escherichia coli* O157:H7 in egg yolk. A 5 log reduction in the population of *E. coli* O157:H7 and *S. enteritidis* was observed at an electric field of 30 kV cm$^{-1}$ and 40 °C.

Exposure of egg shells contaminated with *S.* Enteritidis with UV radiation (1,500 to 2,500 µW/cm$^2$) followed by ozone (5 lb/in$^2$ gauge for 1 min) resulted in an inactivation of 4.6 logs or more in a total treatment time of 2 min (Roriguez-Romo and Yousef, 2005). Although the individual treatments resulted in similar reductions, however exposure time and pressure were comparatively higher. Combined treatment of lactic and acetic acid with super critical $CO_2$ resulted in 2.33 log cfu/cm$^2$ reduction in *S.* Typhimurium in fresh pork which was higher as compared to these treatments being applied individually (Choi et al., 2009b).

Application of PEF (25kV/cm, 250 µs in pulses of 2.12 µs) followed by heat treatment at 55 °C for 3.5 min increased the inactivation of *Salmonella* Enteritidis inoculated into liquid whole egg from 1 logs to 4.3 logs (Hermawan et al., 2004). The combination treatment had no effect on the color, pH, viscosity and brix of the treated samples and had a longer shelf life in comparison to heat treated samples.

High pressure applied in combination with other agents such as heat or antimicrobial agents can be effectively used to increase microbial inactivation. Individual and combined effects of HPP and nisin treatment on relative resistance, viability and cellular components on *S.* Enteritidis (strains: FDA and OSU 799) was evaluated in culture media. High pressure up to 200MPa and nisin (200 IU/ml) when applied separately did not have any effect on the viability of either strain. However, application of high pressure (500 MPa) or a combination of nisin with a pressure of 350MPa (OSU 799 strain) and 400 MPa (FDA strain) resulted in an 8 log reduction (Lee and Kaletunç, 2010). Penetration of nisin into the cells was assisted by the pressure and thereafter the additive effect of two hurdles resulted in inactivation to be achieved at a lower value than when the technique was applied separately. Viedma et al. (2008) studied the synergistic effects of antimicrobial peptide enterocin AS-48 and high-intensity-PEF treatment (35 kV/cm, 150 Hz, 4 µs and bipolar mode) on the inhibition of *S. enterica* CECT 915 in apple juice. A combination of high intensity PEF (1000 µs) and AS-48 (60 µg/ml) and a treatment temperature of 40 °C resulted in 4.5 log reduction. The sequence of the synergistic treatments was an important factor as the inhibition was observed only when HIPEF was applied in the presence of previously-added bacteriocin. Since both, enterocin AS-48 and high pressure PEF, act on the bacterial cytoplasmic membrane, synergism between them could be a result of enhanced permeability of bacterial cytoplasmic membrane.

## 6. Conclusion

With the rise of the concept of "green consumerism", meeting the consumer demand for nutritious and fresh food in addition to providing food safety has increased interest in non thermal preservation methods. The literature described herein gives an account of some of the non-thermal methods used for the elimination of *Salmonella* from foods. Considering the wide range of conditions under which *Salmonella* can easily grow, it is imperative to apply a combination of intervention technologies. With the advent of these novel methods of food preservation, it is hoped that issues of spoilage and contamination of food products, not only with *Salmonella* spp. but also with many other food spoilage or pathogenic micro-organisms could be effectively controlled. Besides, a major impediment in the acceptance of foods processed by these emerging technologies is a lack of information among the consumers. Thus, it is very important to provide proper knowledge to the consumers regarding the benefits of these technologies as a means of food preservation.

## 7. References

Allende, A., McEvoy, J.L., Luo, Y., Artés, F., & Wang, C.Y. (2006). Effectiveness of two-sided UV-C treatment in inhibiting natural microflora and extending the shelf-life of minimally processed 'Red Oak Leaf' lettuce. Food *Microbiology,* Vol. 23, No. 3, (May 2006), pp. 241–249, ISSN 0740-0020

Amiali, M., Ngadi, M.O., Smith, J.P., & Raghavan, G.S.V. (2007). Synergistic effect of temperature and pulsed electric field on inactivation of *Escherichia coli* O157:H7 and *Salmonella enteritidis* in liquid egg yolk. *Journal of Food Engineering*, Vol. 79, No. 2, (March 2007), pp. 689-694, ISSN 0260-8774.

Angsupanich K., & Ledward, D.A. (1998). High pressure treatment effects on cod (*Gadus morhua*) muscle. *Food Chemistry*, Vol. 63, No. 1, (September 1998), pp. 39–50, ISSN 0308-8146

Barbosa-Canovas, G.V., Pierson, M.D., Zhang, Q.H., & Schaffner, D.W. (2001). Pulsed electric fields. *Journal of Food Science*, pp. 65–79 Supplement, ISSN 1750-3841

Bouwknegt, M., Dam-Deisz, W.D.C., Schouten, J.M., Wannet, W.J.B., Van Pelt, W., Visser, G., van de Giessen, A. W., *Surveillance of zoonotic bacteria in farm animals in the Netherlands* (2003) Results from January 1998 until December 2000. (RIVM report 285859013, available from *www.rivm.nl*) Accessed on 2 July 2011, http://www.rivm.nl/bibliotheek/rapporten/285859013.pdf

Bull, M.K., Zerdin, K., Howe, E., Goicoechea, D., Paramanandhan, P., Stockman, R., Sellahewa, J., Szabo, S.A., Johnson, R.L., & Stewart, C.M. (2004). The effect of high pressure processing on the microbial, physical and chemical properties of Valencia and Navel orange juice. *Innovative Food Science and Emerging Technologies*, Vol. 5, No. 2, (June 2004), pp. 135-149, ISSN 1466-8564

Burt, S.A., Fledderman, M.J., Haagsman, H.P., van Knapen, F., & Veldhuizen, E.J.A. (2007). Inhibition of *Salmonella enterica* serotype Enteritidis on agar and raw chicken by carvacrol vapour. *International Journal of Food Microbiology*, Vol. 119, No. 3, (November 2007), pp. 346-350, ISSN 0168-1605

Careaga, M., Fernández, E., Dorantes, L., Mota, L., Jaramillo, M.E., & Hernandez-Sanchez, H. (2003). Antibacterial activity of *Capsicum* extract against Salmonella *typhimurium* and *Pseudomonas aeruginosa* inoculated in raw beef meat. *International Journal of Food Microbiology*, Vol. 83, No. 3, (June 2003), pp. 331-335, ISSN 0168-1605

Cheah, P.B., & Ledward, D.A. (1996). High pressure effects on lipid oxidation in minced pork. *Meat Science*, Vol. 43, No. 2, (June 1996), pp. 123–134, ISSN 0309-1740

Chen, H., Guan, D., & Hoover, D.G. (2006). Sensitivities of food-borne pathogens to pressure changes. *Journal of Food Protection*, Vol. 69, No. 1, (January 2006), pp. 130–136, ISSN 0362-028X

Choi, Y.M., Bae, Y.Y., Kim, K.H., Kim, B.C., & Rhee, M.S. (2009a). Effects of supercritical carbon dioxide treatment against generic *Escherichia coli, Listeria monocytogenes, Salmonella typhimurium*, and *E. coli* O157:H7 in marinades and marinated pork. *Meat Science*, Vol. 82, No. 4, (August 2009), pp. 419–424, ISSN 0309-1740

Choi, Y.M., Kim, O.Y., Kim, K.H., Kim, B.C., & Rhee, M.S. (2009b). Combined effect of organic acids and supercritical carbon dioxide treatments against nonpathogenic *Escherichia coli, Listeria monocytogenes, Salmonella typhimurium* and *E. coli* O157:H7 in fresh pork. *Letters in Applied Microbiology*, Vol. 49, No. 4, (October 2009), pp. 510-515, ISSN 0266-8254.

Chun, H.H., Kim, J.Y., Chung, K.S., Won, M., & Song, K.B. (2009). Inactivation kinetics of *Listeria monocytogenes, Salmonella enterica* serovar Typhimurium, and *Campylobacter jejuni* in ready-to-eat sliced ham using UV-C irradiation. Meat Science, Vol. 83, No. 4, (December 2009), pp. 599-603, ISSN 0309-1740

Chun, H.H., Kim, J.Y., Lee, B.D., Yu, D.J., & Song, K.B. (2010). Effect of UV-C irradiation on the inactivation of inoculated pathogens and quality of chicken breasts during storage. *Food Control*, Vol. 21, No. 3, (March 2010), pp. 276-280, ISSN 0956-7135

de Souza, P.M., & Fernández, A. (2011). Effects of UV-C on physicochemical quality attributes and *Salmonella enteritidis* inactivation in liquid egg products. *Food Control*, Vol. 22, No. 8, (August 2011), pp. 1385-1392, ISSN: 0956-7135

Erkmen, O. (2000). Inactivation of *Salmonella typhimurium* by high pressure carbon dioxide. *Food Microbiology*, Vol. 17, No. 2, (April 2000), pp. 225-232, ISSN: 0740-0020

Erkmen, O., & Karaman, H., (2001). Kinetic studies on the high pressure carbon dioxide inactivation of *Salmonella* typhimurium. *Journal of Food Engineering*, Vol. 50, No. 1, (October 2001), pp. 25–28, ISSN 0260-8774

EFSA (2009). The community summary report on food-borne outbreaks in the European Union in 2007. ESFA Journal, (available at efsa.europa.eu), Accessed on 29 June 2011, http://www.efsa.europa.eu/en/efsajournal/pub/271r.htm

EFSA-ECDC, (2007). EFSA-ECDC report for 2007: Salmonella remains most common cause of food-borne outbreaks, (available at efsa.europa.eu), Accessed on 25 June 2011, http://www.efsa.europa.eu/en/press/news/zoonoses090506.htm

Escriu, R., & Mor-Mur, M. (2009). Role of quantity and quality of fat in meat models inoculated with *Listeria innocua* or *Salmonella Typhimurium* treated by high pressure and refrigerated stored. *Food Microbiology*, Vol. 26, No. 8, (December 2009), pp. 834–840, ISSN 0740-0020

FDA, 2001. Food and Drug Administration (FDA) final rule-66 FR 6137, Hazard analysis and critical control point (HACCP) procedures for the safe and sanity processing of juice. *Federal Register*, date of access 10 July 2011 http://www.fda.gov/Food/FoodSafety/HazardAnalysisCriticalControlPointsHACCP/JuiceHACCP/ucm073594.htm

Goodridge, L.D., Willford, J., & Kalchayanand, N. (2006). Destruction of *Salmonella Enteriditis* inoculated onto raw almonds by high hydrostatic pressure. *Food Research International*, Vol. 39, No. 4, (May 2006), pp. 408–412, ISSN 0963-9969

Govaris, A., Solomakos, N., Pexara, N., & Chatzopoulou, P.S. (2010). The antimicrobial effect of oregano essential oil, nisin and their combination against *Salmonella* Enteritidis in minced sheep meat during refrigerated storage. *International Journal of Food Microbiology*, Vol. 137, No. 2-3, (February 2010), pp. 175-180, ISSN 0168-1605.

Gündüz, G.T., Gönül, S.A., & Karapinar, M. (2010). Efficacy of sumac and oregano in the inactivation of *Salmonella* Typhimurium on tomatoes. *International Journal of Food Microbiology*, Vol. 141, No.1-2, (June 2010), pp. 39-44, ISSN 0168-1605

Gupta, S., Cox, S., Rajauria, G., Jaiswal, A.K., & Abu-Ghannam, N. (2011). Growth inhibition of common food spoilage and pathogenic micro-organisms in the presence of brown seaweed extracts. *Food and Bioprocess Technology*, (DOI: 10.1007/s11947-010-0502-6), ISSN 1935-5130

Hayouni, E.A., Chraief, I., Abedrabba, M., Bouix, M., Leveau, J.Y., Mohammed, M., & Hamdi, M. (2008). Tunisian *Salvia officinalis* L. and *Schinus molle* L. essential oils: Their chemical compositions and their preservative effects against *Salmonella* inoculated in minced beef meat. *International Journal of Food Microbiology*, Vol. 125, No. 3, (July 2008), pp. 242-251, ISSN 0168-1605

Hermawan, N., Evrendilek, G.A., Dantzer, W.R., Zhang, Q.H., & Richter, E.R. (2004). Pulsed electric field treatment of liquid whole egg inoculated with *Salmonella* enteritidis. *Journal of Food Safety*, Vol. 24, No. 1, (April 2004), pp. 71-85, ISSN 0149-6085

Hong, Y.H., Park, J.Y., Park, J.H., Chung, M.S., Kwon, K.S., Chung, K., Won, M., & Song, K.B. (2008). Inactivation of *Enterobacter sakazakii, Bacillus cereus,* and *Salmonella typhimurium* in powdered weaning food by electron-beam irradiation. *Radiation Physics and Chemistry*, Vol. 77, No. 9, (September 2008), pp. 1097-1100, ISSN: 0969-806X

Hvizdzak, A.L., Beamer, S., Jaczynski, J., & Matak, K.E. (2010). Use of electron beam radiation for the reduction of *Salmonella* enteric serovars typhimurium and Tennessee in peanut butter. *Journal of Food Protection,* Vol. 73, No. 2, (February 2010), pp. 353-357, ISSN 0362-028X

Jaiswal, A.K., Gupta, S., Abu-Ghannam, N., & Cox, S. (2011). Application of Baranyi function to model the antibacterial properties of solvent extract from Irish York cabbage against food spoilage and pathogenic bacteria. *Food Science and Technology International,* (DOI 10.1177/1082013210399667), ISSN 1532-1738

Karapinar, M., & Sengun, I.Y. (2007). Antimicrobial effect of koruk (unripe grape—*Vitis vinifera*) juice against *Salmonella typhimurium* on salad vegetables. *Food Control,* Vol. 18, No. 6, (June 2007), pp. 702-706, ISSN 0956-7135

Kim, Y.H., Nam, K.C., & Ahn, D.U. (2002). Color, oxidation–reduction potential, and gas production of irradiated meat from different animal species. *Journal of Food Science,* Vol. 67, No. 5, (June 2002), pp. 1692–1695, ISSN 1750-3841

Kim, S.R., Rhee, M.S., Kim, B.C., Lee, H.J., &Kim, K.H. (2007). Modeling of the inactivation of *Salmonella typhimurium* by supercritical carbon dioxide in physiological saline and phosphate-buffered saline. *Journal of Microbiological Methods,* Vol. 70, No. 1, (July 2007), pp. 132–141, ISSN 0167-7012

Kincal, D., Hill, W.S., Balaban, M.O., Portier, K.M., Wei, C.I., & Marshall, M.R. (2005). A continuous high pressure carbon dioxide system for microbial reduction in orange juice. *Journal of Food Science,* Vol. 70, No. 5, (June 2005), pp. M249–M254, ISSN 1750-3841

Lee, J., & Kaletunç, J. (2010). Inactivation of *Salmonella* Enteritidis strains by combination of high hydrostatic pressure and nisin. *International Journal of Food Microbiology*, Vol. 140, No. 1, (May 2010), pp. 49-56, ISSN 0168-1605

Liang, Z., Mittal, G.S., & Griffiths, M.W. (2002). Inactivation of *Salmonella* Typhimurium in orange juice containing antimicrobial agents by pulsed electric field. *Journal of Food Protection*, Vol. 65, No. 7, (July 2002), pp. 1081–1087, ISSN 0362-028X

Liao, H., Kong, X., Zhang, Z., Liao, X., &, Hu, X. (2010). Modeling the inactivation of *Salmonella typhimurium* by dense phase carbon dioxide in carrot juice. *Food Microbiology,* Vol. 27, No. 1, (February 2010), pp. 94-100, ISSN 0740-0020

Ma, H.J., Ledward, D.A., Zamri, A.I., Frazier, R.A., & Zhou, G.H. (2007). Effects of high pressure / thermal treatment on lipid oxidation in beef & chicken muscle. *Food Chemistry*, Vol. 104, No. 4, (2007), pp. 1575–1579, ISSN 0308-8146

Mahmoud, B.S.M. (2009). Effect of X-ray treatments on inoculated *Escherichia coli* O157:H7, *Salmonella enterica, Shigella flexneri* and *Vibrio parahaemolyticus* in ready-to-eat shrimp. *Food Microbiology, Vol.* 26, No. 8, (December 2009), pp. 860–864, ISSN 0740-0020

Mahmoud, B.S.M., Bachman, G., & Linton, R.H. (2010). Inactivation of *Escherichia coli* O157:H7, *Listeria monocytogenes, Salmonella enterica* and *Shigella flexneri* on spinach leaves by X-ray. *Food Microbiology, Vol.* 27, No. 1 (February 2010), pp. 24–28, ISSN 0740-0020

Mahmoud, B.S.M. (2010). The effects of X-ray radiation on *Escherichia coli* O157:H7, *Listeria monocytogenes, Salmonella enterica* and *Shigella flexneri* inoculated on whole Roma tomatoes. Food microbiology, Vol. 27, No. 8, (December 2010), pp. 1057-1063, ISSN 0740-0020

Maitland, J.E., Boyer, R.R., Eifert, J.D., & Williams, R.C. (2011). High hydrostatic pressure processing reduces *Salmonella enterica* serovars in diced and whole tomatoes. *International Journal of Food Microbiology,* doi:10.1016/j.ijfoodmicro.2011.05.024, ISSN 0168-1605

Martins, C.G., Behrens, J.H., Destro, M.T., Franco, B.D.G.M., Vizeu, D.M., Hutzler, B., & Landgraf, M. (2004). Gamma radiation in the reduction of *Salmonella* spp. inoculated on minimally processed watercress (*Nasturtium officinalis*). *Radiation Physics and Chemistry*, Vol. 71, No. 1-2, (September –October 2004), pp. 89-93, ISSN 0969-806X

McArdle, R.A., Marcos, B., Kerry, J.P., & Mullen, A.M. (2011). Influence of HPP conditions on selected beef quality attributes and their stability during chilled storage. *Meat Science*, Vol. 87, No. 3, (March 2011), pp. 274-281, ISSN 0309-1740

Monfort, S., Gayán, E., Saldaña, G., Puértolas, E., Condón, S., Raso, J., & Álvarez, I. (2010). Inactivation of *Salmonella* Typhimurium and *Staphylococcus aureus* by pulsed electric fields in liquid whole egg. *Innovative Food Science and Emerging Technologies*, Vol. 11, No. 2, (April 2010), pp. 306-313, ISSN 1466-8564

Mosqueda-Melgar, J., Raybaudi-Massilia, R.M., & Martín-Belloso, O. (2007). Influence of treatment time and pulse frequency on *Salmonella* Enteritidis, *Escherichia coli* and *Listeria monocytogenes* populations inoculated in melon and watermelon juices treated by pulsed electric fields. *International Journal of Food Microbiology.* Vol. 117, No.2, (June 2007), pp.192-200, ISSN 0168-1605

Ohene-Adjei, S., Bertol, T., Hyung, Y., Ellis, M., McKeith, F.K., & Brewer, M.S. (2004). Effect of vitamin E, low dose irradiation and display time on the quality of pork. Meat *Science*, Vol. 68, No. 1, (September 2004), pp. 19–26

Park, J.G., Yoon, Y., Park, J.N., Han, I.J., Song, B.S., Kim, J.H., Kim, W.G., Hwang, H.J., Han, S.B., & Lee, J.W. (2010). Effects of gamma irradiation and electron beam irradiation on quality, sensory, and bacterial populations in beef sausage patties. *Meat Science*, Vol. 85, No.2, (June 2010), pp. 368-372, ISSN 0309-1740

Prakash, A., Lim, F.T., Duong, C., Caporaso, F., & Foley, D. (2010). The effects of ionizing irradiation on *Salmonella* inoculated on almonds and changes in sensory properties. *Radiation Physics and Chemistry*, Vol. 79, No. 4, (April 2010), pp. 502-506, ISSN 0969-806X

Risco, S.A.D. (2009). *Risk factors influencing the growth and survival of Salmonella on poultry products*. Ph.D. thesis, Rutgers The State University of New Jersey - New Brunswick. 140 pages

Roriguez-Romo, L.A., & Yousef, A.E. (2005). Inactivation of Salmonella enteric serovar enteritidis on shell eggs by ozone and UV radiation. *Journal of Food Protection*, Vol. 68, No. 4, (April 2005), pp. 711-717, ISSN 0362-028X

Sommers, C. H., Scullen, O. J., & Sites, J. E. (2010). Inactivation of foodborne pathogens on frankfurters using ultraviolet light and GRAS antimicrobials. *Journal of Food Safety*, Vol. 30, No. 3, (August 2010), pp. 668–678, ISSN 0149-6085.

Song, H.J., Lee, J.H., & Song, K.B. (2011). Effects of irradiation and fumaric acid treatment on the inactivation of *Listeria monocytogenes* and *Salmonella typhimurium* inoculated on sliced ham. *Radiation Physics and Chemistry*, doi:10.1016/j.radphyschem.2011.06.012, ISSN 0969-806X

Tahergorabi, R., Matak, K.E., & Jaczynski, J. (2011). Application of electron beam to inactivate *Salmonella* in food: Recent developments. *Food Research International*, doi:10.1016/j.foodres.2011.02.003, ISSN 0963-9969

Teo, A.Y., Ravishankar, S., & Sizer, C.E. (2001). Effect of low-temperature, high-pressure treatment on the survival of *Escherichia coli* O157:H7 and *Salmonella* in unpasteurised fruit juices. *Journal of Food Protection*, Vol. 64, No. 8, (August 2001), pp. 1122–1127, ISSN 0362-028X

Tesfai, A.T., Beamer, S.K., Matak, K.E., & Jaczynski, J. (2011). Microbial radio-resistance of Salmonella Typhimurium in egg increases due to repetitive irradiation with electron beam. *Radiation Physics and Chemistry*, Vol. 80, No. 4, (April 2011), pp. 591-596, ISSN 0969-806X

Uhart, M., Maks, N., & Ravishankar, S. (2006). Effect of spices on growth and survival of Salmonella typhimurium DT 104 in ground beef stored at 4 and 8 °C. *Journal of Food Safety*, Vol. 26, No. 2, (May 2006), pp. 115-125, ISSN 0149-6085.

USFDA, (2007). US Food and Drug Administration, 2007 (http://www.fda.gov/Food/FoodIngredientsPackaging/IrradiatedFoodPackaging/ucm110564.htm#authors) Accessed on 15 June 2011

Viedma, P.M., López, A.S., Omar, N.B., Abriouel, H., López, S.L., Valdivia, E., Belloso, O.M., & Gálvez, A. (2008). Enhanced bactericidal effect of enterocin AS-48 in combination with high-intensity pulsed-electric field treatment against *Salmonella enterica* in apple juice. *International Journal Food Microbiology*, Vol. 128, No. 2, (December 2008), pp. 244-249, ISSN 0168-1605

Wei, C.I., Balaban, M.O., Fernando. S.Y., & Peplow, A.J. (1991). Bacterial effect of high pressure $CO_2$ treatment on foods spiked with *Listeria* and *Salmonella. Journal of Food Protection,* Vol. 54, (1991), pp. 189–193, ISSN 0362-028X

Whitney, B.M., Williams, R., Eifert, J., & Marcy, J. (2007). High- pressure resistance variation of *Escherichia coli* O157:H7 strains and Salmonella serovars in tryptic soy broth, distilled water, and fruit juice. *Journal of* Food *Protection*, Vol. 70, No. 9, (September 2007), pp. 2078–2083, ISSN 0362-028X

Wouters, P., Álvarez, I., &. Raso, J. (2001). Critical factors determining inactivation kinetics by pulsed electric field food processing. *Trends in Food Science & Technology,* Vol. 12, No. 3-4, (March 2001), pp. 112–121, ISSN 0924-2244

Xu, W., Qu, W., Huang, K., Guo, F., Yang, J., Zhao, H., & Luo, Y.B. (2007). Antibacterial effect of Grapefruit Seed Extract on food-borne pathogens and its application in the preservation of minimally processed vegetables. *Postharvest Biology and Technology,* Vol. 45, No. 1, (July 2007), pp. 126-133, ISSN 0925-5214.

# 14

# Use Thyme Essential Oils for the Prevention of Salmonellosis

Abderrahmane Romane[1], Rajae Harrak[2] and Fouad Bahri[3]
[1]*CadiAyyad University/Marrakech*
[2]*Laboratory of Hygiene and Epidemiology/Marrakech*
[3]*University of Abdelhamid Ben Badis/Mostaganem*
[1,2]*Morocco*
[3]*Algeria*

## 1. Introduction

Over sixty percent (60%) of poisoning in the world are caused by Salmonella. Salmonellosis is thus become a public health event which justifies the involvement of the World Health Organization (WHO) in the fight against Salmonella (Salm-Surv, 2005). Salmonellosis is a foodborne illness of the most common and widespread. It represents a significant burden to public health and a considerable cost to society in many countries. Each year, millions of cases are reported worldwide, causing thousands of deaths. This disease is caused by the bacterium Salmonella (Salmonella). We know now more than 2500 types, or serotypes of Salmonella. The genus Salmonella, which belongs to the *Enterobacteriaceae* family, is named by Dr. Daniel Elmer Salmon American Veterinary even if the scientist who discovered the type was Theobald Smith, co-worked with Dr. Salmon in the Bureau of Animal Industry (BAI) in 1884 (Brown, 1935).
In 1880 Eberth discovered the causative agent of typhoid fever. The culture of this bacterium was considered in 1884 by Gaffky. The genus Salmonella was used after the bacteriologist Dr. Daniel Salmon had isolated in 1886 a bacterium from the pig (Salmonella choleraesuis), which was considered the cause of swine fever (hog cholera) (Encarta Encyclopedia 2004). In 1896 Widal showed the antigenic diversity of strains of salmonella. Now, more than 2500 Salmonella serotypes were isolated. Since the first observations reported by Eberth until now, the genus Salmonella has continued to have considerable importance in the veterinary and medical domain, both in economic losses due to animal disease, and by the high incidence on humans, typhoid fever and food poisoning salmonella (Bornert, 2000).

## 2. Taxonomy

| | |
|---|---|
| Domain: | Bacteria |
| Phylum: | Proteobacteria |
| Class: | Gammaproteobacteria |
| Order: | Enterobacteriale |
| Family: | *Enterobacteriaceae* |
| Genre: | *Salmonella* |

The nomenclature of salmonella recognizes that the genre has three *Salmonella* species (Le Minor and Popoff, 1987, Reeves et al. Nov.1989):
*Salmonella bongori; Salmonella enterica* or *Salmonella choleraesuis* and *Salmonella subterranea* (Shelob olina et al., 2004).
The second most important species includes six subspecies (Grimont et al., 2000): *Salmonella enterica* subsp. *Arizonae; Salmonella enterica* subsp. *Diarizonae; Salmonella enterica* subsp. *Enterica; Salmonella enterica* subsp. *Houtenae; Salmonella enterica* subsp. *Indica* and *Salmonella enterica* subsp. *salamae.*
With this division into species and sub-species actually, 2541 serotypes are recognized officially. These result from multiple combinations of somatic O polysaccharide in nature, flagellar H antigens, protein in nature and, finally, capsular (Vi). Genetic determinants of these factors are stable enough to perform reliable epidemiological surveys. The type of classification based on the O and H antigens is called the Kauffmann-White scheme (Grimont et al., 2000). Names of serotypes should necessarily be written in capitalized block characters (not italics): *Salmonella enterica* subsp. *enterica* serotype Typhimurium. However, the following simplifications are allowed: *Salmonella* Typhimurium or *S.* Typhimurium.

## 3. Biology of *Salmonella*

*Salmonella* belongs to the *Enterobacteriaceae* family. On Light microscopy, they appear as Gram-negative, 0,3 to 1µm wide and 1 to 6 µm microns long (Figure 1). They are moving through peritrichous ciliature. Salmonella are mesophilic bacteria, developing at temperatures between 5.2 °C and 47 °C and optimally between 35 ° C and 37 °C, at pH between 4.5 and 9, with water activity (Aw) greater than 0.93.
Salmonella is aero-anaerobic, reduce nitrate to nitrite, can use citrate as single carbon source. She ferments glucose but not lactose or sucrose and she produce gas from glucose (except Salmonella Typhi). Hydrogen sulfide is generally produced from the mid commonly called "triple sugar". The reaction in the oxidase test is negative (Le Minor, 1984 International Commission on Microbiological Specifications for Foods, 1996, Hanes 2003). Like all bacteria stain Gram-negative envelope of Salmonella consists of three elements: the cytoplasmic membrane and outer membrane separated by a periplasmic space consists of peptidoglycan. This structure gives the bacterium its shape and rigidity and allows it to withstand a relatively high osmotic pressure in the environment (Rycroft, 2000)

### 3.1 Habitats

*Salmonella* can be isolated from the intestines of many animal species. They are zoonotic agents. The animals are a reservoir and release into the environment is mainly due to fecal contamination (Berends et al. 1996; Murray, 2000; Hanes, 2003). Salmonella can also survive for very long periods in the environment: a few days to 9 months in soil and surface materials Farm Building (wood, concrete, steel, iron and brick), a few months in dry foods not acidified, on stems and leaves of plants and ensiled over a year in the dust (Gray and Fedorka-Cray, 2001). These bacteria can bind to many substrates, such as, boots, brushes, shovels, wheel barrows, clothes... When cleaning and disinfection of livestock housing and feeding it must consider all inanimate material, which can cause a re-infection of the next batch. Can also be contaminated: spider webs, water, byproducts of agro-food, animal feed, the surrounding farms, fishes and birds (Berends et al., 1996). Rodents and insects can also be an important source of *Salmonella* in livestock (Letellier et al., 1999).

### 3.1.1 Animal reservoir

Serotypes can be classified according to the target animal species. First, some are exclusively adapted to humans, causing serious and very specific diseases. This is essentially *Salmonella* Typhi, Paratyphi, and Sendai, causative agents of typhoid and paratyphoid fevers (Bäumler et al. 1998; Hu and Kopecko, 2003). Second, a number of serotypes can attract animals. Among these are: Choleraesuis, Typhisuis pigs, Abortusequi in horses, sheep Abortusovis, Gallinarum, specific poultry... Finally, most Salmonella serotypes can cross the species barrier. They are present in many animal species, usually in a latent or subclinical disease-causing, and can reach the man, either through food, which is the most common way, either by direct or indirect contact. Any salmonella, with rare exceptions, is potentially dangerous to humans. United States, Salmonella has been associated with collective poisoning from reptiles, which are used as pets (Center for Disease Control, 1999, Mitchell and Shane, 2000). This shows that Salmonella are capable of multiple adjustments and can cause new and various problems to humans, from various sources.

### 3.1.2 Salmonella and human

The specific agents of salmonellosis in humans (Salmonella Typhi, Paratyphi, and Sendai) are the agents of typhoid and paratyphoid fevers. Worldwide, the human deaths caused by typhoid fever are estimated at 600,000 per year (Hu and Kopecko, 2003). The cases are mainly listed in the Third World. In developed countries, cases are usually du to imported food. Five percent of patients infected with S. Typhi become chronic carriers, asymptomatic (Mermin et al., 1999). This poses enormous problems if they are employed by food companies.

### 3.2 Mechanisms of virulence

A considerable number of genes (of the order of hundreds) must be mobilized by Salmonella to counteract the defense mechanisms of the host. All Salmonella serotypes can in theory cause a systemic infection in humans with decreased immune status, although most will generate a febrile diarrhea, vomiting, abdominal pain and in elderly or immuno-défiscients bacteremia, the septicemia and extra intestinal locations, especially vascular (Bäumler et al., 2000). When there is localization of the infection, Salmonella often remain confined to the mesenteric lymph nodes. The first defense mechanisms used by the host are made by the acidity of the stomach and bile salts in the small intestine, which exert a bactericidal effect. Once in the small intestine, Salmonella must as soon as possible adhere to the intestinal mucosa. They will cross at the lymphoid follicles of the ileum (Peyer's patches, located at the bottom of intestinal crypts). At this point in the gut, the epithelium is characterized by the presence among the enterocytes, M cells and the absence of cells secreting mucus. It seems that the fimbriae (adhesins) must be present to allow recognition and binding of Salmonella to Peyer's patches (Dibb-Fuller et al. 1999; Thorns and Woodward, 2000, Vimal et al., 2000).These fimbriae play a critical role in the pathology and the fact that some serotypes are specifically tailored to a particular species. Entry into the Peyer's patches requires the presence of secretion systems of type III. They are encoded by sets of pathogenicity genes ("pathogenicity islands"), known as SPI-1 and SPI-2 (China and Goffaux, 1999; Bäumler et al. 2000; Cornelis, 2000; Jones et al. 2002; Doublet et al., 2005). SPI-1 is normally necessary for passage through M cells of the intestinal mucosa, whereas SPI-2 is involved in the systemic nature of the infection (Hueck, 1998). Subsequent to penetration of salmonella in M cells, the latter will be killed by apoptosis, leading to transmigration across mucosal inflammatory cell type polymorphonuclear (PMN) and acute gastroenteritis.

To survive in the inflammatory process and the development of bactericidal proteins produced by PMN, a set of genes must be activated, especially those in the complex PhoPQ.

## 4. Biochemical characteristics of salmonella

Salmonella possess the general characteristics of the Enterobacteriaceae and intrinsic differential characters.

### 4.1 Family characters

Eight main characters determine the Enterobacteriaceae, they are:

1. Bacilli Gram negative;
2. Often through their mobile ciliature peritrichous (rarely stationary), non-spore forming;
3. Bacteria that grow on ordinary media;
4. Aero-anaerobic bacteria optional;
5. Bacilli that ferment glucose with or without gas production;
6. Bacteria that reduce nitrate to nitrite;
7. Bacilli that do not have cytochrome oxidase (Hanes, 2003; ICMSF, 1996);
8. Bacilli that have a catalase.

Some strains do not obey all these characters, in the case of Erwinia, which does not reduce nitrates, Shigella dysenteriae serotype 1 (SD1) that does not have catalase, Salmonella pullorum-galinarum is immobile.

### 4.2 Differential characters of the genus *Salmonella*

The main biochemical characteristics for identification of Salmonella (Humbert et al., 1998) are:

- The absence of an active urease, tryptophan or phenylalanine deaminase;
- Lack of production of indole and acetoin (Voges-Proskauer test negative);
- The production of hydrogen sulfide from thiosulfate (presence of thiosulfate reductase);
- The frequent decarboxylation of lysine and ornithine;
- The growth on Simmons citrate medium.

## 5. Antigens of Salmonella

Salmonella can have three types of diagnostic antigens of interest (Dumas, 1958).

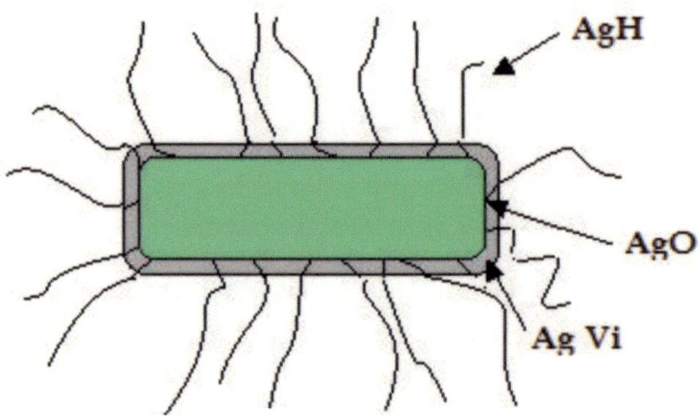


Fig. 1. Salmonella posses a flagellar antigen (H), somatic (O) and a surface antigen Vi

### 5.1 Somatic O antigen (Ag O)

The O antigen is an antigen of the wall. O antigens are carried by chains specific lipopolysaccharide (LPS). The O antigen has properties immunizing is a complex containing a protein, a polysaccharide and a phospholipid compound. We distinguish 67 O factors depending on the nature of the sugars used in the construction of oligosaccharide units of the polysaccharide (Humbert et al., 1998). O antigens are composed of a lipid fraction called lipid A is responsible for toxic effects, or basal part of the core and the support of the specific polysaccharide (Gledel and Corbion, 1991). Antigens are classified as major factors O and O factors accessories. The major factors are related to the presence of certain sugars (abequose for O: 4, tyvélose for O: 9) (Humbert et al., 1998). The somatic antigen is stable and it is resistant to alcohol and phenol for two and a half hours at a 100 ° C (Dumas, 1958).

### 5.2 Flagellar antigen (Ag H)

It is a polymer of flagellin (structural protein of flagella). This antigen is thermolabile, destroyed by heat at 100 ° C by the action of alcohol and by proteolytic enzymes. It is resistant to formalin and loses their agglutinability by antibodies in the presence of alcohol and phenol. Optimum development is achieved on soft liquid media after spending eight hours at 37 ° C (Dumas, 1958). The vast majority of serovars has two genetic systems, and can alternately express two different specificities for their flagellar antigen. It is said that the flagellar antigens of Salmonella are two-phase (Humbert et al., 1998).

### 5.3 The virulence antigen (Vi Ag)

It is an antigen of the envelope; it was identified in three types of serovar: Typhi, Paratyphi C and Dublin, but all strains of these serotypes do not necessarily have this antigen (Humbert et al., 1998). This antigen is considered a surface antigen (Dumas, 1958), it is distinct from the somatic antigen and the flagellar antigen. The Vi antigen makes germs inagglutinable by antibodies O when it is abundant. It does not develop if the cultures are carried out below 25 ° C and above 40 ° C. Heating at 100 ° C destroys the germs and become agglutinating antibodies by O. It is likely glucidolipidopolypeptidique. In addition to these antigens exists in the genus Salmonella, the protein structures from surface pilis pilis which differentiate into common (occurring in mannose-dependent haemagglutination) and sexual pilis (involved in bacterial conjugation) and whose presence is encoded by plasmids (and Gledel Corbion, 1991).

## 6. Isolation and identification of salmonella

### 6.1 Isolation of salmonella

*Salmonella* Typhi, Paratyphi A, B, C are preferably isolated in the blood and feces of typhoid (Dumas, 1958). The *Salmonella* that cause food poisoning or acute gastroenteritis are still being sought in the feces and in food. The detection of *Salmonella* may be direct (bacteriological method) or indirect (serological technique) according to (Humbert et al., 1998). The microbiological analysis of a food is to highlight the microorganisms responsible for the alteration of merchantability and / or health. The analytical methods vary with the type of food, the potential danger it presents, and conservation features, consumption (raw or cooked) and the desired type of germ. Food is supportive environments for the development of a multitude of germs, some of which are pathogenic. Faced with the task of finding a pathogenic bacteria specie in very small proportion of a product heavily contaminated with the bacteria most various conventional methods of analysis, sampling and isolation have been proposed. Several standards govern the detection of Salmonella in food hygiene (Humbert et al., 1998): the horizontal standards applicable to all types of products (ISO6579 December 1993) at international level and industry standards specific to one type of product (NF V59 - 109 for edible gelatin). The detection of Salmonella in a food according to ISO 6579 has four key steps: The pre-enrichment; Enrichment; Isolation and Biochemical and serological identification.

#### 6.1.1 The pre-enrichment

It's a non-selective phase that uses a rich medium in which the sample is diluted to one tenth (1 / 10) and for which the incubation period is about twenty hours at 35 ° C or 37 ° C (Humbert et al ., 1998). The pre-enrichment allows bacteria to sublethal to recover all of their potential at the end of incubation. The media used are liquids, most often using buffered peptone water or lactose broth (Humbert et al., 1998). For dairy products can be used Ringer's solution or phosphate buffer solution.

#### 6.1.2 Enrichment

Enrichment is designed to minimize the growth of other bacteria associated with the collection and continue the selective breeding of Salmonella. 0.1 ml or 1 ml of the solution pre-enrichment was transferred to one or more enrichment media (10 ml of medium). The enrichment media are classified into three families (Humbert et al., 1998):

- selenite broth;
- broths containing tetrathionate (Muller Kauffmann broth) and
- broth containing malachite green and magnesium chloride.

#### 6.1.3 Isolation

This is a phase that uses selective solid media cast in Petri dishes. The isolation media contains a variety of combination of selective factors (Humbert et al., 1998). *Salmonella* colonies appear as features in their form, color and morphology. Solid media used for isolation are: Rambach medium; Hektoen medium; Salmonella agar - Shigella (SS agar); brilliant green agar and phenol red (VB-RP); xylose lysine Tergitol medium (XLT); Compass mid Salmonella; mannitol lysine, crystal violet, brilliant green; deoxycholate citrate agar lactose sucrose (DCLS); xylose lysine deoxycholate agar (XLD) and Bismuth sulfite agar.

With conventional bacteriological diagnostic methods, other unconventional techniques can be used. These are among others: sensitivity to phage 01, and Felix and Callow and standardized systems (API 20 E, 20 E RAPID, Enterotube Rocks, MIS *Enterobacteriaceae*). The lysis by phage 01 (Felix and Callow) that can be used as a confirmatory test for membership of Salmonella that do not provide positive results with all strains (Gledel and Corbion, 1991).

### 6.2 Biochemical identification

Biochemical identification of the colonies tried characteristics is done in two steps:

1. The search for characters of the family: often, the Gram stain, the presence of catalase, the absence of cytochrome oxidase, mobility, respiratory type, the mainstream culture

and fermentation of glucose are sufficient to encourage the search for differential characters.

2. The search for differential characters requires pure cultures. Used for this purpose, the reduced rack of le Minor which is a set of five settings: the mid-Hajna Klinger; the Simmons citrate medium; the lysine iron or Taylor medium; the tryptophan-urea medium and mannitol nitrate mobility medium.

**The mid-Hajna Kliger** (solid medium): The mid-Hajna Kliger has a carmine red color. This medium is only valid for the fermentative bacteria. It is part of the study of carbohydrate metabolism. **The lysine iron medium** or mid-Taylor (purple), enriched with L-lysine and contains low concentrations of glucose. **The Simmons citrate** medium (green), contains citrate as the sole carbon source. Bacteria that are able to use this carbon source, will grow on this agar and cause a pH change at the origin of the middle turn blue. Remains green agar for strains citrate (-). **The urea-indole medium** (liquid medium), the urea -indole or urea -tryptophan medium, is a medium orange, made up of urea and tryptophan. It allows for three enzymatic activities of protein metabolism, including urease, tryptophanase and tryptophan deaminase. **The medium with glycerol** (liquid medium), this medium is green; it is very often added to other settings of Le Minor rack. It helps to distinguish Citrobacter and Salmonella genus. Citrobacter degrades glycerol by causing acidification of the medium (turns to yellow) and Salmonella do not degrade it, the green color is maintained. In summary, the general biochemical characteristics of most serotypes isolated from humans and warm-blooded animals are:

- Lactose (-), ONPG (-)(orthonitrophenyl-β-D-galactopyranoside), $H_2S$ (+), gas (glucose) (+);
- LDC (+)(lysine decarboxylase), ODC (+)(ornithine decarboxylase), ADH (-)(arginine dihydrolase), urease (-), TDA (-)(tryptophane deaminase), indole (-), gelatinase (-) DNase (-);
- No production of acetoin (Voges-Proskauer test (-)), RM (+)(methyl red energy source), Simmons citrate (-), adonitol (-), glycerol (-), galacturonate (-).

It should be noted that there are important exceptions. The serotype Typhi does not decarboxylated ornithine, does not grow on a medium composed of Simmons citrate, it is agazogene and produces only trace amounts of $H_2S$. Serotype Paratyphi A does not decarboxylated lysine and does not grow on Simmons citrate medium. Finally, Salmonella Paratyphi A, Choleraesuis, and Gallinarum do not produce H2S. In this case, the settlements will not have black centers on isolation media consisting of iron citrate and sodium thiosulfate (eg, XLD, Hektoen, SS).

## 7. Economic importance and societal

The economic importance of these diseases is considerable. In the U.S., economists have estimated the annual costs of salmonellosis between 400 million and U.S. $ 3.5 billion for the entire U.S. economy. They took into account the medical costs and lost productivity (Frenzen et al. 1999; Sarwari et al., 2001). Europe, whereas 95% of salmonellosis is food borne, annual costs range between 560 million and 2.8 billion euros. A single case of salmonellosis is estimated, in turn, to a value between EUR 24 and EUR 3.8 million. This estimate refers to cases where the patient dies of infection (European Parliament and Council of the European Union, 2001). In Africa, there are no data on the annual cost of salmonellosis.

## 8. Prophylaxis

Currently, even if the food manufacturing is done according to the standards proposed by the WHO, an important part of the fight against zoonoses must be borne by the consumer, who can be considered an integral link in the chain. We must therefore inform about the risks that may result from errors in food handling. Unfortunately, at present, few initiatives have been undertaken in Africa, unlike the situation in Europe and the United States, where politics at this level is a little more proactive. The operation FightBac ® bases its message on a logo simple and easy to understand for educators, children and operators of processing lines and distribution. CSCC logo are constantly reminded that people must wash their food ("Clean"), separate ("Separate"), Cook ("Cook") and cool ("Chill"). Advice is provided for hand washing, cooking food. The FDA in collaboration with the Center for food Safety and Applied Nutrition (CFSAN) has published a brochure about the risk of salmonellosis associated with eggs (FDA 2002). The CDC ("Centers for Disease Control") has published a leaflet on Salmonella Enteritidis, available on the Internet (Center for Disease Control, 2003). Finally, the educated consumers will, no doubt, more likely to seek medical attention, which will encourage feedback and help to reduce the phenomenon of under-reporting of cases.

## 9. Resistant salmonella

Salmonella is still a topical; it is in any way, a rearguard battle. They are among the first known causes of food borne illness. It is a collective and a real public health problem. Economically, they are crucial, given the casualties they cause. In recent years, problems related to Salmonella have increased significantly, both in terms of the incidence of salmonellosis, that the severity of human cases. While some countries have managed to reverse the upward trend in the incidence of human salmonellosis, new problems were identified. Since the late 90s, Salmonella strains resistant to a range of antimicrobials including major therapeutic agents in human medicine have emerged and are threatening to cause serious public health problem (Mermin et al., 1999). After a very long incubation period, between 7 and 21 days (sometimes up to six weeks), the disease can take many forms (Hu and Kopecko, 2003). The infection may be asymptomatic or cause very mild symptoms in the case of S. Paratyphi or, conversely, cause typhoid fever, severe disease, with fever and sepsis. It mainly affects young children and teenagers (Bäumler et al., 1998). This resistance results from the use of antimicrobials in both human medicine and animal husbandry.

## 10. Essential oils

### 10.1 Introduction

The use of essential oils (EO) dates back to the earliest civilizations: first in the East and the Middle East and later in North Africa and Europe (Franchomme et al., 1990). The Hydrosols (aromatic) were used in India over than 7000 years. Between 3000 and 2000 B.C., the Egyptians made used extensively aromatic plants and other plants to treat the sick. the Persians seem to be the first ones who used the hydrodistillation in 1000 B.C. The use of essential oils was a common practice among the Greeks, several books have been published on the subject. Examples of this literature are "Natural History" by Pliny, "The Aphorisms" by Hippocrates, "odor treatment" by Theophrastus and Dioscorides Pedanius wrote a book on herbal medicine (phytotherapy). The Arabs have made a significant improvement in chemistry and in the distillation of oils by inventing the alembic still by Jaber Ibn Hayan. In the late seventeenth and eighteenth century, more than 10 essential oils were used. In modern history, the therapeutic properties of essential oils have an increasing importance. Aromatherapy has been used to describe the healing properties of essential oils. Actually, we recognize that essential oils have pharmacological, psychological and physiological effects in humans.

Among the plant species estimated by botanists (800 000 to 1 500 00), only 10% are classified as "aromatic". Aromatic plants synthesize and secrete trace amounts of aromatic essence through hair, secretory pockets or channels. Types capable of developing the components of essential oils are distributed in a limited number of families, Myrtaceae, Lauraceae, Rutaceae, Lamiaceae, Asteraceae, Cupressaceae, Poaceae, Zingiberaceae, such as Piperaceae [Bruneton, 1999]. About 20,000 of plant species in the world are used for food, cosmetics, chemical, pharmaceutical and therapeutic food. Among the 4,000 plant species existing in Morocco, more than 280 plants are currently operating.

The AFNOR NF T 75-006 (AFNOR, 1986) defines the essential oil as "a product made from a vegetable raw material, either by steam or by mechanical means from the exocarp, Citrus, or by dry distillation. Essential oils (EO), also called "essences" are aromatic substances, volatile and oily consistency, contained in plants [Balz, 1986 - Lardry and Haberkorn, 2003]. Most plants contain (Eo), but usually in lower quantities. Only plants known as "aromatic" produce essential oils in sufficient quantity. They are usually concentrated in a particular area of the plant such as leaves, bark or fruit, and generally when they occur in various organs from the same plant, they have different compositions (Conner, 1993). The synthesis and accumulation of essential oils, classified as secondary metabolites, are generally in the specialized histological structures, often located on or near the surface of the plant (Brunechon, 1987): pockets (citrus exocarp ) of a storage (eucalyptus), secretory canals or blisters containing resin (conifers), or glands in cuticular (conical epidermal cells on the flowers of Rosaceae), trichomes or secretory glandular trichomes on the leaves of solanaceous or Lamiaceae (Gershenzon, 2000) (Figure 8). It is important to note that several categories of these secretory tissues can coexist simultaneously in the same species, even within the same organ (Fahn, 1979 - Fahn, 1988). For example, to the Lamiaceae family, it is within the secretory hairs, in Myrtaceae in pockets secretory or secretory channels in Asteraceae. Essential oils can be stored in various organs of the plant: flowers (oregano), leaves (lemon grass, eucalyptus), bark (cinnamon), wood (rosewood, sandalwood), roots (vetiver), rhizomes (sweet flag), fruits (star anise) and seeds (caraway). Essential oils are complex mixtures consisting of several compounds, mainly terpenes. Terpenes are formed by one or more isoprene units (Tedder, 1970; Brunechon, 1987), constituting a diverse family both structurally and functionally. Mainly mono-and sesquiterpenes (with 10 and 15 carbon atoms) are the most encountered the diterpenes (20 carbon atoms). Essential oils can also contain aliphatic or aromatic compounds. These terpenoids have an ecological role in plant interactions, such as allelopathic agents. They can be inhibitor of germination, but also during plant-animal interactions, as a protective agent against predators such as insects.

They are also involved, through their characteristic odors in the attraction of pollinators (Langenheim, 1969). Some plants may have an odor similar due to a common molecule present in significant amounts in the essential oil. According to the economic environment, it would be profitable to produce plant species may provide an essential oil with high molecular compound, and therefore generally better (Tedder, 1970).

Herbs that produce essential oils have been the subject of various researches particularly in the field of perfumery. A range of products to smell more or less pronounced depending on the concentration of volatile compounds collected from the essential oils produced by steam distillation or expression of the peel fruit (Tedder, 1970;Brunechon, 1987).

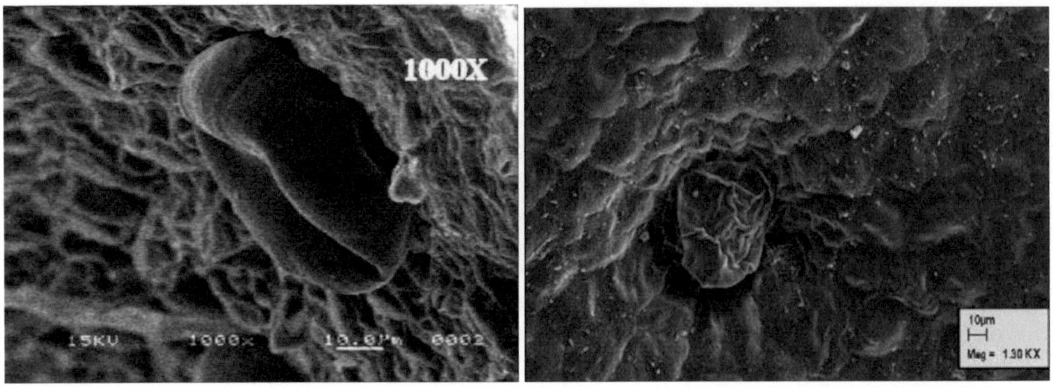


Fig. 2. Glandular trichomes of mint gardens observed in electron microscope scan (1000 ×) before (a) and after (b) extraction by steam distillation [Lucchesi, 2005].

### 10.2 Chemical composition of essential oil

Essential oils are composed of a complex mixture. These compounds mainly belong to two families of chemicals: terpene compounds and aromatic compounds.

The terpene compounds are hydrocarbons of general formula $(C_5H_8)_n$ formed from isoprene units (Figure 3) and are represented in essential oils, mainly monoterpenes, sesquiterpenes and rarely few diterpenes. These compounds may be acyclic, monocyclic, bicyclic or tricyclic [Paris, 1981].

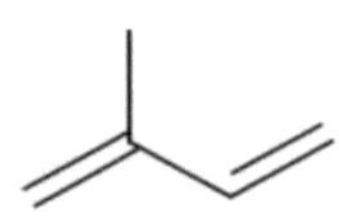

Fig. 3. Isoprene.

The aromatic compounds are derived from phenylpropane, which are characteristic of certain species, such as cinnamaldehyde in cinnamon essential oil, eugenol in the cloves, anethol and aldehyde anasique, in the essential oils of anise and fennel (Fig. 10) (Paris, 1981).

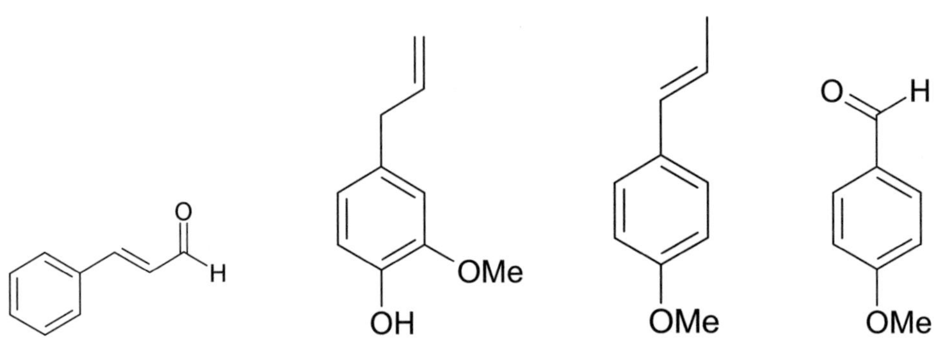


Aldehyde cinnamique Eugenol Anethol Aldehyde anisique

Fig. 4. Examples of aromatic compounds.

The majority of the components of EO are monoterpenes; they represent 90% of most essential oils. They are volatile usually easily driven by steam, have often pleasant odor (Lamart, 1994). By the diversity of their structure, they can be classified into several groups (Bakkali, 2008) (Table 3). Several factors may be responsible of the chemical polymorphism of essential oils. The most important are climate, soil, time harvest and method of storage and retrieval. Genetic factors (Echeverrigaray, 2001) and the growth cycle (Hance, 2003) may also influence this variability…(Bakkali, 2008). The use of essential oils is of great interest in many areas. Thus, the species most studied for their antibacterial and antifungal properties (biological activities) belong to the Lamiaceae family: Thyme, oregano, savory, lavender, mint, rosemary, sage and hyssop.

### 10.3 Biosynthesis of essential oil

Essential oils are very complex natural mixtures that can hold about 20-60 components with very different concentrations. The main group composed by terpenoids or isoprenoids is a family of secondary metabolites widely distributed in the plant kingdom. More than 22000 compounds have been identified (Connolly 1992). Their classification is based on the number of repetition of the basic unit of isoprene: hemiterpene (C5), monoterpene (C10), sesquiterpene (C15), diterpene (C20), sesterpene (C25), triterpene (C30), tetraterpene (C40) and polyterpene. The major terpene components of essential oils are monoterpene and sesquiterpene. Isoprenoid biosynthesis of essential oils can be simplified into three phases: Isopentenyl diphosphate (IPP) Biosynthesis, condensation of IPP units and formation of prenyl diphosphates and Conversion of prenyl-diphosphates. The condensation of isopentenyl diphosphate (nucleophilic entity) to dimethylallyl diphosphate (electrophilicentity) leads to geranyl diphosphate (GPP, C10), precursor of monoterpenes. A further condensation type head-to-tail of IPP on the GPP leads to farnesyl diphosphate (FPP, C15), the precursor of sesquiterpenes. The prenyl transferases allow prenyl chain elongation by addition of one molecule of IPP.

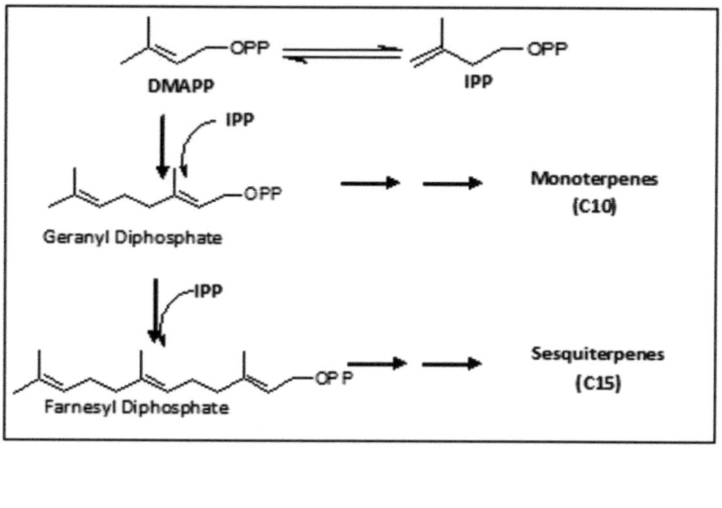


Fig. 5. Biosynthetic precursors of the main metabolic constituents of essential oils

Conversion of prenyl- diphosphates: Under the action of terpene synthases, the acyclic isoprene precursors thus obtained may undergo transformations for the formation of other compounds by hydroxylation, oxidation, inter-conversion alcohol /aldehyde, methylation of the hydroxyl and carboxyl, acylation...

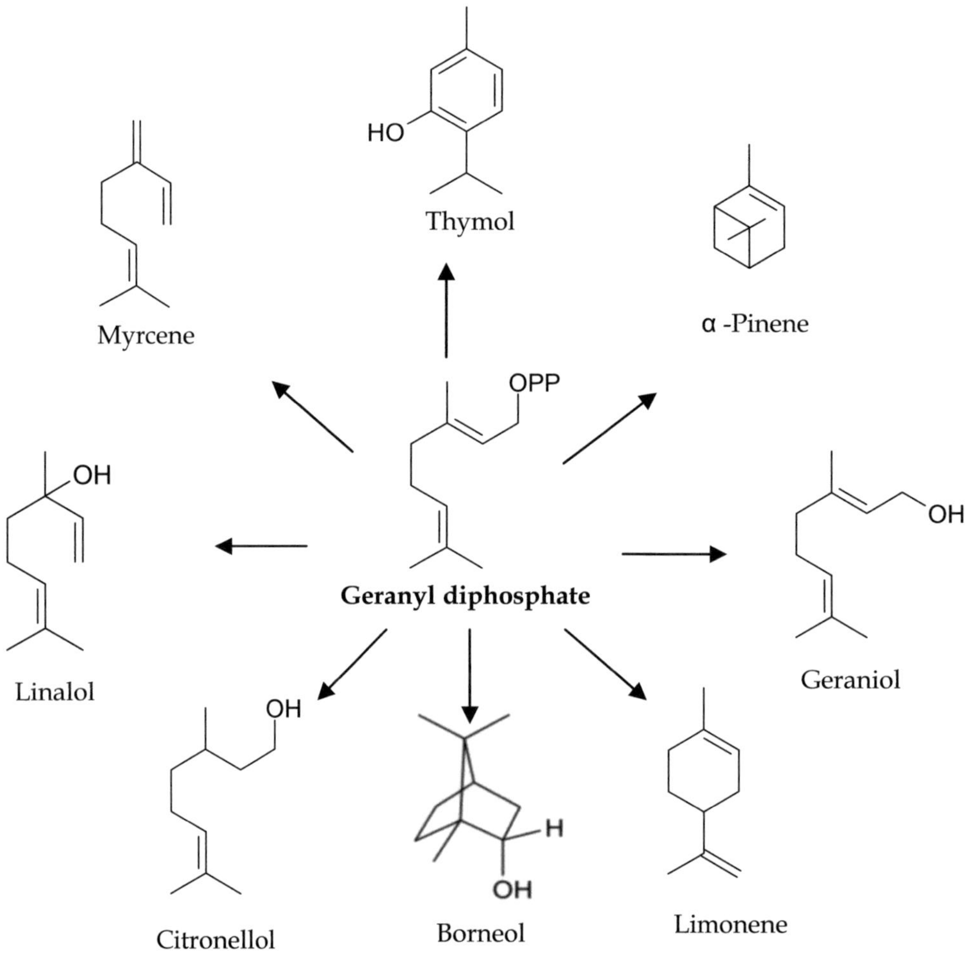


Fig. 6. Structures of monoterpenes derived from geranyl diphosphate.

#### 10.4 Quality control

According to French and European Pharmacopoeia, the control of essential oils can be made by the miscibility of ethanol, the index of refraction, the optical rotation and gravity. The color and smell are also important parameters. The quantitative and qualitative chromatographic profile of an essential oil helps to know exactly the chemical

composition and search for any traces of other undesirable products such as pesticides or chemicals added.
A pure and natural essential oil is characterized by its composition strictly 'vegetable', unlike gasoline, synthetic or "natural identical" fully reconstituted from synthetic chemicals. In aromatherapy, the use of such profiles is essential to differentiate within a species changes induced by chemical factors influencing the plant biosynthesis, such as sunshine, altitude, nature and composition of the soil. Indeed, the observation of a clump of thyme and knowledge of its origin is not sufficient to characterize its essential oil. For example, an essential oil of Thymus vulgaris can be thymol chemotype, linalool, geraniol or thuyanol. Botanically, it is the same plant family Lamiaceae (or Labiatae ).

### 10.5 Economic characteristics of EO

The plant is a concentrate of active ingredients (enzymes, polysaccharides, alkaloids, terpenes, tannins, resins etc.) and often requires large quantities of plants for a few drops of essential oil (100 kilos per 200 grams of EO thyme). If scarcity is one of their attractions, it also makes the price, hence the importance of good conservation: the dark (dark bottles), air and heat. In Morocco, the development of natural resources is the integration of non-food plants in the Moroccan economy, especially their conservation and development in food, cosmetics, industrial and therapeutic. Moroccan products in the areas of essential oils and aromatic extracts are well known on the world market. For some products, Morocco has a privileged position; he is the sole or primary producer, in the case of mint, chamomile wild, thyme, Atlas cedar, etc. For other products, production Moroccan faces other competitors; this was the case for example of rosemary undergoing tough Tunisian and Spanish competition. In other cases, the position of Morocco on the world market is rather high, in the case of myrtle, mint and so on. (Benjilali, 1986).

### 10.6 Methods of extraction of EO

There are several techniques of extraction of essential oils (Sallé, 2004). They can be extracted simply by cold pressing, distillation, by volatile solvent or supercritical fluid such as carbon dioxide. Distillation by steam distillation of water (still) is the method most practiced in the industry. The essential oils obtained are generally low polarity products, volatile, fragrant and usually less dense than water (Valnet, 2005). They are soluble in most organic solvents and poorly soluble in water. (Sallé, 2004). Steam-hydrodistillation is the most common method of recovery of essential oils. Under the action of water vapor, gas is released by the plant tissue and effect of temperature, volatiles products are driven by the steam. The essential oils are recovered by condensing (Bruneton, 1993). Hydrodistillation (steam water 'in situ') method involves by immersing the plant material in water which is then boiled (Bruneton, 1999). The enfleurage, distillation assisted by microwaves, extraction with solvents, extraction with a supercritical fluid are among the methods used to recover the EO of aromatic and medicinal plants (Sallé,2004, Brian, 1995).

## 11. Biological activity of thymus EO

### 11.1 Source of *Salmonella sp*

Salmonella sp. was isolated from soil argan Marrakech (Morocco). The identification was performed according to the methods described above. Inocula were prepared from liquid cultures by 18 h, diluted with saline so as to contain about 108 cells / ml, at a density of between 0.08 and 0.1 at 625 nm (Careaga and al. 2003; Joffin and Leyral,2001). We evaluated the sensitivity of this strain against the essential oils of *thymus broussonetii* and *thymus maroccanus* from the region of Marrakech (Morocco). We used the Mueller Hinton medium for our study. The antimicrobial activity of essential oils, we used the method of diffusion from antibiotic susceptibility discs of pure essential oil (Jacob et al., 1979). The media poured in Petri dishes are inoculated with 1 ml of bacterial suspension of 108 cells / ml and excess inoculum was removed by aspiration (Shunying et al., 2005). The essential oil is deposited in the volume of 10 ml on Whatman sterile paper discs of 6 mm in diameter. In parallel, we use cookies to check the growth of the strain tested. The petri dishes were left 30 min at room temperature to allow complete diffusion of the product (CA-SFM, 1993). The antibacterial activity was determined in terms of diameter of inhibition zone around the discs recorded after 24 h of incubation at 37 ° C. The test is performed in three repetitions in the same experimental conditions.

### 11.2 Essential oils of T. broussonetii and T. maroccanus

*Thymus* (thyme) is an aromatic and medicinal plant belonging to the *Lamiaceae* family. This plant is native to the Mediterranean region. (Duke, 1989; Zargari, 1990; Newall et al., 1996). *Thymus broussonetii* Boiss and *Thymus maroccanus*. are an endemic plants of Morocco. Its species are used for traditional medicine for the treatment of various illnesses (Bellakhdar, 1997; Sijelmassi, 1993). The studies of essential oil of *T. broussonetii* have been published indicating the antimicrobial, anti-inflammatory, the immunological, behavioural effects and antitumor properties (Lattaoui et al., 1994; Lattaoui and Tantaoui-Elaraki, 1994, Ismaili et al. 2001; 2002; 2004, Elhabazi et al., 2006, Jaafari et al, 2007).

*T. broussonetii* and *T. maroccanus* were collected at flowering stage in July 2006 in a High Atlas mountain respectively, in "Ait Ourir" and in "Essaouirra" from the region, Centre and Southwest of Morocco. The inflorescences, leaves and stem were separated by hand. Samples were dried at the shade.

### 11.3 Chemical composition of essential oils of T. broussonetii and T. maroccanus

The identification of 93.1% (36 compounds) of the chemical composition of the essential oil of some leaf of *T. broussonetii* (figure 7) is shown in Table 2. This part produces a yield of 1.6% essential oils. The chemical identity of this oil shows that it consists mainly of monoterpene hydrocarbons which represent more than half of this oil (53.3%). In this class of monoterpenes, p-cymene (21.0%), the α-pinene (11.8%) and camphene (8.5%) are the most important compounds. The class of oxygenated monoterpenes is second with 33%, represented mainly by borneol (16.5%) and thymol (11.3%). The sesquiterpene hydrocarbon represent 6.6% and consist mainly leden (3.2%). The spathulénol is the only oxygenated sesquiterpene identified in this part of the plant with a percentage of 0.2%.

The identification of 96.7% of the chemical composition of the essential oil of some leaf of T. maroccanus (figure 8) is shown in Table 3. The yield of essential oils of this part is 1%. The monoterpene hydrocarbon species represent 49.5% of the leaves of this species. The α-pinene (11.6%) and p-cymene (25.3%) are the most important compounds in this class. The oxygenated monoterpenes represent 37.9%, they consist mainly of carvacrol (33%). The sesquiterpene hydrocarbon represents 6.6% and consists of 2% β-caryophyllene. The oxygenated sesquiterpenes represented only 0.4% of this oil.

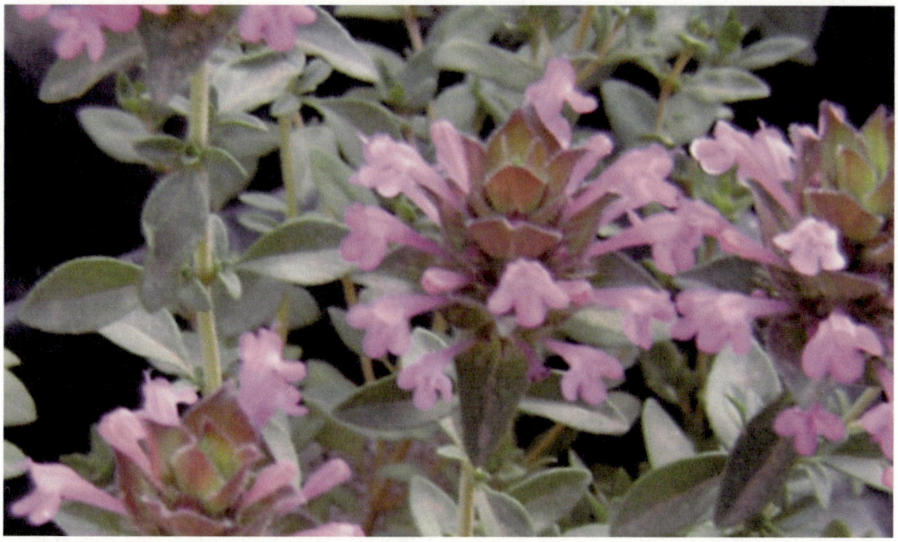

Fig. 7. *T. broussonetii*

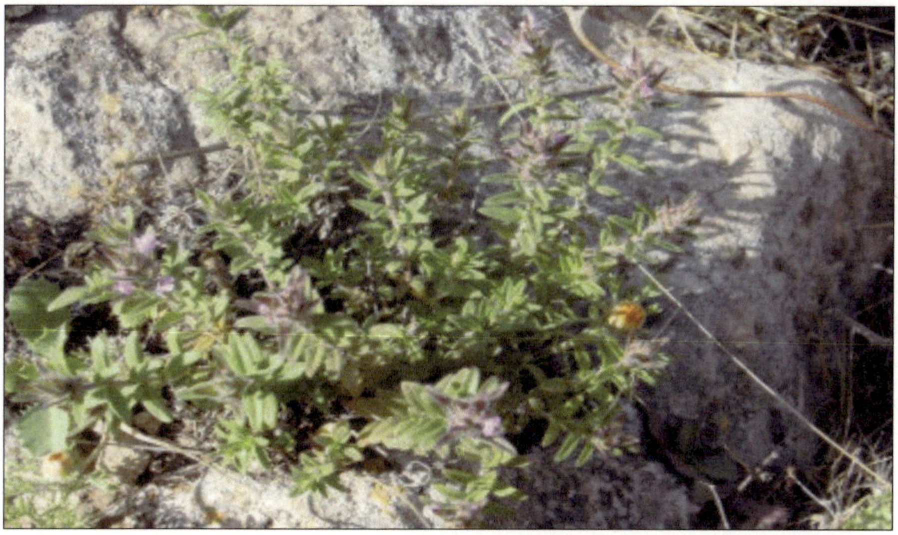

Fig. 8. *T. maroccanus*

| | IRa | IRb | % |
|---|---|---|---|
| **Monoterpenes hydrocarbon** | | | **53.3** |
| Tricyclene | 921 | 1001 | 0.3 |
| α-Thujene | 924 | - | 0.3 |
| α-Pinene | 934 | 1012 | 11.8 |
| Thuja-2,4(10)-diene | 937 | 1112 | 0.1 |
| Camphene | 944 | 1051 | 8.5 |
| Sabinene | 966 | 1105 | 0.2 |
| β-Pinene | 971 | 1093 | 1.9 |
| Myrcene | 984 | 1141 | 2.1 |
| α-phellandrene | 998 | 1185 | 0.2 |
| 3-δ-carene | 1006 | 1128 | 0.1 |
| α-terpinene | 1010 | 1158 | 1.0 |
| *p*-cymene | 1017 | 1244 | 21.0 |
| Limonene | 1024 | 1176 | 2.2 |
| γ-Terpinene | 1052 | 1220 | 2.5 |
| Terpinolene | 1079 | 1254 | 0.2 |
| **Oxygenated Monoterpenes** | | | **33.0** |
| (E)-Sabinene hydrate | 1054 | 1423 | 0.3 |
| Linalol | 1085 | 1510 | 0.2 |
| Camphre | 1122 | 1466 | 0.1 |
| Isoborneol | 1140 | 1651 | tr |
| Borneol | 1148 | 1651 | 16.5 |
| Terpinen-4-ol | 1161 | 1554 | 0.4 |
| Dihydrocarvone 1 | 1171 | 1557 | 0.4 |
| Dihydrocarvone 2 | 1179 | 1579 | 0.1 |
| Carvenone | 1233 | 1676 | tr |
| Thymol | 1268 | 2124 | 11.3 |
| Carvacrol | 1280 | 2151 | 3.7 |
| **Sesquiterpenes hydrocarbon** | | | **6.5** |
| α-Cubebene | 1348 | 1431 | tr |
| β-Bourbonene | 1382 | 1488 | 0.1 |
| α-Gurjunene | 1408 | 1497 | 0.1 |
| β-caryophyllene | 1416 | 1558 | 0.3 |
| Aromadendrene | 1437 | 1570 | 2.1 |
| allo-Aromadendrene | 1456 | 1605 | 0.4 |
| γ-Muurolene | 1469 | 1683 | 0.2 |
| Ledene | 1491 | 1655 | 3.2 |
| Calamenene | 1508 | 1784 | tr |
| **Oxygenated Sesquiterpènes** | | | **0.2** |
| Spathulenol | 1561 | 2059 | 0.2 |

IRa: Index of retention in non-polar chromatographic column HP-1
IRb: Index of retention in the polar chromatographic column HP-20
tr: trace

Table 2. Percentage and chemical composition of the EO part of the leaf of *T. broussonetii*

| | IRa | IRb | % |
|---|---|---|---|
| **Monoterpenes hydrocarbon** | | | **49.5** |
| Tricyclene | 921 | 1001 | tr |
| α-Thujene | 924 | - | 0.8 |
| α-Pinene | 934 | 1012 | 11.6 |
| Thuja-2,4(10)-diene | 937 | 1112 | 0.1 |
| Camphene | 944 | 1051 | 0.8 |
| β-Pinene | 971 | 1093 | 0.4 |
| Myrcene | 984 | 1141 | 1.4 |
| α-phellandrene | 998 | 1185 | 0.3 |
| α-terpinene | 1010 | 1158 | 1.1 |
| *p*-cymene | 1017 | 1244 | 25.3 |
| Limonene | 1024 | 1176 | 2.7 |
| γ-Terpinene | 1052 | 1220 | 4.6 |
| Terpinolene | 1079 | 1254 | 0.1 |
| **Oxygenated Monoterpenes** | | | **37.9** |
| (E)-Sabinene hydrate | 1054 | 1423 | 0.2 |
| Linalol | 1085 | 1510 | 2.3 |
| Camphre | 1122 | 1466 | 0.2 |
| Borneol | 1148 | 1651 | 0.8 |
| Terpinen-4-ol | 1161 | 1554 | 0.5 |
| Dihydrocarvone 1 | 1171 | 1557 | 0.3 |
| Dihydrocarvone 2 | 1179 | 1579 | 0.2 |
| Carvone | 1233 | 1676 | 0.2 |
| Thymol | 1268 | 2124 | 0.4 |
| Carvacrol | 1280 | 2151 | 33.0 |
| Eugenol | 1328 | - | tr |
| **Sesquiterpenes hydrocarbon** | | | **6.6** |
| α-Cubebene | 1348 | 1431 | tr |
| α-ylangene | 1370 | 1461 | tr |
| Copaene | 1375 | 1463 | 0.1 |
| β-Bourbonene | 1382 | 1488 | 0.1 |
| β-Patchoulene | 1386 | - | tr |
| β-caryophyllene | 1416 | 1558 | 2.0 |
| β-Cubebene | 1425 | 1667 | tr |
| Aromadendrene | 1437 | 1570 | 1.4 |
| α-Humulene | 1449 | - | 0.1 |
| allo-Aromadendrene | 1456 | 1605 | 0.2 |
| D-Germacrene | 1474 | 1667 | tr |
| β-Gurjunene | 1484 | 1681 | 0.2 |
| Ledene | 1491 | 1655 | 1.0 |
| γ-Cadinene | 1504 | - | 1.3 |
| Calamenène | 1508 | 1784 | 0.1 |
| (Z)-α-Bisabolène | 1532 | - | tr |
| Guaiazulène | 1652 | - | tr |

| | IRa | IRb | % |
|---|---|---|---|
| **Sesquiterpènes oxygénés** | | | **0.2** |
| Spathulénol | 1561 | 2059 | 0.2 |
| Caryophyllène oxyde | 1567 | 1920 | 0.1 |
| Globulol | 1571 | - | tr |
| **Autres** | | | **2.4** |
| Octen-3-ol | 964 | 1357 | 1.3 |
| Octen-3-one | 980 | 1225 | 0.2 |
| Carvacryl acetate | 1345 | 1690 | Tr |
| Acetovanillone | 1516 | - | 0.9 |

IRa: Index of retention in non-polar chromatographic column HP-1
IRb: Index of retention in the polar chromatographic column HP-20, tr: trace

Table 3. Percentage and chemical composition of the HE part of the leaf of *T. maroccanus*

### 11.4 In vitro effect of essential oils of *T. broussonetii* and *T. maroccanus*

As has been reported in the literature, we considered that an essential oil has bacteriostatic action if the diameter of inhibition is greater than 12 mm (Baudoux, 2001; Sağdac ° 2003) or 15mm (Rossi, 2003). The diameters of inhibition zones obtained with the essential oils of *T. broussonetii* and *T. maroccanus*, from the region of Marrakech (Morocco), are 19 mm and 23 mm respectively. The essential oils acted actively on the growth of *Salmonella sp* responsible for salmonellosis. They have an inhibitory effect on the growth of Salmonella sp.

| | Inhibition Zone (mm) | | | |
|---|---|---|---|---|
| | *Essential oil* | | Standard antibiotics | |
| | *T.b.* | *T.m.* | Gentamicine | Tetracycline |
| *Salmonella sp.* | 19±0.9 | 23±0.4 | 25±0.1 | 15±0.3 |

Table 4. Antibacterial activity of the essential oils of *Thymus broussonetii* (T.b.) and *Thymus maroccanus* (T.m.) and from antibiotic expressed by diameter of inhibition zone.

These values are reported as means ± standard deviations of three separate determinations. Disc diameter. 6mm (Romane et al, 2010).

The major activity of essential oils of *Thyme broussonetii* and *Thyme maroccanus* is due to their richness in phenolic compounds (thymol and carvacrol). Most antimicrobial compounds are phenols (carvacrol, thymol, eugenol), followed by alcohol (cineole, linalool ...) and to a lesser extent alkenes (p-cymene, pinene, terpinene ...) (Burt, 2004, Ultee et al., 2002). Indeed, several studies have shown that high antimicrobial power of essential oils of several species of thyme is attributed to their high phenolic compounds (carvacrol and thymol) (Marino et al. 1999; Mirmostafa and Rasool, 2002; Dafer and Ziogas , 2000; Baranauskiene et al. 2003; Di Pasqua et al. 2005; Di Pasqua et al. 2007; Cristan et al., 2007).

Most of the work that had for its object the study of the mechanism of action of phenolic compounds suggests that their main site of action is the bacterial plasma membrane

(Shunying et al., 2005). They are able to disintegrate the bacterial cell membrane (Ultee et al., 1999). The membrane loses its structure and becomes more permeable to ions (Lambert et al., 2001). Damages to the cell membrane may also allow the dissipation of pH gradient and decreased membrane potential (Ultee et al., 1999).

### 11.5 The antibacterial activity of antibiotics

The study by (Imelouane & ElBachiri, 2010) of the antibiotic susceptibility shows that the strain used is relatively sensitive to Florenfinicol, Spectinomycin, Enrofloxacin, Cotrimoxazole, Flumequine Tiafen, Tetracycline and Gentamycin. This sensitivity varies from one antibiotic to another and from one strain to another

| | Inhibition Zone (mm) antibiotics | | | | |
|---|---|---|---|---|---|
| | $KF_{30}$ | $AMP_{10}$ | $AML_{25}$ | $TPC_{30}$ | $E_{15}$ |
| *Salmonella sp* | 0 | 0 | 0 | 30 | 0 |

| | Inhibition Zone (mm) antibiotics | | | | | |
|---|---|---|---|---|---|---|
| | $UB_{30}$ | $SXT_{25}$ | MY | $ENR_5$ | SH | FFC |
| *Salmonella sp* | 28 | 25 | 0 | 32 | 18 | 34 |

Kf: Cephalothin; AMP: Ampiciline; AML:Amoxycilline; TPC:Tiafen; E:Erythromycine
UB: Fluméquine ,SXT: Cotrimoxazole; MY:Lyncomycine ; ENR:Enrofloxacine ; SH : Spectinomycine; FFC: Florenfinicol

Table 5. Inhibitory effect of different antibiotic discs: Diameter of inhibition zones in mm among Salmonella sp.

The study of antibiotic susceptibility shows that the strain used is sensitive to Florenfinicol, Spectinomycin, Enrofloxacin, Flumequine, Tetracycline and Gentamycin. This sensitivity varies from one antibiotic to another (Table), while the strain is resistant to Cephalothin, Ampicillin, Amoxicillin and Lyncomycine.
Quantitative comparison of the results of EO to antibiotics is difficult because the nature of the activity and composition of the molecules are not comparable. Unlike EO, complex mixtures of volatile compounds that evaporate, but also that diffuse into the agar at different speeds, antibiotics are large non-volatile molecules. There Dissemination takes place probably at the surface and / or volume in the mass of the agar.

| | Inhibition Zone (mm) |
|---|---|
| microorganisms | Thymus pubescens |
| *Salmonella sp* | 08 |

Table 6. Antibioaromatogramme of the essential oil of *Thymus pubenscens*. Diameter of inhibition zone of *Salmonella sp* determined using the diffusion method on solid medium.

## 12. Conclusion

Recently, Salmonella strains resistant to a range of antibiotics, including major therapeutic agents in human medicine have emerged and are threatening to cause serious public health problems.
This resistance results from the use of antibiotics; this situation is getting worse year by year due to misuse or inappropriate use of antibiotics to treat any disease;, hence the importance of direct research into plants that have always been a source of inspiration for new drugs. Thus, the essential oils have a lot of interest as a potential source of bioactive natural molecules which extracts have a strong antimicrobial potency.
The use of essential oils is a serious substitute to treatment with antibiotics in infectious diseases because of their interference with bacteria vital functions. The alteration of the cell membrane including permeability may result in abnormal losses of ions or macromolecules.
Several authors have put the relationship between the antibacterial activity of essential oils with their chemical composition; specially
phenolic and terpenic compounds but some studies have shown that the antimicrobial activity, antiviral, insecticidal, larvicidal and ovicidal essential oils are superior to those of its majority compounds tested separately.

## 13. References


Adams R.P. (1995). Identification of Essential Oil Components by Gas Chromatography / Mass Spectroscopy. *Allured Publishing, Carol Stream, IL.*

Agnihotri S., Vaidya A.D.B. (1996). A novel approach to study antibacterial properties of volatile components of selected Indian médicinal herbs. *Indian J. of Exp. Biol.* 34, 712–715.

Ait M'Barek L., Ait Mouse H., Jaâfari A., Aboufatima R., Benharref A., Kamal M., Bénard J., El Abbadi N., Bensalah M., Gamouh A., Chait A., Dalal A., Zyad A. (2007). Cytotoxic effect of essential oil of thyme (*Thymus broussonettii*) on the IGR-OV1 tumor cells resistant to chemotherapy. *Brazilian Journal of Medical Biological Research.* 40, 1537-1544.

Association Française de Normalisation NF EN ISO 6579. 2002. Microbiologie des aliments - Méthode horizontale pour la recherche des *Salmonella* spp. Association Française de Normalisation : *Saint-Denis, Décembre.* 27 p.

Bakkali F., Averbeck S., Averbeck D., Idaomar M. 2008. Biological effects of essential oils. *Food and Chemistry Toxicology* 46, 446–475.

Baranauskiene R., Venskutoni S.P.R., Viskelis P., Dambrauskiene E. 2003. Influence of nitrogen fertilizers on the yield and composition of thyme (*Thymus vulgaris*). *Journal of Agricultural and Food Chemistry* 51, 7751-7758.

Baudoux D. 2001. L'aromathérapie, se soigner par les huiles essentielles. *2ème éd., Atlantica,* pp. 25-6.

Bäumler A., Tsolis R., Ficht T., Adams L. (1998). Evolution of host adaptation in *Salmonella* enterica. *Infection Immunology* 66, 4579-4587.

Bäumler A., Tsolis R., Heffron F. (2000). Virulence Mechanisms of *Salmonella* and their genetic basis. In: Wray C., Wray A. (Eds.), *Salmonella* in Domestic Animals. *CABI Publishing: Oxon.* 57-72.

Bean N., Goulding J., Daniels M., Angulo F. (1997). Surveillance for foodborne disease outbreaks-United States, 1988- 1992. *Journal of Food Protection* 60, 1265-1286.

Bean N., Griffin P. (1990). Foordborne disease outbreaks in the United States, 1973-1987: pathogens, vehicles, and trends. *Journal of Food Protection* 53, 804-817.

Bellakhdar J. (1997). La pharmacopée marocaine traditionnelle. *Ibiss Press Paris*. 358 p.

Benabid A. (2000). Flore et écosystèmes du Maroc. Evaluation et préservation de la biodiversité. *Ed. Ibis Press. Paris*, 359 p.

Benjilali B., Hammoumi M., Richard H. (1987). Chemical polymorphism of Moroccan thyme essential oils. 1. Compounds characterization. *Sciences des Aliments* 1, 77- 91.

Benjilali B., Tantaoui-Elarki A., Ismaili-Alaoui M., Ayadi A. 1986. Méthode d'étude des propriétés antiseptiques des huiles essentielles par contact direct en milieu gélose. *Plant Médicinal Phytothérapy* 20, 155–167. 129

Berends B., Urlings H., Snijders J., Van Knapen F. (1996). Identification and quantification of risk factors in animal management and transport regarding *Salmonella* spp. In pigs. *International Journal of Food and Microbiology*, 30, 37-53.

Birouk A., Tazi M., Mellas H., Maghnouj M. (1995). Rapport de pays pour la conférence technique internationale de la FAO sur les ressources phytogénetiques.

Bornert G. (2000). Le poulet sans salmonelles : mythe ou réalité ? *Revue de Médecine Vétérinaire* 151(12), 1083-1094.

Bouhdid S., Idaomar M., Zhiri A., Baudoux D., Skali N.S., Abrini J. (2006). *Thymus* essential oils: chemical composition and *in vitro* antioxidant and antibacterial activities *Congrès International de Biochimie. Agadir*, 09-12 Mai 2006.

Bown D. (1996). Encyclopedia of Herbs and their uses, *London Dorling Kindersley*.

Brown D., Mather H., Browning L., Coia J. (2003). Investigation d'infections humaines à *salmonella* enterica sérotype Java en Ecosse : association possible avec de la volaille importée. *EuroSurveillance* 8, 35-40 .

Brown J.H. (1935). *Theobald Smith 1859-1934. Journal of Bacteriol*ogy 30 (1), 1–3.

Burt S.A., Vlielader R., Haagsman H.P., Veldhuizen E.J.A. (2005). Increase in activity of essential oil components carvacrol and thymol against *Escherichia coli* O157:H7 by addition of food stabilizers. *Journal of Food Protection* 68, 919-926.

Burt S.A. (2004). Essential oils: their antibacterial properties and potentiel applications in a foods- rewiew International. *Journal of Food Microbiology* 94, 223-53.

Cantino P.D., Sanders R.W. (1986). Subfamilial classification of Labiatae. *Systematic Botany* 1, 163–185.

Careaga M., Fernández E., Dorantes L., et al. (2003). Antibacterial activity of Capsicum extract against Salmonella typhimurium and Pseudomonas aeruginosa inoculated in raw beef meat International. *Journal of Food Microbiol*ogy 83, 331-5.

Carson C.F., Hammer K.A., Riley T.V. (2006). Melaleuca alternifolia (Tea Tree) Oil: a Review of Antimicrobial and Other Medicinal Properties. *Clinical Microbiology Reviews* 19, 50-62

Carson C.F., Riley T.V. 1995. Antimicrobial activity of the major components of the essential oil of Malaleuca alternifolia. *Journal Applied Bacteriology*78, 264 269.

CA-SFM. (1993). Comité de l'antibiogramme de la société Française de Microbiologie. Paris.

Center for Disease Control Disease Information: *Salmonella* enteritidis. 2003. [en ligne] Adresse URL :http://www.cdc.gov/ncidod/dbmd/diseaseinfo/salment_g. htm. Consulté le 08/09/04.

Center for Disease Control. (1999). Reptile-associated *salmonellosis*: selected states, 1996-1998. *Morbidity and Mortality Weekly Report* 48, 1009-1013.

Chadefaud M., Emberger L. (1960). Traité de Botanique systématique, tome II : les végétaux vasculaires, *fascicule. I et II. Masson, Paris.* 1539 p.

Charai M., Faid M., Chaouch A. (1999). Essential oils from aromatic plants (Thymus broussonetti Boiss., O. compactum Benth., and Citrus limon (L.) N.L. Burm.) as natural antioxidants for olive oil. *Journal of Essential Oil Res*earch 11, 517 521.

China B., Goffaux F. (2000). Secretion of virulence by *Escherichia coli. Vet. Res.* 30, 181-202.

Conner D.E. (1993). Naturally occuring compounds. In P. Davidson & A. L. Branen, Antimicrobials in foods. *New York, NY: Marcel Dekker*, 441–468.

Cornelis G. (2005). Type III secretion: a bacterial device for close combat with cells of their eukaryotic host. *Phil. Trans. R. Soc. Lond.* 355, 681-693.

Cosentino S., Tuberoso C.I.G., Pisano B., Satta M., Mascia V., Arzedi E., Palmas F.(1999). In vitro antimicrobial activity and chemical composition of Sardinian *Thymus* essential oils. *Letters in Applied Microbiology,* 29, 130-135.

Cristani M, D'Arrigo M, Mandalari G, et al. (2007). *Interaction of four monoterpenes contained in essential oils with model membranes: implications for their antibacterial activity. Journal of Agricultural Food and Chem*istry, 55 (15) 6300–8.

Daferera D.J., Ziogas B.N. (2000). Polissiou MG. GC–MS analysis of essential oils from some Greek aromatic plants and their fungitoxicity on *Penicillium digitatum. Journal of Agricultural Food and Chem*istry, 48, 2576-2581.

Daube G., Van loock F., (1997), Surveillance des toxi-infections d'origine alimentaire en Belgique. *Archives of Public Health,* 55, 351-361.

Davies N.W. (1990). Gas chromatographic retention indexes of monoterpenes and sesquiterpenes on methyl silicone and carbowax 20M phases, *Journal of Chromatographic,* 503, 1- 24.

Demetzos C., Perdetzoglou D.K. (2001). Composition and antimicrobial studies of the oils of Origanum calcaratum Juss. and O. scabrum Boiss. et Heldr. From Greece. *Journal of Essential Oil Research* 13, 460–462.

Di Pasqua R, Betts G, Hoskins N, Edwards M, Ercolini D, Mauriello G. (2007). *Membrane toxicity of antimicrobial compounds from essential oils. Journal of Agricutural Food and Chemistry* 55 (12), 4863–70.

Di Pasqua R., De Feo V., Villani F., Mauriello G. (2005). In vitro antimicrobial activity of essential oils from Mediterranean Apiaceae, Verbenaceae and Lamiaceae against foodborne pathogens and spoilage bacteria. *Annals Microbio*logy 55, 139- 143.

Dibb-Fuller M., Allen-Vercoe E., Thorns C., Woodward M. (1999). Fimbriae- and flagella-mediated association with and invasion of cultured epithelial cells by *Salmonella* enteritidis. *Microbiology*. 145, 1023- 1031.

Doublet B., Boyd D., Mulvaym. (2005). CLOECKAERTA. The Salmonella genomic island is an integrative mobilizable element. *Molecular Microbiology*. 143-148.

Dumas J. 1958. Tribu des *Salmonellae,* In: Bactériologie Médicale. Flammarion et Cie, pp. 399-433.

Elhabazi K. (2007). Contribution à l'étude pharmacologique et comportementale des extraits de certaines espèces de thym marocain. *Thèse de Doctorat, Université Cadi Ayyad, Morocco.*

Encyclopedie Encarta. (2004). Salmonelles (*Microsoft*).

ESO. (2000). The Complete Database of Essential Oils, Boelens Aroma Chemical Information Service, *The Netherlands* (1999).

Evans W.C. (1989). Trease and Evans' Pharmacognosy. *Bailliere Tindall, London, 13th Ed.*, 216–217.

Faleiro L., Miguel G., Gomes S., Costa L., Vena^ncio F., Teixeira A., et al. (2005). Antibacterial and antioxidant activities of essential oils isolated from Thymbra capitata L. (Cav.) and Origanum vulgare L. *Journal of Agricultural and Food Chemistry*. 53, 8162–8168.

Fennane M. (1987). Grande encyclopédie du Maroc: Flore et végétation. *Ed. Grupp. Walk. Over Italie, G.E.M. Rabat.* 114-116.

Fisher I. (2004). International trends in *salmonella* serotypes 1998- 2003: a surveillance report the Enter-net international surveillance network. *EuroSurveillance* 9, 9-10.

Food and Drug Administration Playing It Safe With Eggs.(2002). http://www.cfsan.fda.gov/~dms/fs-eggs.html Consulté le 08/09/04.

Frenzen P., Riggs T., Buzby J., Breuer T., Roberts T., Voeltsch D., Reddy S. (1999). FOODNET WORKING GROUP. *Salmonella* cost estimate updated using FoodNet Data. *Food Review*. 22, 10-15

Gibbs R.D. (1974). Chemotaxonomy of Flowering Plants, vol. 3. *McGill-Queen's University of Press, Montreal.*

Gill A. O., Delaquis P., Russo P., Holley R. A. (2002). Evaluation of antilisterial action of cilantro oil vacuum packed ham. *International Journal of Food Microbiology*. 73, 83–92.

Gledel J., Corbion B.E.A. (1991). Le genre Salmonella dans le contrôle Microbiologique, *2ème édition Edition*. 480 p.

Granger R., Passet J. (1971). Types chimiques (chémotypes) de l'espèce, *Thymus vulgaris* L. *Comptes-rendus de l'Académie des Sciences, Paris*. 273, 2350-2353.

Gray J., Fedorka-Cray P. (2001). Survival and infectivity of *Salmonella* Choleraesuis in swine feces. *Journal of Food Protection*, 64, 945-949.

Grimont P., Grimont F., Bouvet P. (2000), Taxonomy of the genus *Salmonella.*, In: Wray C., W.A. (Ed.) Salmonella in Domestic Animals. *CABI Publishing, Oxon*, pp. 1-17.

Haeghebaert S., Le QuerreC F., Bouvet P., Gallaya., Espie E., Vaillant V. (2002), Les toxi-infections alimentaires collectives en France en 2001. *B.E.H.* 50, 249-253.

Hanes D. (2003). Nontyphoid *Salmonella*, Bier J. (Eds) International Handbook of Foodborne Pathogens *Edition. Milotis N., New york*, 137-149 pp.

Hazzit M., Baaliouamer A., Faleiro M. L., Miguel M. G. (2006). Composition of the essential oils of Thymus and Origanum species from Algeria and their antioxidant and antimicrobial activities. *Journal of Agriculture and Food Chemistry*, 54, 6314–6321.

Hegnauer R. (1989). Chemotaxonomie der pflanzenEine Übersicht über die Verbreitung und die systematische Bedeutung der Pflanzenstoffe, *vol. 8. Birkhauser Verlag, Basel.*

Helander I.M., Alakomi H.L., Latava-Kala K., Mattila-Sandholm T., Pol I., Smid E. J., Gorris L.G.M., Von Wright A. (1998). Characterisation of the action of selected essential oil components on gram-negative bacteria. *Journal of Agriculture and Food Chemistry,* 3590- 3595.

Hmamouchi M. (1998). Country Profil of Morocco in Wild Food and Non–Food plants. *Cahiers OPTIONS. Méditerranéennes.* 38, 263-275.

Hu L., Kopecko D. (2003). Typhoid *Salmonella.* In: Miliotis N., Bier J. (Eds.), International Handbook of Foodborne Pathogens. *Marcel Dekker: New York,* 151-165.

Hueck C. (1998). Type III protein secretion systems in bacterial pathogens of animals and plants. *Microbiology and Molecular Biology Rev*eviews 62, 379-433.

Humbert F., SAutra L., Federighi M., Jouve J.L. (1998). Les salmonelles, In: *Manuel de bacteriologie alimentaire.* pp. 27-52.

Humphrey T. (2000). Public-health aspects of *Salmonella* infection. In: Wray C., Wray A. (Eds.), *Salmonella* in Domestic Animals. *CABI Publishing*: Oxon. 245-263.

Ibn Tattou M., Fennane M. (1989). Apercu historique et état actuel des connaissances sur la flore vasculaire du Maroc. *Bullettin Institue Scientifique* 13, 85–94.

Imelouane B. & ElBachiri A. (2010). Contribution à la valorisation de trois plantes médicinales et aromatique du Maroc oriental *: Lavandula dentata, Artemisia herba alba* et *Thymus vulgaris:* Etude chimique et biologique, Thèse de doctorat, Universty Mohamed 1ier Oujda, Morocco.

International Commission on Microbiological Specifications for Foods *Salmonella*e. (1996). In: ICMSF (Ed.), Microorganisms in Foods 5. Characteristics of Microbial Pathogens. *Blackie Academic & Professional: London,* 192, 217-264.

Jacob M., Pellecuer J., Tomei R. (1979) Centre régional d'étude et de développement des plantes à usage pharmaceutique. *Rivista Italiana EPPOS 11,* 26-30.

Joffin J.N., Leyral G. (2001) Microbiologie technique 1 dictionnaire des techniques. *3e éd. Biologie technique,* p. 58.

Jones M., Wigley P., Page K., Hulme S., Barrow P.( 2002). The role of Type-III secretion in the virulence of *Salmonella enterica* serovar Gallinarum and *Salmonella enterica* serovar Pullorum. In: *Colin P., Clement G. (Eds.*), Proceedings of International *Salmonella* and Salmonellosis, 29-31 may 2002, *Ploufragan, France.* Zoopole développement: *Ploufragan, 2002. Ispaia* : *Ploufragan.* 145-149.

Joulain D., König W.A. (2001). The Atlas of Spectra Data of Sesquiterpene Hydrocarbone. E.B.-Verlag, Hamburg, (1998). Joulain D., König W.A., Hochmuth D.H., Terpenoids and Related Constituents of Essential Oils. *Library of MassFinder* 2. 1. 134

Juven B.J., Kanner J., Schved F. & Weisslowiez H. (1994). Factors that interact with the antibacterial action of thyme essential oil and its active constituents. *Journal of Applied Bacteriology* 76, 626-631.

Kokkini S., Karousou R., Hanlidou E. (2003). Herbs of the Labiatae. In: *Cabarello B., Trugo L., Finglas P., Encyclopedia of Food Sciences and Nutrition. Academic Press, London.*

Lahlou M. (2004). Methods to study phytochemistry and bioactivity of essential oils. *Phytotherapy Research* 18, 435-448.

Lambert R.J.W., Skandamis P.N., Coote P. & Nychas G.J.E. (2001). A study of the minimum inhibitory concentration and mode of action of oregano essential oil, thymol and carvacrol. *Journal of Applied Microbiology* 91, 453-462.

Lambert R.J.W., Skandamis P.N., Coote P.J., Nychas G.-J.E. (2001). A study of the minimum inhibitory concentration and mode of action of oregano essential oil, thymol and carvacrol. *Journal of. Applied Bacteriology* 91, 453-462.

Lataoui N., Tantaoui-Elaraki A. (1994). Individual and combined antibacterial activity of the main components of three thyme essentials oils. *Rivista Italiana EPPOS.* 13, 13–19.

Lawrence B.M. (1992). Chemical components of Labiatae oils and their exploitation. In: *Harley R.M., Reynolds T., Advances in Labiatae Science. The Royal Botanical Gardens, Kew*, 399–436.

Le Floc'h E. (1983). Contribution à une étude ethnobotanique de la flore tunisienne. *Ed. Ministère de l'enseignement supérieur et de la recherche scientifique.*

Le Minor L. (1984). Genus III. *Salmonella,* In: *Krieg N., Holt, J. (Eds.) Bergey's Manual of Systematic Bacteriology (volume 1), Williams and Wilkins: Baltimore*, 427- 458.

Le Minor L., Popoff M.Y. (1987). Request for an Opinion. Designation of Salmonella Enterica sp. Nov. nom. rev, as the type and only species of the genus Salmonella. *International Journal of Systimatic Bacteriology* 37, 465-468.

Letellier A., Messier S., Paré J., Ménard J, Quessy S. (1999). Distribution of *Salmonella* in swine herds in Quebec. *Veterinary Microbiology* 67, 299-306.

Marino M., Bersani C. And Comi G. (1999). Antimicrobial activity of the essential oils of *Thymus vulgaris* L. measured using a bioimpedometric method. *Journal of Food Protection*, 62, 1017-23.

McLafferty F.W., Stauffer D.B. (1989). The Wiley/NBS Registry of Mass Spectral Data. *J. Wiley & Sons*, New York

Mead P., Slutsker L., Dietz V., McCaig L., Bresee J, Shapiro C., Griffin P., Tauxe R. (1999), Food-related illness and death in the United States. *Emerging Infectious Diseases Journal*, 5, 607-625.

Mermin J., VIllar R., Carpenter J., Roberts L., Samaridden A., Gasanova L., Lomakina S., Bopp C., Hutwagner L., Mead P., Ross B., Mintz E. (1999). A massive epidemic of multidrug-resistant typhoid fever in Tajikistan associated with consumption of municipal water. *Journal of Infectious Diseases* 179, 1416-1422.

Miquel J.D., Richard H.M., Sandret F.G. (1976). Volatile constituents of Moroccan Thyme oil, *Journal of Agricultural and Food Chemistry* 24, 833-835.

Mitchell M., Shane S. (2000). Preliminary findings of *Salmonella* spp. in captive green iguanas (Iguana iguana) and their environment. *Preventive Veterinary Medicine* 45, 297-304.

Morales R. (1997). Synopsis of the genus *Thymus* L. in the Mediterranean area. *Logascalia.* 19, 249–262.

Morales R. (2002). The history, botany and taxonomy of the genus *Thymus*. In: *Thyme: the genus Thymus*, 1–43.

Murray C. (2000). Environmental aspects of *Salmonella*. In: *Wray C., Wray A. (Eds.), Salmonella in Domestic Animals. CABI Publishing: Oxon*, 265-283.

Organisation Mondiale de la Santé (OMS). (1999). *Monographs on selected medicinal plants. Geneva, Switzerland: OMS.*

Ozcan G, Sagdic O, Ozcan M. (2003). Note: Inhibition of pathogenic bacteria by essential oils at different concentrations. *International Journal of Food Science & Technology.* 9, 85-88.

Panizzi L., Flamini G., Cioni P.L., Morelli I.(1993). Composition and antimicrobial activity of essential oils of four mediterranean Lamiaceae. *Journal of Ethnopharmacology.* 39, 167- 170.

Parlement Europeen et Conseil de l'Union Europeenne. (2001). Report to the European Parliament and to the Council on the measures to be put in force for the control and prevention of zoonoses - Proposal for a Directive of the European Parliament and of the Council 193 on the moniroting of zoonoses and zoonotic agents, amending Council Decision 90/424/EEC and repealing Council Directive 92/117/EEC - *Proposal for a Regulation of the European Parliament and of the Council on the control of salmonella and other food-borne zoonotic agents and amending Council Directives 64/432/EEC, 72/462/EEC and 90/539/EEC, COM (2001) 452 final, 01.08.2001.*

Pedersen J.A. (2000). Distribution and taxonomic implications of some phenolics in the family Lamiaceae determined by ESR spectroscopy. *Biochemical Systematics Ecology*, 28, 229- 253.

Pellecuer J., Jacob M., Simeon D.M., Dusart G., Attisto M., Barthez M., Gourgas L., Pascal B., Tomei R. (1980). Essais d'utilisation d'huiles essentielles de plantes aromatiques méditerranéennes en odontologie conservatrice. *Plantes Médicinnales Phytothérapie,* 14, 83–98.

Pibiri M.C. (2006). Assainissement microbiologique de l'air et des systèmes de ventilation au moyen d'huiles essentielles. *Thèse no 3311, Ecole polytechnique fédérale de Lausanne, Suisse.*

Quezel P., Medail F. (1994). La région circum-méditerranéenne. Centre mondial majeur de biodiversité végétale. *Actes 6èmes Rencontres de l'A.R.P.E.* 152-161. *Gap. France.*

Quezel P., Santa S. (1963). Nouvelle flore de l'Algérie et des régions désertiques méridionales. Ed. *du Centre National de la Recherche Scientifique. T. II, Paris.* 781- 801.

Rasooli I., Mirmostafa S.A. (2002). Antibacterial properties of *Thymus pubescens* and *Thymus serpyllum* essential oils. *Fitoterapia.* 73, 244-250.

Reeves M.W., Evins G.M., Heiba A.A., Plikaytis B.D., Farmer J.J. (1989). Clonal nature of Salmonella Typhi and its genetic relatedness to other Salmonella as shown by multilocus enzyme electrophoresis and proposal of Salmonella bongori comb. *Journal of Clinical Microbiology* 27, 313-320.

Romane A., Belaqziz R. Harrak R., Oufedou K. ElAlaoui ElFels M.A., (2010) Antimicrobial and Insecticidal Activities of the Endemic *Thymus broussonetti* Boiss. and *Thymus maroccanus* Ball., *Records Natural Products,* 4; 230-237.

Rossi P.G. (2003). Caractérisation et valorisation des produits issus de la biomasse : activité biologique des huiles essentielles. *Université de Corse*, p. 2

Rycroft A. (2000). Structure, function and synthesis of surface polysaccharides in *Salmonella.* In: Wray C., Wray A. (Eds.), *Salmonella* in Domestic Animals. CABI Publishing: Oxon, 19-33.

Sağdac O. 2003. Sensitivity of four pathogenic bacteria to Turkish thyme and oregano hydrosols. *Lebensmittel-Wissenschaft und–Technologie* 36, 467-73.

Salm-Surv G. (2005). Un réseau de l'OMS pour la surveillance des maladies d'origine alimentaire. In *note d'information INFOSAN N°6 / - Programme Global Salm-Surv de l'OMS.*

Sarwari A., Magder L., Levine P., McNamaraa., Knower S., Armstrong G., Etzel R., Hollingsworth J., Morris G. (2001). Serotypes distribution of *Salmonella* isolates from food animals after slaughter differs from that of isolates found in humans. *Journal of Infectious Diseases* 183, 1295-1299.

Scientific Committee on Veterinary Measures Relating to Public Health Opinion of the SCVMPH on *Salmonellae* in Foodstuffs (adopted on 14-15April 2003): http://europa.eu.int/comm/food/fs/sc/scv/out66_en.pdf Consulté le 07/06/04.

Shelobolina E.S., Sullivan S.A., O'neill K.R., Nevin K.P., Lovley D.R. (2004). Isolation, characterization, and U (VI)-reducing potential of a facultatively anaerobic, acid-resistant bacterium from low-pH, nitrate- and U (VI)-contaminated subsurface sediment and description of Salmonella subterranea sp . *Applied and Environmental Microbiology* 70, 2959-2965.

Shunying Z., Yang Y., Huaidong Y., et al. (2005). Chemical composition and antimicrobial activity of the essential oils of Chrysanthemum indicum. *Journal of Ethnopharmacology* 96, 151-8.

Sijelmassi A. (1993). Les plantes médicinales du Maroc. *Ed. Le Fennec, Casablanca*, 286 p.

Sthal-Biskup E., Laakso I.(1990). Essential oil Polymerphism in finish Thymus species. *Planta Medica* 56, 464-468.

Tahiri B. (1996). Étude biosystématique et chimique du genre *Thymus* L. (Labiatae) au Maroc. *Thèse de 3ème cycle, Université Mohamed V, Rabat. Maroc.*

Tantaoui Elaraki A., Lattaoui N., Errifi A. (1993). Composition and antimicrobial activity of the essential oil of *Thymus broussonetti, T. Zygis* and *T. Satureoïde. Journal of Essential Oil. Research,* 5, 45-53.

Taskova R., Mitova M., Evstatieva L., Ancev M., Peev D., Handjieva N., Bankova V., Popov S. (1997). Iridoids, flavonoids and terpenoids as taxonomic markers in Lamiaceae, Scrophulariaceae and Rubiaceae. *Bocconea*. 5, 631–636.

Thorns J., Woodward M. (2000). Fimbriae of *Salmonella*. In : Wray C., Wray A. (Eds.), *Salmonella* in Domestic Animals. *CABI Publishing : Oxon*. 35-55.

Trombetta D., et al. (2005). Mechanisms of antibacterial action of three monoterpenes. *Antimicrobial Agents and Chemotherapy*, 49(6), 2474-2478.

Ultee A., Kets E.P.W., Smid E., et al. (1999). Mechanisms of action of carvacrol on the Food-borne pathogen Bacillus cereus. *Applied Environmental Microbiology*. 65, 4606-10.

Ultee A., Bennink M. H., Moezelaar R. (2002). The phenolic hydroxyl group of carvacrol is essential for action against the foodborne pathogens Bacillus cereus. *Applied Environmental Microbiology*. 68, 1561–1568.

USAID (United States Agency for International Development). (2005). Filière des plantes aromatiques et médicinales. *Note de Synthèse.*

Van Den Broucke C.O., Lemli J.A. (1981). Pharmacological and chemical investigation of thyme liquid extracts. *Planta Medica*. 41, 129-135.

Vardar-Unlu G., Candan F., Sokem A., Daferera D., Polissiou, M., Sokmen M., et al. (2003). Antimicrobial and antioxidant activity of the essential oil and methanol extracts of Thymus pectinatus Fisch, et Mey. var. pectinatu (Lamiaceae). *Journal of Agricultural and Food Chemistry*. 51, 63–67.

Varnam A., Evans M. (1996). Chapter 4 – *Salmonella*. In: Varnam A., Evans, M. (Eds.) Foodborne pathogens – an illustrated text 2nd ed. *Manson Publishing : London*. 51-86.

Vimal D., Khullar M., Gupta S., Ganguly N. (2000). Intestinal mucins: the binding sites for *Salmonella* typhimurium. *Molecular Cellular Biochemistry,* 204, 107-17.

Walsh, S.E., Maillard J.Y., Russell A.D., Catrenich C.E., Charbonneau D.L., Bartolo R.G. (2003). Activity and mechanisms of action of selected biocidal agents on Gram positive and negative bacteria. *Journal of Applied Bacteriology*, 94, 240 247.

Wybo I., Wildemauwe C., Godard C., Bertrand S., Collard J.M. (2002). Antimicrobial drug resistance in nontyphoid human *Salmonella* in Belgium: Trends for the period 2000-2002. *Acta Clinica Belgica* 59, 152-160.

Zargari A. (1990). Medicinal Plants, Vol. 4. *Tehran University Publications, Tehran*. 28–42.

# 15

# Inhibitory Effect of Plant Extracts on *Salmonella* spp.

Krittika Norajit and Gi-Hyung Ryu
*Kongju National University*
*South Korea*

## 1. Introduction

*Salmonella* spp., facultatively anaerobic gram-negative rod-shaped bacteria (Krieg & Holt, 1984), is one of the most important food borne pathogens. If present in food, the bacteria do not affect the taste, smell or appearance of the food. Frequent hand washing, throwing out expired food, avoid eating raw or undercooked eggs, meats, seafood or poultry are the key to preventing *Salmonella* food poisoning. Antibiotics (such as ampicillin, chloramphenicol, streptomycin, sulfonamides and tetracycline) may be prescribed for moderate to severe cases of *Salmonella* food poisoning or when it occurs in a person who is at risk for complications. However, probably as a consequence of the extensive use of antibiotics, that the incidence and severity of human diseases related to *Salmonella* caused by antimicrobial resistant *Salmonella* is rising in many countries (Breuil et al., 2000). Furthermore, illness caused by resistant *Salmonella* can be more severe and difficult to control (Oliveira et al., 2006).

Presence of the bacterium *Salmonella* in food and the disease *Salmonella* food poisoning and typhoid fever continue to be a major public health problem worldwide. Millions of human cases are reported worldwide every year and the disease results in thousands of deaths. The increasingly resistance to antibiotics of food borne *Salmonella* (Breuil et al., 2000) drive much of the current interest on plant antimicrobial molecules. At the same time, increasingly consumer demand for more natural products has led to the food industry to consider the incorporation of the natural preservative in a range of products (Dorman & Deans, 2000; Elgayyar et al., 2001). Plants are complex chemical storehouses of undiscovered biodynamic compounds with unrealized potential for use in modern medicine (Plotkin, 1988). Several antimicrobial agents were isolated from plant including secondary metabolites as essential oil, terpenoides, phenols, alkaloids and flavanoids (Kazmi et al., 1994; Cosentino et al., 1999; Omulokoli et al., 1997). An important characteristic of these compounds is their hydrophobicity, which enables them to partition in the lipids of the bacterial cell membrane and mitochondria, disturbing the structures and rendering them more permeable (Burt, 2004). This chapter is undertake in order to investigate inhibitory effect of plant extracts on *Salmonella* spp., including a prevalence and control of *Salmonella* in foods and incidence of antibiotic resistant strains of *Salmonella*. Information on extraction methods and phytochemical compositions of medicinal plants can be found in this chapter. The current knowledge on potential of plant extracts for antibacterial activity against *Salmonella* spp. and its application in food processing or packaging will be discussed.

## 2. Prevalence of *Salmonella* in foods

Most *Salmonella* can survive for extended periods in food stored at refrigeration to ambient room temperatures (2-25°C). Some *Salmonella* strains can grow in high temperature as 54°C (Montville & Matthews, 2008). The *Salmonellla* are generally transmitted to humans through consumption of contaminated food of animal origin, mainly meat, poultry, eggs and milk. The prevalence of pathogenic serotypes associated with food-borne disease varies by geographical location (Watie & Yousef, 2010). The *Enteritidis, Typhimurium, Newport* and *Javiana* were the most prevalence serotypes in the United States in 2007. The symptoms and sign of *Salmonella* infection include diarrhea, abdominal pains, nausea, vomiting and chills, leading to dehydration and headaches (Richard et al., 2008).

### 2.1 *Salmonella* in egg

In eggs, various *Salmonella* serovars can be found in the egg content, principally *S. enteritidis*, is the serovar most frequently with egg infection (Gast & Beard, 1990; Humphrey et al., 1991; de Louvois 1993). A few reported in human on outbreaks of *Salmonella* food poisoning related egg caused by *S. typhimurium* (EFSA, 2010a). Other *Salmonella* serovars, e.g., *S. mbandaka, S. livingstone, S. heidelberg, S. hadar, S. infantis* and *S. virchow*, also occur with low frequency in layers and consequently on egg surfaces (Chemaly et al., 2009). The risk assessment estimates the probability of human illness due to *Salmonella* following the ingestion of a single food serving of internally contaminated shell eggs, either consumed as whole eggs, egg meals, or product containing these ingredients such as cake or mayonnaise. The growth of *Salmonella* in egg albumen is eased at 20°C, while it is unable to grow at temperature less than 10°C (Gantois et al., 2009). Recently, an average prevalence of 0.5% eggs contaminated with *Salmonella* was reported across the member states of the European Commission (EFSA, 2010b).

### 2.2 *Salmonella* in meat

Pork and pork products are also recognized as one of the major sources of human *Salmonella* food poisoning. The commonly isolated non-typhoid *Salmonella* serovars in pigs, pork and humans is *S. typhimurium* (Astorga Marquez et al., 2007; Boyen et al., 2008; Perugini et al., 2010). During further processing of meat, such as cutting and mincing, *S. typhimurium* from contaminated pork cuts may then spread into pork preparations (Gonzales-Barron et al., 2010). The proportion of human *Salmonella* food poisoning attributable to pork has been estimated to be between 9 and 15% in Denmark and around 21% in Netherlands (EFSA, 2008; Hald et al., 2004). In Ireland, the pork meat has been identified as a significant source of *Salmonella* with an incidence of 2.9% as surveyed in processing plants (Gonzales-Barron, 2010b). A Belgian survey from 2000 to 2003 indicated that the mean prevalence values of *Salmonella* in 25 g samples of pork meat cuts and minced meat were 17.3% (95% CI: 15.0–19.7%) and 11.1% (95% CI: 9.4–13.0%) (Ghafir et al., 2007, 2005), respectively.

### 2.3 *Salmonella* in poultry

In the European Union, three of the top four serovars (*S. infantis*: 29.2%, *S. enteritidis*: 13.6%, *S. kentucky*: 6.2% and *S. typhimurium*: 4.4%, respectively) isolated from poultry are also found in the top four serovars (*S. enteritidis*: 58.0%, *S. typhimurium*: 21.9%, *S. infantis*: 1.1%

and *S. virchow*: 0.7%, respectively) isolated from humans (EFSA, 2010c). The *S. sofia* has rarely been reported to be isolated from poultry in Australia, which the very low prevalence of *Salmonella* food poisoning linked to *S. sofia* suggests low virulence for humans (Duffy et al., 2011). A large percentage of poultry is colonized by salmonellas during grow-out, and the skin and meat of carcasses are frequently contaminated by the pathogen during slaughter and processing. In Brazil, the remarkable increase in the incidence of *S. enteritidis* from foodborne outbreaks, human infections, nonhuman sources, broiler carcasses and other poultry materials has been reported since the 1990s (Peresi et al., 1998; Fuzihara et al., 2000; Tavechio et al., 2002). Of the 281 chicken meat samples in Austria, 46 were positive for the occurrence of *Salmonella* (prevalence of 16.4%) as described by Mayrhofer et al., 2004.

### 2.4 *Salmonella* in milk

One route of *Salmonella* transmission is via raw/unpasteurized milk and products made from raw milk (e.g. cheese) (Cody 1999). In a 2000 study of New York dairy herds, *Salmonella* were isolated from 1.5 percent of 404 milk filters. *Salmonella* contamination of bulk milk most likely occurs through fecal contamination, and mitigation through improved hygiene practices may be possible (Karns et al., 2005). Consumption of cheese contaminated with the mentioned pathogens can lead to serious health problems, which the outbreaks of *Salmonella* spp. in Mozzarella cheese can be seen since 1981 in Italy and USA (De Buyser et al., 2001). In 1985, D'Aoust et al. found that *S. typhimurium* was linked to Canadian foodborne outbreaks associated with the consumption of Cheddar cheese.

### 2.5 *Salmonella* in other food

A recent *Salmonella* outbreak is also occur with other food products (Waite & Yousef, 2010). In United States, Columbia and Canada in 2008, there are estimated more than 1000 case of *Salmonella* food poisoning outbreaks by *S. saintpaul* in raw tomatoes, fresh cilantro, fresh jalapeno peppers and fresh Serrano peppers, whereas in 2007, the foodborne outbreaks was found in peanut butter, frozen pot pie and puffed vegetable snack in United States and boxed lunch in Japan. Other fruit product such as fruit salad and orange juice has been associated with occasional outbreaks of *Salmonella* food poisoning.

## 3. Control of *Salmonella* in foods

High temperatures used in cooking and in pasteurization processes have been regarded as the treatment of choice for the destruction of *Salmonella* in eggs, milk and meat products. Humphrey et al. (1980) showed that to kill *Salmonella* present in the egg yolk, the yolk temperature had to be raised to >8O°C. Boiling for over 6 to 10 min was required inactivate approximately $10^7$ cfu *S. enteritidis* in the yolk of shell eggs, depending on the method of boiling (Chantarapanont et al., 2000). Kuo et al. (1997) determined that UV radiation significantly reduced *S. typhimurium* inoculated on shell eggs. Directional microwave technology resulted in more than 2-log reduction of *S. enteritidis* in shell eggs without causing any detrimental effects to quality reviewed by Lakins et al. (2008). The effectiveness of steam treatments on meat and poultry has been investigated, which the presence of a number of pathogens may be reduced by the application of steam to meat surfaces, mostly gram negative enteric pathogens, such as *Escherichia coli* O157:H7 and a number of

*Salmonella* serotypes (James et al., 2000; Phebus et al., 1997; Whyte et al., 2003). Following the published report by Porto-Fett et al., 2010, the fermentation and drying and/or high pressure processing of contaminated dry sausage or pork are effective for inactivating *Salmonella* spp. High-pressure treatment of milk is considered to be the most promising alternative to traditional thermal treatments. Metrick et al., (1989) indicated that the pressure treatments of 310 and 379MPa/15 min at ambient temperature were required for a 3-log reduction in colony forming units (cfu) of *S. seftenberg* 775W.

## 4. Antibiotic resistance *Salmonella*

The first reports on antibiotic resistant *Salmonella* had been indicated since 1960s and describe mainly case with monoresistance strain (Helmuth, 2000). In the late 1980s, the appearance multiple resistances against ampicillin, chloramphenicol, streptomycin, sulfonamides and tetracycline were found in serovar *Thyphimurium* definitive type 104 (DT 104) (Montville & Matthews, 2005). The main mechanism of bacteria exhibit resistance to antimicrobial agents can be due to many factors including drug inactivation, reduced drug accumulation, alteration of metabolic pathway and target site (Barbosa & Levy, 2000; Schwarz & Chaslus-Dancla, 2001). Much of the resistance to penicillins and cephalosporins by *Salmonella* spp. is attributable to the acquired ability of the strains to produce β-lactamase that can degrade the chemical structure of the antimicrobial agents (Bush, 2003).

In recent years, the prevalence of multidrug resistant *Salmonella* in foods has been reported in many parts of the world. Several clinical treatment failures with fluoroquinolones (such as ciprofloxacin) in cases of *S. typhi* showed in Europe, Asia, and Africa (Butt et al., 2003; Nkemngu et al., 2005). Shirakawa et al. (2006) claims that the resistance to nalidixic acid and decreased susceptibility to fluoroquinolone in the *S. enterica* serovar *Typhi* isolated in Katmandu, Nepal, in 2003 were completely correlated to the mutation at codon 83 of gyrA. Most antimicrobial-resistant *Salmonella* infections are acquired from eating contaminated foods of animal origin. During 2000-2006 in Taiwan, it was found that 30.5% of the raw chicken meat was contaminated with multidrug resistant *S. enterica* serovar *Schwarzengrund* (Chen et al., 2011). Among the 88 *Salmonella* isolated from 300 meat products (raw beef, chicken meat and street foods) in Kuala Lumpur, the highest resistance was to tetracycline (73.8%), followed by sulfonamide (63.6%), streptomycin (57.9%), nalidixic acid (44.3%), trimethoprim sulfamethoxazole (19.3%), ampicillin (17.0%), chloramphenicol (10.2%) (Thong & Modarressi, 2011). The most antimicrobial resistance *S. enteritidis* isolates from South of Brazil reported by de Oliveir et al. (2005) was found in poultry related samples, where all strains were resistant to at least one antimicrobial agent.

The prevalence of extraintestinal *salmonella* infections caused by antibiotic resistant *Salmonella* spp. in several geographic areas of the world is increasing. Pokharel et al. (2006) demonstrated a 5% prevalence of multidrug resistance among *S. enterica* at a tertiary care hospital in Kathmandu, Nepal, with a higher rate of multidrug resistance among *S. paratyphi A* (7%) compared to *S. typhi* (3%). Rotimi et al. (2008) reported the serious problem of drug resistance in *Salmonella* spp. in Kuwait and United Arab Emirates that the non-typhoidal *Salmonella* spp. isolates from fecal samples of patients had 5-fold rise in resistant to cefotaxime and ceftriaxone compared with reported earlier.

## 5. Plant extract

Plant contain a variety of substance called "phytochemicals" (divided into two groups; primary and secondary metabolite), which are naturally occurring biochemicals in plants that give plants their color, flavor, smell and texture. Plant secondary metabolite differ from ubiquitous primary metabolite (e.g. carbohydrate, proteins, fats, nucleic acid) (Bako and Aguh, 2007), that have a scientifically proven effect on human health. The most important of these bioactive constituents of plants are alkaloids, tannins, flavonoids, anthraquinone, other phenolic compound and essential oil (Kisangau et al, 2007).

Extraction is the first important step for the recovery and purification of active ingredients of plant materials. Several extraction techniques and solvents are used for obtain antioxidant and antimicrobial extract from plant origin. The general techniques of medicinal plant extraction include maceration, percolation, hot continuous extraction (Soxhlet), solvent extraction, counter-current extraction, microwave-assisted extraction, ultrasound extraction (sonication), supercritical fluid extraction (Chen et al., 1992; Bicchi et al., 2000; Kaufmann and Christen, 2002). For solvent extraction method, polar solvents (such as organic acids), solvents of intermediate polarity (such as methanol, ethanol, acetone, and dichloromethane) and solvents of low polarity (such as hexane and chloroform) are used to extract plant secondary metabolites, which the extracts obtained from the same plant material with different solvent characteristics have distinct physical and biological properties. Lapornik, et al. (2005) reported that ethanol and methanol extracts of red and black currant contain twice more anthocyanins and polyphenols than water extracts, extracts made from grape marc had seven times higher values than water extracts. Among the five different Indian medical plants, methanol extract showed more antibacterial activity and moderate activity with aqueous, ethyl acetate and chloroform extract (Ashokkumar et al., 2010), while the more-polar solvent extracts (BuOH and water extracts) in Korean herbal medicines gave higher antioxidant activity than that of non-polar solvent extracts (hexane and EtOAC extracts) (Kang et al., 2003). Moreover, the chemical compound of extracts from particular plant species can vary according to the geographic origin, harvesting period and parts of the plant use. Nwokocha et al. (2011) found that all secondary metabolites analyzed were present in all tissues (leaf, stem, root and seed) studied but at different concentrations. A spatial and seasonal impact on the total phenolic content has been reported for *Poacynum henersonii* collected at three sites in China (Hong et al., 2003).

Essential oils are a volatile liquid aromatic compound which extracted from plant cell. The cells are location in specific parts of the plant such as bark, flowers, leave, seed, peel and root. Table 1 shows the plant organ contains essential oil and their essential oil constitutes. Distillation (water distillation, water and steam distillation, steam distillation) is the most commonly used method for produces essential oils on the commercial basis (Rasooli, 2007). Some volatile oils cannot be distilled without decomposition are thus are usually obtained by expression (such as lemon oil or orange oil). The effect of diffrent distillation methods on oil content and composition of aromatic plants have been reported. The water-distillation of the rose-scented geranium (*Pelargonium* sp.) gave a higher oil yield (0.16–0.22%) than did water-steam-distillation (0.09–0.12%) or steam-distillation methods (0.06–0.18%) (Kiran et al., 2005). The oil of *Satureja rechingeri* Jamzad in full flowering stage obtained by hydro-distillation, water- and steam-distillation and direct steam-distillation consisted of twenty, seventeen and twenty-two compounds, respectively, which the major constituents were carvacrol and p-cymene (Sefidkon et al., 2007).

| Plant organ | Plant | Main chemical composition |
|---|---|---|
| Flower | Neroli, rose, jasmine, rosemary, lavender, chamomile | Linalool, citronellol, bezyl acetate, α-pinene, α-bisabolol |
| Leaves | Eucalyptus, tea tree, patchouli, verbena | Eucalyptol, 1,8-cineole, terpinen-4-ol, patchoulol, geranial |
| Aerial part | Basil, peppermint, spearmint | Linalool, manthol, carvone |
| Fruit | Bergamot, juniper, lemon, mandarin | Limonene, α-terpineol, citral, limonene |
| Seed | Coriander, caraway, nutmeg, fennel, angelica | linalool, carvone, sabinene, (E)-anethole, β-Phellandrene |
| Bark and wood | Cinnnamon, cedarwood, sandalwood, pine | Cinnamaldehyde, Thujopsene, α-santalene, α-pinene |
| Rhizomes | Ginger, galanga, calamus, curcuma, kaempferia, | Zingiberene, 1,8-cineole, β-asarone, turmerone, methylcinnamate |
| Roots | Vetiver, saussurea, valerian | Khusimol, α-selinene, bornyl acetate |

Table 1. Essential oils in each plant organ (Base on Krishnasamy, 2008)

## 6. Anti-*Salmonella* activity of plant extract

Chemical compound of the plant extract or essential oils has revealed the presence of several ingredients, most of which posses important antimicrobial properties (Botsoglou et al., 2003; Exarchou et al., 2002). Many studied claim that the phenolic compound in herb and spice significantly contributed to their properties (Hara-Kudo et al., 2004). Twenty-five extracts (accounting for 54% of the 46 test extract as 20 dietary spices and 26 medical herbs) reported by Shan et al. (2007) showed inhibitory activity against *S. anatum* (mean=7.2 mm; 4.7–19.2 mm) with correlate the content of phenolic compound at $R^2$ value of 0.86. Based on the results of chemical composition of the essential oil from *Zataria multiflora* Boiss, can also conclude that the anti-*S. typhi* ATCC 19430 nature of the essential oil studied is apparently related to its high phenolic contents, particularly carvacrol and thymol (Sharififar et al., 2007). Acidic environment enhanced the antibacterial activity of *Filipendula ulmaria* extract when it was tested against *S. enteritidis* PT4, which water-methanol extract from *F. ulmaria* contains a variety of phenolic compounds, such as caffeic, p-coumaric, vanillic acid and myricetin, etc, which demonstrate antibacterial activity (Boziaris et al.,2011).

Out of all the three solvent (hexane, dichloromethane and methanol) used for extract Mauritians flora, the methanol extracts showed relative good anti-bacterial activities, most particularly against *S. enteritidis* (Rangasamy et al., 2007). The aqueous extract of leaf of *Coccinia indica* could be used against *Salmonella*, while no activity was shown by solvent extract (ethanol, petroleum ether and chloroform) (Hussain et al., 2010). From twenty-two medicinal herb species traditionally used in Korea to treat gastrointestinal infections studied, only the aqueous and methanolic extracts of *Schizandrae fructus* exhibited antibacterial activity against all three *Salmonella* serotypes (*S. typhi* ATCC 19943, S. *paratyphi* A and *S. gallinarum* ATCC 9184) (Lee et al., 2006).

In India, Mahida & Mohan (2007) described that the methanol *Manilkara hexandra, Wrightia tomentora* and *Xanthium strumarium* extracts displayed MIC value of 2 mg/mL for *S. paratyphi* A whereas the methanol *Schrebera swietenoiides* and *Wrightia tomentora* showed MIC value of 4 mg/mL for *S. typhi*. The result studied by N'guessan et al. (2007) showed bactericidal effect of the aqueous extract of *Thonningia sanguinea* for all the multiple drug resistance *Salmonella* strains (*S. typhi, S. hadar* and *S. typhimurium)* and sensitive tested strains (*S. enteritidis*). The *S. typhimurium* strain was also found to be sensitive to extracts of *Acacia nilotica, Syzygium aromaticum* and *Cinnamum zeylanicum,* in Khan et al. (2009). The petroleum ether extract of *Pedalium murex* Linn exhibits the activity at 300-500 mg/disc against the *S. paratyphi A* and at 500 mg/disc against the *S. paratyphi B* (Nalini et al., 2011). Furthermore, the root of the *Euphorbia balsamifera* has high activity against the *S. typhimurium* when compared with the leaves and stems extracts (Kamba & Hassa, 2010). In contrast, the extract of eucalyptus from root, leave and stem had exhibited activity against *S. typhi* (Evans et al., 2002).

## 7. *Salmonella* control in food product and food packaging by plant extract

Nowadays, the foodborne outbreaks *Salmonella* food poisoning and the prevalence of antibiotic resistant *Salmonella* in humans, animals and food are increasing (Rabsch et al., 2001; Angulo et al., 2000; O'Brien, 2002). Consumers are also concerned about the safety of food containing synthetic preservative. Therefore, there has been growing interesting in using natural antibacterial extract from herb or spice for food conservation (Smid & Gorris, 1999; Fasseas et al., 2008; Gutierrez et al., 2008). Particular interest has been focused on the potential application of plant extract or essential oils as safer additives for meat, poultry, milk, fruit and vegetable.

The combination of the oregano essential oil at 0.6% with nisin at 500 IU/g showed stronger antimicrobial activity against *S. enteritidis* in minced sheep meat than the oregano EO at 0.6% but lower than the combination with nisin at 1000 IU/g (Govaris et al., 2010). The minimum inhibitory concentration of the Capsicum extract to prevent the growth of *S. typhimurium* in minced beef was 1.5 mL/100 g of meat; the addition of 1%, 2%, 3% and 4% w/w of sodium chloride did not have any additional inhibitory effect on *Salmonella* (Careaga et al., 2003). Ravishankar et al. (2009) suggest that the food industry and consumers could use apple-based edible films containing cinnamaldehyde or carvacrol as wrappings to control surface contamination by foodborne pathogenic microorganisms, which at 23°C on chicken breasts, films with 3% antimicrobials showed the highest reductions (4.3 to 6.8 log cfu/g) of both *S. enterica* and *E. coli* O157:H7. Moreover, the lowest concentration of trans-cinnamaldehyde (10 mM) reducing *S. enteritidis* populations inoculated on chicken cecal contents by approximately 6.0 log(10) cfu/mL after 8 h and >8.0 log(10) cfu/mL after 24 h of incubation (Johny et al., 2010). The carvacrol vapour was effective at preventing growth of *Salmonella* on agar and in significantly reducing viable numbers on raw chicken at temperatures ranging from 4°C to 37 °C (Burt et al., 2007). The results by Shan et al. (2011) showed that the five spice and herb extracts (cinnamon stick, oregano, clove, pomegranate peel, and grape seed) were effective against *S. enterica* in cheese at room temperature (~23°C), which the clove showed the highest antibacterial activity.

Tornuk et al. (2011) indicated that the thyme hydrosol (contain carvacrol: 48.30% and thymol: 17.55%) was the most efficient agent on the carrot samples with resulted in 1.48 log cfu/g reduction in *S. typhimurium* number. The antimicrobial effect of essential oil components (monoterpenes e.g. thymol, menthol and linalyl acetate) might be due to a perturbation of the lipid fraction of bacterial plasma membranes, resulting in alterations of membrane permeability and in leakage of intracellular materials (Trombetta et al., 2005). Both concentrations of carvacrol and trans-cinnamaldehyde, and 0.75% eugenol decreased *Salmonella* counts on tomatoes by ~6.0 log cfu/mL at 1 min (Mattson et al., 2011). Treatment of seeds at 50 degrees C for 12 h with acetic acid (100 and 300 mg/L of air) and thymol or cinnamic aldehyde (600 mg/L of air) significantly reduced *Salmonella* populations on seeds (>1.7 log10 cfu/g) without affecting germination percentage (Weissinger et al., 2001).
The use of edible films to release antimicrobial constituents in food packaging is a form of active packaging. Seydium & Sarikus (2006) reported that the whey protein based edible films containing oregano essential oil was the most effective against *S. enteritidis* (ATCC 13076), at 2% level than those containing garlic and rosemary extracts ($P < 0.05$). Incorporation of garlic oil up to 0.4% v/v in alginate film, the clear zone of inhibition was not observed with *S. typhimurium*. However, incorporation of garlic oil at higher than 0.1% v/v revealed a weak inhibitory effect, indicated by minimal growth underneath film discs (Pranoto et al., 2005).

## 8. Conclusion

Prevalence of *Salmonella* infection has increased markedly in both humans and domestic animals. Probably as a consequence of the extensive use of antibiotics surveillance networks have indicated that the incidence of human *Salmonella* food poisoning caused by antimicrobial resistant *Salmonella* is rising in many countries. In present, the anti-*Salmonella* spp. properties of plant extract/essential oils from a variety of plant have been assessed. It is clear from these studies that these secondary plant metabolites have potential as alternative antibacterial in food conservation. The phenolic compounds are most active and appear to act principally as membrane permeabilisers. In addition, consumers are also demand for food preservation from natural source. Therefore, the incorporating plant extracts in or onto food packaging materials to against foodborne pathogen, especially *Salmonella* spp., is of increasing interest.

## 9. Reference

Angulo, F.J.; Johnson, K.R.; Tauxe, R.V., & Cohen, M.L. (2000). Origins and Consequences of Antimicrobial-Resistant Nontyphoidal *Salmonella*: Implications for the Use of Fluoroquinolones in Food Animals. *Microbial Drug Resistance*, Vol.6, No.1, pp. 77–83, ISSN 1076-6294

Ashokkumar, P.; Fajkumar, & Kanimozhi, M. (2010). Phytochemical Screening and Antimicrobial Activity from Five Indian Medicinal Plant Against Human Pathogens. *Middle-East Journal of Scientific Research*, Vol. 5, No.6, pp. 477-482, ISSN 1990-9233

Astorga Marquez, R.J.; Salaberria, A.E.; Maldonado Garcia, A.; Valdezate Jimenez, S.; Carbonero Martinez, A.; Aladuena Garcia, A., & Casas, A.A. (2007). Surveillance and Antimicrobial Resistance of Salmonella Strains Isolated from Slaughtered Pigs in Spain. *Journal of Food Protection*, Vol.70, No.6, pp. 1502–1506, ISSN 0362-028x

Bako, S.P., & Aguh, B.I. (2007). Qualitative Evaluation of Phytochemical Profiles in *Loranthacean mistletoes* (*Tapinanthus* sp.) as Related to their Hosts. *Nigerian Journal of Botany*, Vol.20, pp. 297-305, ISSN 0795-0128

Barbosa, T.M., & Levy, S.B. (2000). The Impact of Antibiotic Use on Resistance Development and Persistence. *Drug Resistance Updates*, Vol.3, No.5, pp. 303–311, ISSN 1368-7646

Bicchi, C.; Binello, A., & Rubiolo, P. (2000). Determination of Phenolic Diterpene Antioxidants in Rosemary (*Rosmarinus officinalis* L.) with Different Methods of Extraction and Analysis. *Phytochemical Analysis*, Vol.11, No.4, pp. 236-242, ISSN 0958-0344

Botsoglou, N.A.; Govaris, A.; Botsoglou, E.N.; Grigoropoulou, S., & Papageorgiou, G. (2003). Antioxidant Activity of Dietary Oregano Essential Oil and α-tocopheryl Acetate Supplementation in Long-Term Frozen Stored Turkey Meat. *Journal of Agricultural and Food Chemistry*, Vol.51, No.10, pp. 2930–2936, ISSN 0021-8521

Boyen, F.; Haesebrouck, F.; Maes, D.; Van Immerseel, F.; Ducatelle, R., & Pasmans, F. (2008). Non-Typhoidal Salmonella Infections in Pigs: a Closer Look at Epidemiology, Pathogenesis and Control. *Veterinary Microbiology*, Vol.130, No.1-2, pp. 1–19, ISSN 0378-1135

Boziaris, I.S.; Proestos,C.; Kapsokefalou, M., & Komaitis, M. (2011). Antimicrobial Effect of *Filipendula ulmaria* Plant Extract Against Selected Foodborne Pathogenic and Spoilage Bacteria in Laboratory Media, Fish Flesh and Fish Roe Product. *Food Technology and Biotechnoogy*. Vol.49, No.2, pp. 263–270, ISSN 1330-9862

Breuil, J.; Brisabois, A.; Casin, I.; Armand-Lefevre, L.; Fremy, S., & Collatz, E. (2000). Antibiotic Resistance in Salmonellae Isolated from Humans and Animals in France: Comparative Data from 1994 and 1997. *Journal of Antimicrobial Chemotherapy*, Vol.46, No.6, pp. 965-971, ISSN 0305-7453

Burt, S.A.; Fledderman, M.J.; Haagsman, H.P.; van Knapen, F., & Veldhuizen, E.J.A. (2007). Inhibition of *Salmonella enterica* Serotype *Enteritidis* on Agar and Raw Chicken by Carvacrol Vapour. *International Journal of Food Microbiology*, Vol.119, No.3, pp. 346–350, ISSN 0168-1605

Bush, K. (2003). Beta-lactam antibiotics: Penicillins. In: *Antibiotic and chemotherapy: Anti-infective agents and their use in therapy,* R.G. Finch, D. Greenwood, S.R. Norrby, & R.J. Whitley (Eds.), 224–258, Churchill Livingstone, ISBN 0-443071-29-2, Edinburgh, UK

Butt, T.; Ahmad, R.N.; Mahmood, A., & Zaidi, S. (2003). Ciprofloxacin Treatment Failure in Typhoid Fever Case, Pakistan. *Emerging Infectious Diseases*, Vol.9, No.12, pp. 1621–1622, ISSN 1080-6040

Careaga, M., Ferna´ndez, E., Dorantes, L.; Mota, L.; Jaramillo, M.E., & Hernandez-Sanchez, H. (2003). Antibacterial activity of Capsicum extract against Salmonella typhimurium and Pseudomonas aeruginosa inoculated in raw beef meat. *International Journal of Food Microbiology*, Vol. 83, No.3, pp. 331–335, ISSN 0168-1605

Chantarapanont, W.; Slutsker, L.; Tauxe, R.V., & Beuchat, L.R. (2000). Factors Influencing Inactivation of *Salmonella enteritidis* in Hard-Cooked Eggs. *Journal of Food Protection*, Vol.63, No.1, pp. 36–43, ISSN 0362-028x

Chemaly, M.; Huneau-Salaun, A.; Labbe, A.; Houdayer, C.; Petetin, I., & Fravalo, P. (2009). Isolation of Salmonella Enterica in Laying-Hen Flocks and Assessment of Eggshell

Contamination in France. *Journal of Food Protection*, Vol.72, No.10, pp. 2071–2077, ISSN 0362-028x

Chen, M.H.; Hwang, W.Z; Wang, S.W.; Shih, Y.C., & Tsen, H.Y. (2011). Pulsed Field Gel Electrophoresis (PFGE) Analysis for Multidrug Resistant *Salmonella enterica* Serovar *Schwarzengrund* Isolates Collected in Six Years (2000-2005) from Retail Chicken Meat in Taiwan. *Food Microbiology*, Vol.28, No.3, pp. 399-405, ISSN 0740-0020

Chen, Q.Y.; Shi, H., & Ho, C.T. (1992). Effects of Rosemary Extracts and Major Constituents on Lipid Oxidation and Soybean Lipoxygenase Activity. *Journal of the American Oil Chemists' Society*, Vol.69, No.10, pp. 999-1002, ISSN 0003-021x

Cody, S.H. (1999). Raw-Milk Products May Contain Salmonella. *The Journal of the American Medical Association*, Vol.281, No.19, pp. 1805–1810, ISSN 0098-7484

Cosentino, S.; Tuberoso, C.I.G.; Pisano, B.; Satta, M.; Mascia, V.; Arzedi, E., & Palmas, F. (1999). In Vitro Antimicrobial Activity and Chemical Composition of Sardinian Thymus Essential Oils. *Letters in Applied Microbilogy*, Vol.29, No.3, pp. 130-135, ISSN 0266-8254

D'Aoust, J.Y.; Warburton, D.W., & Sewell, A.M. (1985). *Salmonella typhimurium* Phage-Type 10 from Cheddar Cheese Implicated in a Major Canadian Foodborne Outbreak. *Journal of Food Protection*. Vol.48, No.12, pp. 1062-1066, ISSN 0362-028x

De Buyser, M. L.; Dufour, B.; Maire, M., & Lafarge, V. (2001). Implication of Milk and Milk Products in Food-Borne Diseases in France and in Different Industrialised Countries. *International Journal of Food Microbiology*, Vol.67, No.1-2, pp. 1–17, ISSN 0168-1605

Delhalle, L.; Saegerman, C.; Farnir, F.; Korsak, N.; Maes, D., Messens, W.; De Sadeleer, L.; De Zutter, L., & Daub, G. (2009). Salmonella Surveillance and Control at Post-Harvest in the Belgian Pork Meat Chain. *Food Microbiology*, Vol.26, No.3, pp. 265–271, ISSN 0740-0020

De Louvois, J. (1993). Salmonella Contamination of Eggs: A Potential Source of Human Salmonellosis. *PHLS Microbiology Digest*, Vol.10, No.3, pp. 158–162, ISSN 0265-3400

De Oliveira, S.D.; Flores, F.S.; Dos Santos, L.R., & Brandelli, A. (2005). Antimicrobial Resistance in Salmonella enteritidis Strains Isolated from Broiler Carcasses, Food, Human and Poultry-Related Samples. *International Journal of Food Microbiology*, Vol. 97, No.3, pp. 297-305, ISSN 0168-1605

Dorman, H.J.D., & Deans, S.G. (2000). Antimicrobial Agents from Plants: Antibacterial Activity of Plant Volatile Oils. *Journal of Applied Bacteriology*, Vol.88, No.2, pp. 308-316, ISSN 0021-8847

Duffy, L.L.; Dykes, G.A., & Fegan, N. (2011). A Review of the Ecology, Colonization and Genetic Characterization of Salmonella Enterica Serovar Sofia, a Prolific but Avirulent Poultry Serovar in Australia. *Food Research International*, doi:10.1016/j.foodres.2011.04.024, ISSN 0963-9969

Elgayyar, M.; Draughon, F.A.; Golden, D.A., & Mount, J.R. (2001). Antimicrobial Activity of Essential Oils from Plants Against Selected Pathogenic and Saprophytic Microorganisms. *Journal of Food Protection*, Vol.64, No.7, pp. 1019-1024, ISSN 0362-028x

Evans, C.E.; Banso, A., & Samuel, O.A. (2000). Efficacy of Some Nupe Medicinal Plants Against *Salmonella typhi*: An in Vitro Study. *Journal of Ethnopharmacology*, Vol.80, No.1, pp. 21–24, ISSN 0378-8741

European Food Safety Authority. (2008). A Quantitative Microbiological Risk Assessment on Salmonella in Meat: Source Attribution for Human Salmonellosis from Meat. *The EFSA Journal,* Vol.625, pp. 1-32, ISSN 1831-4732

European Food Safety Authority. (2010a). Scientific Opinion on a Quantitative Estimation of the Public Health Impact of Setting a New Target for the Reduction of Salmonella in Laying Hens. *EFSA Journal*, Vol.8, No.4, pp. 1546, ISSN 1831-4732

European Food Safety Authority (2010b). Trends and Sources of Zoonoses and Zoonotic Agents and Food-Borne Outbreaks in the European Union in 2008. *EFSA Journal,* Vol.8, No.1, pp. 1–368, ISSN 1831-4732

European Food Safety Authority. (2010c). Analysis of the Baseline Survey on the Prevalence of Campylobacter in Broiler Batches and of Campylobacter and Salmonella on Broiler Carcasses in the EU, 2008, Part A; Campylobacter and Salmonella Prevalence Estimates. *EFSA Journal*, Vol.8, No.3, pp. 1503, ISSN 1831-4732

Exarchou, V.; Nenadis, N.; Tsimidou, M.; Gerothanassis, I. P.; Troganis, A., & Boskou, D. (2002). Antioxidant Activities and Phenolic Composition of Extracts from Greek Oregano, Greek sage, and Summer savory. *Journal of Agriculture and Food Chemistry,* Vol.50, No.19, pp. 5294–5299, ISSN 0021-8561

Fasseas, M.K.; Mountzouris, K.C.; Tarantilis, P.A.; Polissiou, M., & Zervas, G. (2008). Antioxidant Activity in Meat Treated with Oregano and Sage Essential Oils. *Food Chemistry*, Vol.106, No.3, pp. 1188–1194, ISSN 0308-8146

Fuzihara, T.O.; Fernandes, S.A., & Franco, B.D. (2000). Prevalence and Dissemination of Salmonella Serotypes Along the Slaughtering Process in Brazilian Small Poultry Slaughter-Houses. *Journal of Food Protection*, Vol.63, No.12, pp. 1749–1753, ISSN 0362-028x

Gantois, I.; Ducatelle, R.; Pasmans, F.; Haesebrouck, F.; Gast, R.; Humphrey, T.J., & Immerseel, F.V. (2009). Mechanisms of Egg Contamination by Salmonella Enteritidis. *FEMS Microbiology Reviews*, Vol.33, No.4, pp. 718–738, ISSN 0168-6445

Gast, R.K., & Beard, C.W. (1990). Production of Salmonella Enteritidis-Contaminated Eggs by Experimentally Infected Hens. *Avian Diseases*, Vol.4, No. 2, pp. 438–446, ISSN 0005-2086

Ghafir, Y.; China, B.; Korsak, N.; Dierick, K.; Collard, J.M.; Godard, C.; De Zutter, L., & Daube, G. (2005). Belgian Surveillance Plans to Assess Changes in Salmonella Prevalence in Meat at Different Production Stages. *Journal of Food Protection,* Vol. 68, No. 11, pp. 2269–2277, ISSN 0362-028x

Ghafir, Y.; China, B.; Dierick, K.; De Zutter, L., & Daube, G. (2007). Hygiene Indicator Microorganisms for Selected Pathogens on Beef, Pork and Poultry Meats in Belgium. *Journal of Food Protection,* Vol. 71, No.1, pp. 35-45, ISSN 0362-028x

Gonzales-Barron, U.A.; Redmond, G., & Butler, F. (2010a). A Consumer-Phase Exposure Assessment of Salmonella Typhimurium from Irish Fresh Pork Sausages: I. Transport and Refrigeration Modules. *Food Control,* Vol.21, No. 12, pp. 1683-1692, ISSN 0956-7135

Gonzales-Barron, U.A.; Redmond, G., & Butler, F. (2010b). A Risk Characterization Model of *Salmonella typhimurium* in Irish Fresh Pork Sausages. *Food Control,* doi:10.1016/j.foodres.2010.04.036, ISSN 0956-7135

Govaris, A; Solomakos,N.; Pexara, A., & Chatzopoulou, P.S. (2010). The Antimicrobial Effect of Oregano Essential Oil, Nisin and Their Combination Against *Salmonella enteritidis* in Minced Sheep Meat During Refrigerated Storage. *International Journal of Food Microbiology*, Vol.137, No.2-3, pp. 175–180, ISSN 0168-1605

Gutierrez, J.; Barry-Ryan, C., & Bourke, P. (2008). The Antimicrobial Efficacy of Plant Essential Oil Combinations and Interactions with Food Ingredients. *International Journal of Food Microbiology*, Vol.124, No.1, pp. 91–97, ISSN 0168-1605

Hald, T.; Vose, D.; Wegener, H.C., & Koupeev, T. (2004). A Bayesian Approach to Quantify the Contribution of Animal-Food Sources to Human Salmonellosis. *Risk Analysis*. Vol.24, No.1, pp. 255–269, ISSN 0272-4332

Hara-Kudo, Y.; Kobayashi, A.; Sugita-Konishi, Y. & Kondo, K. (2004). Antibacterial Activity of Plants Used in Cooking for Aroma and Taste. *Journal of Food Protection*, Vol.67, No.12, pp. 2820–2824, ISSN 0362-028x

Helmuth, R. (2000). Antibiotic Resistance in Salmonella, In: *Salmonella in Domestic Animals*, C. Wary & A. Wray (Eds.), 89-116, CABI Publishing, ISBN 0-85199-261-7, Wallingford, UK

Humphrey, T.J.; Greenwood, M.; Gilbert, R.J.; Rowe, B., & Chapman, P.A. (1989). The Survival of Salmonellas in Shell Eggs Cooked Under Simulated Domestic Conditions. *Epidemiology and Infection*, Vol.103, No. 1, pp. 35-45, ISSN 1469-4409

Humphrey, T.J.; Whitehead, A.; Gawler, A.H.L.; Henley, A., & Rowe, B. (1991). Numbers of Salmonella Enteritidis in the Contents of Naturally Contaminated Hens' Eeggs. *Epidemiology and Infection*, Vol.106, No.3, 489–496, ISSN 0950-2688

Hussain, A.; Wahab, S.; Zarin, I., & Hussain, M.D.S. (2010). Antibacterial Activity of the Leaves of Coccinia indica (W. and A) Wof India. *Advances in Biological Research*, Vol. 4, No.5, pp. 241-248, ISSN 1992-0067

James, C.; Go¨ksoy, E.O.; Corry, J.E.L., & James, S.J. (2000). Surface Pasteurisation of Poultry Meat using Steam at Atmospheric Pressure. *Journal of Food Engineering*, Vol.45, No.2, pp. 111–117, ISSN 0260-8774

Johny, A.K.; Darre, M.J.; Donoghue, A.M.; Donoghue, D.J., & Venkitanarayanan, K. (2010). Antibacterial Effect of Trans-Cinnamaldehyde, Eugenol, Carvacrol, and Thymol on *Salmonella enteritidis* and *Campylobacter jejuni* in Chicken Cecal Contents in Vitro. *Journal of Applied Poultry Research*, Vol.19, pp. 237–244, ISSN 1056-6171

Kamba, A.S., & Hassan, L.G. (2010). Phytochemical Screening and Antimicrobial Activities of Euphorbia balasamifera Leaves Stems and Root against Some Pathogenic Microorganisms, *The African Journal of Pharmaceutical Sciences and Pharmacy*, Vol.1, No.1, 57-64, ISSN 2152-7849

Kang, D.G.; Yun, C.K., & Lee, H.S. (2003). Screening and Comparison of Antioxidant Activity of Solvent Extracts of Herbal Medicines Used in Korea. *Journal of Ethnopharmacology*. Vol.87, No. 23, pp. 231–236, ISSN 0378-8741

Karns, J.S.; Van Kessel, J.S.; McCluskey, B.J., & Perdue, M.L. (2005). Prevalence of Salmonella enterica in Bulk Tank Milk from US Dairies as Determined by Polymerase Chain Reaction. *Journal ofDairy Science*. Vol.88, No.10, pp. 3475–3479, ISSN 1525-3158

Kaufmann, B., & Christen, P. (2002). Recent Extraction Techniques for Natural Products: Microwave-Assisted Extraction and Pressurised Solvent Extraction. *Phytochemical Analysis*, Vol.13, No.2, pp. 105-113, ISSN 0958-0344

Kazmi, M.H.; Malik, A.; Hameed, S.; Akhtar, N., & Noor Ali, S. (1994). Plant Products as Antimicrobial Agents. *Phytochemistry*, Vol.36, No.3, pp. 761-763, ISSN 0031-9422

Khan, R.; Islam, B.; Akram, M.; Shakil, S.; Ahmad, A.; Ali, S.M.; Siddiqui, M., & Khan, A.U. (2009). Antimicrobial Activity of Five Herbal Extracts Against Multi Drug Resistant (MDR) Strains of Bacteria and Fungus of Clinical Origin. *Molecules,* Vol.14, No.2, pp. 586-597, ISSN 1420-3049

Kiran, G.D.; Babu, V., & Kaul, K. (2005). Variation in Essential Oil Composition of Rose-Scented Geranium (Pelargonium sp.) Distilled by Different Distillation Techniques. *Flavour and Fragrance Journal*, Vol.20, No.2, pp. 222–231, ISSN 0882-5734

Kisangau, D.P.; Hosea, K.M.; Joseph, C.C., & Lyaruu, H.V.M. (2007). In Vitro Antimicrobial Assay of Plants Used in Traditional medicine in Bukoba Rural District, Tanzania. *African Journal of Traditional, Complementary Alternative medicines*, Vol.4, No.4, pp. 510-523, ISSN 0189-6016

Krieg, N.R., & Holt, J.G. (Eds.). (1984). *Bergey's Manual of Systematic Bacteriology Volume 1.* Williams and Wilkins, ISBN 0-683-04108-8, Baltimore, USA

Krishnasamy, G. (2008). *Extraction Technologies for Medicinal and Aromatic Plants,* International centre for science and high technology, Trieste, Italy

Kuo, F.L.; Carey, J.B., & Ricke, S. (1997). UV Irradiation of Shell Eggs: Effect on Populations of Aerobes, Molds, and Inoculated *Salmonella typhimurium. Journal of Food Protection,* Vol.60, No.6, pp. 639-643, ISSN 0362-028x

Lakins, D.G.; Alvarado, C.Z.; Thompson, L.D.; Brashears, M.T.; Brooks, J.C., & Brashears, M.M. (2008). Reduction of Salmonella Enteritidis in Shell Eggs using Directional Microwave Technology. *Poultry Science,* Vol.87, No.5, pp. 985–991, ISSN 0032-5791

Lapornik, B.; Prosˇek, M., & Wondra, A.G. (2005). Comparison of Extracts Prepared from Plant By-Products using Different Solvents and Extraction Time. *Journal of Food Engineering*. Vol.71, No.2, pp. 214–222, ISSN 0260-8774

Lawley, R.; Curtis, L., & Davis, J. (2008). *The Food Safety Hazard Guidebook*, RSC Publishing, ISBN 978-0-85404-460-3, Cambridge, UK

Lee, M.H.; Kwon, H.A.; Kwon, D.Y.; Park, H.; Sohn, D.H.; Kim, Y.C.; Eo, S,K.; Kang, H.Y.; Kim, S.W., & Lee, J.H. (2006). Antibacterial Activity of Medicinal Herb Extracts Against Salmonella. *International Journal of Food Microbiology,* Vol.111, No.3, pp. 270 –275, ISSN 0168-1605

Mahida, Y., & Mohan, J.S.S. (2007). Screening of Plants for Their Potential Antibacterial Activity Against Staphylococcus and Salmonella spp. *Natural Product Radiance,* Vol.6, No.4, pp. 301-305, ISSN 0972-592x

Ma, M.; Hong, C.L.; An, S.Q., & Li, B. (2003). Seasonal, Spatial, and Interspecific Variation in Quercetin in Apocynum venetum and Poacynum hendersonii, Chinese Traditional Herbal Teas. *Journal of Agricultural and Food Chemistry,* Vol. 51, No.8, pp. 2390-2393, ISSN 0021-8561

Mattson, T.E.; Johny, A.K.; Amalaradjou, M.A.R.; More, K.; Schreiber, D.T.; Patel, J. & Venkitanarayanan, K. (2011). Inactivation of Salmonella spp. on Tomatoes by Plant Molecules. *International Journal of Food Microbiology,* Vol.144, No.3, pp. 464–468, ISSN 0168-1605

Mayrhofer, S.; Paulsen, P.; Smulders, F.J.M., & Hilbert, F. (2004) Antimicrobial Resistance Profile of Five Major Food-Borne Pathogens Isolated from Beef, Pork and Poultry, *International Journal of Food Microbiology,* Vol.97, No.1, pp. 23–29, ISSN 0168-1605

Metrick, C.; Hoover, D.G., & Farkas, D.F. (1989). Effects of High Hydrostatic Pressure on Heat-Resistant and Heat-Sensitive Strains of Salmonella. *Journal of Food Science*, Vol.54, No.6, pp. 1547–1551, ISSN 0022-1147

Montville, T.J., & Matthews, K.R. (2005). *Food Microbiology: An Introduction*, 1st ed., ASM Press, ISBN 1-55581-308-9, Washington, DC

Montville, T.J., & Matthews, K.R. (2008). *Food Microbiology: An introduction, 2nd ed.*, ASM press, ISBN 978-1-55581-396-3, Washington, DC

Nalini, K.; Ashokkumar, D., & Venkateswaran, V. (2011). Antimicrobial Activity of Petroleum Ether and Methanol Extracts of Pedalium murex Leaves. *International Journal of Pharmaceutical Frontier Research*, Vol. 1, No.1, pp. 1-10, ISSN 2249-1112

N'guessan, J.D.; Coulibaly, A.; Ramanou, A.A.; Okou, O.C.; Djaman,A.J., & Guédé-Guina, F. (2007). Antibacterial Activity of *Thonningia sanguinea* Against Some Multi-Drug Resistant Strains of *Salmonella enteric*. *African Health Sciences*, Vol. 7, No.3, pp. 155–158, ISSN 1680-6905

Nkemngu, N.J.; Asonganyi, E.D., & Njunda, A.L. (2005). Treatment Failure in aTyphoid Patient Infected with Nalidixic Acid Resistant *S. enterica* Serovar *Typhi* with Reduced Susceptibility to Ciprofloxacin: A Case Report from Cameroon. *BMC infectious diseases*, Vol. 5, pp. 49, ISSN 1471-2334

O'Brien, T.F. (2002). Emergence, Spread, and Environmental Effect of Antimicrobial Resistance: How Use of an Antimicrobial Anywhere Can Increase Resistance to Any Antimicrobial Anywhere Else. *Clinical Infectious Diseases*, Vol.34, No.3, pp. S78–S84, ISSN 1058-4838

Oliveira, F.A.; Brandelli, A., & Tondo, E.C. (2006). Antimicrobial Resistance in Salmonella Enteritidis from Foods Involved in Human Salmonellosis Outbreaks in Southern Brazil. *The New Microbiologica*, Vol.29, No.1, pp. 49-54, ISSN 1121-7138

Omulokoli, E.; Khan, B., & Chhabra, S.C. (1997). Antiplasmodial Activity of Four Kenyan Medicinal Plants. *Journal of Ethnopharmacology*, Vol.56, No.2, pp. 133-137, ISSN 0378-8741

Plotkin, M.J. (1988). Conservation, Ethnobotany and the Search for New Jungle Medicines: Pharmacognosy Comes of Ageagain. *Pharmacotherapy*, Vol.8, No.5, pp. 257-262, ISSN 0277-0008

Perugini, A.G.; Carullo, M.R.; Esposito, A.; Caligiuri, V.; Capuano, F.; Galiero, G., & Giuseppe, L. (2010). Characterization of Antimicrobial Resistant Salmonella Enterica Serovars Enteritidis and Typhimurium Isolates from Animal and Food in Southern Italy. *Veterinary Research Communications*, Vol.34, No.4, pp. 387–392, ISSN 1573-7446

Phebus, R.K.; Nutsch, A.L.; Schafer, D.E.; Wilson, R.C.; Riemann, M.J.; Leising, J.D.; Knaster, C.L.; WOLF, J.R., & Prasai, R.K. (1997). Comparison of Steam Pasteurisation and Other Methods for Reduction of Pathogens on Surfaces of Freshly Slaughtered Beef. *Journal of Food Protection*, Vol. 60, No.5, pp. 476-484, ISSN 0362-028x

Pokharel, B.M.; Koirala, J.; Dahal, R.K.; Mishra, S.K.; Khadga, P.K., & Tuladhar, N.R. (2006). Multidrug-Resistant and Extended-Spectrum Beta-Lactamase (ESBL)-Producing Salmonella enterica (Serotypes Typhi and Paratyphi A) from Blood Isolates in Nepal: Surveillance of Resistance and a Search for Newer Alternatives. *International Journal of Infectious Diseases*, Vol.10, No.6, pp. 434-438, ISSN 1201-9712

Porto-Fett, A.C.S.; Call, J.E.; Shoyer, B.E.; Hill, D.E.; Pshebniski C.; Cocoma, G.J., & Luchansky, J.B. (2010). Evaluation of Fermentation, Drying, and/or High Pressure

Processing on Viability of Listeria monocytogenes, Escherichia coli O157:H7, Salmonella spp., and Trichinella spiralis in Raw Pork and Genoa Salami. *International Journal of Food Microbiology*, Vol.140, No. 1, pp. 61–75, ISSN 0168-1605

Pranoto, Y.; Salokhe, V.M., & Rakshit, S.K. (2005). Physical and Antibacterial Properties of Alginate-Based Edible Film Incorporated with Garlic Oil. *Food Research International*. Vol.38, No.3, pp. 267–272, ISSN 0963-9969

Rabsch, W.; Tschäpe, H.; Andreas, J., & Bäumler, A.J. (2001). Review, Non-Typhoidal Salmonellosis: Emerging Problems. *Microbes and Infection*, Vol.3, No.3, pp. 237–247, ISSN 1286-4579

Rangasamy, O.; Raoelison,G.; Rakotoniriana, F.E.; Cheuk, K.; Urverg-Ratsimamanga, S.; Quetin-Leclercq, J.; Gurib-Fakim, A., & Subratty, A.H. (2007). Screening for Anti-infective Properties of Several Medicinal Plants of the Mauritians flora. *Journal of Ethnopharmacology*, Vol.109, No.2, pp. 331–337, ISSN 0378-8741

Rasooli, I. (2007). Food Preservation-A Biopreservative Approach. *Food*, Vol. 1, No.2, pp. 111-136, ISSN 1749-1740

Ravishankar, S.; Zhu, L.; Olsen, C.W.; McHugh, T.H., & Friedman, M. (2009). Edible Apple Flm Wraps Containing Plant Antimicrobials Inactivate Foodborne Pathogens on Meat and Poultry Products. *Journal of Food Science*, Vol.74, No.8, pp. 440–445, ISSN 0022-1147

Rotimi, V.O.; Jamal, W.; Pal, T.; Sonnevend, A.; Dimitrov, T.S., & Albert, M.J. (2008). Emergence of Multidrug-Resistant Salmonella spp. and Isolates with Reduced Susceptibility to Ciprofloxacin in Kuwait and the United Arab Emirates. *Diagnostic Microbiology and Infectious Disease*, Vol.60, No.1, pp. 71-77, ISSN 0732-8893

Schwarz, S., & Chaslus-Dancla, E. (2001). Use of Antimicrobials in Veterinary Medicine and Mechanisms of Resistance. *Veterinary Research*, Vol.32, No.3-4, pp. 201–225, ISSN 0928-4249

Sefidkon, F.; Abbasi, K.; Jamzad, Z., & Ahmadi, S. (2007). The Effect of Distillation Methods and Stage of Plant Growth on the Essential Oil Content and Composition of Satureja rechingeri Jamzad. *Food Chemistry*, Vol. 100, No.3, pp. 1054–1058, ISSN 0308-8146

Seydim, A.C. & Sarikus, G. (2006). Antimicrobial Activity of Whey Protein Based Edible Films Incorporated with Oregano, Rosemary and Garlic Essential Oils. *Food Research International*, Vol.39, No.5, pp. 639–644, ISSN 0963-9969

Shan, B.; Cai, Y.Z.; Brooks, J.D., & Corke, H. (2011). Potential Application of Spice and Herb Extracts as Natural Preservatives in Cheese. *Journal of Medicinal Food*. Vol.14, No.3, pp. 284-290, ISSN 1096-620x

Shan, B.; Cai, Y.Z.; Brooks, J.D., & Corke, H. (2007). The in Vitro Antibacterial Activity of Dietary Spice and Medicinal Herb Extracts . *International Journal of Food Microbiology*, Vol.117, No.1, pp. 112-119, ISSN 0168-1605

Sharififar, F.; Moshafi, M.H.; Mansouri, S.H.; Khodashenas, M., & Khoshnoodi, M. (2007). In Vitro Evaluation of Antibacterial and Antioxidant Activities of the Essential oil and Methanol Extract of Endemic Zataria multiflora Boiss. *Food Control*, Vol.18, No.7, pp. 800–805, ISSN 0956-7135

Shirakawa, T.; Acharya, B.; Kinoshita, S.; Kumagai, S.; Gotoh, A., & Kawabata, M. (2006). Decreased Susceptibility to Fluoroquinolones and gyrA Gene Mutation in the Salmonella enterica Serovar Typhi and Paratyphi A Isolated in Katmandu, Nepal, in 2003. *Diagnostic Microbiology and Infectious Disease*, Vol.54, No.4, pp. 299–303, ISSN 0732-8893

Smid, E.J., & Gorris, L.G.M. (1999). Natural Antimicrobials for Food Preservation. In: *Handbook of Food Preservation*, M.S., Rahman, (Ed.), 285–308, Marcel Dekker, ISBN 978-0-824-70209-0, New York, USA

Tavechio, A.T.; Ghilardi, A.C.; Peresi, J.T.; Fuzihara, T.O.; Yonamine, E.K.; Jakabi, M., & Fernandes, S.A. (2002). Salmonella Serotypes Isolated from Nonhuman Sources in Sa˜o Paulo, Brazil, from 1996 through 2000. *Journal of Food Protection*, Vol.65, No. 6, pp. 1041-1044, ISSN 0362-028x

Thong, K.L., & Modarressi, S. (2011). Antimicrobial Sesistant Genes Associated with Salmonella from Retail Meats and Street Foods. Food Research International, doi:10.1016/j.foodres.2011.05.013, ISSN 0963-9969

Tornuk, F.; Cankurt, H.; Ozturk, I.; Sagdic, O.; Bayram, O., & Yetim, H. (2011). Efficacy of Various Plant Hydrosols as Natural Food Sanitizers in Reducing *Escherichia coli* O157:H7 and *Salmonella typhimurium* on Fresh Cut Carrots and Apples. *International Journal of Food Microbiology*. Vol. 148, No.1, pp. 30–35, ISSN 0168-1605

Trombetta, D.; Castelli, F.; Sarpietro, M.G.; Venuti, V.; Cristani, M.; Daniele, C.; Saija, A.; Mazzanti, G., & Bisignano, G. (2005). Mechanisms of Antibacterial Action of Three Monoterpenes. *Antimicrobial Agents and Chemotherapy*, Vol.49, No.6, pp. 2474–2478, ISSN 0066-4840

Waite, J.G., & Yousef, A.E. (2010). Overview of Food Safety, In: *Processing Effects on Safety and Quality of Foods*, E. Ortega-Rivas, (Ed.), 11-65, CRC Press, ISBN 978-1-4200-6112-3, Boca Raton, FL.

Weissinger, W.R.; McWatters, K.H., & Beuchat, L.R. (2001). Evaluation of Volatile Chemical Treatments for Lethality to Salmonella on Alfalfa Seeds and Sprouts. *Journal of Food Protection*, Vol.64, No.4, pp. 442–450, ISSN 0362-028x

Whyte, P.; McGill, K., & Collins, J. D. (2003). An Assessment of Steam Pasteurization and Hot Water Immersion Treatments for the Microbiological Decontamination of Broiler Carcasses. *Food Microbiology*, Vol.20, No.1, pp. 111–117, ISSN 0740-0020

# 16

# Laboratory Typing Methods for Diagnostic of Salmonella Strains, the "Old" Organism That Continued Challenges

Ben Salem Imen, Mzoughi Ridha and Aouni Mahjoub
*Laboratory of Infectious Diseases and Biological Agents*
*Faculty of Pharmacy, Monastir, Tunisia*
*Monastir University*
*Tunisia*

## 1. Introduction

*Salmonella* are enteric gram negative organisms that are widely dispersed in nature. These organisms can reside as common commensals in the gastrointestinal tracts of animals and man or cause disease states that range from self-limited diarrhea to bacteremia with enteric fever or invasion of vascular structures, bone or other localized sites (Hook, 1990).
Organisms can be highly host adapted, where they infect only a limited number of species, or can be much more ubiquitous. The most significant human host-adapted organism is *S. typhi*, the cause of typhoid fever. Man remains the only known reservoir for these isolates. Similarly, *S. pullorum* and *S. gallinarum* are poultry associated organisms that are so host-adapted that even upon transmission to man they usually remain non-pathogenic (Ziprin & Hume, 2001). More frequently, animal host-adapted organisms can be transmitted to man causing symptomatic disease. *S. choleraesuis* is normally a porcine organism though it can cause gastroenteritis and enteric fever, when transmitted to man (especially in children). Other organisms, such as *S. typhimurium*, have a broad host range and these serotypes are responsible for the majority of human infections.
Thus, *Salmonella* strains, the well and "old" pathogens, continued threat to public health. In fact, despite that, the incidence of salmonellosis has decreased substantially especially in developed country, recent events and several articles illustrate continued challenges in *Salmonella* control. The first challenge in *Salmonella* control is the widespread distribution of food; in fact contaminated food produced in one country may cause illness far away demonstrating the importance of robust control programmes. Likewise, this organism cause substantial economic loss resulting from mortality, morbidity, poor growth of infected animals, poultry and human beings; hazardous of transmitting food poisoning with gastroenteritis to human and so represents a serous problem for the food industry (Khan et al., 2007).
The second challenge is traceability, in fact, the complexity of the food supply chains and/ or the lack of identifying markers on foods can make it extremely difficult to trace back to their origin.

The third is antimicrobial resistance; in fact, over the last decade, strains of *Salmonella enterica* with multiples drug resistance have been distributed widely in many countries.
The fourth is capacity building to enhance outbreak detection through routinely subtyping certain *Salmonella* using molecular methods.
To contain this organism, it is essential to maintain continued vigilance, including rapid identification of similar strains and the immediate sharing of information within the public health community. Many nations have established extensive surveillance systems to track *Salmonella* infections and disrupt epidemic spread. Most of these surveillance projects rely on traditional serotype and phage type analyses to identify trends and potential outbreaks. Many clinical outbreaks cluster among a few serotypes so further discrimination is often needed.
Molecular epidemiological techniques have been used to enhance surveillance and discriminate outbreak strains within these common serotypes. The institution of these techniques has led to enhanced detection of outbreaks worldwide. In this chapter, we review the theoretical and practical basis of laboratory typing method for diagnostic of *salmonella* strains with emphasis on molecular methods which would contribute to the monitoring of human and animal *Salmonella* infections. Overall, traditional serotype surveillance in association with one or several molecular typing techniques, appears to provide the most reproducible and comparable discrimination of epidemiologically-linked isolates.

## 2. General properties of the genus *Salmonella*

*Salmonella* are Gram negative, short plump shaped rods, nonsporeforming, noncapsulated, aerobic and facultatively anaerobic organisms and classified under the family Enterobacteriaceae (Freeman, 1985).
*Salmonella* nomenclature has changed many times and still is not stable. The genus *Salmonella* was previously differentiated into two species: *Salmonella enterica* and *Salmonella bongori*. However, a new species, *Salmonella subterranea* was identified and validated (Shelobolina et al., 2004; Validation List No: 102, 2005). Among them, the species *Salmonella enterica (S. enterica)* is further divided into the six subspecies *S. enterica* subsp. *enterica* (I), *S. enterica* subsp. *salamae* (II), *S. enterica* subsp. *arizonae* (IIIa), *S. enterica* subsp. *diarizonae* (IIIb), *S. enterica* subsp. *houtenae* (IV), and *S. enterica* subsp. *indica* (VI). Formerly, *S. bongori* was the subspecies V, but later considered as a separate species (Fluit, 2005).
Fermentation of selected substances, such as dulcitol, malonate, sorbitol, d-tartrate, galacturonate, mucate, salicine, ONPG, and lactose, as well as production of enzymes such as gelatinase, β-glutamyl-transferase or β-glucuronidase, but also lysis by phage O1 allow a differentiation between the different species and subspecies (Le Minor 1984).
Furthermore, the genus composed of over 2500 serotypes differentiated according to three different types of surface antigens discussed bellow in more detail. 99% of these serotypes belong to *S. enterica* and nearly 60% of them are in *S. enterica* subsp. *enterica*. The average DNA sequence similarity between *Salmonella* serotypes is 96-99% (Edwards et al., 2002).

## 3. Bacterial isolations

A standard technique was used to isolate *Salmonella* strains in many laboratories. The technique is explained bellow.

### 3.1 Food samples

Samples were analysed according to French Norm for *Salmonella spp.* NFV 08-052/97. From each sample, 25 g was pre-enriched in 275 ml buffered peptone water (Oxoid, Dardilly Cedex, France) at 37°C for 24h. Afterwards, 0.1 ml of the pre-enrichment sample was incubated in 9.9 ml of buffered Rappaport-Vassiliadis medium (Oxoid, Dardilly Cedex, France) and 2 ml in 20 ml of buffered selenite cystine medium for another 24 h at 42 °C and 37 °C, respectively. The enrichment samples were then applied onto Hecktoen and Kampelmacher agar. Both selective media were incubated during 24 h at 37 °C.

Suspicious colonies were identified by Gram staining performed according to the conventional method and also with biochemical test (oxydase reaction). Both Gram-negative and oxidase-negative isolates were further tested. Biochemical tests other than oxidase test were done by using API 20E test kit (bioMérieux, Inc., France).

The plastic strips holding twenty mini-test tubes were inoculated with the saline suspensions of the cultures according to manufacturer's directions. This process also rehydrated the desiccated medium in each tube. A few tubes were completely filled (CIT, VP and GEL), and some tubes were overlaid with mineral oil such that anaerobic reactions could be carried out (ADH, LDC, ODC, H2S, URE) **(Figure 1)**.

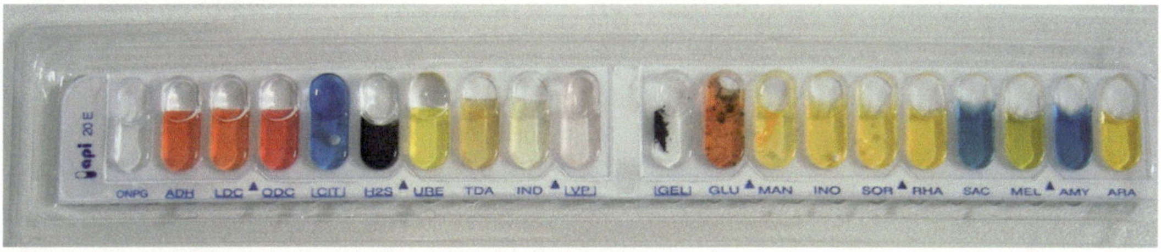


Fig. 1. Typical *Salmonella* reaction of API 20E test kit.

After incubation in a humidity chamber for 18-24 hours at 37°C, the colour reactions were read (some with the aid of added reagents as supplied by the kit). The data were analysed by the manufacturer's software and positive results with ≥89% probabilities were confirmed as *Salmonella*. The list of the biochemical tests performed by API 20E test kit and typical reactions exhibited by *Salmonella spp.* are given in **Table 1**.

### 3.2 Stool sample

Each stool sample was streaked onto Hecktoen agar and pre-enriched in selenite broth at 37 °C for 24 h. The pre-enrichment sample was streaked onto Hecktoen agar, and after incubation at 37 °C for another 24 h, the suspicious colonies were identified with biochemical test (as mentioned above).

### 3.3 Environmental water samples

From each sample, 100 ml was pre-enriched in 100 ml double concentrated buffered peptone water (Oxoid, Dardilly Cedex, France) at 37 °C for 24 h. Afterwards, 0.1 ml of the pre-enrichment sample was incubated in 9.9 ml of buffered Rappaport-Vassiliadis medium (Oxoid, Dardilly Cedex, France) and 1 ml in 9 ml of buffered selenite cystine medium for another 24 h at 37 °C; The enrichment samples were then applied onto Hecktoen and

Kampelmacher agar. Both selective media were incubated during 24 h at 37 °C. The suspicious colonies were identified with biochemical test (as mentioned above).

| Tests | Substrate | Reaction | (-) Results | (+) Results | *Salmonella spp.* |
|---|---|---|---|---|---|
| **ONPG** | ONPG | betagalactosidase | colorless | yellow | - |
| **ADH** | arginine | Arginine dihydrolase | yellow | red/orange | - |
| **LDC** | lysine | Lysine decarboxylase | yellow | red/orange | + |
| **ODC** | ornithine | Ornithine decarboxylase | yellow | red/orange | + |
| **CIT** | citrate | Citrate Utilization | pale to green/yellow | blue-green/ blue | - |
| **H2S** | Na thiosulfate | H2S production | colorless/gray | black deposit | + |
| **URE** | urea | Urea hydrolysis | yellow | red/orange | - |
| **TDA** | tryptophan | deaminase | yellow | brown-red | - |
| **IND** | tryptophan | Indole production | yellow | red (in 2 min) | - |
| **VP** | Na-pyruvate | Acetoin production | colorless | pink/red (in 10 min) | - |
| **GEL** | charcoal gelatin | Gelatinase | no diffusion of black | black diffusion | - |
| **GLU** | glucose | fermentation/oxidation | blue/ blue-green | yellow | + |
| **MAN** | mannitol | fermentation/oxidation | blue/ blue-green | yellow | + |
| **INO** | inositol | fermentation/oxidation | blue/ blue-green | yellow | - |
| **SOR** | sorbitol | fermentation/oxidation | blue/ blue-green | yellow | + |
| **RHA** | rhamnose | fermentation/oxidation | blue/ blue-green | yellow | + |
| **SAC** | sucrose | fermentation/oxidation | blue/ blue-green | yellow | - |
| **MEL** | melibiose | fermentation/oxidation | blue/ blue-green | yellow | + |
| **AMY** | amygdalin | fermentation/oxidation | blue/ blue-green | yellow | - |
| **ARA** | arabinose | fermentation/oxidation | blue/ blue-green | yellow | + |

Table 1. Biochemical reactions involved in API 20E (bioMérieux, Inc., France) test kits and typical *Salmonella* reactions.

## 4. Laboratory typing methods

The determination of the relatedness of strains within a *Salmonella* serotype is a prerequisite for the identification of the sources of infection and for tracing the routes of *Salmonella* dissemination in outbreaks. Since biochemical analysis did not further differentiate between the bacteria assigned to the same *S. enterica* subspecies, other phenotypic and molecular methods have been used (Riley, 2004).

### 4.1 Phenotypic methods

#### 4.1.1 Serotyping

Serotyping is the initial step for routine diagnostics of *Salmonella* strains and performed with commercially available omni-, poly- and monovalent antisera. Up to date, over 2500 serotypes of *Salmonella* has been identified and classified in the Kaufmann-White scheme. This scheme differentiates between O (=somatic) antigens of the cell surface, H1 and H2 (=flagellar) antigens of the phase 1 or phase 2, respectively (Selander et al., 1996) and the Vi (=capsular) antigens which, however, may only be present in very few serotype, such as *Typhi, Paratyphi C* or *Dublin*.

Each *Salmonella* serogroup has a group specific O-antigen. Within each O-group, different serovars are distinguished by the combination of O- and H-antigens that are present. Each serotype has a specific antigenic formula where the O-antigens are indicated by Arabic numbers, the H1-antigens by lower case letters and the H2- antigens again by Arabic numbers. In these formulas, underlined antigens may only be expressed once the culture is lysogenised by the corresponding converting phage whereas letters or numbers in brackets indicate antigens which may be present or absent without relation to phage conversion (Le Minor, 1984).

For most of the isolates assigned to *S. enterica* and the subspecies I, antigenic formula corresponds to a serotype name. In contrast, serotypes identified after 1996 in the subspecies *salamae*, *houtenae* and *indica* and in the subspecies *bongori* are designated only by antigenic formula (Brenner et al., 2000).

| Serotype | O-antigen(s) | H1-antigen(s) | H2-antigen(s) |
|---|---|---|---|
| ***S. Enteritidis*** | 1, 9, 12 | [f], g, m, [p] | [1, 7] |
| ***S. Dublin*** | 1, 9, 12 [Vi] | g, p | - |
| ***S. Gallinarum*** | 1, 9, 12 | - | - |
| ***S. Typhimurium*** | 1, 4, 5, 12 | i | 1, 2 |
| ***S. Virchow*** | 6, 7 | r | 1, 2 |
| ***S. Infantis*** | 6, 7, 14 | r | 1, 5 |

Table 2. Examples for the antigenic formulas of *Salmonella enterica* subsp. *enterica* serotypes according to Kaufmann-White scheme (Poppoff and Le Minor, 2001).

The detection of the presence of *Salmonella* O- and H- antigens were tested by slide agglutination with the commercially available antisera. One loop of appropriate antisera was dropped onto a cleaned glass slide. One loop of overnight culture grown on agar was dispersed in the drop to obtain a homogeneous and turbid suspension. The slide was rocked gently for 30 s and clumping was monitored by a magnifying glass. The scheme to obtain the serotype was given in **Figure 2.**

Serotyping is easy to perform and standardized antisera are commercially available. However, it only allows the assignment of *Salmonella* strains to a specific serotype, and no further differentiation between strains of the same serotype is achieved.

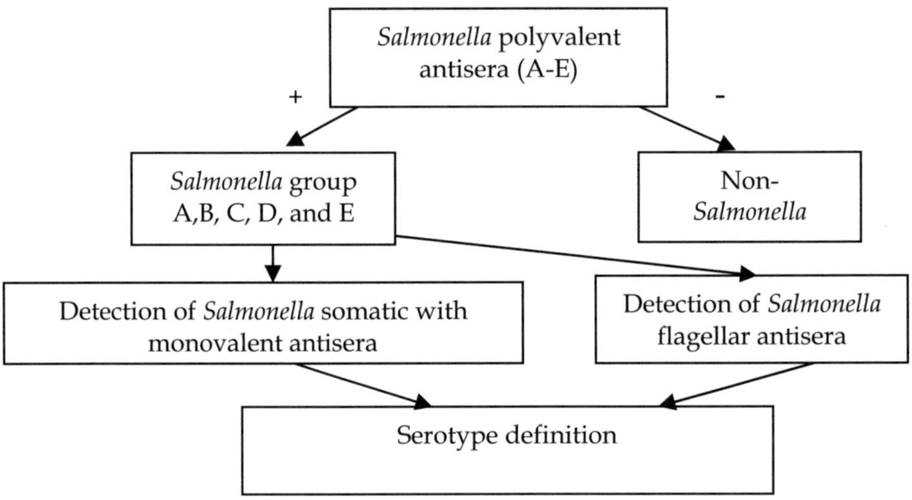


Fig. 2. Serotyping analysis scheme for *Salmonella*

During the 1980's, a tremendous increase in *S. enteritidis* was identified, particularly in the Northeastern U.S. (Rodrigue et al.,1990). Studies linked *S. enteritidis* to contaminated shell eggs or foods that contained eggs (Mishu et al., 1994). During 1987-1997, five serotypes accounted for 66% of all clinical infections in which a *Salmonella* isolate was identified to the serotype level. *S. typhimurium* accounted for 24% of these isolates, *S. enteritidis* (22%), *S. heidelberg* (9%), *S. newport* (5%) and *S. hadar* (4%) followed (Olsen et al., 2001). When clinical outbreaks were distinguished from sporadic infections, *S. enteritidis* was implicated in 55% of *Salmonella* cases associated with a clinical outbreak (Olsen et al., 2001).

In Tunisia, from 1994 to 2004, 16.214 *Salmonella* isolates were reported to the national Centre of Enteropathogenic bacteria at Pasteur Institute, Tunis, Tunisia. (Ridha et al., 2007). The largest proportion of *Salmonella* isolates was from human origin (n=6815) followed by isolates from food (n=5539). During the surveillance period, the top five reported *Salmonella* serotypes were: *Enteritidis, Anatum, Corvallis, Braenderup,* and *Livingstone.* These five serotypes accounted for 3479 strains of all *Salmonella* isolates from food. (Ridha et al., 2007). Finally, *Salmonella* isolates reported from environmental origin cam in last position (n=1611) after isolates from animal origin (n=2249) (Ridha et al., 2007).

Serological analysis usually remains the first step in an epidemiological investigation of *Salmonella* and may be sufficient for epidemiological investigations associated with uncommon serotypes (Threlfall & Frost, 1990). However, smaller labs often do not have access to the pools of serum required for this analysis and may need to rely on other techniques to analyze isolates. The multiplex PCR, an easier molecular method, has been developed to differenciate between the most common serotypes of *Salmonella enterica* subsp. *enterica* (Imen et al. 2010).

#### 4.1.2 Phage typing

Individual isolates of many *Salmonella* serotypes vary in their susceptibility to lysis by different bacteriophages and this has led to a typing scheme based on reactivity to a panel of bacteriophage. Therefore, a *Salmonella* strain is subjected to a specified set of typing phages and the lytic pattern obtained commonly allows the assignment to a specific phage type. The strains exhibiting a lytic pattern that does not correspond to a known phage type are classified as RDNC (= Reacting with the typing phage, but lytic pattern Did Not Correspond to any recognized phage types).

Phage typing is mostly performed for serotypes such as *S. Typhimurium, S. Enteritidis, S. Typhi* or *S. Paratyphi*, although phage typing systems are also available for a number of additional serotypes, including *S. Virchow*. Phage typing has led to the discrimination of over 200 *S. typhimurium* phage types (Threlfall & Frost, 1990) and, together with antimicrobial susceptibility analyses, led to detection of several large-scale, international epidemics including the dissemination of a multi-drug resistant clone of *S. typhimurium* DT104, (definitive phage type, DT, 104) (Threlfall, 2000). In Denmark, phage typing as described by the World Health Organization (WHO) Collaborative Centre for phage typing of Salmonella (Health Protection Agency (HPA), Colindale, United Kingdom) has been applied for surveillance of S. Enteritidis and S. Typhimurium in humans, food and food production animals. Phage typing has proven to be an important tool for strain characterisation and the results obtained have been used since the mid-90s in surveillance, source attribution and outbreak investigations (Baggesen & Wegener, 1994; Hald et al., 2007)

In general, phage typing is only performed by the National Reference Centers, since only these institutions have access to the defined sets of typing phages. The interpretation of the results requires considerable experience (Riley, 2004). Although, phage typing in *Salmonella* epidemiology has been used since the 1950s, the stability of phage types can be limited by phage type conversion (Rabsch et al., 2002), even during an outbreak (Mmolawa et al., 2002). This is due to the acquisition of a temperate phage or a plasmid. Besides, host-controlled phage defence mechanisms such as restriction/modification systems and phage adsorption inhibition are also responsible for the phage typing difficulties of a *Salmonella* strain.

By means of a sterile inoculation loop, the test culture was inoculated into a test tube containing 4 mL double strength nutrient broth with a special care for heavy inoculum to give visible turbidity for *S. Enteritidis* and a very light inoculum for *S. Typhimurium* to give a barely visible turbidity.

The culture was incubated by shaking at 200 rpm at 37°C for 1-1.5 h for *S. Enteritidis* and for *S. Typhimurium* 1.5 h without agitation to obtain a very light growth in early log phase. After incubation, it was flooded over the surface of double strength nutrient agar using a flooding pipette and the excess of culture was removed. As soon as the surface of agar dried, the appropriate typing phages at routine test dilutions were applied to the dried surface by a multipoint inoculation loop. When the phage spots dried, the agar plate was incubated at 37°C for 18 h. At the end of the incubation, the agar plate was read using a magnifying glass through the bottom of the plate (Ward et al., 1987).

Phage susceptibilities were evaluated by means of the plaque number, size and transparency. The pattern was compared with known phage type patterns in the database and defined. If the culture did not react with any of the typing phages, it was defined as non-typable (NT); and if the culture reacted with the typing phages, but gave a different pattern other than those in the database, it was considered as reacting with the typing phages, but lytic pattern did not correspond to any recognized phage types, so called RDNC (= Reacting with the typing phage, but lytic pattern Did Not Correspond to any recognized phage types). But, we must note that phage typing analyses needs typing phage sets to be performed.

In bref, phage typing can play an important role in surveillance and control of the common *Salmonella* serotypes. However, this requires strengthened efforts to make the system available to more laboratories internationally, possibly a simplification of the system to enhance its robustness even though this may slightly compromise its discriminatory power, and finally improved external and internal quality assurance systems.

### 4.2 Molecular methods

Phenotypic typing methods requiring enough time, personnel and reagent have led to the development of typing methods based on genotypic information. Currently used molecular typing methods are based on restriction endonuclease digestion, nucleic acid amplification, or nucleotide sequencing techniques.

#### 4.2.1 Plasmid profiling

Plasmid profile analysis was one of the earliest DNA-based subtyping schemes. It is particularly important, since most of the plasmids harbour virulence and antimicrobial resistance properties in *Salmonella*. Plasmid content of the host within the same serotype reveals the differentiation according to the profile (the number and molecular sizes of plasmids) obtained. The different plasmid profiles within a serotype points the lateral transfer by gaining or loosing the plasmid(s). The plasmids found in *Salmonella* differ in size 2 - 200 kb with different functionalities (Rychlik et al., 2006).

The detection method is based on the isolation of plasmids followed by agarose gel electrophoresis. Different protocols can be used (Helmuth et al., 1985). To view the plasmid pattern, agarose gel must be stained with ethidium bromide solution and then visualised under UV light.

Plasmid analysis has several limitations. Plasmids can rapidly be acquired or lost. Also, single predominant plasmids have become endemic within various serotypes. In sporadic isolates of *S. enteritidis* from Maryland, 88% of isolates contained a single 36-Mda plasmid (Morris et al., 1992). Similarly, only 1 of 56 *S. typhimurium* isolates failed to encode a 90 kb plasmid, which is thought to be a serotype specific virulence plasmid. Despite the ubiquitous nature of the 90 kb plasmid, profiling of the entire complement of plasmids in each strain was able to discriminate *S. typhimurium* strains isolated from a single poultry flock or closely related flocks (Millemann et al.,1995).

Plasmid analysis was also able to identify a multi-state outbreak of chloramphenicol resistant *S. newport* in humans that could be traced back to contaminated beef and to dairy farms (Riley et al.,1983). In a testament to the power of combining a strong traditional epidemiological analysis with serological and genotypic tests, a peak of *S. muenchen* was noted in Ohio, Michigan, Georgia and Alabama. Epidemiological studies failed to identify a common food source responsible for this outbreak, but a strong correlation with marijuana use was identified. Marijuana obtained from affected households was contaminated with *S. muenchen* and the isolates from the different states showed a similar plasmid fingerprint suggesting interstate transfer of the contaminated drug (Taylor et al., 1982).

Plasmid profiling is most useful in an outbreak setting that is limited temporally and geographically (Mendoza & Landeras, 1999). Furthermore, this technique will only be successful if the serotype of interest carries multiple plasmids of differing sizes.

### 4.2.2 PFGE (pulsed field gel electrophoresis)

PFGE has been considered as the "gold standard" among other molecular typing methods. By cutting the bacterial DNA with rare-cutting restriction endonucleases and running with special electrophoresis separation technique which use pulsed currents that change polarity at defined intervals, it separates the large fragments of DNA up to 12000 kb and yields strain specific patterns.

The choice of restriction endonuclease is somewhat empiric, but the most commonly used enzymes in *Salmonella* have been XbaI, SpeI and NotI. Comparisons of patterns from multiple enzymes can elucidate new subtypes and increase the discriminatory power of this technique (Liebisch & Schwarz, 1996).

PFGE of 60 *S. enteritidis* isolates revealed 28 different XbaI restriction profiles and 26 with SpeI, yet when the patterns generated from both enzymes were combined, 32 different pulsed-field types could be identified (Ridley et al., 1998). PFGE was used to determine whether molecular subtyping was able to detect unsuspected clusters or outbreaks of *S. typhimurium* (Bender et al., 2001). In fact, during a four-year period, 16% of isolates were linked to common source outbreaks. Of these, the authors felt that 62% of outbreak strains would have been missed without the use of PFGE molecular subtyping (Bender et al., 2001). PFGE has also been used to track outbreak strains occurring across national boundaries (Lyytikainen et al., 2000).

PFGE is characterized by a high degree of reproducibility both within and between laboratories (Swaminathan et al., 2001). The recent introduction of computerized gel-based data collection and analysis systems allows better standardization between laboratories thus creating the ability to rapidly compare restriction fragment patterns from isolates analyzed from remote locations (Swaminathan et al., 2001). Large databanks that house PFGE patterns from isolates around the world will greatly enhance *Salmonella* outbreak detection. PulseNet, a molecular subtyping network for foodborne bacterial disease surveillance, has been active in developing standardized PFGE protocols and establishing a national database. An outbreak of *S. agona* linked to contaminated cereal was identified in 1998. PFGE, in association with PulseNet, was used to identify cases in adjoining states that were not initially thought to be at risk (Swaminathan et al., 2001). In fact, combining typing methods such as PFGE and information from food chains, it was possible to identify related strains and common source of contamination. This type of approach may be useful in order to improve Salmonella spp. surveillance systems.

PFGE, however, is not always successful. Some serotypes, especially those with certain distinct phage types, can be so genetically homogeneous that multiple genotypic techniques fail to discriminate outbreak from non-outbreak strains. Ahmed et al. (Ahmed et al., 2000) evaluated PFGE to differentiate *S. enteritidis* DT8 strains that developed during a Canada-wide outbreak of gastroenteritis that was eventually traced to contaminated cheese. Successful discrimination was only achieved with a combination of intensive epidemiological, genotypic and phenotypic methods (Ahmed et al., 2000). Additionally, certain serotypes may be more susceptible to genetic rearrangements that can alter the PFGE pattern, even within an outbreak (Echeita & Usera, 1998).

Despite that PFGE is usually considered as the method of choice to determine the molecular relatedness among *Salmonella* strains; this method is relatively slow, often taking three days to complete, and requires the presence of expensive specialized equipment, high quality chemicals, and a considerable experience in the preparation of the DNA-containing agarose slices. Moreover, single genetic events, such as point mutations, integration, deletion or recombination events, can result in differences in the fragment patterns (Herschleb et al., 2007).

#### 4.2.3 Ribotyping

The Fingerprinting of rRNA coding sequences, termed ribotyping, describes the hybridization of restriction-digested DNA fragments with probes specific for rDNA.

Multiple copies of the rRNA operon are present within the *Salmonella* chromosome (Mendoza & Landeras, 1999). The rRNA genes themselves are quite homologous among these copies and between isolates, but the intervening sequences vary in length and nucleotide composition.

Ribotyping begins with separating endonuclease-digested chromosomal DNA on agarose gels, DNA then is transferred to a membrane and fragments are hybridized to a probe that recognizes 16S and 23S rRNA. Analysis of multiple restriction endonucleases can improve the discriminatory powers of ribotyping (Millemann et al., 1995).

Ribotype analysis is clearly able to subtype some of the isolates that fall within some common serotypes and phage types (Landeras et al., 1996). Lin et al. (Lin et al., 1996) detected 7 different ribotypes among 17 *S. enteritidis* PT 8 isolates when chromosomal DNA was digested with SphI. Using rRNA gene restriction patterns to investigate the relatedness of S. Enteritidis strains isolated in São Paulo, from 1975 to 1995; Fernandes et al. showed that ribotyping is a genomic profiling method that is reproducible and suitable for tracing the spread of S. Enteritidis. They found that the restriction endonuclease SphI discriminated best between subtypes of this serotype. Dambaugh et al. presented evidence suggesting that the ribotyping of Salmonella using the restriction enzyme PvuII increased the incidence of discreet ribotype patterns for the most common Salmonella serovars. This study evaluates the potential of PvuII to generate serotype-specific DNA fingerprints. However, studies have identified isolates that belong to different phage types yet demonstrate identical ribotypes (Fontana et al., 2002). Therefore, ribotyping is considered not suitable for local epidemiological studies or surveillance studies in a restricted region (Riley, 2004).

Comparisons of ribotyping with PFGE have been somewhat unpredictable and often depend on the enzymes used for digestion as well as the nature of the population being tested. Several studies have found PFGE to be more discriminating than ribotype analysis (Fontana et al., 2002) while others have found the two procedures equivalent (Navarro et al., 1996) or ribotype analysis superior (Liebana et al., 2001). Ribotype analysis using two restriction enzymes, Pst I -SphI or HindIII - EcoRV, can improve discrimination (Liebana et al., 2001). Particular care must be taken when analyzing chromosomal patterns of *S. typhi*. The rapid genomic reassortment that occurs in *S. typhi* can affect ribotype analysis (Ng et al., 1999).

Though most laboratories continue to perform ribotyping manually, machinery has been developed to perform this entire procedure in an automated fashion. Data is stored electronically and the banding pattern from a particular organism can be compared to the entire databank stored in the computer. In contrast to PFGE, the time required to perform automated ribotyping is minimal; hybridization results can be obtained within 4 hours. A recent study tracking the rise of a multi-drug resistant, cephalosporin-resistant *S. newport* proposes to use automated ribotyping as a way to rapidly identify the *newport* serotype and PFGE to further evaluate strain associations (Fontana et al., 2002). The major drawbacks of automated ribotyping are the high reagent costs per isolate and the cost of the automated riboprinter itself.

Laconha et al. and Ridley et al. investigated the genotypic differences between strains of *Salmonella* by plasmid analysis, ribotyping and pulsed-field gel electrophoresis (PFGE). The results obtained by those researchers indicated that PFGE may offer a better level of discrimination of *S. Enteritidis* types than other genotypic methods. Conversely, other epidemiological studies of *S. Enteritidis* have demonstrated that PFGE methodology has a lower discriminatory capacity than ribotyping (Olsen et al. 1994; Thong et al. 1998).

#### 4.2.4 Insertion sequence (IS) typing

IS200 is a mobile element found in a variety of eubacterial genera, such as *Salmonella, Escherichia, Shigella, Vibrio, Enterococcus, Clostridium, Helicobacter,* and *Actinobacillus.* IS200 elements are very small (707-711 bp) and contain a single gene. Unlike typical mobile elements, IS200 transposes rarely. A consequence of IS200 self-restraint is that the number and distribution of IS200 elements remain fairly constant in natural populations of bacteria. This stability makes IS200 a suitable molecular marker for epidemiological and ecological studies, especially when the number of IS200 copies is high. IS200 typing, has been used to evaluate the molecular relationships between *Salmonella* isolates. In *Salmonella enterica,* IS200 fingerprinting is extensively used for strain discrimination. It is a 708 bp insertion sequence that is present in multiple copies within the *Salmonella* chromosome (Lam & Roth, 1983). Hybridization of digested chromosomal DNA with an IS200 probe has been useful in describing the clonal heritage of *Salmonella* from various serotypes, but has not been as discriminating as phage typing itself for *S. enteritidis, S. typhi* and others (Threlfall et al., 1994). For certain phage types of *S. typhimurium,* such as the multidrug resistant DT204c and 193 types common in the U.K., IS200 typing can result in strain discrimination and in some studies has been superior to PFGE and ribotyping (Jeoffreys et al., 2001). More frequently, PFGE has performed better than IS200 typing (Amavisit et al., 2001).

#### 4.2.5 RAPD (randomly amplified polymorphic DNA)

The standard RAPD technology (Williams et al., 1990) utilises short synthetic oligonucleotides (10 bases long) of random sequences as primers to amplify nanogram amounts of total genomic DNA under low annealing temperatures by PCR. Amplification products are generally separated on agarose gels and stained with ethidium bromide. Decamer primers are commercially available from various sources (e.g., Operon Technologies Inc., Alameda, California). PCR amplification with primers shorter than 10 nucleotides [DNA amplification fingerprinting (DAF)] has also been used producing more complex DNA fingerprinting profiles (Caetano-Annoles et al., 1991).

Although these approaches are different with respect to the length of the random primers, amplification conditions and visualisation methods, they all differ from the standard PCR

condition (Erlich, 1989) in that only a single oligonucleotide of random sequence is employed and no prior knowledge of the genome subjected to analysis is required.
At an appropriate annealing temperature during the thermal cycle, oligonucleotide primers of random sequence bind several priming sites on the complementary sequences in the template genomic DNA and produce discrete DNA products if these priming sites are within an amplifiable distance of each other.
The profile of amplified DNA primarily depends on nucleotide sequence homology between the template DNA and oligonucleotide primer at the end of each amplified product. Nucleotide variation between different sets of template DNAs will result in the presence or absence of bands because of changes in the priming sites. Recently, sequence characterised amplified regions (SCARs) analysis of RAPD polymorphisms (Bardakci & Skibinski, 1999) showed that one cause of RAPD polymorphisms is chromosomal rearrangements such as insertions/deletions. Therefore, amplification products from the same alleles in a heterozygote differ in length and will be detected as presence and absence of bands in the RAPD profile.
Although the RAPD method is relatively fast, cheap and easy to perform in comparison with other methods that have been used as DNA markers, the issue of reproducibility has been of much concern since the publication of the technique. In fact, ordinary PCR is also sensitive to changes in reaction conditions, but the RAPD reaction is far more sensitive than conventional PCR because of the length of a single and arbitrary primer used to amplify anonymous regions of a given genome. This reproducibility problem is usually the case for bands with lower intensity. The most important factor for reproducibility of the RAPD profile has been found to be the result of inadequately prepared template DNA (Welsh & McClelland, 1994). Differences between the template DNA concentration of 2 individuals' DNA samples result in the loss or gain of some bands (Bardakci, 1996).
Since RAPD amplification is directed with a single, arbitrary and short oligonucleotide primer, DNA from virtually from all sources is amenable to amplification. Therefore, DNA from the genome in question may include contaminant DNA from infections and parasites in the material from which the DNA has been isolated. Special care is needed for keeping out the DNA to be amplified from other sources of DNA.
Finally, due to the amplification conditions, RAPD method is sensitive to slight changes within amplification parameters, thus it is hard to achieve reproducibility. However, ribotyping is a supplementary tool in conjunction with other typing methods (Yan et al., 2003).

#### 4.2.6 AFLP (amplified fragment length polymorphism)

Also termed infrequent restriction site PCR (IRS PCR). It, has been developed by Vos et al. (1995). L'AFLP analysis belongs to the category of selective restriction fragment amplification techniques, which are based on the ligation of adapters (i.e., linkers and indexers) to genomic restriction fragments followed by a PCR-based amplification with adapterspecific primers.
The optimal number of scorable bands (50–100) can easily be set by selection of the appropriate AFLP primers and restriction enzymes. These characteristics make AFLP a powerful fingerprinting technique which can be used in identification, epidemiology and taxonomy (Folkerstma et al. 1996; Huys et al. 1996; Janssen et al. 1996). In addition, the technique can be used to generate large numbers of molecular markers for linkage studies (Ballvora et al. 1995; Becker et al. 1995; van Eck et al. 1995).

For AFLP analysis, only a small amount of purified genomic DNA is needed; this is digested with two restriction enzymes, one with an average cutting frequency (like EcoRI) and a second one with a higher cutting frequency (like MseI or TaqI).

Double-stranded oligonucleotide adapters are designed in such a way that the initial restriction site is not restored after ligation, which allows simultaneous restriction and ligation, while religated fragments are cleaved again.

An aliquot is then subjected to two subsequent PCR amplifications under highly stringent conditions with adapter-specific primers that have at their 39 ends an extension of one to three nucleotides running into the unknown chromosomal restriction fragment.

An extension of one selective nucleotide amplifies 1 of 4 of the ligated fragments, whereas three selective nucleotides in both primers amplify 1 of 4,096 of the fragments. The PCR primer which spans the average-frequency restriction site is labeled.

After polyacrylamide gel electrophoresis a highly informative pattern of 40 to 200 bands is obtained. The patterns obtained from different strains are polymorphic due to (i) mutations in the restriction sites, (ii) mutations in the sequences adjacent to the restriction sites and complementary to the selective primer extensions, and (iii) insertions or deletions within the amplified fragments.

Optimization of restriction enzymes and adapter-specific primers is ongoing for the *Salmonella* (Garaizar et al., 2000), but the technique appears more reproducible than ribotyping techniques (Savelkoul et al., 1999). Some of the studies have shown specificity to the serotype level with occasional subserotype discrimination (Garaizar et al., 2000).

Alternative AFLP typing procedures are based on one enzyme with a single adapter and analysis by agarose gel electrophoresis (Gibson et al., 1998). A major improvement has been obtained using a fluorescent amplified fragment length polymorphisms (FAFLP) technique that followed the same principles of AFLP yet the adapter-specific primers were tagged with a fluorescent moiety (Tamada et al., 2001). Fluorescent tagged fragments are then accurately sized on an automated sequencer.

FAFLP analysis of *S. typhimurium* generated 45-50 fragments ranging in size from 80-430 bp, though only a subset of these fragments were polymorphic among the strains. FAFLP grouped the isolates into four distinct clusters while PFGE generated three clusters.

Sizing was enhanced by incorporation of a fluorescent internal marker (Tamada et al., 2001). This accurate sizing, combined with the ability to acquire and analyze the data as a gel image, electrophorogram or in a tabular data format will allow comparison of patterns among different laboratories or within databanks (Savelkoul et al., 1999).

FAFLP appears quite promising. Disadvantages include the need for a greater technical expertise. In fact, despite that AFLP has been considered as a highly discriminative method, it remains a labour- and cost-intensive technique (Riley, 2004). Set up costs may be prohibitive until automated sequencers become more affordable.

### 4.2.7 MLST (multilocus sequence typing)

A recently developed methodology (Maiden et al., 1998) called multilocus sequence typing (MLST) may provide an ideal balance of high discriminatory power and a powerful data analysis capability requiring minimal human input. Multilocus sequence typing (MLST) is a molecular typing strategy that compares DNA sequences from portions of housekeeping or virulence genes and/or rRNA sequences which varies due to mutation or recombination events (Maiden et al., 1998). Nucleotide differences in the individual genes are combined and used to determine the differentiation of strains (Yan et al., 2003). MLST provides data similar to those obtained by multilocus enzyme electrophoresis, but in substantively greater detail, because it has the ability to assess individual nucleotide changes rather than to screen for changes in the overall charge and expression of the enzyme under study (Maiden et al., 1998).

This method is extremely useful for long-term epidemiological studies or phylogenetic analyses. Over 230 *Salmonella* isolates were recently characterized by MLST based on sequences from the 16S RNA, pduF, glnA and manB genes (Kotetishvili et al., 2002). These results were compared to PFGE and serotype analysis. MLST was able to differentiate strains better than PFGE, though not all genes performed equally. Among the four loci, only manB demonstrated clusters among the clinical and environmental strains. As expected, the 16S rRNA locus showed significant homogeneity among the isolates and grouped most isolates together.

MLST shows great promise for accurate strain discrimination with data that can be accurately shared between laboratories. However, like FAFLP, the universal appeal of this technique will be improved when automated sequence machinery becomes more affordable and labs can develop familiarity with complicated DNA sequence analysis and statistical software

### 4.2.8 Multiplex PCR

**Theoretical basis of multiplex PCR method: Critical Parameters**

Multiplex polymerase chain reaction (PCR) is a variant of PCR in which two or more loci are simultaneously amplified in the same reaction. Since its first description in 1988 (Chamberlain et al., 1988), this method has been successfully applied in many areas of DNA testing, including analyses of deletions (Henegariu et al., 1994), mutations (Shuber et al., 1993) and polymorphisms (Mutirangura et al., 1993), or quantitative assays (Mansfield et al., 1993) and reverse transcription PCR (Crisan, 1994).

The role of various parameters that may influence the performance of standard (uniplex) PCR has been discussed (Robertson & J., 1998). However, fewer publications discuss multiplex PCR (Henegariu et al., 1997).

The optimization of multiplex PCRs can pose several difficulties, including poor sensitivity or specificity and/or preferential amplification of certain specific targets (Polz & C. M., 1998). The presence of more than one primer pair in the multiplex PCR increases the chance of obtaining spurious amplification products, primarily because of the formation of primer dimers (Brownie et al., 1997). These nonspecific products may be amplified more efficiently than the desired target, consuming reaction components and producing impaired rates of annealing and extension. Thus, the optimization of multiplex PCR should aim to minimize or reduce such non-specific interactions.

Compatibility among the primers within the reaction mixture such that there is no interference, is of great technical importance. Primer selection followed simple rules (i) primer length of 18–24 bp or higher and (ii) a GC content of 35%–60%, thus having an annealing temperature of 55 °C-58 °C or higher. Longer primers (28-30 bp) allowed the reaction to be performed at a higher annealing temperature and yielded less unspecific products.

Combining the primers in various mixtures and amplifying many loci simultaneously required alteration/optimization of some of the parameters of the reaction. When the multiplex reaction is performed for the first time, it is useful to add the primers in equimolar amounts. The results will suggest how the individual primer concentration and other parameters need to be changed. Special attention to primer design parameters such as homology of primers with their target nucleic acid sequences, their length, the GC content, and their concentration have to be considered (Robertson & J., 1998). Ideally, all the primer pairs in a multiplex PCR should enable similar amplification efficiencies for their respective target. This may be achieved through the utilization of primers with nearly identical optimum annealing temperatures and should not display significant homology either internally or to one another (Henegariu et al., 1997). Also, the extension rate of specific primer-target hybrids depends on the activity of the enzyme, availability of essential components such as deoxyribonucleoside triphosphates (dNTPs), and the nature of the target DNA. Thus, the majority of modifications to improve PCR performance have been directed towards the factors affecting annealing and/or extension rates. Therefore, in multiplex PCR, as more loci are simultaneously amplified, the pool of enzyme concentrations, PCR buffer constituents and nucleotides becomes a limiting factor and more time is necessary for the polymerase molecules to complete synthesis of all the products (Chamberlain et al., 1989).

Variation in concentrations of reaction components above those used in uniplex PCR probably reflects the competitive nature of the PCR process. The desired target DNA can be outcompeted by the more efficient amplification of other targets (including nonspecific products), leading to decreases in the efficiency of the amplification of the desired targets and hence sensitivity of the reaction (Raeymaekers, 1995).

Various authors recommend dimethyl sulfoxide (DMSO) and glycerol to improve amplification efficiency (higher amount of product) and specificity (no unspecific products) of PCR, when used in concentrations varying between 5%-10% (vol/vol) (Innis & D.H., 1990). Also bovine serum albumin, or betaine, has been reported to be of benefit in multiplex PCRs (Jackson et al., 1996). The components may act to prevent the stalling of DNA polymerization, which can occur through the formation of secondary structures within regions of template DNA during the extension process (Hengen, 1997). Also it can act as destabilizing agents, reducing the melting temperature of GC-rich sequences, or as osmoprotectants, increasing the resistance of the polymerase to denaturation (Hengen, 1997).

A straightforward solution to difficulties encountered in the development of multiplex PCR has been the use of hot start PCR (Chou et al., 1992) and/or nested PCR (Zheng et al., 1995). The former often eliminates nonspecific reactions (particularly production of primer dimers) caused by primer annealing at low temperature (4 to 25°C) before commencement of thermocycling (Chou et al., 1992). The procedure has recently been made more practicable through the use of a nonmechanical hot start methodology which involves the use of a form of Taq polymerase, for example, Ampli Taq Gold (Roche Diagnostics), which is activated only if the reaction mixture is heated in first denaturation step at approximately 94°C for 10 min (Kebelmann-Betzing et al., 1998).

Nested PCR increases the sensitivity and specificity of the test through two independent rounds of amplification using two discrete primer sets. Although this adaptation is undoubtedly effective in most cases, it also considerably complicates the practical application of PCR. The second round of amplification delays results, increases the possibility of cross-contamination, and may complicate automation.

## Practical test of multiplex PCR method: Application and results in *Salmonella* serotyping

During the last decade, a number of studies have demonstrated the practicality of identifying *Salmonella* serovars using multiplex PCR (mPCR) (Kim et al., 2006). In addition, the technique has been shown to be a powerful and cost-effective tool for *Salmonella* serotyping. For these reasons, we optimize a mPCR protocole to type the most common *Salmonella enterica* subsp. *enterica* serovars. This method is based on detection of genes present in specific serotypes. These genes were selected from analysis of previous work including whole-genome sequencing (Porwollik et al., 2004, 2005).

The first step is to extract bacterial DNA. In this study, it was prepared by boiling (Agarwal et al. 2002). Then, we prepared the final PCR volume (34µl) that included: dNTPs mixture (0.2 mM); MgCl2 (2 mM); TaqDNA polymerase (5.0 units); primer(s) (50 ng each); genomic DNA template (5µl) and deionised water to make up the volume (Imen et al. 2010).

All assays used the same cycling parameters under the following conditions: enzyme activation at 94°C for 5 min and then an additional 40 cycles with heat denaturation at 94°C for 30 s, primer annealing at 62°C for 30 s, and DNA extension at 72°C for 1 min. After the last cycle, samples were maintained at 72°C for 5 min to complete the synthesis of all strands.

The PCR products (10µl) were separated by electrophoresis on 2% Tris-acetate EDTA agarose gel stained with ethidium bromide, visualized with UV induced fluorescence, and photographed (Imen et al. 2010).

The first multiplex PCR for *Salmonella* serotyping was applied using five primer sets in the same reaction mixture. Using these five STM primers with the 19 *Salmonella* serovars, we can identify four distinct groups (Imen et al. 2010). In a second approach, we validated the mPCR for *Salmonella* serovars detection by using STY primers. Thus, the 19 different tested *Salmonella* serovars could be classified into three groups on the basis of scoring the presence or absence of appropriately size amplicons (Imen et al. 2010). To further evaluate the discriminatory method for *Salmonella* serotyping and to increase identified serovars, we combined molecular results of both the STM and STY primers (Imen et al. 2010).

In this study, using suitable primers for the two five-plex PCRs methods for molecular *Salmonella* serotyping, we could easily discriminate all the tested *Salmonella* serotypes that represented 100% of all *Salmonella* isolates in our laboratory. Also, a high rate of correlation was found between traditional and molecular serotyping. However, one exception was found with *Salmonella Anatum* serotype (Imen et al. 2010).

These results have been found elsewhere (Perch et al. 2003). Whereas, we have noted a resemblance in molecular amplicon code in some *salmonella* serovars that can be explained by the presence of a very similar region in these serovars. It can also be explained by deletion problems that can concern a specific region and so the absence of appropriately sized amplicons with specific primers (Garaizar et al. 2002). A secondary discrimination problem that was interesting to note was that for *Anatum* serovar more than one amplicon code can be detected which may reflect intraserovar variation.

To further discriminate each serovar, we can associate to this multiplex PCR serotyping the PFGE analysis, or the 16 S\23 S r RNA ribotyping. These methods provided a high degree of intraserovar discrimination.

In this way, we describe the mPCR as a rapid, specific, and cost-effective molecular method that has demonstrated its efficient discrimination in serotyping of the most common clinical and food isolates of *S. enterica* subsp. *enterica* in our region. This technique can be used as an alternative method of standard serotyping in many clinical laboratories.

## 5. Conclusions and perspectives

Overall the *Salmonella* demonstrate significant phenotypic diversity. Several phenotypic typing techniques have been developed and have been used successfully for decades. Over the years, serotype and phage type analyses have been particularly useful as evidenced by the success of the National *Salmonella* Surveillance System, and many other national surveillance projects throughout the world. However, these techniques have often been relegated to reference laboratories making rapid analysis by an individual laboratory difficult. An ideal typing method should fulfil the following six criteria: typeability, reproducibility, discriminatory power, and ease of interpretation, easy to use, and low cost. It is clear, that any method used currently for typing of *Salmonella* strains is an ideal method alone in terms of these criteria, but all methods exhibit benefits and also limitations. It is obvious that it is difficult to find a single method, which is most suitable for typing of *Salmonella* strains. As a consequence, the best discrimination has resulted from combinations of techniques, often a combination of phenotypic and genotypic techniques. At this time, major reference institutions rely on serotype analysis followed by PFGE as the gold standard for strain discrimination. PCR-based techniques, though, are more rapid and within a particular laboratory can be used as a primary screening tool for strain discrimination. Better standardization between laboratories will be required before any of the PCR techniques can become the method of choice. Additionally, validation in outbreak situations involving varied serotypes will be required to prove these techniques effective in the field.

## 6. References

Agarwal, A.; Makker, A. & Goel, SK. (2002). Application of the PCR technique for a rapid, specific and sensitive detection of *Salmonella spp.* in foods. *Mol Cell Probes*, 16, 243–250.

Ahmed, R.; Soule, G.; Demczuk, W. H.; Clark, C.; Khakhria, R.; Ratnam, S.; Marshall, S.; Ng, L. K.; Woodward, D. L.; Johnson, W. M. & Rodgers, F. G. (2000). Epidemiologic typing of *Salmonella enterica* serotype *enteritidis* in a Canada-wide outbreak of gastroenteritis due to contaminated cheese. *J Clin Microbiol*, 38, 2403-6.

Amavisit, P.; Markham, P. F.; Lightfoot, D.; Whithear, K. G. & Browning, G. F. (2001). Molecular epidemiology of *Salmonella Heidelberg* in an equine hospital. *Vet Microbiol*, 80, 85-98.

Baggesen, DL. & Wegener, HC. (1994). Phage types of *Salmonella enterica ssp. enterica* serovar *typhimurium* isolated from production animals and humans in Denmark. *Acta Vet Scand*, 35(4), 349-54.

Ballvora, A., Hesselbach, J., Niewo¨hner, J., Leister, D., Salamini, F. and Gebhardt, C. (1995) Marker enrichment and high-resolution map of the segment of potato chromosome VII harbouring the nematode resistance gene Gro1. Molecular General Genetics 249, 82–90.

Bardakci, F. (1996). Applications of the random amplified polymorphic DNA (RAPD) technique in tilapia: species, subspecies and sex identification. Ph.D. Thesis, University of Wales Swansea.

Bardakci, F. & Skibinski, D:O.F. (1999). A polymorphic SCAR-RAPD marker between species of tilapia. *Animal Genetics*, 30, 78-79.

Becker, J., Vos, P., Kuiper, M., Sallamini, F. and Heun, M. (1995) Combined mapping of AFLP and RFLP markers in barley. Molecular General Genetics 249, 65–73.

Ben Aissa, Ridha.; Al-Galas, Nazek.; Troudi, Hinda.; Belhadj, Nabiha. & Belhadj, Abderazzaque. (2007). Trends in *Salmonella enterica* serotypes isolated from human, food, animal, and environment in Tunisia, 1994-2004. *Journal of infection*, 55: 324-339.

Bender, J. B.; Hedberg, C. W.; Boxrud, D. J.; Besser, J. M.; Wicklund, J. H.; Smith, K. E. & Osterholm, M. T. (2001). Use of molecular subtyping in surveillance for *Salmonella enterica* serotype *typhimurium*. *N Engl J Med*, 344, 189-95.

Ben Salem, Imen.; Aouni, Mahjoub. & Mzoughi, Ridha. (2010). Two five-plex PCRs methods for identification of common *Salmonella spp*. serotypes. *Ann Microbiol*, 60:135–141

Brenner F. W.; Villar R. G.; Angulo F. J.; Tauxe R. & Swaminathan B. (2000). *Salmonella* nomenclature. *Journal of Clinical Microbiology*, 38:2465- 2467.

Brownie, J.; Shawcross, S.; Theaker, J.; Whitcombe, D.; Ferrie, R.; Newton, C. & Little, S. (1997). The elimination of primer-dimer accumulation in PCR. *Nucleic Acids Res*, 25:3235–3241.

Caetano-Annoles, G.; Bassam, B.J & Gresshoff, P.M. (1991). DNA amplification fingerprinting using very short arbitrary oligonucleotide primers. *Bio/Technology*, 9, 553-557.

Dambaugh, T. R.; Mangiaterra, E. & Fritschel, S. (1997). Ribotype characterization of *Salmonella* and *E. coli* O157:H7 with PvuII on the RiboPrintert microbial characterization system. Abstr. *American Society for Microbiology, Washington, D.C.* , 439. P-14.

Erlich, H.A. (1989). PCR Technology Principles and Applications for DNA amplification. *Stockton Press*, New York.

Fernandes, S.A. et al. (2003). Phenotypic and molecular characterization of *Salmonella enteritidis* strains isolated in São Paulo, Brazil. *Rev Inst Med Trop*, 45: 59-63.

Chamberlain, J.S.; Gibbs, R.A.; Ranier, J.E.; Nguyen, P.N. & Caskey, C.T. (1988). Deletion screening of the Duchenne muscular dystrophy locus via multiplex DNA amplification. Nucleic Acids Res, 16:11141- 11156.

Chamberlain, J. S.; Gibbs, R. A.; Ranier, J. E.; Nguyen, P. N. & Caskey, C. T. (1989). Multiplex PCR for the diagnosis of Duchenne muscular dystrophy. *In D. H*, 272–281.

Chou, Q.; Russel, M.; Birch, D. E.; Raymond, J. & Bloch. W. (1992). Prevention of pre-PCR mis-priming and primer dimerization improves lowcopy- number amplifications. *Nucleic Acids Res*, 11:1717–1723.

Crisan, D.(1994). Molecular diagnostic testing for determination of myeloid lineage in acute leukemias. *Ann. Clin. Lab. Sci*, 24:355-363.

Echeita, M. A. & Usera, M. A. (1998). Chromosomal rearrangements in *Salmonella enterica* serotype *typhi* affecting molecular typing in outbreak investigations. *J Clin Microbiol*, 36, 2123-6.

Edwards R. A.; Olsen G. J. & Maloy S. R. (2002). Comparative genomics of closely related *salmonella. Trends in Microbiology*, 10:94-99.

Fluit, A. C. 2005. Towards more virulent and antibiotic-resistant *Salmonella*? FEMS Immunology and Medical Microbiology, 43:1-11.

Folkertsma, R.T.; Rouppe van der Voort, J.N.A.M.; de Groot, K.E. *et al.* (1996). Gene pool similarities of potato nematode populations assessed by AFLP analysis. *Molecular Plant–Microbe Interactions,* 9: 47–54.

Fontana, J.; Stout, A.; Tyndall, M.; Bolstorff, B.; Rossiter, S. & Timperi, R. The use of pulsed field gel electrophoresis and automated ribotyping to monitor the increased prevalence of a multidrug resistant *Salmonella* serotype *newport* in Massachusetts associated with cows. *International Conference on Emerging Infectious Diseases,* Atlanta, GA (2002)

Freeman BA (1985). Burrows Textbook of Microbiology. 22nd edn. W. B. Saunders Company, Philadelphia, 464-472.

Garaizar, J.; Lopez-Molina, N.; Laconcha, I.; Lau Baggesen, D.; Rementeria, A.; Vivanco, A.; Audicana, A. & Perales, I. (2000). Suitability of PCR fingerprinting, infrequent-restriction-site PCR, and pulsed-field gel electrophoresis, combined with computerized gel analysis, in library typing of *Salmonella enterica* serovar *enteritidis, Appl Environ Microbiol,* 66, 5273-81.

Garaizar, J.; Porwollik, S.; Echeita, A.; Rementeria, A.; Herrera, S.; Wong, RM.; Frye, J.; Usera, MA. & McClelland M. (2002). DNA microarraybased typing of an atypical monophasic *Salmonella enterica* serovar. *J Clin Microbiol*, 40:2074–2078

Gibson, J.; Slater, R. E.; Xerry, J.; Tompkins, D. S. & Owen, R. J. (1998). Use of an amplified-fragment length polymorphism technique to fingerprint and differentiate isolates of *Helicobacter pylori. J. Clin. Microbiol.* 36:2580– 2585.

Hald, T.; Lo Fo Wong, DM. & Aarestrup, FM. (2007). The Attribution of Human Infections with Antimicrobial Resistant *Salmonella* Bacteria in Denmark to Sources of Animal Origin. *Foodborne Pathog Dis.* 4(3):313-26

Helmuth, R.; Stephan, R.; Bunge, C.; Hoog, B.; Steinbeck, A. & Bulling, E. (1985). Epidemiology of virulence-associated plasmids and outer memrane protein pattenrs within seven common *Salmonella* serotypes. *Infection and Immunity*, 48: 175-182.

Henegariu, O.; Heerema, N. A.; Dlouhy, S. R.; Vance, G. H. & Vogt, P. H. (1997). Multiplex PCR: critical parameters and step-by-step protocol. *Bio- Techniques,* 23:504–511.

Henegariu, O.; Hirschmann, P.; Kilian, K.; Kirsch, S.; Lengauer, C.; Maiwald, R.; Mielke, K. & Vogt, P. (1994). Rapid screening of the Y chromosome in idiopathic sterile men, diagnostic for deletions in AZF, a genetic Y factor expressed during spermatogenesis. *Andrologia,* 26:97-106.

Hengen, P. N. (1997). Optimizing multiplex and LA-PCR with betaine. *Trends Biol. Sci.,* 22:225–226.

Herschleb, J.; Ananiev, G. & Schwartz, D. C. (2007). Pulsed-field gel electrophoresis. *Nature Protocols*, 2:677-684.

Hook, E. W. (1990). *Salmonella* species (including typhoid fever), p. 1700-1715. In G. L. Mandell, Douglas, R. G. & J. E. Bennett (ed.), Principles and Practices of Infectious Diseases. *Churchill Livingstone*, New York.

Huys, G.; Coopman, R.; Janssen, P. & Kersters, K. (1996). High resolution genotypic analysis of the genus *Aeromonas* by AFLP fingerprinting. *International Journal of Systematic Bacteriology*, 4: 572–580.

Innis, M.A. & Gelfand, D.H. (1990). Optimization of PCRs, p 3-13. In M.A. Innis, Gelfand, D.H.; Sninsky, J.J. & White (Eds.), T.J. PCR Protocols. *A Guide to Methods and Applications. Academic Press*, San Diego.

Jackson, R.; Morris, D. J.; Cooper, R. J.; Bailey, A. S.; Klapper, P. E. & Cleator, G. M. (1996). Multiplex polymerase chain reaction for adenovirus and herpes simplex virus in eye swabs. *J. Virol. Methods*, 56:41–48.

Janssen, P.; Coopman, R.; Huys, G. et al. (1996). Evaluation of the DNA fingerprinting method AFLP as a new tool in bacterial taxonomy. *Microbiology*, 142: 1881–1893.

Jeoffreys, N. J.; James, G. S.; Chiew, R. & Gilbert, G. L. (2001). Practical evaluation of molecular subtyping and phage typing in outbreaks of infection due to *Salmonella enterica* serotype *typhimurium*. *Pathology*, 33, 66-72.

Kebelmann-Betzing, C.; Seeger, S.; Dragon, G.; Schmitt, A.; Moricke, T. A.; Schild, G.; Henze. & B. Beyermann. (1998). Advantages of a new Taq DNA polymerase in multiplex PCR and time-release PCR. *BioTechniques*, 24: 154–158.

Khan, AA.; Melvin, CD. & Dagdag, EB. (2007). Identification and molecular characterization of *Salmonella spp*. from unpasteurized orange juices and identification of new serotype *Salmonella* strain *S. enterica* serovar Tempe. *Food Microbiology*, 24: 539-543.

Kim, S.; Frye, JG.; Hu, J.; Fedorka-Cray, PJ.; Gautom, R. & Boyle, DS. (2007). Multiplex PCR-based method for identification of common clinical serotypes of *Salmonella enterica* subsp. *enterica*. *J Clin Microbiol*, 44:3608–3615.

Kotetishvili, M.; Stine, O.C.; Kreger, A.; Morris, J.G. & Sulakvelidze, A. (2002). Multilocus sequence typing for characterization of clinical and environmental *Salmonella* strains. *J. Clin. Micro.*, 40, 1626-1635

Laconha, I. et al. (2000). Genotypic characterization by PFGE of *Salmonella enterica* serotype *enteritidis* phage types 1, 4, 6, and 8 isolated from animal and human sources in three European countries. *Vet Microbiol.*, 75, 155-65.

Lam, S. & Roth, J. R. (1983). IS200: a *Salmonella*-specific insertion sequence. *Cell*, 34, 951-60.

Landeras, E.; onzalez-Hevia, M. A.; Alzugaray, R. Mendoza, M. C. (1996). Epidemiological differentiation of pathogenic strains of *Salmonella enteritidis* by ribotyping. *J Clin Microbiol*, 34, 2294-6.

Le Minor L. (1984). Facultative anaerobic gram-negative rods. In: Holt J. G. and Krieg N. R. (eds.), Bergey's Manual of Systematic Bacteriology. Williams and Wilkins, Baltimore, 9th edition, vol:1, pp. 427-458.

Liebana, E.; Garcia-Migura, L.; Breslin, M. F.; Davies, R. H. & Woodward, M. J. (2001). Diversity of strains of *Salmonella* enterica serotype *enteritidis* from English poultry farms assessed by multiple genetic fingerprinting. *J Clin Microbiol*, 39, 154-61.

Liebisch, B. & Schwarz, S. (1996). Molecular typing of *Salmonella enterica* subsp. *enterica* serovar *Enteritidis* isolates. *J Med Microbiol*, 44, 52-9.

Lin, A. W.; Usera, M. A.; Barrett, T. J. & Goldsby, R. A. (1996). Application of random amplified polymorphic DNA analysis to differentiate strains of *Salmonella enteritidis*. *J Clin Microbiol*, 34, 870-6.

Lyytikainen, O.; Koort, J.; Ward, L.; Schildt, R.; Ruutu, P.; Japisson, E.; Timonen, M. & Siitonen, A. (2000). Molecular epidemiology of an outbreak caused by *Salmonella enterica* serovar *Newport* in Finland and the United Kingdom. *Epidemiol Infect*, 124, 185-92.

Maiden, M. C. J.; ygraves, J.A.; Feil, E.; Morelli, G.; Russell, J.E.; Urwin, R.; Zhang, Q.; Zhou, J.; Zurth, K; Caugant, D.A.; Feavers, I.M.; Achtman, M. & Spratt, B. G. (1998). Multilocus sequence typing: a protable approach to the identification of clones within populations of pathogenic microorganisms. *Proc. Natl. Acad. Sci.* USA, 95, 3140- 3145

Mansfield, E.S.; Robertson, J.M.; Lebo, R.V.; Lucero, M.Y.; Mayrand, P.E.; Rappaport, E.; Parrella, T.; Sartore, M.; Surrey, S. & Fortina, P. (1993). Duchenne/Becker muscular dystrophy carrier detection using quantitative PCR and fluorescence-based strategies. *Am. J. Med. Genet*, 48:200-208.

Mendoza, M. C. & Landeras, E. (1999). Molecular epidemiological methods for differentiation of *Salmonella enterica* serovar *Enteritidis* strains in humans and animals: epidemiology, pathogenesis, and control. Saeed, A. M., Gast, R.E., Potter, M.E. and Wall, P.G., Ed., Iowa University Press, Ames, IA, pp. 125-140

Millemann, Y.; Lesage, M. C.; Chaslus-Dancla, E. & Lafont, J. P. (1995). Value of plasmid profiling, ribotyping, and detection of IS200 for tracing avian isolates of *Salmonella typhimurium* and *S. enteritidis*. *J Clin Microbiol*, 33, 173-9.

Mishu, B.; Koehler, J.; Lee, L. A.; Rodrigue, D.; Brenner, F. H.; Blake, P. & Tauxe, R. V. (1994). Outbreaks of *Salmonella enteritidis* infections in the United States, 1985- 1991. *J Infect Dis*, 169, 547-52.

Mmolawa, P. T.; Willmore, R.; Thomas, C. J. & Heuzenroeder, M. W. (2002). Temperate phages in *Salmonella enterica* serovar *Typhimurium*: implications for epidemiology. *International Journal of Medical Microbiology*, 291:633-644.

Morris, J. G.; Dwyer, Jr.; Hoge, D. M.; Stubbs, C. W.; Tilghman, A. D.; Groves, D.; Israel, C. E. & Libonati, J. P. (1992). Changing clonal patterns of *Salmonella enteritidis* in Maryland: evaluation of strains isolated between 1985 and 1990. *J Clin Microbiol*, 30, 1301-3.

Mutirangura, A.; Greenberg, F.; Butler, M.G.; Malcolm, S.; Nicholls, R.D.; Chakravarti, A. & Ledbetter, D.H. (1993). Multiplex PCR of three dinucleotide repeats in the Prader-Willi/Angelman critical region (15q11-q13): molecular diagnosis and mechanism of uniparental disomy. *Hum. Mol. Genet*, 2:143-151.

Navarro, F.; Llovet, T.; Echeita, M. A.; Coll, P.; Aladuena, A.; Usera, M. A. & Prats, G. (1996). Molecular typing of *Salmonella enterica* serovar *typhi*. *J Clin Microbiol*, 34, 2831-4.

Ng, I.; Liu, S. L. & Sanderson, K. E. (1999). Role of genomic rearrangements in producing new ribotypes of *Salmonella typhi*. *J Bacteriol*, 181, 3536-41.

Olsen, S. J.; Bishop, R.; Brenner, F. W.; Roels, T. H.; Bean, N.; Tauxe, R. V. & Slutsker, L. (2001). The changing epidemiology of *salmonella*: trends in serotypes isolated from humans in the United States, 1987-1997. *J Infect Dis*, 183, 753-61.

Olsen, J.E. et al. (1994). Clonal lines of *Salmonella enterica* serotype *enteritidis* documented by IS200-, ribo-, pulsed-field gel electrophoresis and RFLP typing. *J Med Microbiol*, 40, 15-22.

Perch, M.; Braden, C.R.; Bishop, R.; Fields, P.; Plikaytis, R. & Tauxe, R.V. (2003). *Salmonella* surveillance summary, 2003. U.S. Department of Health and Human Services, Centers for Disease Control and Prevention, Atlanta, Ga.

Polz, M. F. & C. M. Cavanaugh. (1998). Bias in template-to-product ratios in multitemplate PCR. *Appl. Environ. Microbiol*. 64:3724–3730.

Poppoff M. Y. & Le Minor L. (2001). Kauffmann-White Scheme. WHO Collaborating Centre for Reference and Research on Salmonella, Institut Pasteur, Paris, France.

Porwollik, S.; Boyd, EF.; Choy, C.; Cheng, P.; Florea, L.; Proctor, E. & McClelland, M. (2004). Characterization of *Salmonella* enterica subspecies I genovars by use of microarrays. *Bacteriol*, 186:5883–5898.

Porwollik, S.; Santiviago, CA.; Cheng, P.; Florea, L. & McClelland, M. (2005). Differences in gene content between *Salmonella* enterica serovar *Enteritidis* isolates and comparison to closely related serovars *Gallinarum* and *Dublin*. *J Bacteriol*, 187:6545–6555

Rabsch, W.; Mirols, S.; Hard, W. D. & Tschape, H. (2002). The dual role of wild phages for horizontal gene transfer among *Salmonella* strains. Berliner und Münchener Tierarztliche Wochenschrift, 115:335-359.

Raeymaekers, L. (1995). A commentary on the practical applications of competitive PCR. *Genome Res*. 5:91–94.

Ridley, A. M.; Threlfall, E. J. & Rowe, B. (1998). Genotypic characterization of *Salmonella enteritidis* phage types by plasmid analysis, ribotyping, and pulsed-field gel electrophoresis. *J Clin Microbiol*, 36, 2314-21.

Riley L. W. 2004. Molecular epidemiology of infectious diseases: principles and practices. ASM Press, Washington, p.337.

Riley, L. W. DiFerdinando, G. T., Jr.; DeMelfi, T. M. & Cohen, M. L. (1983). Evaluation of isolated cases of *salmonellosis* by plasmid profile analysis: introduction and transmission of a bacterial clone by precooked roast beef. *J Infect Dis*, 148, 12-7.

Robertson, J. M. & Walsh-Weller, J. (1998). An introduction to PCR primer design and optimisation of amplification reactions. *Methods Mol. Bio,*. 98:121–154.

Rodrigue, D. C.; Tauxe, R. V. & Rowe, B. (1990). International increase in *Salmonella enteritidis*: a new pandemic?. *Epidemiol Infect*, 105, 21-7.

Rychlik, I.; Gregorova, D. & Hradecka, H. (2006). Distribution and function of plasmids in *Salmonella enterica*. *Veterinary Microbiology*, 112:1-10.

Savelkoul, P. H.; Aarts, H. J.; de Haas, J.; Dijkshoorn, L.; Duim, B.; Otsen, M.; Rademaker, J. L.; Schouls, L. & Lenstra, J. A. (1999). Amplified-fragment length polymorphism analysis: the state of an art. *J Clin Microbiol*, 37, 3083-91.

Selander, R. K.; Li, J. & Nelson, K. (1996). Evolutionary genetics of *Salmonella enterica*. In: Neidhardt F. C. (eds.), *Escherichia coli* and *Salmonella*. *Cellular and Molecular Biology*. ASM Press, Washington D. C., pp.2691-2707.

Shelobolina, E. S.; Sullivan, S. A.; O'Neill, K. R.; Nevin, K. P. & Lovely, D. R. (2004). Isolation, characterization, and U(VI)-reducing potential of a facultatively anaerobic, acid-resistant bacterium from low-pH, nitrateand U(VI)-contaminated subsurface sediment and description of *Salmonella subterranea* sp. *nov*. *Applied and Environmental Microbiology*, 70:2959-2965.

Shuber, A.P.; Skoletsky, J.; Stern, R. & Handelin, B.L. (1993). Efficient 12-mutation testing in the CFTR gene: a general model for complex mutation analysis. *Hum. Mol. Genet*, 2:153-158.

Swaminathan, B.; Barrett, T. J.; Hunter, S. B. & Tauxe, R. V. (2001). PulseNet: the molecular subtyping network for foodborne bacterial disease surveillance, United States, *Emerg Infect Dis*, 7, 382-9.

Tamada, Y.; Nakaoka, Y.; Nishimori, K.; Doi, A.; Kumaki, T.; Uemura, N.; Tanaka, K.; Makino, S. I.; Sameshima, T.; Akiba, M.; Nakazawa, M. & Uchida, I. (2001). Molecular typing and epidemiological study of *Salmonella enterica* serotype *Typhimurium* isolates from cattle by fluorescent amplified- fragment length polymorphism fingerprinting and pulsed-field gel electrophoresis. *J Clin Microbiol*, 39, 1057-66.

Taylor, D. N.; Wachsmuth, I. K.; Shangkuan, Y. H.; Schmidt, E. V.; Barrett, T. J.; Schrader, J. S.; Scherach, C. S.; McGee, H. B.; Feldman, R. A. & Brenner, D. J. (1982). Salmonellosis associated with marijuana: a multistate outbreak traced by plasmid fingerprinting, *N Engl J Med*, 306, 1249-53.

Thong, K-L.; Puthucheary, S. & Pang, T. (1998). Outbreak of *Salmonella enteritidis* gastroenteritis: investigation by pulsed-field gel electrophoresis. Int J Infect Dis, v. 2, n. 3, p. 159-63.

Threlfall, E. J. & Frost, J. A. (1990). The identification, typing and fingerprinting of *Salmonella*: laboratory aspects and epidemiological applications. *J Appl Bacteriol*, 68, 5- 16.

Threlfall, E. J. (2000). Epidemic *salmonella typhimurium* DT 104-a truly international multiresistant clone. *J Antimicrob Chemother*, 46, 7-10.

Threlfall, E. J.; Torre, E.; Ward, L. R.; Davalos-Perez, A.; Rowe, B. & Gibert, I. (1994). Insertion sequence IS200 fingerprinting of *Salmonella typhi*: an assessment of epidemiological applicability. *Epidemiol Infect*, 112, 253- 61.

Validation List No:102. (2005). Validation of publication of new names and new combinations previously effectively published outside the IJSEM. *International Journal of Systemic and Evolutionary Microbiology*, 55:547-549.

Van Eck, H.J., Rouppe van der Voort, J., Draaistra, J. et al. (1995) The inheritance and chromosomal localization of AFLP markers in a non-inbred potato off-spring. Molecular Breeding 1, 397–410.

Vos, P.; Hogers, R.; Bleeker, M. et al. (1995). AFLP: a new technique for DNA fingerprinting. *Nucleic Acid Research*, 23: 4407–4414.

Ward, L. R.; de Sa J. D. H. & Rowe, B. (1987). A phage typing scheme for *Salmonella enteritidis*. *Epidemiology and Infection*, 99: 291-294.

Williams, J.G.K.; Kubelik, A.R.; Livak, K.J.; Rafalski, J.A. & Tingey, S.V. (1990). DNA polymorphisms amplified by arbitrary primers are useful as genetic markers. *Nucleic Acids Res.*, 18, 6531-6535.

Yan, S. S.; Pendrak, M. L.; Abela-Ridder, B.; Punderson, J. W.; Fedorko, D. P. & Foley, S. L. (2003). An overview of *Salmonella* typing public health concern. *Clinical and Applied Immunology Reviews*, 4:189-204.

Ziprin, R. L. & Hume, M.H. (2001). Human Salmonellosis: General Medical Aspects, in Foodborne Disease Handbook, Vol. Volume 1, Hui, Y. H., Pierson, M.D., Gorham, J.R., Ed., Marcel Dekker, Inc., New York, 285-321

# 17

# *Salmonella* Detection Methods for Food and Food Ingredients

Joseph A. Odumeru and Carlos G. León-Velarde
*University of Guelph, Guelph, Ontario*
*Canada*

## 1. Introduction

*Salmonella* is the etiologic agent of Salmonellosis in humans causing severe illness in infants, the elderly, and immunocompromised patients (Cross et al. 1989; Tauxe 1991; Smith 1994; Baumler et al. 2000). Salmonellosis symptoms include watery diarrhea, abdominal pain, nausea, fever, headache and occasional constipation with hospitalization required in cases of severe infections. The genus currently contains two species, *Salmonella bongori and Salmonella enterica* (including six subspecies: *enterica* (I), *salamae* (II), *arizonae* (IIIa), *diarizonae* (IIIb), *houtenae* (IV), and *indica* (VI). However, there are more than 2,500 serovars of *Salmonella* based on the Kauffmann-White antigenic scheme for the classification of Salmonellae (Popoff et al. 1994). *Salmonella* is a gram-negative, non-spore forming rod and facultative anaerobe that can ferment glucose belonging to the family Enterobacteriaceae. Most strains are motile with peritrichous flagella and can reduce nitrate to nitrite (Grimont et al. 2000). The organism is mesophilic with optimum growth temperature in the range of 32 - 37°C but capable of growth within a wide temperature range of 6 - 46°C. *Salmonella* is ubiquitous in the environment originating from the gastrointestinal tracts of domesticated and wild animals and can be present without causing apparent illness. Most infections result from the ingestion of foods of animal origin contaminated with *Salmonella* species such as beef, chicken, turkey, pork, eggs, and milk (D'Aoust 1997; D'Aoust 2000; Olsen et al. 2000). Other vehicles, including non-animal foods such as fresh fruits and vegetables (Mahon et al. 1997), reptiles (Friedman et al. 1998), water (Angulo et al. 1997), and direct person-to-person transmission (Lyons et al. 1980), have also been implicated. However, certain serotypes of *Salmonella* such as *S.* Enteritidis, which can penetrate poultry reproductive organs resulting in the contamination of egg contents has been a prominent cause of human illness for several decades (Gantois et al. 2009). In addition to faecal contamination, cross-contamination of foods by *Salmonella* during food preparation can be an important source of foodborne illness.

Generally, detection methods are based on physiological and biochemical markers of the organism (Williams 1981). Cultural methods are based on nutrient acquisition, biochemical characteristics, and metabolic products unique to *Salmonella* spp. (Ricke et al. 1998). More rapid immunological and molecular screening methods of detection have been devised to detect cell surface markers and nucleic acids, respectively. This chapter will provide an overview of various culture based methods and rapid methods currently available for the detection of *Salmonella* in foods and food ingredients. We will focus our discussion on advances introduced for the improvement of conventional culture methods, the use of Polymerase Chain Reaction (PCR) technology, immunology-based methods, and bacteriophage based assays. Whenever possible, examples from the academic literature as well as from commercial applications will be considered. The importance of sample preparation will be examined throughout as it relates to its impact on sensitivity and turn-around time for detection. Specific *Salmonella* serovars will be named according to the nomenclature of Leminor and Popoff (2001), e.g. *Salmonella* Enteritidis or *S.* Enteritidis.

## 2. Culture methods

Culture based methods are still the most widely used detection techniques and remain the gold standard for the detection of *Salmonella* due to their selectivity and sensitivity. For instance, the US Food and Drug Administration (FDA) and the Food Safety and Inspection Service (FSIS) of the US Department of Agriculture (USDA), requires an isolated organism as unambiguous proof of contamination (Alocilja and Radke 2003). Depending on the approach, standard culture methods typically require 5–7 days to obtain a result as they rely on the ability of *Salmonella* to multiply to visible colonies, which can then be characterized by performing additional biochemical and or serological tests. Due to their widespread use, numerous and varied bacteriological media (selective enrichment broths and selective agar plates) are applied to best monitor for *Salmonella* in food and food ingredients. The media may contain inhibitors in order to stop or delay the growth of non-target organisms, or particular substrates that only the target bacteria can degrade, or that confer a particular colour to the growing colonies (Manafi 2000).
Cultural methods typically involve the enrichment of a portion of the food sample to recover sub-lethally injured cells due to heat, cold, acid, or osmotic shock (Sandel et al. 2003; Gracias and McKillip 2004) in a non-selective pre-enrichment media, such as Buffered Peptone Water (BPW), and to increase the number of target cells as these are generally not uniformly distributed in foods, typically occur in low numbers, and may be present in a mixed microbial population. Next, primary enrichment cultures are typically inoculated into secondary selective enrichment broths, such as Selenite Cystine broth (SC), Rappaport Vasiliadis Soy broth (RVS), Tetrathionate Broth (TT), or Muller-Kauffmann Tetrathionate-Novobiocin broth (MKTTn) and incubated at elevated temperatures (37°C or 42°C for 18-24 hours) before being struck onto selective agars such as Xylose Lysine Deoxycholate agar (XLD agar), Bismuth Sulphite agar (BIS), Brilliant Green agar (BG) with or without the addition of sulfadiazine or sulfapyridine (BGS), modified semisolid Rappaport Vasiliadis (MSRV), Salmonella Shigella Agar, or Hektoen Enteric agar. There are several published standard methods utilizing combinations of media such as the current ISO horizontal method, ISO 6579:2002 (updated in 2007) for the detection *Salmonella*, including *Salmonella* Typhi and *Salmonella* Paratyphi applicable to products intended for human consumption and the feeding of animals, and to environmental samples in the area of food production and food handling. Similar standard methods have been published elsewhere, most notably in the FDA Bacteriological Analytical Manual (BAM).
Typical *Salmonella* colonies based on morphology and or indicative biochemical reactions on selective agars are then cultured onto non-selective media prior to confirmatory testing. There are well-established confirmations and identification procedures for *Salmonella*. Preliminary identification is traditionally performed using classical biochemical and serological tests. Key biochemical tests include the fermentation of glucose, negative urease

reaction, lysine decarboxylase, negative indole test, $H_2S$ production, and fermentation of dulcitol. Serological confirmation tests typically utilize polyvalent antisera for flagellar (H) and somatic (O) antigens. Isolates with a typical biochemical profile, which agglutinate with both H and O antisera are identified as *Salmonella* species. Where results are inconclusive, it may be necessary to perform additional biochemical tests. Positive isolates are often sent for further serotyping to identify the serovar using specific antisera as per the Kauffman-White (KW) typing scheme recognizing 46 O antigens, and 119 H antigens, thereby permitting the characterization of 2,541 serotypes (Shipp and Rowe 1980). Serotyping is a useful epidemiological tool in identifying circulating serotypes and to characterize outbreaks. The antigenic formulae of Le Minor and Popoff (2001) is a standard method for naming the serovars. However, serotyping is normally undertaken at reference laboratories and is rarely performed in routine food or clinical laboratories. Reference laboratories are also able to further type isolates using techniques such a phage typing (Anderson and Williams 1956; Callow 1959; Anderson 1964; Anderson et al. 1977), antibiotic susceptibility (Bauer et al. 1966), pulsed-field gel electrophoresis (PFGE), or other emerging genetic typing technologies such Multiple-Locus Variable Number Tandem Repeat Analysis (MLVA) and Multilocus sequence typing (MLST) (Kruy et al. 2011).

Although standard culture methods are excessively time-consuming, there is potential for further improvements, and thus many attempts have been made to maximize their efficiency by introducing new technologies, making reliability of detection more convenient, user friendly, as well as by reducing the costs of materials and labour (de Boer and Beumer 1999; Weenk, 1992). For example, biochemical confirmatory tests may be easily replaced by commercial identification kits such as the API 20E (BioMérieux) or other commercially available bacterial identification kits. The detection of sub-lethally damaged cells is of utmost importance as these may still pose a risk to human health and may lead to false negative results. Strategies for the recovery of injured bacteria are based on overlay methods such as tryptic soy agar (TSA) overlayed on XLD selective agar (Kang and Fung 2000) and other approaches also include the development of single enrichment broths where multiple step enrichments are usually required (Baylis et al. 2000). Other novel approaches include the addition of bacteriophages for the elimination of background microflora that may out-compete the target organism. For example, RapidChek® SELECT™ Salmonella (Strategic Diagnostics Inc.) employs a primary enrichment media supplemented with a bacteriophage cocktail as a selective agent, which reduces the level of background flora in high burden samples allowing *Salmonella* to grow with minimal competition. In addition, there is also the development of enrichment broths for the concurrent enrichment of pathogens thereby reducing laboratory workloads with respect to the preparation of sample homogenates since different enrichment broths would no longer be required, and multiple analyses could be performed from a single universal enrichment culture (Kim and Bhunia 2008). Amendments to media have also been performed such as the addition of novobiocin (Restaino et al. 1977; Devenish et al. 1986), and cycloheximide to decrease fungal overgrowth (Ricke et al. 1998). Lastly, and perhaps the most important advancement is the use of chromogenic or fluorogenic substrates in selective agars, permitting identification to be performed directly on the isolation plate, thereby expediting or eliminating the use of subculture media or additional biochemical tests as these media provide highly specific reactions, and help reduce the workload for unnecessary examination of suspect colonies arising from poor specificity of conventional agars (Manafi 1996; Manafi 2000). A number of selective chromogenic agar media specifically designed for the differentiation of *Salmonella* colonies are commercially available with varying success of adoption by regulatory agencies such as: Salmonella SMS (AES Chemunex), BBL CHROMagar (CHROMagar), RAPID'Salmonella (Bio-Rad Laboratories, S.A.), chromID Salmonella (BioMerieux), Harlequin Salmonella ABC (Lab M), Oxoid Brilliance Salmonella Agar (Oxoid), and Rambach Agar (Merck), among others.

It is evident that the multitude of options for isolation of *Salmonella* and the lack of inter-laboratory consistency make *Salmonella* isolation one of the most variable procedures in laboratories with new media available every year, promising to be more sensitive, specific, and rapid (Hyatt and Weese 2004). With this myriad of choice, laboratories must chose culture approaches which efficiently and accurately provide timely results via the development of standard methods and participation in proficiency quality assurance programs.

### 2.1 Immunomagnetic separation

In an attempt to reduce the length of routine microbiological analysis and to minimize the problems associated with rapid detection systems such as interference from foods and food ingredients debris, background micro-organisms, and lack of sensitivity, there has been a lot of interest in the development of separation and concentration techniques prior to detection. Various techniques have been utilized for this purpose including: centrifugation (Basel et al. 1983), filtration (Farber and Sharpe 1984), and lectin-based biosorbents (Payne et al. 1992). However, the most successful of approaches for the separation and concentration of target organisms has been the use of immunomagnetic separation (IMS). The advantages of IMS are that it reduces the total analysis time and improves the sensitivity of detection. IMS is rapid, technically simple, and specific method for the isolation of the target organisms (Shaw et al. 1998). Paramagnetic particles are coated with antibodies specific to the target organism and added to a post enrichment culture. The target organism is captured onto the magnetic particles and the whole complex is then removed from the system by the application of a magnetic field. Target organisms are thus removed from food debris and competing microorganisms, which may otherwise interfere with the detection system. If required, the isolated complex may be re-suspended in an enrichment broth so that cell numbers can be rapidly increased to improve the sensitivity of detection assays. In addition, IMS by design can be used in conjunction with other rapid detection methods, including ELISA, conductance microbiology, electrochemiluminescence, and polymerase chain reaction (PCR) to further increase its analytical sensitivity (Fluit et al. 1993; Cudjoe et al. 1994; Cudjoe et al. 1995; Sapanova et al. 2000). It has been reported that IMS is more sensitive than conventional culture methods and is able to reduce the total culture analysis time by one to two days (Lynch et al. 2004; Ten Bosch et al. 1992).

The most commonly used commercial IMS bead for the recovery of *Salmonella* from food samples is Dynabeads™ anti *Salmonella* (Invitrogen). Similar magnetic beads specific for *Salmonella* are available such as Captivate Salmonella (Lab M), Tecra Salmonella Unique (3M), as wells as for specific serovars such as *S.* Enteritidis, via Rapidchek Confirm *S.* Enteritidis IMS kit (SDIX). IMS can also be automated using automated IMS separators such as the BeadRetriever (Invitrogen) capable of processing up to fifteen 1 mL enrichments volumes per cycle (23 minutes), to larger scale instruments such as the Kingfisher IMS separator (Thermofisher) or Mag Max (Life Technologies) capable of processing up to 100 samples with the capability of re-suspending the IMS target complex in microtitre plates for further testing by PCR, or ELISA. For instance, the VIDAS ICS test (BioMérieux) uses automated immunoconcentration prior to analysis by an automated ELISA instrument for the detection of *Salmonella* from food and food ingredients. Another IMS variation was also developed by Pathatrix (Matrix MicroScience Ltd) combining IMS and a recirculation step (Flow Through Immunocapture or FTI), to further increase the sensitivity of detection since larger enrichment volumes can be reacted with IMS beads. For example Warren et al. (2007) investigated FTI, using the Pathatrix device, followed by plating on XLD agar (FTI-XLD) or analysis by real-time PCR (FTI-PCR) for the detection of *Salmonella* on smooth tomato surfaces and in potato salad and ground beef. The FTI-XLD method demonstrated the ability to isolate presumptive *Salmonella* colonies up to 48 h faster than did the standard modified BAM *Salmonella* culture method and the FTI-PCR was able to detect *Salmonella* within 8h.

Among the problems associated with IMS is non-target carryover where non-target organisms adhere to the walls of glass test tubes (Meadows 1971). Protamine as well as the use of mild detergents is commonly used to minimize non-target carryover since it adheres to the glass and to the bacteria in the sample reducing the net negative charge to prevent adherence. IMS also suffers in that it requires small sample sizes, organisms may be lost from beads during separation from samples with high fat content, and non specific binding of *Citrobacter freundii* and coliforms with mucoid layers has also been observed (Coleman et al 1995).

## 3. Immunological based methods

### 3.1 Rapid agglutination assays

Several rapid latex agglutination assay tests are widely used for the rapid detection of *Salmonella*. These assays however, are primarily used as a confirmation screen for presumptive *Salmonella* colonies after culture isolation from selective agar plates, with further confirmation and identification work carried out on those organisms giving a positive latex reaction. An aliquot of a colony suspension or enrichment broth is simply mixed with the latex reagent and after a few minutes rotation, the results are clearly visible. If the test is negative, the latex remains in smooth suspension and retains its original colour. A positive result is indicated by distinct colour agglutination against an altered background. By reducing the number of samples requiring further confirmatory testing, these tests save time and resources and allow negative results to be reported at least 24 hours earlier than by conventional culture methods. However, depending on the antibodies used they may lack specificity due to non-specific agglutination of some organisms (Cheesbrough and Donnelly, 1996). Some commercial kits include Remel Wellcolex Colour tests for the presumptive identification of *Salmonella* serogroups A, B, C, D, E, and G, and the $V_i$ antigen using just two reagents. Similar tests include Oxoid Salmonella latex test, Microgen Salmonella Latex test, and Denka-Seiken, among others.

### 3.2 Enzyme-linked immunosorbent assay (ELISA)

Enzyme-linked immunosorbent assay (ELISA) also known as an enzyme immunoassay (EIA), is a biochemical technique used to detect the presence of an antibody or an antigen in a sample. In the context of *Salmonella* detection, a sample with an unknown amount of antigen is immobilized on a solid support (usually a polystyrene microtitre plate) either non-specifically (via adsorption to the surface) or specifically (via capture by another antibody specific to the same antigen, in a "Sandwich" ELISA). After the antigen is immobilized, a detection antibody linked to an enzyme such as Horse Radish Peroxidase (HRP) is added, forming a complex with the antigen. Between each step, the plate is typically washed with a mild detergent solution to remove any proteins or antibodies that are not specifically bound. After the final wash step, the plate is developed by adding an enzymatic substrate (ABTS or 3,3′,5,5′-tetramethylbenzidine) to produce a visible signal (colorimetric or fluorescent product) due to the enzymatic cleavage of the substrate. Colorimetric equipment is used to measure the signal indicating colorimetric equipment indicating the presence of target antigen in the sample.

ELISAs are highly specific, sensitive, rapid, easy to perform, and scalable, allowing laboratories to easily adopt the technology for routine microbiological testing. The ELISA reactivity however, is influenced by various components of the enrichment medium and incubation conditions used. With most ELISA methods, negative results can be obtained within 24 h after an overnight incubation in selective broth. Positive results may still require further cultural isolation and serological and biochemical confirmation depending of regulatory requirements.

Currently, there are numerous ELISA plate based assay systems for the detection on *Salmonella: Salmonella* ELISA (BIO ART SA), TRANSIA® PLATE *Salmonella* Gold (BioControl), and RIDASCREEN® *Salmonella* ELISA (R-Biopharm AG). Some of these tests have the advantage of being able to process numerous samples at once in 96 well microtitre plates, and some such as the Tecra™ *Salmonella* Visual Immunoassay (3M), provide a visual indication of detection without the use of colorimetric equipment. In addition ELISA systems have been automated to facilitate routine laboratory testing such as the EIAFoss (Foss Electronics) and the VitekImmuno Diagnostic Assay System (VIDAS) (BioMerieux). For example, the VIDAS®SLM assay (BioMérieux), is intended for use with the VIDAS as an automated qualitative enzyme-linked fluorescent immunoassay (ELFA) for the detection of *Salmonella* in food and food ingredients. The VIDAS instrument performs all of the assay steps automatically. In contrast to the manual manipulation required for microtitre plate based systems, a pipette tip-like disposable unit (a solid phase receptacle or SPR) serves as the solid phase as well as a pipetter during the process. The SPR is coated with polyclonal anti-*Salmonella* antibodies and reagents for the assay are sealed in reagent strips. An aliquot of the enrichment broth is placed into the reagent strip and the sample and reagents are sequentially cycled in and out of the SPR for a specific length of time until the instrument detects fluorescence.

Nevertheless, ELISA methods are not without disadvantages, some of which include high limits of sensitivity of $>10^5$ cfu/mL (Cox 1988) variable cell surface antigen production (Peplow et al. 1999); cross reactivity (Westerman et al. 1997), and changes to antigens due to acetylation and changing recognition by assay antibodies (Kim and Slauch, 1999). Newer ELISA-like techniques utilize fluorogenic, electrochemiluminescent, and real-time PCR reporters to create quantifiable signals. However, given that the general principles in these assays are largely similar, they are often grouped in the same category as ELISAs.

### 3.3 Lateral flow immunoassays

Lateral flow immunoassays typically use a sandwich type ELISA and the majority use polyclonal antibody as a capture antibody and a monoclonal antibody as the detection antibody. The antibodies are fixed on a hydrophobic polyvinylidine difluoride-based membrane. A drop of an enrichment sample is placed in a reaction window and travels by capillary action across the membrane to react with the antibodies and provide a colour change. Results are often available within 24 hours. False positive results may be observed during the reaction because of denaturation or degradation of the capture antibody and it is likely that detection antibody or enzyme-conjugated antibody may also bind non-specifically to denatured capture antibody. Commercially available lateral flow immunoassays for the detection of *Salmonella* include: DuPont™ Lateral Flow System *Salmonella*, Singlepath *Salmonella* (Merck), Reveal® *Salmonella* lateral flow (Neogen), VIP Gold (BioControl), and RapidChek® SELECT (SDIX). Recently, serotype specific lateral flow immunoassays for the detection of *S.* Enteritidis have also been introduced to serve the egg and poultry industry such as RapidChek® SELECT *S.* Enteritids (SDIX) and Reveal *S.* Enteritidis (Neogen). In general, these types of immunoassays are ideally suited where a low testing throughput is expected. The implementation of these tests is beneficial in that they require low technical expertise, and minimal capital expenditure.

## 4. Molecular methods

### 4.1 Polymerase chain reaction (PCR)

Over the past 15 years there has been an important evolution in molecular approaches for the rapid detection of food borne pathogens rather than relying on their biochemical and phenotypic characteristics. Foremost among these tools is the Polymerase Chain Reaction (PCR), a technique based on the specific amplification of a short target DNA sequence (Mullis et al. 1986). Briefly, extracted DNA is first subjected to heat denaturation into single stranded DNA. Next, specific short DNA fragments (primers) are annealed to the single DNA strands, followed by extension of the primers complementary to the single stranded DNA with the aid of a thermostable DNA polymerase, such as Taq polymerase, an enzyme originally isolated from the bacterium *Thermus aquaticus* (Chien et al. 1976). Each new double-stranded DNA is then a targeted during a new thermal cycle and thus the exponential amplification of the specific DNA sequence is achieved. The amplified product is then separated by gel electrophoresis and visualized by staining with fluorescent ethidium bromide. This type of conventional or endpoint PCR, although sensitive and specific under optimized conditions, is time consuming and labour intensive due to post-amplification steps, not sensitive enough to measure the accumulated DNA copies accurately, and can only provide a qualitative result. Nevertheless, PCR techniques have expedited the process of pathogen detection and in some cases, replaced traditional methods for bacterial identification, characterization, and enumeration in foods (McKillip and Drake 2004).

### 4.2 Real-time PCR

The development of novel chemistries and instrumentation platforms enabling detection of PCR products on a real-time basis has led to widespread adoption of real-time PCR as the method of choice for detection of *Salmonella* (Espy et al. 2006). This method combines amplification and detection stages of the process so that nucleic acid amplification is monitored and recorded continuously hence eliminating the need for post-amplification steps such as gel electrophoresis. The detection of PCR products is accomplished via the generation of a fluorescent signal by any of the commercially available chemistries for real-time PCR: TaqMan® (Applied Biosystems®), Molecular Beacons, Scorpions®, and SYBR® Green (Molecular Probes), among others.

The simplest approach involves the use of the intercalating fluorescent dye SYBR® Green. This fluorogenic dye exhibits little fluorescence when in solution, but emits a strong fluorescent signal upon binding to double-stranded DNA. Thus, as a PCR product accumulates, fluorescence increases. The advantages of SYBR® Green are that it is inexpensive, simple, and sensitive. The disadvantage is that SYBR® Green will bind to any double-stranded DNA in the reaction, which may result in an overestimation of the target concentration. A second, more accurate and reliable method is to use fluorescent reporter probes (TaqMan®, Molecular Beacons, Scorpions®). These probes depend on Förster Resonance Energy Transfer (FRET) to generate the fluorescence signal via the coupling of a fluorogenic dye molecule and a quencher moeity to the same or different oligonucleotide substrates. The main advantage of TaqMan probes, Molecular Beacons and Scorpions is that they allow for multiplex PCR assays by using spectrally separated fluor/quench moieties for each probe. Multiplex PCR allows internal controls to be co-amplified and permits allele discrimination in single-tube, homogeneous assays. These hybridization probes afford a level of discrimination impossible to obtain with SYBR® Green, since they will only hybridize to true targets in a PCR and not to primer-dimers or other spurious products. However these probes can be expensive to synthesize, with a separate probe needed for each target being analyzed.

Commercial real time PCR assays employ a high degree of automation to reduce the number of operations involved and reduce the risk of contamination. The reaction usually takes place inside a combined thermocycler-fluorescence detection instrument and uses pre-prepared reagents, often in a dehydrated tablet form. The thermo-cycling and detection are controlled by software that also calculates and interprets the results. Total time for an analysis for the detection of *Salmonella* species is normally 20 to 48 hours but can be as little as 12 hours depending on the food matrix, enrichment conditions, and instrument run time. The main advantage of these PCR systems over other methods is in time saving, both in the total time from sampling to result and in the technical time needed to set up and run the assay. In addition many available real time PCR assays have achieved a variety of certifications via AOAC, AFNOR, NORDVAL, and ISO 16140 validation. However, capital costs for automated PCR systems are relatively high and consumable costs are also high by comparison to culture based techniques. There is a clear cost benefit in rapid test results allowing faster HACCP verification and release of finished food products particularly where the prevalence of *Salmonella* is known to be low, thus reducing additional culture confirmation tests or where pooling of samples is permitted. Numerous assays are commercially available using real time PCR for the detection of *Salmonella.* The BAX PCR detection system (DuPont-Qualicon Inc.), a platform adopted by USDA-FSIS as a screening tool offers a detection kit for the detection of *Salmonella* in a variety of food and food ingredients. Other systems offering similar testing capabilities include: ADIAFOOD Rapid Pathogen Detection System (AES Chemunex), the Assurance Genetic Detection System GDS (Biocontrol Inc.) utilizing a post enrichment IMS step followed by real time PCR, iQ-Check™ Salmonella II (BioRad Laboratories, S.A.), and R.A.P.I.D. LT system (Idaho Technology Inc.), among others.

Lastly, real time PCR systems have sufficient flexibility to allow for the rapid development of new assays targeting specific *Salmonella* serovars of clinical significance. More recently in 2010, in order to minimize the potential for foodborne illness from eggs containing *S.* Enteritidis, the FDA implemented new regulations for the egg industry, which included requiring large-scale egg producers to begin SE monitoring programs in their poultry houses and potentially on their products. In response to the industry testing needs, a 27 hour commercial real time PCR assay for the detection of *S.*Enteritidis was developed by Applied Biosystems®, the TaqMan® *Salmonella* Enteritidis Detection Kit.

### 4.3 Multiplex PCR

In multiplex PCR (mPCR), several specific primer sets are combined into a single PCR assay for the simultaneous amplification of more than one target DNA sequence (Chamberlain et al. 1988). As with conventional or endpoint PCR, the amplified DNA targets are separated by agarose gel electrophoresis and visualized by ethidium bromide staining. Depending on the number of targets, the analysis is carried out by a single amplification reaction of four–to five targets, or could take place via a two-step amplification reaction for five–six targets or more (Settanni and Corsetti 2007). For example, Malorny et al. (2007) developed an assay for the specific detection of *S.* Enteritidis in whole chicken carcass rinses and consumption eggs. The assay used specifically designed primers and a TaqMan probe to target the *Prot6e* gene located on the *S.* Enteritidis 60-kb virulence plasmid. As an internal amplification control to monitor *Salmonella* DNA in the sample, a second primer/TaqMan probe set detected simultaneously the *Salmonella* specific *invA* (invasion protein A) gene. It must be considered however, that the majority of the articles in the scientific literature deal with mPCR methods developed to identify and or characterize *Salmonella* serotypes from pure cultures, or in controlled artificial inoculation experiments, with only a minority of studies providing results from *in situ* detection of pathogens in foods or environmental samples. Soumet et al. (1999) developed a multiplex PCR assay for the simultaneous identification of *Salmonella* species, *S.* Enteritidis and *S.* Typhimurium from environmental swabs of poultry houses. Similarly, O'Regan et al. (2008) developed a real-time multiplex PCR assay for the detection of multiple *Salmonella* serotypes in chicken samples. Poultry-associated serotypes detected in the assay included *S.* Enteritidis, *S.* Gallinarum, *S.* Typhimurium, *S.* Kentucky and *S.* Dublin. Generally, the 16S rRNA gene is the most common target for mPCR as it is routinely used to establish phylogenetic distinctions among bacteria (Rossello-Mora and Amman 2001). However, other target genes are also considered in order to achieve a high specificity. For example, Rajtak et al. (2011) developed a two step real-time mPCR assay for the rapid screening of 19 *Salmonella* serotypes frequently encountered in humans, animals, and animal-associated meat products within the European Union. Specific primers for serotype differentiation were designed to target the genes encoding either phase 1 and 2 flagellar antigens *fliC* and *fljB* or unique serotype-specific loci. In addition, the assay simultaneously screened for the presence of the ampicilin-amoxicillin, chloramphenicol-florfenicol, streptomycin-spectinomycin, sulfanomides, and tetracycline (ACSSuT)-type multidrug resistance pattern, indicated by the *floR* gene, and for the *Salmonella* virulence plasmid encoded by the svp operon in *S.* Typhimurium. The assay represents a more rapid and reliable method for identification of large numbers of serotypes than assays using phenotypic serotyping methods. Multiplex PCR is thus quite versatile and numerous other assays have been published for the rapid detection and characterization of specific *Salmonella* serotypes (Alvarez et al. 2004; Woods et al. 2008; Kim et al. 2006; Chiu et al. 2006) analogous to mPCR approaches used for the differentiation of multiple species belonging to single genera such as gastroenteritis causing themotolerant *Campylobacter* species (Korolik et al. 2001;Klena et al. 2004; Wang et al. 2002; Yamazaki-Matsune et al. 2007) or for the differentiation of the major *L. monocytogenes* serovars (1/2a, 1/2b, 1/2c, and 4b) commonly implicated in food borne listeriosis (Doumith et al. 2004; Zhang and Knabel 2005; Chen and

Knabel 2007). Lastly, and perhaps the largest impact that mPCR may provide in a near future is in the rapid and simultaneous detection of *Salmonella* concurrently with other bacterial pathogens. For instance, Gilbert et al. (2003) established a mPCR assay in order to detect *Salmonella* along with *Campylobacter jejuni*, and *E. coli* O157:H7 in a variety of raw and ready-to-eat food products. The primers amplified a single product from each target bacterium. More recently, Kim et al. (2007) developed a novel mPCR assay for the simultaneous screening of five foodborne pathogenic bacteria including *Salmonella*. Specific primers for mPCR amplification of the Shiga-like toxin gene (*Stx2*), *femA* (cytoplasmic protein), *toxR* (transmembrane DNA binding protein), *iap* (invasive associative protein), and *invA* genes were designed to allow simultaneous detection of *E. coli* O157:H7, *S. aureus*, *Vibrio parahaemolyticus*, *L. monocytogenes*, and *Salmonella* spp., respectively. Furthermore, the detection of all five food borne pathogenic bacteria could be completed in less than 24 h. Similar approaches have been described by others utilizing various primer sets for a variety of pathogens (Li and Mustapha 2004; Park et al. 2006).

### 4.4 Reverse transcriptase PCR (RT-PCR)

Thus far, there is no correlation between viability and detection as provided by PCR assays. The amplification of genomic DNA by PCR has been shown to be inappropriate for distinguishing viable from non-viable bacteria owing to DNA stability over time (Masters et al. 1994). Furthermore, the detection of pathogens by PCR in food samples often requires additional evidence of viability before risk can be assigned. In an effort to address the issue of viability, many researchers turned to RNA amplification methods using mRNA as a target since it is a molecule with a very short half-life of 0.5 to 2 minutes due to the rapid degradation by endogenous RNases (King et al. 1986). The outcome was the development of an amplification technique for detecting mRNA termed reverse transcriptase PCR (RT-PCR). To date however, due to the variable persistence of nucleic acids in cells post-death, the correlation between the presence of DNA and RNA and viability is still not clear (Cenciarini-Borde et al. 2009). In RT-PCR, an RNA strand is first reverse transcribed into its DNA complement (complementary DNA, or cDNA) using the enzyme reverse transcriptase, and the resulting cDNA is then amplified using conventional, multiplex, or real-time PCR. For example, Rijpens et al. (2002) targeted the housekeeping *rpoD* gene of *Salmonella.* Overall, the assay could not detect viable *Salmonella* in heat or ethanol killed *Salmonella* cells. However, conventional RT-PCR techniques are labour intensive since the amplicon can be visualized only after the amplification ends, requires the rapid extraction of RNA due to its short half-life, suffers from an increased cross-contamination risk of the samples thus requiring DNase treatments, and the target genes must demonstrate abundant transcript expression, expression throughout the growth cycle, and negligible or no transcriptional regulation (Klein and Juneja 1997; Deisingh and Thompson 2004; Yaron and Matthews 2002). Due to these difficulties, the development of RT-PCR applications focusing on the detection of food-borne pathogens, including *Salmonella* in foods and environmental samples has been limited. D'Souza et al. (2009) developed a RT-PCR for the rapid detection of *Salmonella* using *invA* primers. Park et al. (2011) evaluated immunomagnetic beads and a RT-PCR method for the detection of *Salmonella* inoculated into poultry feed demonstrating that the *hilA* gene is a candidate for use in RT-PCR. Techathuvanan and D'Souza (2011) optimized a rapid *Salmonella* detection assay in liquid whole eggs by SYBR® Green based real-time RT-PCR targeting the *invA* gene as described previously for the detection of

*Salmonella* from jalapeno and serrano peppers, and Pork (Miller et al. 2010; Techatuvanan et al. 2010). To further address the issue of viability of the species detected in a complex matrix such as foods, perhaps the best alternative could be the development and validation of real time and multiplexed PCR assays targeting mRNA, also termed multiplex RT-PCR (Gonzalez-Escalona et al. 2009; Settanni and Corsetti 2007). Thus far however, no commercial PCR assay is available utilizing reverse-transcriptase technology for detecting *Salmonella* in foods.

It is evident that molecular methods offer improved sensitivity and potential reduction in assay time. It has now become possible to rapidly detect and confirm the presence of foodborne *Salmonella* spp. in a wide array of food and environmental samples by commercial amplification detection systems. The primary challenges remaining are to develop more reliable recovery and extraction procedures for routine processing of samples from a wider variety of feed and environmental matrices and apply molecular techniques for further characterizing *Salmonella* spp.

### 4.5 Nucleic acid hybridization

Endpoint PCR is commonly utilized for the detection of amplified PCR products. However, DNA hybridization has also been described for detection (Chan et al. 1988; Hill and Keasler 1991; Hill and Lampel 1990). Probes directed to specific gene regions of the *Salmonella* genome provide a powerful tool for use in DNA hybridization assays. Such methods of detection have proven to be more sensitive than agarose gel electrophoresis and more specific than culture or immunological based assays (Ten Bosch et al. 1992; Manzano et al. 1998). For example, Maciorowski et al. (1998) was able to detect PCR products from *S.* Typhimurium inoculated animal feeds by hybridization with biotin and fluorescently labeled probes. Such specificity eliminates the need for serological confirmation and incidences of false-positive identification caused by antibody cross-reactivity with other organisms. Also, unlike biochemical differentiations, probe reactions do not rely on enzymatic activities and are therefore unaffected by media interference or the presence of bacteria with similar phenotypes. The majority of DNA based hybridization assays have exploited this specificity for DNA microarray assay targeting multiple genes with few applications related to the detection of *Salmonella* from food and environmental samples. Probes complimentary to amplified gene products have been used for the detection of *Salmonella* in oysters and chicken meat as well as from environmental poultry house drag swabs (Cohen et al. 1994; Doran et al. 1994; Jones et al. 1993; Bej et al. 1996). Commercial hybridization assays for the detection of *Salmonella* include the GeneQuence *Salmonella* assay (Neogen) utilizing probes previously evaluated by D'Aoust et al. (1995). This test employs Salmonella-Specific DNA probes, which are directly labeled with horseradish peroxidase. A colorimetric endpoint is then used for the detection of *Salmonella* spp. in food samples following broth culture enrichment with results available within 24 h.

## 5. Phage based detection methods

Bacteriophages are viruses infecting bacteria and by definition obligate intracellular parasites lacking their own metabolism, are extremely host-specific, and able only to infect specific species or even strains. Virulent phages with a broad host range within the *Salmonella* genus are ideally suited for detection purposes since they are unable to integrate into the host genome, with the successful infection always resulting in the death of their host (Hagens and Loessner 2007). Since the first report of the use of phage for detection by Ulitzur and Kuhn (1987), different strategies have been described for the detection of *Salmonella*. Generally, the majority of methods described involve measuring the activity of a reporter gene (generally, the luciferase *lux* genes from *Vibrio fisherii*), cloned into a vector carried by a phage, and expressed only after infection (Kuhn et al. 2002; Thouand et al. 2008). Luciferase genes have the enormous advantage in that background noise or photon emission is absent from food samples and the luminescence, when detected, reflects the presence of viable target bacteria. Other approaches include use of an ice nucleation reporter phage (Wolber and Green 1990); concentration by IMS followed by phage mediated release of adenylate kinase (AK) (Blasco et al. 1998; Wu et al. 2001); fluorescently labelled phage (Jiang et al 2009); and an IMS-bacteriophage plaque formation assay requiring the addition of a virucide to inactivate free phage particles (Fravrin et al. 2001). The usefulness of phage-based cell wall recognition proteins for magnetic capture has also been recently described utilizing cell-wall-binding domains (CBDs) highly specific for recognition and binding to target cells surfaces (Kretzer et al. 2007; Korndoerfer et al. 2006; Loessner et al. 2002). Paramagnetic beads coated with CBD molecules were shown to outperform commercially available antibody-based magnetic beads with respect to sensitivity and percent recovery (Kretzer et al. 2007). An extension to this approach has been the use of phage-tail-associated recognition proteins for the immobilization of gram-negative cells (Galikowska et al. 2011). For example, BioMerieux. has recently introduced *Salmonella* Up, an automated ELISA based VIDAS assay using a phage recombinant protein derived from specific bacteriophage tail fibers for the detection of *Salmonella* in food and food ingredients within 18-24 hours after enrichment in a non-selective broth.

Although at present commercial phage based detection systems are limited, the technology may circumvent the problem of viability presented by PCR, while promising to be more rapid than standard culture methods.

## 6. Conclusions and future perspectives on *Salmonella* detection methods

A wide range of methods for the detection of *Salmonella* has been developed in the last decade and significant progress has been made in sample preparation techniques for improved isolation and detection of *Salmonella* in foods and food ingredients. The use of immunomagenetic separation technique which separates target organisms from background flora, is now routinely applied in various diagnostic labs for a variety of foodborne pathogens including *Salmonella*. This technique has increased the sensitivity of the detection of *Salmonella* in various types of food and food ingredients as well as environmental samples with high levels of background. Similarly, the application of molecular methods, immunological methods, and bacteriophage detection systems for *Salmonella* is now routine in many diagnostic food microbiology labs. Novel technologies such as the application of biosensors, microarrays, and nanotechnology are currently in the research stage and these are likely to become available for routine testing of food and food ingredients within the next decade.

The application of rapid methods for the detection, identification, and characterization of *Salmonella* provides a useful tool for assessment of the safety of food products when used in conjunction with foodsafety programs such as the Hazard Analysis Critical Control Point (HACCP) program for the assessment of raw materials and food ingredients used in food processing and production. Further improvements to rapid methods for isolation and detection of *Salmonella* and other microbial pathogens will continue to focus on sample enrichment and preparation procedures to reduce test turn around times and increase the sensitivity of detection, and also on the application of novel technologies such as biosensors, microarrays and nanotechnology for pathogen detection in foods.

## 7. References

Alocilja E.C., and Radke S.M. 2003. Market analysis of biosensors for food safety, Biosensors & bioelectronics, 18(5-6):841-846.

Alvarez J., Sota M., Vivanco A.B., Perales I., Cisterna R., Rementeria A., Garaizar J. 2004. Development of a multiplex PCR technique for detection and epidemiological typing of salmonella in human clinical samples. J Clin Microbiol, 42(4):1734-8.

Anderson E.S., and Williams R.E.O. 1956. Bacteriophage typing of enteric pathogens and staphylococci and its use in epidemiology. J. Clin. Pathol. 9:94– 114.

Anderson E.S. 1964. The phagetyping of Salmonella other than S. typhi. In: Van Oye, E. (Ed.), The World Problem of Salmonellosis. Dr W. Junk Publishers, The Hague, The Netherlands, pp. 89–100.

Anderson, E.S., Ward L.R., de Saxe M.J., 1977. Bacteriophage typing designations of Salmonella typhimurium. J. Hyg. 78:297– 300.

Angulo F.J., Tippen S., Sharp D.J. 1997. A community waterborne outbreak of salmonellosis and the effectiveness of a boil water order. Am J Public Health 87:580-4.

Basel R.M., Richter E.R., and Banwart G.J. 1983. Monitoring microbial numbers in food by density centrifugation. Appl Environ Microbiol, 45(3):1156-9.

Bauer, A.W., Kirby J.C., Turck M. 1966.Antibiotic susceptibility testing by a standardized single disk method. Am. J. Clin.Apthol. 45:493– 496.

Baumler A.J., Tsolis R.M. and Heffron F. 2000. Virulence mechanisms of Salmonella and their genetic basis. In: C Wray and A Wray (eds), Salmonella in Domestic Animals, (CAB International, Wallingford, UK), pp.52-57.

Baylis C.L., MacPhee S., Betts R.P. 2000. Comparison of methods for the recovery and detection of low levels of injured salmonella in ice cream and milk powder. Letters in Applied Microbiology, 30:320-324.

Bej A.K., Southworth J.P., Law R., Mahbubani M.H., Jones D.D. 1996. Detection of *Salmonella* in chicken meat using PCR. *Food Testing & Analysis.* 2:17–20.

Blasco R., Murphy M.J., Sanders M.F., Squirrell D.J.1998. Specific assays for bacteria using phage mediated release of adenylate kinase. J Appl Microbiol, 84:661–666

Callow B.R. 1959. A new phage-typing scheme for *Salmonella typhimurium*. J. Hyg. 57: 347–359.

Campylobacter lari, and Campylobacter upsaliensis by a multiplex PCR developed from the nucleotide sequence of the lipid A gene lpxA", *Journal of clinical microbiology,* vol. 42, no. 12, pp. 5549-5557.

Chamberlain, J.S., Gibbs, R.A., Ranier, J.E., Nguyen, P.N.&Caskey, C.T. 1988, "Deletion screening of the Duchenne muscular dystrophy locus via multiplex DNA amplification", *Nucleic acids research,* vol. 16, no. 23, pp. 11141-11156.

Chan, S.W., Wilson, S., Hsu, H.-Y., King, W., Halbert, D.H., and Klinger, J.D. 1988. Model non-isotopic hybridization systems for detection of food- borne bacteria:

preliminary results and future prospects, in *Biotechnology and Food Quality,* S. Kung, D.D. Bills and R. Quatrano, Eds., Boston, MA: Butterworths, 219–237.

Cheesbrough S., and Donnely C. 1996. The use of a rapid Salmonella latex serogrouping test (Spectate) to assist in the confirmation of ELISA-based rapid Salmonella screening tests.Lett Appl Microbiol. 22(5):378-80.

Chen, Y. &Knabel, S.J. 2007, "Multiplex PCR for simultaneous detection of bacteria of the genus Listeria, Listeria monocytogenes, and major serotypes and epidemic clones of *L. monocytogenes*", Applied and Environmental Microbiology, vol. 73, no. 19, pp. 6299-6304.

Chien, A., Edgar, D.B. &Trela, J.M. 1976, "Deoxyribonucleic acid polymerase from the extreme thermophile Thermusaquaticus", Journal of Bacteriology, vol. 127, no. 3, pp. 1550-1557.

Chiu C.H., Su L.H., Chu C.H., Wang M.H., Yeh C.M., Weill F.X., Chu C. 2006. Detection of multidrug-resistant *Salmonella enterica* serovar typhimurium phage types DT102, DT104 and U302 by multiplex PCR.J Clin Microbiol. 2006 Jul; 44(7):2354-8.

Cohen, N.D., Wallis, D.E., Neibergs, H.L., McElroy, A.P., McGruder, E.D., DeLoach, J.R., Corrier, D.E., and Hargis, B.M. 1994b. Comparison of the polymerase chain reaction using genus-specific oilgonucleotide primers and microbiologic culture for the detection of *Salmonella* in drag-swabs from poultry houses. *Poult. Sci.* 73, 1276–1281.

Coleman D.J., Nye K.J., Chick K.E. and Gagg C.M. 1995. A comparison of immunomagnetic separation plus enrichment with conventional salmonella culture in the examination of raw sausages. Letters in Applied Microbiology 21:249-251.

Cox N.A. 1988. Salmonella methodology update. Poultry Science 67:921-927.

Cross J.H., George R.H., Booth I.W., and Mayne A.J. 1989. Life-threatening Salmonella enteritidis phage type 4 gastroenteritis in infancy. Lancet 8638:625-626.

Cudjoe, K.S., Hagtvedt, T., Dainty, R., 1995.Immunomagnetic separation of Salmonella from foods and their detection using immunomagnetic particle (IMP)-ELISA.Int. J.Food Microbiol. 27, 11–25.

Cudjoe, K.S., Krona, R., Grøn, B., Olsen, E., 1994. Use of ferrous sulphate andimmunomagnetic separation to recover *Salmonella enteritidis* from raw eggs.Int.J. Food Microbiol. 23, 149–158.

D'Aoust, J.Y. (1997). Salmonella species. In Food Microbiology. Fundamentals and Frontirers (eds. Doyle, M.P., Beuchat, L.R., and Montville, T.J.) ASM Press, Washington, D.C., 129-158.

D'Aoust, J.Y. (2000). Salmonella. In The Microbiological Safety and Quality of Food, Volume II (eds. Lund, B.M., Baird-Parker, T.C., and G. W. Gould) Aspen Publishers, Inc, Gaithersburg, Maryland, 1233-1299.

D'Aoust, J.-Y., Sewell, A.M., Greco, P., Mozola, M.A., and Colvin, R.E. 1995. Performance assessment of the GENE-TRAK colorimetric probe assay for the detection of foodborne *Salmonella* spp. *J. Food Prot.* 58, 1069–1076.

De Boer, E. &Beumer, R.R. 1999, "Methodology for detection and typing of foodborne microorganisms", International Journal of Food Microbiology, vol. 50, no. 1-2, pp. 119 130.

Deisingh, A.K. & Thompson, M. 2004, "Biosensors for the detection of bacteria", Canadian Journal of Microbiology, vol. 50, no. 2, pp. 69-77.

Devenish J.A., Ciebin B.W., and Brodsky M.H. 1986. Novobiocin-brilliant green-glucose agar: new medium for isolation of salmonellae. Applied and Environmental Microbiology, 52, 539-545.

Doran, J.L., Collinson, S.K., Kay, C.M., Banser, P.A., Burian, J., Munro, C.K., Lee, S.H., Somers, J.M., Todd, E.C., and Kay, W.W. 1994. *FimA* and *tctC* based DNA diagnostics for *Salmonella. Mol. Cell. Probes.* 8, 291–310.

Doumith, M., Buchrieser, C., Glaser, P., Jacquet, C. & Martin, P. 2004, "Differentiation of the major Listeria monocytogenes serovars by multiplex PCR", Journal of Clinical Microbiology, vol. 42, no. 8, pp. 3819-3822.

D'Souza D.H., Critzer F.J., Golden D.A. 2009. Real-time reverse-transcriptase polymerase chain reaction for the rapid detection of Salmonella using invA primers. Foodborne Pathog Dis. 2009 Nov; 6(9):1097-106.

Espy, M.J., Uhl, J.R., Sloan, L.M., Buckwalter, S.P., Jones, M.F., Vetter, E.A., Yao, J.D., Wengenack, N.L., Rosenblatt, J.E., Cockerill, F.R.,3rd & Smith, T.F. 2006, "Real-time PCR in clinical microbiology: applications for routine laboratory testing", Clinical Microbiology Reviews, vol. 19, no. 1, pp. 165-256.

Farber J.M., and Sharpe A.N. 1984. Improved bacterial recovery by membrane filters in the presence of food debris. Appl Environ Microbiol. 1984 Aug;48(2):441-3.

Favrin S.J., Jassim S.A., Griffiths M.W. (2001). Development and optimization of a novel immunomagnetic separation-bacteriophage assay for detection of Salmonella enterica serovar enteritidis inbroth. Appl Environ Microbiol 67:217–224

Fluit, A.C., Widjojoatmodjo, M.N., Box, A.T.A., Torensma, R., and Verhoef, J. 1993. Rapid detection of salmonellae in poultry with the magnetic immunopolymerase chain reaction assay. Appl. Environ. Microbiol. 59, 1342–1346.

Friedman C.R., Torigian C., Shillam P.J., et al. An outbreak of salmonellosis among children attending a reptile exhibit at a zoo. J Pediatr 1998;132:802-7

Galikowska E., Kunikowska D., Tokarska-Pietrzak E., Dziadziuszko H., Loś J.M., Golec P., Węgrzyn G., Loś M. 2011. Specific detection of *Salmonella enterica* and *Escherichia coli* strains by using ELISA with bacteriophages as recognition agents. Eur J Clin Microbiol Infect Dis. 2011 Feb 15. [Epub ahead of print]

Gantois I., Ducatelle R., Pasmans F., Haesbrouck F., Gast R. Humphrey T.J., VanImmerseel F. 2009. Mechaniosms of egg contamination by Salmonella Enteritidis. FEMS Microbiolo Rev 33(4):718-38.

Gilbert, C., Winters, D., O'Leary, A. & Slavik, M. 2003. "Development of a triplex PCR assay for the specific detection of *Campylobacter jejuni*, *Salmonella* spp., and *Escherichia coli* O157:H7", Molecular and Cellular Probes, vol. 17, no. 4, pp. 135-138.

Gonzalez-Escalona, N., Hammack, T.S., Russell, M., Jacobson, A.P., De Jesus, A.J., Brown, E.W. &Lampel, K.A. 2009, "Detection of live Salmonella sp. cells in produce by a TaqMan based quantitative reverse transcriptase real-time PCR targeting invA mRNA", Applied and Environmental Microbiology, vol. 75, no. 11, pp. 3714-3720.

Gracias, K.S. &McKillip, J.L. 2004, "A review of conventional detection and enumeration methods for pathogenic bacteria in food", Canadian Journal of Microbiology, vol. 50, no. 11, pp. 883-890.

Grimont P.A.D., Grimont F. and Bouvet P. 2000. Taxonomy of the genus Salmonella. In

Hagens S., and Loessner M. Application of bacteriophages for detection and control of foodborne pathogens. Appl Microbiol Biotechnol (2007) 76:513–519.

Hill, W.E., and Keasler, S.P. 1991. Identification of foodborne pathogens by nucleic acid hybridization. *Int. J. Food Microbiol.* 12, 67–76.

Hill, W.E., and Lampel, K.A. 1990. Gene probes used in food microbiology, in *Biotechnology and Food Safety,* D.D. Bills and S.-D. Kung, Eds., Boston, MA: Butterworth-Heinemann, 139–165.

Hyatt D.R., and Weese J.S. 2004. Salmonella Culture: sampling procedures and laboratory techniques. Vet Clin North Am Equine Pract, 20(3):577-85.

Jiang L., Jiang Q., Huang K., Zhang C., Tang T. 2009. Rapid detection of Salmonella in food by using fluorescently labeled phage O-I. Wei Sheng Wu Xue Bao. 4;49(3):372-7.

Jones, D.D., Law, R., and Bej, A.K. 1993. Detection of *Salmonella* spp. in oysters using polymerase chain reactions (PCR) and gene probes. *J. Food Sci.* 58, 1191–1197.

Kang D.H., and Fung D.Y.C. 2000. Application of thin agar layer method for recovery of injured *Salmonella typhymurium* . In International Journal of Food Microbiology, 54, 127-32.

Kim M.L., Slauch J.M. 1999. Effect of acetylation (O-factor 5) on the polyclonal antibody response to *Salmonella typhimurium* O-antigen. FEMS Immunol Med Microbiol.1999 Oct;26(1):83-92.

Kim S., Frye J.G., Hu J., Fedorka-Cray P.J., Gautom R., Boyle D.S. 2006. Multiplex PCR-based method for identification of common clinical serotypes of Salmonella enterica subsp. enterica. Appl Environ Microbiol. 2006 Sep;72(9):6142-51.

Kim, H. &Bhunia, A.K. 2008. "SEL, a selective enrichment broth for simultaneous growth of Salmonella enterica, Escherichia coli O157:H7, and Listeria monocytogenes", Applied and Environmental Microbiology, vol. 74, no. 15, pp. 4853-4866.

Kim, J.S., Lee, G.G., Park, J.S., Jung, Y.H., Kwak, H.S., Kim, S.B., Nam, Y.S. & Kwon, S.T. 2007. "A novel multiplex PCR assay for rapid and simultaneous detection of five pathogenic bacteria: *Escherichia coli* O157:H7, *Salmonella* spp., *Staphylococcus aureus, Listeria monocytogenes,* and *Vibrio parahaemolyticus*", *Journal of food protection,* vol. 70, no. 7, pp. 1656-1662.

King, T.C., Sirdeskmukh, R. &Schlessinger, D. 1986. "Nucleolytic processing of ribonucleic acid transcripts in procaryotes", Microbiological Reviews, vol. 50, no. 4, pp. 428-451.

Kitazato, M., Nukina, M., Misawa, N. & Tsukamoto, T. 2007. "Development of a multiplex PCR assay for identification of *Campylobacter coli, Campylobacter fetus, Campylobacter hyointestinalis* subsp. hyointestinalis, *Campylobacter jejuni, Campylobacter lari* and *Campylobacter upsaliensis*", Journal of Medical Microbiology, vol. 56, no. Pt 11, pp. 1467-1473.

Klein, P.G. &Juneja, V.K. 1997. "Sensitive detection of viable Listeria monocytogenes by reverse transcription-PCR", Applied and Environmental Microbiology, vol. 63, no. 11, pp. 4441 4448.

Klena, J.D., Parker, C.T., Knibb, K., Ibbitt, J.C., Devane, P.M., Horn, S.T., Miller, W.G. & Konkel, M.E. 2004. "Differentiation of Campylobacter coli, Campylobacter jejuni,

Korndoerfer, I.P., Danzer J., Schmelcher M., Zimmer M., Skerra A., Loessner M.J. (2006). The crystal structure of the bacteriophage PSA endolysin reveals a unique fold responsible for specific recognition of Listeria cell walls. J Mol Biol 364:678–689

Korolik, V., Friendship, D.T., Peduru-Hewa, T., Alfredson, D.A., Fry, B.N. &Coloe, P.J. 2001. "Specific identification, grouping and differentiation of Campylobacter jejuni among thermophilic campylobacters using multiplex PCR", Epidemiology and Infection, vol. 127, no. 1, pp. 1-5.

Kretzer J.W., Lehmann R., Banz M., Kim K.P., Korn C., Loessner M.J. 2007. Use of high affinity cell wall-binding domains of bacteriophage endolysins for immobilization and separation of bacterial cells. Appl Environ Microbiol 73:1992–2000

Kruy S.L., van Cuyck H., Koeck J.L. 2011. Multilocus variable number tandem repeat analysis for Salmonella entericasubspecies.Eur J Clin Microbiol Infect Dis. 1 Apr;30(4):465-73. Epub 2010 Dec 11.

Kuhn J., Suissa M., Wyse J., Cohen I., Weiser I., Reznick S., Lubinsky-Mink S., Stewart G., Ulitzur S (2002) Detection of bacteria usingforeign DNA: the development of a bacteriophage reagent for Salmonella. Int J Food Microbiol 74:229–238

Le Minor, L., Popoff, M.Y., 2001. Antigenic formulas of the Salmonella serovars. WHO Collaborating Centre for Reference and Research on Salmonella, Paris, 8th ed.

Li, Y. & Mustapha, A. 2004, "Simultaneous detection of Escherichia coli O157:H7, Salmonella and Shigella in apple cider and produce by a multiplex PCR", Journal of food protection, vol. 67, no. 1, pp. 27-33.

Loessner M.J., Kramer K., Ebel F., Scherer S. (2002). C-terminal domains of Listeria bacteriophage peptidoglycan hydrolases determine specific recognition and high affinity binding to bacterial cell wall carbohydrates. Mol Microbiol 44:335–349

Lynch M.J., Leon-Velarde C.G., McEwen S., Odumeru J.A. 2004. Evaluation of an automated immunomagnetic separation method for therapid detection of *Salmonella* species in poultry environmental samples J MicrobiolMethods.2004 Aug;58(2):285-8.

Lyons R.W., Samples C.L., DeSilva H.N., Ross K.A., Julian E.M., Checko P.J. An epidemic of resistant Salmonella in a nursery: animal-to-human spread. JAMA 1980;243:546-7

Maciorowski, K.G., Pena, J., Pillai, S.D., and Ricke, S.C. 1998. Application of gene amplification in conjunction with a hybridization sensor for rapid detection of *Salmonella* spp. and fecal contamination indicators in animal feeds. *J. Rapid Meth. Auto. Microbiol.* 6, 225–238.

Mahon B.E., Ponka A., Hall W.N., et al. An international outbreak of Salmonella infections caused by alfalfa sprouts grown from contaminated seeds. J Infect Dis 1997;175:876-82.

Malorny B., Bunge C., Helmuth R. 2007. A real-time PCR for the detection of Salmonella Enteritidis in poultry meat and consumption eggs. J Microbiol Methods.2007 Aug;70(2):245-51.

Manafi, M. 1996. "Fluorogenic and chromogenic enzyme substrates in culture media and identification tests", International Journal of Food Microbiology, vol. 31, no. 1-3, pp. 4558.

Manafi, M. 2000. "New developments in chromogenic and fluorogenic culture media", International Journal of Food microbiology, vol. 60, no. 2-3, pp. 205-218.

Manzano, M., Cocolin, L., Astori, G., Pipan, C., Botta, G.A., Cantoni, C., and Comi, G. 1998. Development of a PCR microplate—capture hybridization method for simple, fast and sensitive detection of *Salmonella* serovars in food. *Mol. Cell. Probes.* 12, 227–234.

Masters, C.I., Shallcross, J.A. & Mackey, B.M. 1994. "Effect of stress treatments on thedetection of *Listeria monocytogenes* and enterotoxigenic *Escherichia coli* by the polymerase chain reaction", The Journal of Applied Bacteriology, vol. 77, no. 1, pp. 73-79.

McKillip, J.L. & Drake, M. 2004. "Real-time nucleic acid-based detection methods for pathogenic bacteria in food", Journal of Food Protection, vol. 67, no. 4, pp. 823-832. reaction for *Salmonella enterica* detection from jalapeño and serranopeppers. Foodborne Pathog Dis. 2010 Apr;7(4):367-73.

Meadows P.S. 1971. The attachment of bacteria to solid surfaces. Arch Mikrobiol, 75(4):374-81.

Mullis, K., Faloona, F., Scharf, S., Saiki, R., Horn, G. &Erlich, H. 1986. "Specific enzymaticamplification of DNA in vitro: the polymerase chain reaction", Cold Spring Harbor Symposia on Quantitative Biology, vol. 51 Pt 1, pp. 263-273.

Olsen S.J., MacKinnon L., Goulding J., Bean N.H., Slutsker L. Surveillance for foodborne-disease outbreaks: United States, 1993–1997. Morbidity and Mortality Weekly Report CDC Surveillance Summary 2000;49(SS-1):1-62

O'Regan E., McCabe E., Burgess C., McGuinness S., Barry T., Duffy G., Whyte P., Fanning S. 2008. Development of a real-time multiplex PCR assay for the detection of multiple Salmonella serotypes in chicken samples. BMC Microbiol. 2008 Sep 21;8:156.

Park S.H., Jarquin R., Hanning I., Almeida G., Ricke S.C.2011. Detection of Salmonella spp. survival and virulence in poultry feed by targeting the hilA gene. J Appl Microbiol. 2011 Aug;111(2):426-32.

Park, Y.S., Lee, S.R. & Kim, Y.G. 2006. "Detection of *Escherichia coli* O157:H7, *Salmonella* spp., *Staphylococcus aureus* and *Listeria monocytogenes* inkimchi by multiplex polymerase chain reaction (mPCR)", Journal of Microbiology (Seoul, Korea), vol. 44, no. 1, pp. 92-97.

Payne M.J., Campbell S., Patchett R.A., Kroll R.G. 1992. The use of immobilized lectins in the separation of *Staphylococcus aureus*, *Escherichia coli*, *Listeria* and *Salmonella* spp. from pure cultures and foods. J Appl Bacteriol. 1992 Jul;73(1):41-52.

Peplow M.O., Correa-Prisant M., Stebbins M.E., Jones F., Davies P. 1999. Sensitivity, specificity, and predictive values of three Salmonella rapid detection kits using fresh and frozen poultry environmental samples versus those of standard plating. Appl Environ Microbiol. 1999 Mar; 65(3):1055-60.

Popoff M.Y., Bockemuhl, J., and McWhorter-Murlin A. 1994. Supplement 1993 (no. 37) to the Kauffmann-White scheme. Res. Microbiol. 145:711-716

Rajtak U., Leonard N., Bolton D., Fanning S. 2011. A Real-Time Multiplex SYBR Green I Polymerase Chain Reaction Assay for Rapid Screening of Salmonella Serotypes Prevalent in the European Union. Foodborne Pathog Dis. 2011 Jul;8(7):769-80.

Restaino L., Grauman G.S., McCall W.A., Hill W.M. 1977. Effects of varying concentrations of novobiocin incorporated into two Salmonella plating media on the recovery of four Enterobacteriaceae. Applied and Environmental Microbiology, 33, 585-589.

Ricke S.C., Pillai S.D., Norton R.A., MAciorowski K.G., and Jones F.T. 1998. Applicability of rapid methods for detection of Salmonlla spp. in poultry feeds: a review. Journal of Rapid Methods and automation in Microbiology, 6, 239-258.

Rijpens N., Herman L., Vereecken, Jannes G., De Smedt J., and De Zutter L. 1999. Rapid detection of stressed salmonella spp in dairy and egg products using immunomagnetic separation and PCR. International Journal of Food Microbiology 46, 37-44.

Rossello-Mora, R. &Amann, R. 2001. "The species concept for prokaryotes", FEMS microbiology reviews, vol. 25, no. 1, pp. 39-67.

Sandel, M.K., Wu, Y.F. &McKillip, J.L. 2003. "Detection and recovery of sublethally-injured enterotoxigenic *Staphylococcus aureus*", Journal of Applied Microbiology, vol. 94, no. 1, pp. 90-94.

Settanni, L. &Corsetti, A. 2007. "The use of multiplex PCR to detect and differentiate food- and beverage-associated microorganisms: a review", Journal of Microbiological Methods, vol. 69, no. 1, pp. 1-22.

Shaw, S.J., Blais, B.W., Nundy, D.C., 1998. Performance of the Dynabeads anti-Salmonella system in the detection of *Salmonella* species in foods, animal feeds, and environmental samples. J. Food Prot. 61, 1507–1510.

Shipp, C.R., Rowe, B., 1980. A mechanised microtechnique for Salmonella serotyping. J. Clin. Pathol. 33, 595–597.

Smith J.L. 1994. Arthritis and foodborne bacteria. Journal of Food Protection 57:935-941.

Soumet C., Ermel G., Rose V., Rose N., Drouin P., Salvat G., Colin P. 1999. Identification by a multiplex PCR-based assay of *Salmonella typhimurium* and *Salmonella enteritidis* strains from environmental swabs of poultry houses. Lett Appl Microbiol. 1999 Jul;29(1):1-6.

Spanová, A., Rittich, B., Karpisková, R., Cechová, L., Skapová, D., 2000. PCR identification of Salmonella cells in food and stool samples after immunomagnetic separation. Bioseparation 9, 379–384.

Tauxe R.V. 1991. Salmonella: a postmodern pathogen. Journal of Food Protection, 54:563-568.

Techathuvanan C., Draughon F.A., D'Souza D.H. Real-time reverse transcriptase PCR for the rapid and sensitive detection of *Salmonella typhimurium* from pork. J Food Prot. 2010 Mar; 73(3):507-14.

Techathuvanan C., D'Souza D.H. 2011. Optimization of rapid Salmonella enterica detection in liquid whole eggs by SYBR green I-based real-time reverse transcriptase-polymerase chain reaction. Foodborne Pathog Dis. 2011 Apr;8(4):527-34. Epub 2011 Mar 7.

Ten Bosch C., Van der Plas J., Havekes M., Geurts J., Van der Palen C., Huis in 'T Veld, J.H.J. and Hofstra, H. 1992. Salmonella PCR: implementation of a screening method in meat and meat products. In. Reports and Communications: Salmonella and Salmonellosis, (Ploufragan, saint-Brieuc, France).

Thouand G., Vachon P., Liu S., Dayre M., Griffiths M.W. 2008. Optimization and validation of a simple method using P22::luxAB bacteriophage for rapid detection of *Salmonella enterica* serotypes A, B, and D in poultry samples. J Food Prot. 71(2):380-385.

Ulitzur S., Kuhn J (1987). Introduction of lux genes into bacteria, a new approach for specific determination of bacteria and their antibiotic susceptibility. In: Schlomerich J, Andreesen R, Kapp A, Ernst M, Woods WG (eds) Bioluminescence and chemiluminescence new perspectives. Wiley, New York, pp 463–472

Wang, G., Clark, C.G., Taylor, T.M., Pucknell, C., Barton, C., Price, L., Woodward, D.L. & Rodgers, F.G. 2002. "Colony multiplex PCR assay for identification and differentiation of *Campylobacter jejuni, C. coli, C. lari, C. upsaliensis*, and *C. fetus* subsp. fetus", Journal of Clinical Microbiology, vol. 40, no. 12, pp. 4744-4747.

Warren B.R., Yuk H.G., Schneider K.R. J Food Prot. 2007. Detection of salmonella by flow-through immunocapture real-time PCR in selected foods within 8 hours. J Food Prot. 2007 Apr;70(4):1002-6.

Weenk G.H. 1992. Microbiological assessment of culture media: comparison and statistical evaluation of methods. Int J Food Microbiol.17(2):159-81.

Westerman R.B., He Y., Keen J.E., Littledike E.T., Kwang J. Production and characterization of monoclonal antibodies specific for the lipopolysaccharide of *Escherichia coli* O157. J Clin Microbiol. 1997 Mar;35(3):679-84.

Williams, J.E. 1981. Salmonellas in poultry feeds—a worldwide review. Part II: Methods in isolation and identification. *World's Poult. Sci. J.* 37, 19–25.

Wolber P.K., Green R.L. (1990). Detection of bacteria by transduction of ice nucleation genes. Trends Biotechnol 8:276–279

Woods D.F., Reen F.J., Gilroy D., Buckley J., Frye J.G., Boyd E.F. Rapid multiplex PCR and real-time TaqMan PCR assays for detection of Salmonella enterica and the highly virulent serovarsCholeraesuis and Paratyphi C. J Clin Microbiol. 2008 Dec;46(12):4018-22.

Wray and A. Wray (eds), Salmonella in Domestic Animals (CAB International, Wallingford, UK), 1-17.

Wu Y., Brovko L., Griffiths M.W. (2001). Influence of phage population on the phage-mediated bioluminescent adenylate kinase (AK) assay for detection of bacteria. Lett Appl Microbiol 33:311–315

Yamazaki-Matsune, W., Taguchi, M., Seto, K., Kawahara, R., Kawatsu, K., Kumeda, Y., Yaron, S. & Matthews, K.R. 2002. "A reverse transcriptase-polymerase chain reaction assay for detection of viable *Escherichia coli* O157:H7: investigation of specific target genes", Journal of Applied Microbiology, vol. 92, no. 4, pp. 633-640.

Zhang, W. &Knabel, S.J. 2005. "Multiplex PCR assay simplifies serotyping and sequence typing of *Listeria monocytogenes* associated with human outbreaks", J Food Protection, vol. 68, no. 9, pp. 1907-1910.

18

# Detection of *Salmonella* spp. Presence in Food

Anna Zadernowska and Wioleta Chajęcka
*University of Warmia and Mazury in Olsztyn, Faculty of Food Sciences*
*Chair of Industrial and Food Microbiology*
*Poland*

## 1. Introduction

The analysis of food products for presence of pathogenic microorganisms is one of the basic steps to control safety and quality of food. Development of new, fast, and reliable identification methods for biological threats are necessary to meet the safety standards of food products and risk management. *Salmonella* spp., a marker of food products safety, is widely distributed foodborne pathogen.

The standard culture methods to detect the presence of microorganisms in food products are well developed; although these methods require 4 to 5 days to obtain presumptive positive or negative results. These tests are time-consuming and can take up to 7 days depending on the realization of biochemical and serological confirmations. In addition, sensitivity of cultures can be affected by antibiotic treatment, inadequate sampling, and a small number of viable microorganisms in samples.

Standardized classical culture methods are still in use by many labs, especially by regulatory agencies, because they are harmonized methods, looked at as the "gold standards" in food diagnostics and thus overall well accepted. These are important aspects in international trade and compliance testing. A serious drawback is that, although they demand no expensive infrastructure and are rather cheap in consumables, they are laborious to perform, demand large volumes usage of liquid and solid media and reagents, and encompass time-consuming procedures both in operation and data collection.

As an alternative to time-consuming culture methods, several approaches have been developed to accelerate detection of pathogenic microorganisms in food products. In the present work, besides the standard method of *Salmonella* spp. detection in food products (ISO 6579:2003) some alternative detection methods have been presented.

## 2. Taking samples for tests

The first stage of microbiological analysis of food consists in taking and preparing a sample for analyses. Incorrect sampling can lead to obtaining false negative or false positive results. When talking about taking samples, the term "representative sample" is often used. The sample should reflect the image of the product from which it originates as precisely as possible. It is quite easy to take a representative sample from liquid products, e.g. milk, if the milk has been sufficiently mixed before taking the sample. On the other hand, when the subject of examination is a product of high viscosity, with slow flow or of a heterogeneous structure, then it is very difficult to assess the microbiological quality of the entire batch (e.g. a barrel or a truckload) by examining only one 25-gram sample. The answer to the question concerning the required number of single samples is extremely difficult. In view of the high costs of microbiological tests, the number of samples is generally limited. In a microbiological laboratory, samples are taken with the use of sterile tools, e.g. spoons, scalpels, knives, spatulas and pipettes. Frozen products should be first thawed at below 5°C (for not longer than 12 hours). In the case of deeply frozen samples, sterile drills are used for sampling.

Determination of *Salmonella* sp. in food products always consists in detecting the presence of those bacteria in a specified amount of the product (generally 25g/ml, very rarely 10g/ml), but the number of those microorganisms in food is not determined. Both in the classical method and in its modifications, the first stage of detection is non-selective enrichment. This is crucial, since food production involves its technological treatment, e.g. heating, which can cause the death of most cells or cause sub-lethal injured. Omission of the stage of pre-enrichment of the sample and inoculating the material directly on the solid medium can give false negative results. If the examined material includes a very low number of living cells, or the cells have been sub-lethally damaged during the technological processes, we may not receive macroscopically-visible colonies on the solid medium. In such a case there is a risk of releasing the product to market although it does not satisfy safety criteria. During the storage of such a product, damaged cells can be repaired and bacteria can proliferate to a level that would be hazardous for the consumers.

There are many methods to determine *Salmonella sp.* in food and, for this reason, the present study focuses on the classical culture method – the application of a Vidas device – as the only fully automated one. Additionally, the PCR method (a commonly-applied alternative to the plate method) and the FISH method (which is still not popular, although work on its optimization is ongoing) are also described.

## 3. A classical culture method of detecting *Salmonella*

Detection of the presence of *Salmonella* pursuant to Commission Regulation (EC) No 2073/2005 (microbiological criteria for foodstuff) as amended, is carried out according to the ISO 6579 standard - Microbiology of food and animal feeding stuffs - Horizontal method for detection of *Salmonella spp.*(ISO, 2002). Pursuant to the above regulation, detection of *Salmonella* in food should be carried out for such products as raw meat, meat products intended for consumption in the raw state, gelatine, cheese, butter, cream, unpasteurized milk, powdered milk, eggs and products containing raw eggs, crustaceans, molluscs, fruit and vegetables, unpasteurized juice, powdered infant formulas and dietary food for special medical purposes.

Standard ISO 6579 2003 (Microbiology of food and animal feeding stuffs - Horizontal method for detection of *Salmonella* spp.)includes four stages of the detection process and depending on the need to obtain confirmations, it lasts from 5 to 7 days:

- Pre-enrichment in non-selective liquid medium
- Selective enrichment in liquid media
- Plating on selective media
- Serological and biochemical identification of suspected colonies

During the first stage, in order to proliferate and regenerate damaged cells, the culture is performed on liquid peptone water at 37°C for 18±2 hours. **Buffered peptone water** is applied for non-selective enrichment of *Salmonella* sp. For such products as cocoa or chocolate products, peptone water is applied with an addition of casein or skimmed milk and brilliant green in order to inhibit the growth of Gram-positive bacteria. In the case of acid and soured food products, peptone water should be used with double concentration of components, while for meat and food of high fat content, pre-enrichment should be performed in lactose broth with the addition of Triton X-100.

| | |
|---|---|
| **Non-selective pre-enrichment** | |
| 25 g food in 225ml of 10% buffered pepton water | 37°C, 24 h |
| ↓ | |
| **Selective enrichment** | |
| 0.1 ml in 10 ml Rappaport-Vassiliadis Soy Broth | 37°C, 24 h |
| 1 ml in 10 ml Tetrathionate broth (Müller-Kauffman) | 41.5°C, 24 h |
| ↓ | |
| **Isolation** | |
| XLD with an inoculation loop | |
| BGA or Hektoen or other selective agar plates with an inoculation loop | 37°C, 24 h |
| ↓ | |
| **Streaking on nutrient agar** | 37°C, 24 h |
| ↓ | |
| **Biochemical confirmation** | 37°C, 24 h |
| ↓ | |
| TSI | |
| Urea broth | |
| LDC | |
| ONPG | |
| VP | |
| Indole | |
| ↓ | |
| **Serotyping** | |
| O-antigens | |
| H-antigens | |

Fig. 1. Flow diagram for detection of *Salmonella*.

After the non-selective pre-enrichment stage, a $0.1cm^3$ sample is taken from the culture and inoculated on $10cm^3$ of selective medium, Rappaport-Vassiliadis with soya, and on **Muller-Kauffmann** medium in the amount of 1 $cm^3$. **Rappaport-Vassiliadis (RVS)** medium is solid, strongly selective and contains malachite green and sodium chloride (inhibiting the growth of accompanying microflora). Soya peptone, pH 5.2, and increased temperature of incubation (41.5°C) favour the growth of *Salmonella* sp. strains. The medium is dark blue and clear. *Salmonella* sp. strains grow on this medium in the form of milky residue, while the colour of the medium itself does not change. The other selective medium, **Muller-Kauffmann broth (MKTTn)**, contains sodium thiosulphate and potassium iodide, which react to form a compound known as sodium tetrathionate, inhibiting the growth of the coliforms. *Salmonella* sp. are able to reduce this compound. The broth also contains brilliant green, which, in turn, inhibits the growth of Gram-positive bacteria.

After incubation at 37°C for 48±3 hours, cultures are inoculated on two selective media, so as to receive individual colonies. The first of them is XLD (xylose lysine deoxycholate) agar. The other can be chosen by the laboratory, and it can be BGA (brilliant green agar), Hektoen or Wilson-Blair agar for example.

**XLD agar** contains lactose, saccharose, L-lysine, sodium thiosulphate, sodium deoxycholate, ferric ammonium citrate (III) and phenol red. Differential agents of the agar include: lactose, saccharose, xylose, lysine and sodium thiosulphate, from which hydrogen sulfide is released, forming in reaction with iron salts (III) black residue of iron sulfide in the centre of the colony. The pH indicator is phenol red. The agar makes it possible to determine the sugar fermentation ability. Incubation is carried out at 37°C for 24±3 hours. Typical colonies can be colourless, very light, slightly shiny and transparent (colour of the medium) with a dark tinted centre, surrounded by a light red area and yellow edge, or of pink to red colour, with a black centre or without a black centre. $H_2S$ (-) colonies are colourless or light pink with darker centres, and lactose (+) colonies are yellow or without the characteristic blackening.

**BGA**. Differential factors of this agar are sugars: saccharose and lactose. Brilliant green is a selective agent. Typical colonies are transparent, colourless or light pink, and the colour around colonies changes from pink to light red.

**Hektoen agar**. Selective agents include bile salts, inhibiting the growth of Gram (+) bacteria Differential factors are three sugars: lactose, saccharose and salicin. Increased lactose content ensures that bacteria fermenting this sugar with a delay are not omitted. Bacteria colonies producing hydrogen sulfide had a dark centre as a result of the reaction between hydrogen sulfide and iron (III). Typical colonies of *Salmonella* sp. are green, with or without a black centre.

**Wilson-Blair agar**. This is a strongly selective and differential medium for *Salmonella*, including *S.* Typhi isolated from food. *Salmonella spp.*, depending on the strain, grow in the form of black colonies surrounded with an area of black medium or dark brown and brown without this area. A characteristic feature of *Salmonella spp*. colonies is a metallic, shining surface as a result of produced hydrogen sulfide, forming a metallically-black residue in reaction with iron ions. The growth of Gram-positive bacteria and other *Enterobacteriaceae*, including *Shigella spp.*, is strongly inhibited by brilliant green and bismuth sulfite present in the medium.

**Rambach-agar chromogenic medium** – with sodium deoxycholate, proplylene glycol and chromogenic mix. Colonies of *Salmonella* sp. are red as a result of glycol fermentation, lactose positive bacteria from the coli group, due to the activity of galactosidase, destroy a bound between the components of chromogenic mix and released chromophore gives those colonies a blue-violet or blue-green colouring. *Salmonella* Typhi and *Salmonella* Paratyphi form colourless or yellowish colonies on this medium.

New selective media have been developed based on biochemical characteristic of *Salmonella* such as α-galactosidase activity in the absence of β-galactosidase activity, C8-esterase activity, catabolism of glucuronate, glycerol and propylene glycol, hydrolysis of X-5-Gal, and $H_2S$ production. e.g. SMID agar (BioNerieux, France), Rainbow *Salmonella* agar (Biolog, USA), CHROMagar *Salmonella* (CHROM agar, France), chromogenic *Salmonella* esterase agar (PPR Diagnostics Ltd, UK), Compass *Salmonella* agar (Biokar diagnostics, France), and chromogenic ABC medium (Lab M. Ltd., UK) (Maciorowski et al., 2006; Manafi, 2000; Perry et al., 2007; Schonenbrucher et al., 2008)

| MEDIUM | REACTIONS/ENZYMES | RESULTS | |
|---|---|---|---|
| | | NEGATIVE | POSITIVE |
| TSI[a] | Acid production (if the butt is yellow, and the slope is red, acid production is only from glucose) | Butt red | Butt yellow |
| TSI[a] | Acid production from lactose and/or sucrose | Surface red | Surface yellow |
| TSI[a] | Gas production | No air bubbles in butt | Air bubbles in butt |
| TSI[a] | $H_2S$ production | No black colour | Black colour |
| UREA BROTH | Urease | Yellow | Rose pink - deep cerise |
| LCD TEST | Lysine decarboxylase | A yellow/brown colour | A purple colour (and a yellow/brown colour in the LDC control medium if used) |
| ONPG | β-Galactosidase | Remain colourless | Yellow |
| VOGES PROSKAUER | Acetoin production | Remain colourless | A pink/red colour |
| INDOLE | Indole production | Yellow ring | Red / pink ring |

Table 1. Interpretation table. [a]Regarding TSI: Read the colour of the butt and of the surface of the medium; ALK: A red colour corresponding to no acid production; NC: No change in the colour of the medium ; A: A yellow colour corresponding to acid production; G: Gas production in the butt; $H_2S$ production; +: Black colour; -: No black colour

After 48 h incubation at 37°C, a preliminary identification is made on the basis of the appearance of colonies grown on selective media. Five characteristic colonies are selected from each plate and are plating on the nutrient agar medium, followed by biochemical examinations. In order to perform these examinations, biochemical tests are carried out on the following media:

- TSI medium (Triple-sugar iron agar)
- Christensen medium with urea (urease production)
- peptone medium with tryptophan (indole production)
- medium with lysine (lysine decarboxylation)
- Clark medium (V-P reaction)
- ONPG medium (β-galactosidase detection)

| Test | Positive or negative reaction | Percentage of *Salmonella* inoculations showing the reaction[1)] |
|---|---|---|
| TSI glucose (acid formation) | + | 100 |
| TSI glucose (gas formation) | + | 91.9[2)] |
| TSI lactose | - | 99.2[3)] |
| TSI sucrose | - | 99.5 |
| TSI hydrogen sulfide | + | 91.6 |
| Urea splitting | - | 99 |
| Lysine decarboxylation | + | 94.6[4)] |
| β-Galactosidase reaction | - | 98.4[3)] |
| Voges-Proskauer reaction | - | 100 |
| Indole reaction | - | 98.9 |

[1)] These percentages indicate only that not all strains of *Salmonella* show the reactions marked + or -. These percentages may vary from country to country and from food product to food product.
[2)] *Salmonella* Typhi is anaerogenic.
[3)] The *Salmonella* subspecies III (Arizona) gives positive or negative lactose reactions but is always β-galactosidase positive. The *Salmonella* subspecies II gives a negative lactose reaction, but gives a positive β-galactosidase reaction. For the study of strains, it may be useful to carry out complementary biochemical tests.
[4] *S.* Paratyphi A is negative.

Table 2. Biochemical results for *Salmonella.*

**Triple-sugar iron agar** is used for differentiation of *Enterobactericeae* according to their ability to ferment lactose, sucrose and glucose. The colour of the slope and the butt and gas production are noted. Acid production from fermentation of one or more of the sugars results in a yellow colour because the phenol red indicator turns yellow at low pH. Very little glucose is present in the medium, so if a bacteria, like *Salmonella,* only ferments glucose then only a little acid will be formed. On the slope, the acid will be oxidised by the air and by the breakdown of protein in the medium and the colour will remain red while the butt is yellow. $H_2S$ production from thiosulphate will be seen as black areas in the medium due to FeS production. Gas production from fermentation of sugars will be seen as gas bubbles in the medium. The medium is only lightly inoculated.

**Christensen medium with urea.** Urea medium tests for high urea activity. It is the most common method to detect urease production by Enterobacteriaceae (1):

$$(NH_2)_2CO + H_2O \rightarrow 2NH_3 + CO_2 \tag{1}$$

The phenol red turns red at alkaline pH so a positive reaction is shown as the development of a red-pink colour.

**Tryptone/tryptophane medium for indole reaction.** The media is used for testing the liberation of indole from tryptophane. When Kovacs reagent containing amyl alcohol and p-dimethylaminobenzaldehyde is added, indole can be extracted into the amyl alcohol layer by shaking a little. Indole and p-dimethylaminobenzaldehyde produces a red or pink colour.

**L-Lysine decarboxylation medium for the LDC test.** The LDC broth is used for the test of production of lysine decarboxylase. This enzyme decarboxylates lysine to yield the alkaline compound cadaverin and $CO_2$. A paraffin oil layer is added after inoculation to keep the pH alkaline. Often glucose is metabolised in the beginning of the incubation period and a yellow colour develops in the media after some hours of incubation, but later the media turns purple if the lysin decarboxylase is present because of formation of the alkaline compound cadaverin. As other compounds in the media could be broken down to alkaline compounds, the LDC control media without lysine is also inoculated, a layer of paraffin oil added and it is incubated at the same time. If both the LDC media and the LDC control media turn purple, it cannot be shown that lysine decarboxylase is present and the test is evaluated as negative.

**Medium VP.** This is a test for acetoin production from glucose. The acetoin produced is oxidised to diacetyl, which produces a red colour with α-naphtol at alkaline pH. A positive reaction is seen as a very pale red colour.

**ONPG medium.** This medium shows the presence of β-galactosidase producing bacteria. β-galactosidase liberates o-nitrophenol, which is yellow at alkaline pH, from ONPG. The reaction is positive if a yellow colour develops.

**API.** Determination of biochemical features of the examined bacteria can also involve the application of API 20E tests (Biomerieux), aimed at identification of bacteria from the family *Enterobacteriaceae*. The API 20E system facilitates the 24-hour identification of *Enterobacteriaceae* as well as 24 or 48-hour identification of other Gram negative bacteria. The API 20E strip consists of microtubes containing dehydrated substrates for the demonstration of enzymatic activity and carbohydrate (CHO) fermentation. The substrates are reconstituted by adding a bacterial suspension. After incubation, the metabolic end products are detected by indicator systems or the addition of reagents. CHO fermentation is detected by colour change in the pH indicator.

**Serological tests**. These tests are carried out for strains of bacteria which have been classified into the *Salmonella* genus on the basis of their biochemical features, in order to detect the presence of somatic O, capsular Vi and flagellar H antigens. The examinations are carried out by slide agglutination on the basis of Kauffmann-White antigenic schema. Polyvalent and monovalent serums should be used to determine somatic antigens, and anti-Vi and anti - H serums to detect the presence of Vi and H antigen. Determination of flagellar antigens makes it possible to determine the serological type of the examined bacteria.

Culture methods are labor intensive and time consuming when handling many samples. In addition, detection can be prevented by the presence of other competing microorganisms during cultural enrichment, and the selective agar media have a very poor specificity creating an abundance of false positives (such as *Citrobacter* or *Proteus*) (Manafi, 2000). Therefore, there is a need for *Salmonella* detection methods that provide results more rapidly with sensitivity similar to or greater than, the conventional methods.

## 4. Polymerase chain reaction

Due to its high sensitivity, specificity, and rapid results, PCR is an efficient alternative to conventional microbiological culture methods to detect specific types of microorganisms in foods, water, and environmental samples (Moganedi et al., 2007; Glynn et al., 2006; Piknova´et al., 2002). The International Standardization Organization (ISO) recently published standards which address the PCR methodology for the detection of food-borne pathogens (Tomás et al., 2009).

| Gene Target | Matrices | Enrichment | Limit of detection | Primers (1-forward; 2-reverse; 3-probe) | References |
|---|---|---|---|---|---|
| *ttrBCA* | chicken<br>minced meat<br>fish | 20 h | < 3 CFU/ml | 1: CTC ACC AGG AGA TTA CAA CAT GG<br>2: AGC TCA GAC CAA AAG TGA CCA TC<br>3: CAC CGA CGG CGA GAC CGA CTT T | Malorny et al., 2004 |
| *fimC* | ice cream | without | $10^3$ CFU/ml | 1: ATA AAT CCG GCG GCC TGA TG<br>2: TGG TAT CGA CGC CTT TAT CTG AGA<br>3: TTA CAC CGG AGT GGA TTA AAC GGC TGG G | Seo et al., 2006 |
| *invA* | salmon<br>chicken meat<br>milk | 16h | 2,5-5 CFU/25g (salmon, chicken)<br>5 CFU/25 ml (milk) | 1: GTG AAA TAA TCG CCA CGT TCG GGC AA<br>2: TCA TCG CAC CGT CAA AGG AAC CGT AA<br>3: TTA TTG GCG ATA GCC TGG CGG TGG GTT TTG TTG | Hein et al., 2006 |
| *invA* | chili powder<br>shrimp | 35°C-24h (pre-)<br>41°C-24h (selective) | 0,04 CFU/g | 1: AAC GTG TTT CCG TGC GTA AT<br>2: TCC ATC AAA TTA GCG GAG GC<br>3: TGG AAG CGC TCG CAT TGT GG | Cheng et al., 2008 |
| *oriC* | cheddar<br>turkey meat<br>cooked turkey meat | 48 h (selective) | 6,1 x $10^1$ CFU/ml | 1: TCACCTGCGACAGCCATGA<br>2: TGAGCATCGCCATCGGCAT<br>3: ATTCCAGCAGTCGGCCATAGCTG (Set I)<br>1: CATTGATGCCATGGGTGACART<br>2: CGTGACGATAATCCGTGTAC<br>3: TACACGAGTCACTAAATCCTTCAGT (Set II) | McCarthy et al., 2009 |

Table 3. Detection of *Salmonella* using real-time PCR.increase of the released dye concentration). Consequently, we are able to monitor, in real time, whether the product of reaction has been obtained.

### 4.1 Conventional PCR

PCR – polymerase chain reaction – is an enzymatic reaction replicating a DNA molecule. A critical condition of the PCR course is the presence of an enzyme, thermostable DNA polymerase. Substrates of the reaction are deoxyribonucleotides (building blocks of newly synthesized DNA molecules) and oligonucleotides (starters), which on a complementary basis attach to the replicated DNA strand. Polymerase chain reaction is a thermal process, with cyclically changing temperatures. One cycle leading to synthesis of one copy of DNA from one matrix molecule is composed of the following stages: DNA denaturation (90-95°C), attachment of starters (the so-called annealing, 50-65°C) and strand elongation. Reaction under laboratory conditions is carried out in a device known as thermocycler. Usually, one PCR reaction is made of 35-40 cycles, which result in creating billions of copies of an individual DNA molecule (with a logarithmic increase of the product in each cycle).

### 4.2 Real–time PCR

Real-time PCR is a polymerase chain reaction observed in real time, is an improvement of the classical PCR method (Al-Soud et al., 2005; Bansal et al., 2006). A real-time PCR thermocycler is equipped with an optical system which collects information about the course of reaction, cycle by cycle. TaqMan® probes labelled with fluorescent dyes make an additional component of PCR real time reactions. A probe is an oligonucleotide designed to bind highly specifically to a replicated fragment of DNA, therefore – in case of the analysed application in food microbiology – to "detect" a sequence which is characteristic for the required pathogen. The probe should bind specifically and strongly, which can be ensured by special protein molecules (a MGB molecule in TaqMan® Applied Biosystems probes). Polymerase, while synthesising a new strand, moves along the matrix, encountering a probe on its way. Because of its exonucleolytic activity, the enzyme starts to "unstick" the probe from the matrix and afterwards to destroy it, releasing a fluorescent dye. An optical system of the thermocycler triggers and then receives dye glow, which becomes more intense with each cycle (a logarithmic increase of the amount of product results in a logarithmic

A forty-cycle real-time PCR reaction lasts about 1.5 hours. After adding the time needed to isolate DNA from the analysed sample (up to 30 minutes), the entire determination of the presence or the lack of pathogen lasts 2 hours (while using the Applied Biosystems TaqMan® Pathogen Detection System). Samples for determination are taken from pre-enrichment cultures on buffered peptone water after 18 h incubation at 37°C, so the total time from the collection of a sample to the final results does not exceed 24 hours.

Chen *et al.* (2000) evaluated the TaqMan system for the detection of *Salmonella* that utilizes primers and probes developed from a novel target sequence (*inv*A). The detection limit was below 3 CFU/25 g or 25 ml when raw milk, ground beef and ground pork inoculated with *Salmonella* were pre-enriched overnight. Malorny *et al.* (2004) used specifically designed primers and a probe target within the ttrRSBCA locus, and included internal amplification control, which is coamplified with the same primers as the *Salmonella* DNA in the assay. The diagnostic accuracy was shown to be 100% compared to the traditional culture method when 110 various food samples (chicken rinses, minced meat, fish, and raw milk) were investigated for *Salmonella* by real-time PCR including a pre-enrichment step in buffered peptone water.

A very frequent target of species-specific *Salmonella* PCR assays is the invasion protein *inv*A gene, and several *inv*A-based PCR assays have been already developed and validated (Malorny et al. 2003a; b).

Validated PCR methods are available from Bio-Rad, Roche, Qualicon/Oxoid, Genesystems, AES Chemunex, Applied BioSystems, Idaho Technology Inc., Lantmännen, IEH Laboratries and Consulting Group, ADNucleis and BioControl systems. Validation is an important step in the process of standardizing a method because it provides evidence that the new method gives similar results and is in agreement with the currently used reference method (Patel et al., 2006).
One major difficulty with PCR is the presence of compounds that inhibit the PCR reaction. These compounds can contaminate the DNA templates extracted from food samples and may in turn generate false-negative results (Elizaquivel et al., 2008). Therefore, evaluation and elimination of PCR inhibitory compounds are important steps in the development of PCR and real-time PCR assays (Abu Al-Soud et al., 2000). The PCR procedure is sufficiently sensitive such that, in theory, only a few template molecules are required to initiate the synthesis reactions (Uyttendaele et al., 2003). However, an enrichment step is still required to detect small numbers of *Salmonella* in food samples. This step may consist of non-selective enrichment with buffered peptone water (BPW) and selective enrichment with Rappaport-Vassiliadis. These enrichment broth have been directly utilized for *Salmonella* DNA template preparation. However, limited research has been conducted to quantitatively evaluate the effects of the enrichment broths using conventional PCR assays and even less using a real-time PCR protocol. Therefore, identifying and eliminating the PCR inhibitory effects of the enrichment broths is key to enhancing the performance of PCR assays in detecting *Salmonella* in foods.

### 4.3 Multiplex polymerase chain reaction (PCR)

Multiplex PCR is a variant of the PCR technique in which two or more loci are simultaneously amplified in the same reaction. Multiplex PCR can be described as a specific and sensitive in vitro amplification of DNA with distinguishable size products from the same or different organisms in a single reaction (Jasson et al., 2010; Fitzgerald et al., 2007). In this methodology several specific primer sets are combined into a single PCR assay. MPCR is undoubtedly useful to rapidly establish simultaneous detection of multiple virulence factors (Fach et al., 2009) or combined detection of multiple isolates (Kawasaki et al., 2009; Settanni & Corsetti, 2007). A convened format for MPCR is the GeneDisc (PALL) (Beutin et al., 2009).
Recently, multiplex real-time PCR assays have been applied to detect more than two gene sequences in a single reaction by using spectrally distinct dye-labeled probes (TaqMan system) (Elizaquivel et al., 2008). This technology could potentially save time and effort in the laboratory and thus may lower testing-related costs incurred by the food industry (Elizaquivel et al., 2008).

## 5. Fish (fluorescent *in situ* hybridization)

The literature provides a limited number of reports concerning the application of the FISH technique for food examination (Ootsubo et al., 2003), while it is broadly applied in microbiology of environment, histopathology, histoimmunology, cytogenetics. Initially, it was developed in order to identify and to determine the number of bacterial cells in water ecosystem environments (Skowrońska & Zmysłowska, 2006), deposits, rhizosphere and soil.

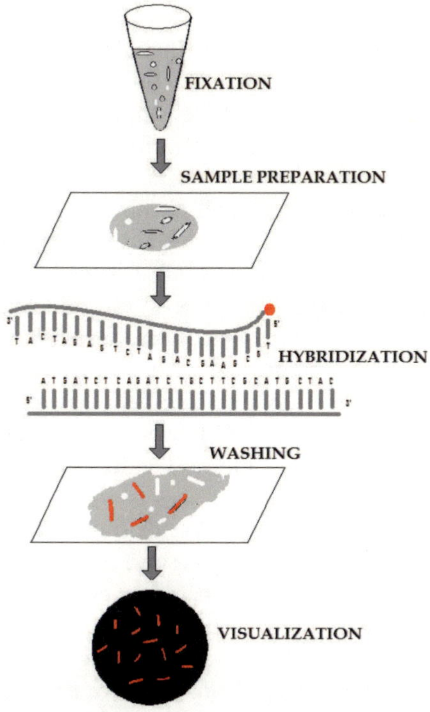


Fig. 1. Flow chart of a typical FISH procedure.

The FISH technique consists in hybridization of the rRNA sequence of immobilized cells by a fluorescently-labelled 16S rRNA oligonucleotide probe (Zwirglmaier, 2005; Baudart et al., 2005). Oligonucleotide probes are short fragments of deoxyribonucleic acid which hybridize or are paired with complementary sequences of DNA or RNA extracted from the analysed microorganisms. They are paired in the same way as double-stranded DNA forms (adenine with thymine and guanine with cytosine). If the sequence of bases on the DNA probe is complementary to the sequence characteristic for the determined microorganism, the probe binds only with the DNA of the identified microorganism. Probes are most often marked on one or on both ends with a fluorescent dye. Molecular probes bind specifically to rRNA in ribosomes of the target cells, identifying them on various taxonomic levels. Such a solution significantly increases the sensitivity of determination - since rRNA is an integral part of bacterial ribosome, it is found in the cell in large number of copies (between 1,000 and 10,000). Another advantage of this solution is the availability of vast information concerning rRNA sequences originating from various microorganisms which are often very closely genetically related, which allows probes to have very high specificity (Sakai et al., 2004; Ercoloni et al., 2005) Due to the range of probe specificity, the following probes can be distinguished: universal, e.g. EUB338 (GCTGCCTCCCGTAGGAGT), specific for *Bacteria* domain, except for the *Planctomycetales* order, antisense, e.g. NON388 (CGACGGAGGGCATCCTCA) designed to detect non-specific probe binding, and specific probes, e.g. for *Salmonella* sp.: Sal3 (5'-AATCACTTCACCTACGTG-3').

The FISH method with the application of fluorescently labelled 16S rRNA oligonucleotide probes is used for determining only the number of physiologically active cells, since rRNA has a shorter half-life than DNA, which makes rRNA a potentially better indicator of their activity. Ribosomes of quickly-growing cells include a certain number of rRNA copies, usually over 1,000, which is sufficient for inducing a light signal after the labelled probe binds (Bottari et al., 2006). After the death of the cell, rRNA disintegrates, and the rate of this process depends, among others, on the concentration of enzymes - RNAz, as well as on the continuity of the cytoplasmic membrane (Vieira-Pinto et al., 2007). Slowly growing or metabolically inactive cells, containing a small number of ribosome copies, emit light of low intensity. New, more sensitive modifications of the FISH technique lead to amplification of the signal (TSA-FISH also known as CARD-FISH), becoming a useful tool for contemporary microbiology (Fang et al., 2003). 16S rRNA oligonucleotide probes labelled with fluorophores of various molecular weight (e.g. horseradish peroxidase - 44 kDa, fluorescein - 330 kDa) provide a visual assessment of the degree of cell wall permeabilization, on the basis of differences in dye permeation into the cell. An extreme advantage of the FISH technique is the possibility to detect VBNC (viable but not culturable) cells which do not grow on solid media, which makes this method more sensitive in comparison to the plate methods (Pisz et al., 2007, Oliver, 2005)

The most frequent used dyes for the detection of the FISH signals are FITC (fluorescein isothiocyanate) that emits a green fluorescence and dyes with orange or red fluorescence, such as Cy3™ , or TexasRed™. Another commonly used fluorochrome in FISH experiments is Cy5™ that emits in the far red/close infrared. Since this fluorescence is not visible by eye it would need detection by an infrared sensitive camera mounted on the microscope. (Hoefel et al., 2003; Gatti et al., 2006)There are various other dyes with similar characteristics available from various different vendors. For example, FITC can well be replaced by Rhodamin 110, and Cy3™ by TAMRA (carboxytetramethyl- rhodamine) depending on the actual price and for some dyes, depending on the quality of the currently distributed lot (Table 4).

| | **Dyes** | **Ex.Max.** | **Em.Max.** |
|---|---|---|---|
| **Blue** | DAPI | 358 | 461 |
| **Turquoise** | DEAC | 426 | 480 |
| **Green** | FITC/R110 | 494/500 | 517/525 |
| **Yellow** | R6G | 524 | 550 |
| **Orange** | TAMRA/Cy3™ | 552/550 | 575/570 |
| **Red** | TexRed/Cy3.5™ | 590/581 | 612/596 |
| **Near Infrared** | Cy5™ | 649 | 670 |
| **Infrared** | Cy5.5™ | 675 | 694 |

Table 4. Characteristics of selected fluorescent dyes.

A standard FISH methodology includes preparation and permeabilization of cells, hybridization, washing off the excess unbound probe and detecting the signal with the application of fluorescence microscopy (Jasson et al., 2010; Ootsubo et al., 2003)

Reports concerning the use of fluorescent *in situ* hybridization in food research indicate the possibility of its application of *Salmonella* spp. detection and recommend this method as very sensitive, fast and cheap.

Vieira-Pinto et al., (2005) compared FISH methods with the classical plate method for detection of *Salmonella* spp. Out of 47 samples of pork tonsils, 16 (34%) were positive for *Salmonella* spp detection by the FISH method with the application of 23S rRNA Sal3 probe. Out of 31 negative results obtained by FISH method, one sample was positive for *Salmonella* spp. detection by the plate method. Similar results were obtained by Fang et al., (2003), who detected *Salmonella* sp. species in 56 samples of food products by the FISH method (23S rRNA Sal3), while 28 samples were not positive for *Salmonella* spp. detection by the plate method. Huge number of positive results can derive from the presence of cells slightly damaged or occurrence of factors inhibiting their growth in food products, which can transfer cells to VBNS state. The authors suggest that FISH method seems to be less prone to diverse physical-chemical properties of preserved food products (temperature, concentration of NaCl, pH), which can work as a stress factor for *Salmonella* spp. cells. Presence of microflora can be another reason of high number of positive results obtained by the FISH method as compared to the plate methods.

The conclusions drawn from the research show the need for continuous improvement of the methodology and selecting and/or designing more specific probes. This is related to the varied chemical and microbiological composition of food (the so-called matrix), which can lead to errors in reading. Therefore, a relatively fast assessment of the quality and safety of food requires not only the selection of probes for individual species of microorganisms, but first of all optimal preparation of food samples for examination purposes on the basis of the matrix. Preparation of samples is understood as proper filtration and centrifugation at various parameters in order to eliminate large particles, and also the choice of optimal digestion conditions or permeabilization of the cell wall of microorganisms (e.g. with lysozyme, proteinase K, achromopeptidase, paraformaldehyde, ethanol etc.) occurring in the examined food. Proper preparation of samples and cells prevents non-specific absorption of the probe on cell elements and easier penetration of cell cytoplasm.

## 6. VIDAS

VIDAS™ (BioMérieux) is an automated enzyme-linked fluorescent assay (ELFA) method based on the detection of *Salmonella* by using specific antibodies coated on the inner surface of a tip-like disposable pipette which is introduced into the VIDAS system along with the VIDAS *Salmonella* strip containing the boiled *Salmonella* culture.

VIDAS Immuno-concentration *Salmonella* (ICS) is a fully automated method for the concentration of *Salmonella* from foods. It replaces traditional selective enrichment procedures with an automated immunological capture and specific release process (Yeh et al., 2002). The method is based on multistage reaction. The kit contains so called reagent stripes, that is a set of wells with reagents sealed tightly inside, and pipettes, which inner sides are coated with antibodies against specific antigens. The amount of 500 μl of the sample after selective enrichment stage on RVS is introduced to the first well and a strip is placed in the immunoanalyser chamber. Reaction suspension is cyclically pulled up and down by pipettes. A pipet tip-like device, the solid-phase receptacle (SPR) serves as the solid phase as well as the pipet for the assay. The SPR is coated with anti-*Salmonella* antibodies absorbed on the surface. A final enzymatic step releases the captured *Salmonella* into a well.

Detection of *Salmonella* antigens is based on enzyme-linked fluorescent immunoassay performed in the automated VIDAS instrument. ASPR serves as the solid phase as well as the pipet for the assay. The SPR is coated with a cocktail of highly specific monoclonal antibodies. All of the assay steps are performed automatically by the VIDAS instrument. For the detection of *Salmonella by* VIDAS SLM, the sample is inoculated into lactose broth and incubated for 18 h at 37°C (non-selective pre-enrichment). Subsequently, 0.1 ml of this medium is inoculated into Rappaport–Vassiliadis broth and 1 ml into tetrathionate broth, and then incubated for 8 h at 42°C and 8 h at 37°C, respectively. Then, 1 ml of each broth is inoculated separately into 10 ml of M-broth and incubated at 42°C for 18 h. Finally, 1 ml of each broth is placed in a tube, which is heated for 15 min at 100°C. Following pre-enrichment, immuno-concentration, and postenrichment of test portions, an aliquot of the boiled test suspension is placed into the reagent strip and is cycled in and out of the SPR for a specific length of time. *Salmonella* antigens, if present, bind to the monoclonal antibodies coating the interior of the SPR. All other unbound material is washed away. Antibodies conjugated with alkaline phosphatase are cycled in and out of the SPR, binding to any *Salmonella* antigen bound to the SPR wall. The final wash step removes unbound conjugate. The substrate, 4-methyl umbelliferyl phosphate, is converted by the enzyme on SPR wall to the fluorescent product, 4-methyl umbelliferone.

The intensity of fluorescence is measured by the optical scanner in VIDAS. The fluorescence intensity is measured twice at 450 nm. The first result is related to the background, the second it the value after incubation of the substrate with enzyme. Based on that, the apparatus calculates the result of the test and interprets it as a positive or negative one. RFV (Relative Fluorescence Value) is calculated as the difference between the sample and background fluorescences. The printed report contains the RFV value of the sample, RFV value of the standard, and test value (TV), which is a quotient of the sample value and standard value. A result was interpreted by the apparatus as positive, if TV $\geq$ 0.23, while as negative if TV $\leq$ 0.23. Results are interpreted after the test values and control are compared to thresholds stored in the computer. A positive result requires confirmation with classical culture methods, that is streak plating on two plates with selection growth medium. For confirmation, previously prepared and stored under cold conditions broth culture of the investigated sample is used.

Based on the comparative studies with the standard plate method, it can be concluded that the VIDAS system can be use to get fast results; however, because these results can be false positive then they have to be confirmed by culture method (Yeh et al., 2002; Zadernowska et al., 2010; Walker et al., 2001)

Problems with detection of some *Salmonella* spp. serotypes were observed during detection by the immunoenzymatic method. This may be caused by weak binding of antibodies, which is confirmed by results obtained by other authors. Vitek Immunodiagnostic Assay System (VIDAS, BioMérieux) are currently used in the meat and poultry processing industries (Maciorowski et al., 2006). Several validation studies have been reported that the detection rate of VIDAS systems were comparable to that of culture method (Yeh et al., 2002) and real-time PCR (Uyttendaele et al., 2003) for detecting of *Salmonella* in food.

**VIDAS Salmonella Xpress** (VIDAS SLMX) is most rapid method for the detection of *Salmonella than VIDAS SLM.* The results are obtained as little as 17 hours. The method has been simplified with a single enrichment in buffer peptone water and just one pipeting step. A broad incubation time of 16 to 24 hours simplifies the laboratory workflow, enabling all samples to be processed as they arrive during the day. This test is validated for raw beef and veal meats (including frozen), not flavoured and pasteurized egg products.

**VIDAS UP Salmonella** is a new generation of assay based on **the latest technology** available for pathogen screening: Phage recombinant protein. Bacteriophages are viruses infecting bacteria. Phages are extremely host-specific. Most bacteria can be infected by particular phages and it is common that a given phage can recognize and infect only one or a few strains or species of bacteria (Hagens & Loessner, 2007). The specificity of these phages is partly mediated by tail-associated proteins that distinctively recognize surface molecules of susceptible bacteria (Kretzer et al., 2007). Bacteriophages or proteins of bacteriophages have been included in various ways in detection methods for pathogens (Favrin et al., 2003)

Although there is a need to perform a collaborative study to further evaluate the methods before it can be concluded that their performances are equal, both the PCR and the ELFA-based assay could provide a rapid and user-friendly screening method for detection of *Salmonella* in food (Uyttendaele et al., 2003; Priego et al., 2009; Kumar et al., 2008; Szabo et al., 2008)

## 7. Conclusion

Numerous and diverse alternative methods for microbial analysis of foods, as described above, exist (Bohaychuk et al., 2005; Wu, 2008) . They are currently brought to the market by various suppliers in a variety of formats as a result of recent developments, particularly in the field of biotechnology, microelectronics and related software development. Many of them have been proven to be equivalent to the "golden standard" reference methods with regard to the performance characteristics of the method.

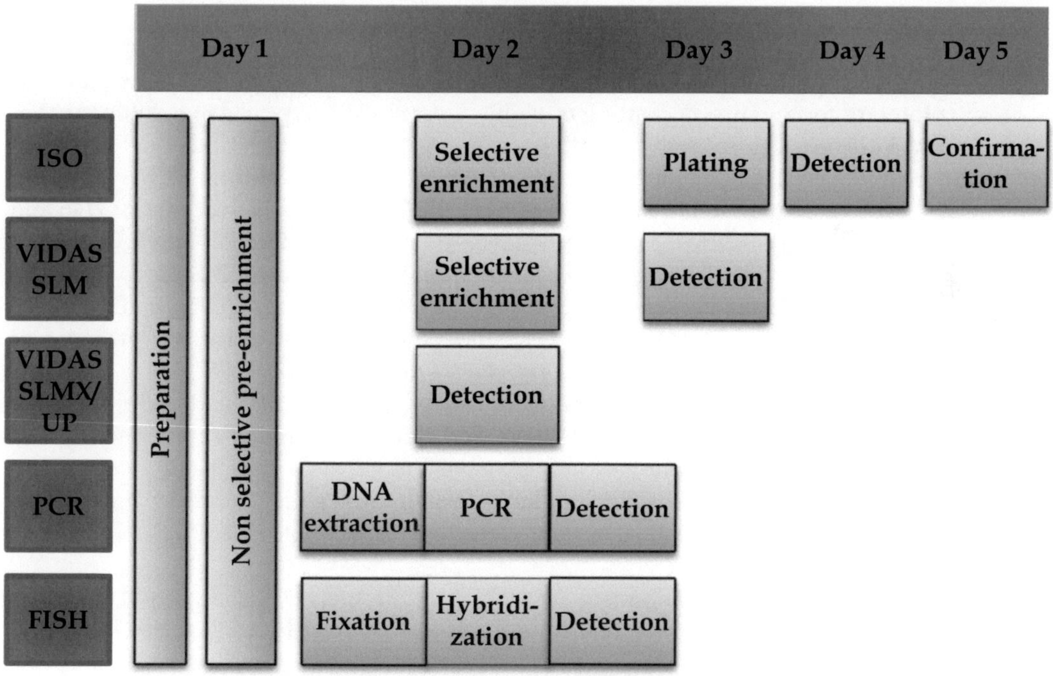


Fig. 2. Detection of *Salmonella* spp. from food.

Due to an overload of alternative methods and/or formats on the market, food business operators or competent authority, for which microbial analysis of food is only a supporting tool in the assurance of food safety, have difficulties in deciding which method is best fit for their purpose in their particular context. (Jasson et al., 2010)
Evolution in alternative rapid methods, mainly immunological and molecular methods, focus on the combination of available techniques e.g. combination of immunocapture and PCR and/or by elaboration of new formats optimizing reading and registration software rather than introducing new principles of detection or enumeration.

## 8. Acknowledgment

This study was supported by the Grant N N312 491340 from the National Science Centre, Poland.

## 9. References

Al-Soud, W. A., Ouis I. S., Ljungh, D. Q. Li., Wadström, S. T. (2005). Characterization of the PCR inhibitory effect of bile to optimize real-time PCR detection of *Helicobacter* species. *FEMS Immunology & Medical Microbiology* 44:177-182

Al-Soud, W. A.; & Radstrom, P. (2000). Effects of amplification facilitators on diagnostic PCR in the presence of blood, feces, and meat. *Journal of Clinical Microbiology*, Vol. 38, pp. 4463-70

Bansal, N. S., Gray, V., & McDonell, F. (2006). Validated PCR assay for the routine detection of *Salmonella* in food. *Journal Food Protection*, Vol. 69, pp. 282-7

Baudart, J., Olaizola, A., Coallier, J., Gauthier V., Laurent P. (2005). Assessment of a new technique combining a viability test, whole-cell hybridization and laser-scanning cytometry for the direct counting of viable *Enterobacteriaceae* cells in drinking water. *FEMS Microbiology Letters.*, Vol. 243,pp. 405-409

Beutin, L., Jahn, S., Fach, P. (2009). Evaluation of the 'GeneDisc' real-time PCR system for detection of enterohaemorrhagic *Escherichia coli* (EHEC) O26, O103, O111, O145 and O157 strains according to their virulence markers and their O- and Hantigen-associated genes. *Journal of Applied Microbiology*. Vol. 106, pp.1122-1132

Bohaychuk, V.M., Gensler, G.E., King, R.K.,Wu, J.T., McMullen, L.M. (2005). Evaluation of detection methods for screening meat and poultry products for the presence of foodborne pathogens. *Journal Food Protection*. Vol. 68, pp. 2637-2647

Bottari, B., Ercolini, D., Gatti, M., Neviani, E. (2006). Application of FISH technology for microbiological analysis: current state and prospects. *Applied Microbiology and Biotechnology*. Vol. 73, pp. 485-494

Chen, W., G. Martinez, and A. Mulchandani. (2000). Molecular beacons: a real-time polymerase chain reaction assay for detecting *Salmonella*. *Analytical Biochemistry* Vol. 280, pp. 166-72

Cheng, C. M., Lin, W., Van, K. T., Phan, L., Tran, N. N. & Farmer, D. (2008). Rapid detection of *Salmonella* in foods using real-time PCR. *Journal Food Protection*, Vol.71, No.12, pp. 2436-41

Elizaquivel, P., & Aznar, R. (2008). A multiplex RTi-PCR reaction for simultaneous detection of *Escherichia coli* O157:H7, *Salmonella* spp. and *Staphylococcus aureus* on fresh, minimally processed vegetables. *Food Microbiology*, Vol.25, No.5, pp. 705-13

Ercolini, D., Hill, P.J., Dodd, C.E.R. (2005). Development of a fluorescence *in situ* hybridization method for cheese using a 16S rRNA probe. *Journal of Microbiological Methods*. Vol.52, pp. 267-271

Fach, P., Micheau, P., Mazuet, C., Perelle, S., Popoff, M. (2009). Development of real-time PCR tests for detecting botulinum neurotoxins A, B, E, F producing *Clostridium botulinum, Clostridium baratii* and *Clostridium butyricum*. *Journal of Applied Microbiology*, Vol.107, pp. 465-473

Fang, Q.; Brockmann, S.; Botzenhart, K., Wiedenmann, A. (2003). Improved detection of *Salmonella* sp. in foods by fluorescent *in situ* hybridization with 23S rRNA probes: a comparison with conventional cultural methods. *Journal of Food Protection*, Vol.66, pp.723-731

Favrin, S.J., Jassim, S.A., Griffiths, M.W. (2003). Application of a novel immunomagnetic separation-bacteriophage assay for the detection of *Salmonella* enteritidis and *Escherichia coli* O157: H7 in food. *International Journal of Food Microbiology*. Vol.85, pp. 63-71

Fitzgerald, C.; Collins, M.; van Duyne, S.; Mikoleit, M.; Brown, T.; Fields, P. (2007). Multiplex, bead-based suspension array for molecular determination of common *Salmonella* serogroups. *Journal of Clinical Microbiology*, Vol.45, No.10, pp.3323-3334

Gatti M., Bernini V., Lazzi C., Neviani E.: Fluorescence microscopy for studying the viability of micro-organisms in natural whey starters. *Letters of Applied Microbiology*. 2006, 42, 338–343

Glynn, B., Lahiff, S.,Wernecke, M., Barry, T., Smith, T.J., Maher, M. (2006). Current and emerging molecular diagnostic technologies applicable to bacterial food safety. *International Journal of Dairy Technology*. Vol.59, pp.126-139

Hagens, S., Loessner, M.J. (2007). Application of bacteriophages for detection and control of foodborne pathogens. *Applied Microbiology and Biotechnology*. Vol.76, pp. 513-519

Hein, I., Flekna, G., Krassnig, M. & Wagner, M. (2006). Real-time PCR for the detection of *Salmonella* spp. in food: An alternative approach to a conventional PCR system suggested by the FOOD-PCR project. *Journal of Microbiological Methods*. Vol. 66(3), pp. 538-47

Hoefel D., Grooby W.L., Monis P.T., Andrews S., Saint C.P. (2003). A comparative study of carboxyfluorescein diacetate and carboxyfluorescein diacetate succinimidyl ester as indicators of bacterial activity. *Journal of Microbiological Methods*, Vol.52, pp. 379– 388

International Standards Organization. ISO 6579 Microbiology of food and animal feeding stuffs - Horizontal method for detection of *Salmonella spp*. 6579:2002

Jasson, V.; Jacxsens, L., Luning P., Rajkovic, A., Uyttendaele, M. (2010). Alternative microbial methods: An overview and selection criteria. *Food Microbiology*, Vol.27, pp. 710-730

Kawasaki, S.; Fratamico, P.M.; Horikoshi, N.; Okada, Y.; Takeshita, K., Sameshima, T.; Kawamoto, S. (2009). Evaluation of a multiplex PCR system for simultaneous detection of *Salmonella* spp., *Listeria monocytogenes*, and *Escherichia coli* O157: H7 in foods and in food subjected to freezing. *Foodborne Pathogens and Disease*. Vol.6, pp. 81-89

Kretzer, J.W., Lehmann, R., Schmelcher, M., Banz, M., Kim, K.P., Korn, C., Loessner, M.J. (2007). Use of high-affinity cell wall-binding domains of bacteriophage endolysins for immobilization and separation of bacterial cells. *Applied and Environmental Microbiology*. Vol.73, pp. 1992-2000

Kumar, R., Surendran, P.K., Thampuran, N. (2008). Evaluation of culture, ELISA and PCR assays for the detection of *Salmonella* in seafood. *Letters. in Applied. Microbiology*. Vol.46, pp. 221-226

Maciorowski, K. G., Herrera, P., Jones, F. T.,Pillai, S. D., Ricke, S. C. (2006). Cultural and immunological detection methods for *Salmonella* spp. in animal feeds - A Review. *Veterinary Research Communications*, Vol. 30, pp.127-37

Malorny, B, Tassios, P.T., Rådström, P., Cook, N., Wagner, M., Hoorfar, J. (2003b). Standardization of diagnostic PCR for the detection of foodborne pathogens. *Applied and Environmental Microbiology*, Vol.83, No.1, (May 2003), pp.39-48

Malorny, B., Hoorfar, J., Bunge, C., Helmuth, R. (2003a). Multicenter Validation of the Analytical Accuracy of *Salmonella* PCR: towards an International Standard. *Applied and Environmental Microbiology*, Vol. 69, No. 1,(January 2003), pp. 290-296

Malorny, B., Paccassoni, E., Fach, P., Bunge, C., Martin, A., Helmuth, R. (2004). Diagnostic real-time PCR for detection of *Salmonella* in food. *Applied and Environmental Microbiology*, Vol.70, pp.7046-52

Manafi, M. (2000). New developments in chromogenic and fluorogenic culture media. *International Journal of Food Microbiology*, Vol. 60, pp. 205-18

McCarthy, N., Reen, F. J., Buckley, J. F., Frye, J. G., Boyd, E. F. & Gilroy, D. (2009). Sensitive and rapid molecular detection assays for *Salmonella enterica* Serovars Typhimurium and Heidelberg. *Journal of Food Protection*, Vol.72, No.11, pp. 2350-7

Moganedi, K. L. M., Goyvaerts, E. M. A., Venter, S. N., Sibara, M. M. (2007). Optimisation of the PCR-*invA* primers for the detection of *Salmonella* in drinking and surface waters following pre-cultivation step. *Water SA* 33, 196-202

Oliver J.D. (2005). The viable but nonculturable state in bacteria. *Journal of Microbiology*, 43, 93-100

Ootsubo M., Shimizu T., Tanaka R., Sawabe T., Tajima K., Ezura Y. (2003). Seven-hour fluorescence *in situ* hybridization technique for enumeration of *Enterobacteriaceae* in food and environmental water sample. Journal of Applied Microbiology. Vol.95, pp.1182–1190

Patel, J. R., Bhagwat, A. A., Sanglay, G. C., and Solomon, M. B. (2006). Rapid detection of *Salmonella* from hydrodynamic pressure-treated poultry using molecular beacon real-time PCR. *Food Microbiology*. Vol.23, pp.39–46

Perry, J.D., Freydiere, A.M. (2007). The application of chromogenic media in clinical microbiology. *Journal of Applied. Microbiology*. Vol.103, pp.2046-2055

Piknova , L., Stefanovicova´, A., Drahovska´ , H., Sa´sik, M., & Kuchta, T. (2002). Detection of *Salmonella* in food, equivalent to ISO 6579, by a three-days polymerase chain reaction-based method. *Food Control*, Vol.13, pp.191–194.

Pisz, J. M.; Lawrence, J. R.; Schafer, A. N.; Siciliano, S. D. (2007). Differentiation of genes extracted from non-viable versus viable micro-organisms in environmental samples using ethidium monoazide bromide. *Journal of Microbiological Methods*, Vol.71, No.3, pp. 312-318

Priego, R., Medina, L. M., Jordano, R. (2009). Comparison between the Vitek Immunodiagnostic Assay System and PCR for the detection of pathogenic microorganisms in an experimental dry sausage during its curing process. *Journal Food Protection*. Vol.72 , No.9, pp.1977-81

Sakai, K., Mori, M., Fujii, A., Iwami, Y., Chukeatirote E., Shirai Y. (2004). Fluorescent *in situ* hybridization analysis of open lactic acid fermentation of kitchen refuse using rRNA-targeted oligonucleotide probes. *Journal of Bioscience and Bioengineering*, Vol.98, pp. 48-56

Schonenbrucher, V., Mallinson, E.T., Bulte, M. (2008). A comparison of standard cultural methods for the detection of foodborne *Salmonella* species including three new chromogenic plating media. *International Journal of Food Microbiology*. 123, 61e66.

Seo, K. H., Valentin-Bon, I. E. & Brackett, R. E. (2006). Detection and enumeration of *Salmonella* Enteritidis in homemade ice cream associated with an outbreak: comparison of conventional and real-time PCR methods. *Journal Food Protection*, Vol.69, No.3, pp. 639-43

Settanni L, Corsetti A. (2007). The use of multiplex PCR to detect and differentiate food- and beverage-associated microorganisms: a review. *Journal of Microbiological Methods* Vol.69, No.1, pp.1-22

Skowrońska A., Zmysłowska I. (2006). Współczesne metody identyfikacji bakterii stosowane w ekologii mikroorganizmów wodnych - fluorescencyjna hybrydyzacja *in situ* (FISH). *Postępy Mikrobiologii.*, Vol.45, pp.183-193

Szabo, I., Scherer, K., Roesler, U., Appel, B., Nockler, K., Hensel, A., (2008). Comparative examination and validation of ELISA test systems for *Salmonella* typhimurium diagnosis of slaughtering pigs. *International Journal of Food Microbiology*. 124, 65e69.

Tomás, D, Rodrigo, A., Hernández, M., Ferrús, M. A. (2009). Validation of Real-Time PCR and Enzyme-Linked Fluorescent Assay-Based Methods for Detection of *Salmonella* spp. in Chicken Feces Samples. *Food Analytical Methods*. Vol2: pp: 180–189

Uyttendaele, M., K., Vanwildemeersch, Debevere, J. (2003). Evaluation of real-time PCR vs automated ELISA and a conventional culture method using a semi-solid medium for detection of *Salmonella*. *Letters Applied Microbiology*. Vol. 37 , pp; 386-91

Vieira-Pinto, M., Oliveira, M., Bernardo, F., Martins, C. (2005). Evaluation of Fluorescent in situ Hybridization (FISH) as a rapid screening method for detection of *Salmonella* in tonsils of slaughtered pigs for consumption: a comparison with conventional culture method. *Journal of Food Safety*. Vol. 25, pp: 109–119

Vieira-Pinto, M.; Oliveira, M., Bernardo, F., Martins, C. (2007). Rapid detection of *Salmonella* sp. in pork samples using fluorescent *in situ* hybridization: a comparison with VIDAS®-SLM system and ISO 6579 cultural method. *Arquivo Brasileiro de Medicina Veterinária e Zootecnia*, Vol.59, No.6, pp.1388-1393

Walker, R. L., Kinde, H., Anderson, R. J., Brown, A. E. (2001). Comparison of VIDAS enzyme-linked fluorescent immunoassay using more swab sampling and conventional culture method for *Salmonella* detection in bulk tank milk and in-line milk filters in California dairies. *International Journal of Food Microbiology*. Vol.67, pp. 123-9

Wu, V.C.H. (2008). A review of microbial injury and recovery methods in food. *Food Microbiology*. Vol. 25, pp: 735-744

Yeh, K. S., C. E. Tsai, S. P. Chen, and C. W. Liao. (2002). Comparison between VIDAS automatic enzyme-linked fluorescent immunoassay and culture method for

*Salmonella* recovery from pork carcass sponge samples. *Journal of Food Protection.* Vol. 65, pp. 1656-9

Zadernowska, A., Łaniewska-Trokenheim, Ł., Chajęcka,W. (2010) Detection of *Listeria monocytogenes* and *Salmonella* sp. rods in fish and fish products using the mini Vidas system. *Medycyna Weterynaryjna.* Vol.66, No 4, pp. 264-267

Zwirglmaier, K. (2005). Fluorescence *in situ* hybridization (FISH) - the next generation. *FEMS Microbiology Letters,* Vol.246, pp. 151-158

# 19

# Studies on PCR-Based Rapid Detection Systems for *Salmonella* spp.

Jeongsoon Kim
*Food Research & Development Center, Samsung Everland Inc.*
*Mabuk-dong, Giheung-gu, Yongin*
*South Korea*

## 1. Introduction

### 1.1 Using molecular biological methods to identified *Salmonella* spp.

As the industrialization had made food supply to exceed demand, more and more consumers were interested in 'Delicious food' than 'Good quality food' today and they ask for not only taste but also safety. Microbiological safety is one of the most critical factors for ensuring safe food supply. Fig 1. is a flow chart of traditional detection procedure for *Salmonella* spp., showing that it takes about one week. Therefore, a rapid screening method using PCR is the basis of most molecular diagnostic laboratories. As the field of molecular pathology becomes more accessible to practicing pathologists, a working knowledge of PCR techniques is necessary related to biological safety of food is very essential in food industry. *Salmonella* spp. are an important cause of food-borne infections throughout the world, and the availability of rapid and simple detection techniques is critical for the food industry.

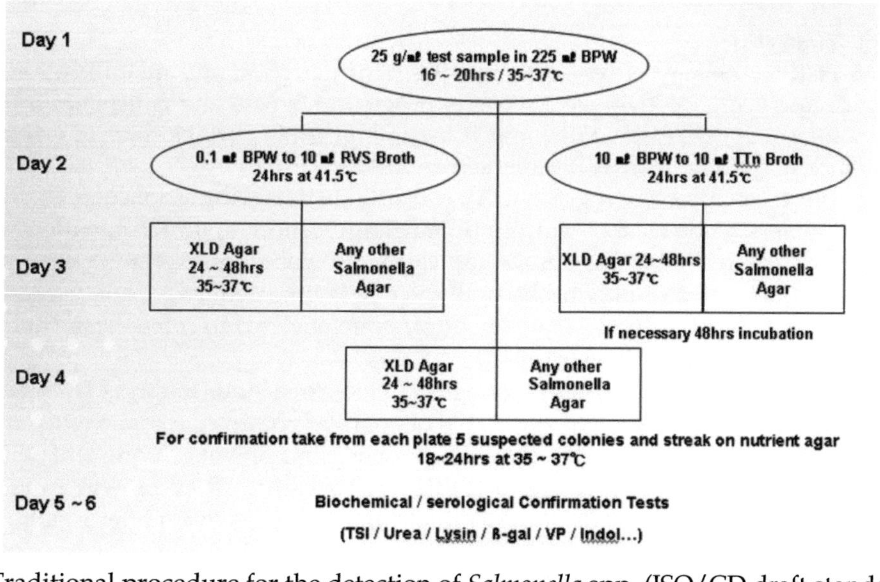


Fig. 1. Traditional procedure for the detection of *Salmonella* spp. (ISO/CD draft standard 6575 revision 2000)

Present commercial detection system for *Salmonella* spp. can be classified into four categories. The first, traditional method which uses culture medium and observe colony morphology formed on it. This requires at least four days and experienced skill to perform biological tests, but it is the only common method authorized throughout the world for now.

The second, Enzyme-Linked Immuno-Sorbent Assay (ELISA) detects certain bacteria using immune reaction between antibody and antigen specific for them. This method is easy to use because it makes color change or forms lines but it can be applied only for those which has specific toxin protein and requires more than $10^6$ CFU / ml for detection which needs 16 hours of incubation. The third, Adenosine triphosphate (ATP) detection kit detects level of bacterial contamination by the amount of ATP in sample. This method can not be used for identification of bacteria because it can only tell including the total amount of ATP from food. This is usually used for comparing hygiene level before and after washing. The fourth, genetic method which is based on PCR is highly specific and sensitive enough to detect 100 CFU / ml of bacteria, but at the same time it can detect even the dead cells after processing or cooking food because of the high sensitivity.

### 1.2 Advanced PCR technologies

#### 1.2.1 Multiplex PCR

Multiplex PCR can amplify two or more amplicons in a single PCR reaction. For multiplex PCR, each primer set is designed to amplify its target gene and make a PCR product of certain size to the target gene. To perform a multiplex PCR, the concentration of primers, $Mg^{2+}$, free dNTPs and polymerase must be optimized to allow synthesis of the genes of interest, And also the PCR reaction temperature parameters must be optimized to the best average for amplicon production for all primer sets. This technique saves time and labor more than one target DNA sequence can be detected in each reaction, It might not be optimal if the PCR products are limited in certain sizes and agarose gel staining with ethidium bromide (John Maurer, 2006). Therefore, it is possible to detect multiple pathogens in a sample with a single PCR test (Panicker *et al.*, 2004)

#### 1.2.2 Real-Time PCR

Real-Time PCR technology is based on the ability of detection and quantification of PCR products, or amplicons, as the reaction cycles progress. Higuchi and colleagues introduced this technology (Higuchi *et al.*, 1993) and it became possible by including of a fluorescent dye that binds to the amplicon as it is made (Fig. 2. A).

Initially, a fluorescent dye, SYBR green I (A), was used to detect the amplicons. SYBR green I binds the double stranded, DNA amplicon and fluorescences upon illumination with UV light. In TaqMan PCR (B), the oligoprobe contains a fluorescent marker and chemical group that quenches fluorescent of oligoprobe until the dye is liberated by 3' exonuclease activity of the Taq DNA polymerase (Source http://cafe.naver.com/solgent.cafe?iframe_url=/ArticleRead.nhn%3Farticleid=38&)

In TanMan PCR, an intact, "internal" fluorogenic oligoprobe binds to target DNA sequence, internal to the PCR primer binding sites. This oligoprobe possesses a reporter dye that will fluorescence and a suppressor dye known as quencher that prevent fluorescent activity via Fluorescence Resonance Energy Transfer (FRET). After each PCR cycle, when the double-stranded DNA products are made, a measure of fluorescence is taken after the fluorogenic probe is hydrolytically cleaved from the DNA structure by exonuclease activity of the *Thermus aquaticus* DNA polymerase (Heid *et al.*, 1996; Holland *et al.*, 1991). Once cleaved, the probe's fluorescent activity is no longer suppressed (Fig. 2. B). FAM (6-Carboxyfluorescein) and TAMRA(6-Carboxy-Tetramethyl-Rhodamin) are most frequently used as reporter and quencher, respectively. This PCR is often referred to as 5′ exonuclase-based, real-time PCR or TaqMan PCR (Mullah *et al.*, 1998).

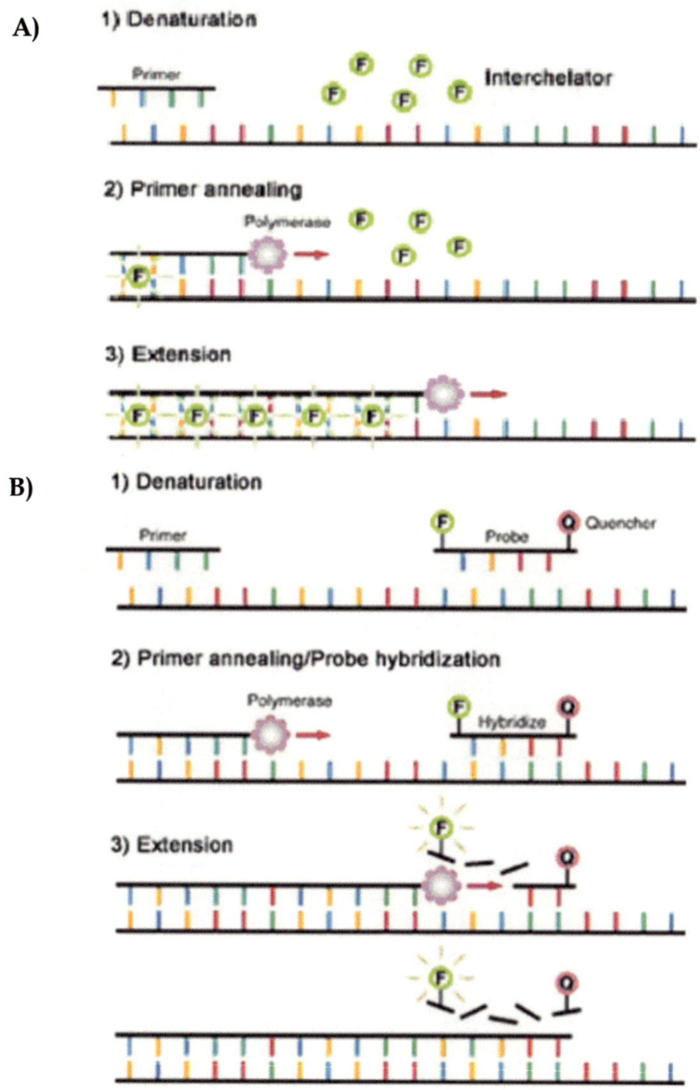


Fig. 2. Real-Time PCR detection of amplicons

### 1.2.3 Isothermal PCR

Recently, Jung *et al.* (2010) developed a new highly sensitive and specific isothermal amplification and detection system called isothermal target and probe amplification (iTPA) by employing DNA-RNA-DNA chimeric primers and a FRET (fluorescence Resonance Energy Transfer) probe. The iTPA method is based on a combination of novel isothermal chain amplification (ICA) and FRET cycling probe technology (CPT) (Fig. 3).

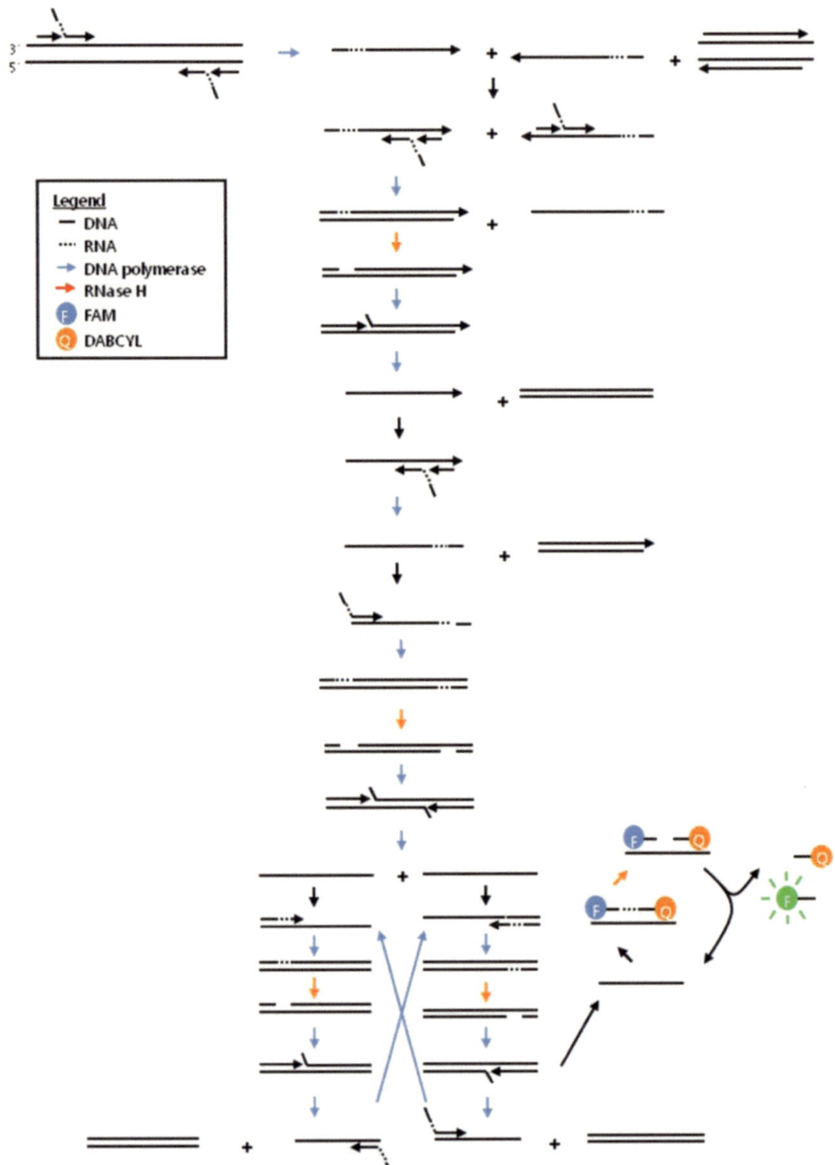


Fig. 3. Scheme of the Isothermal Target and Probe Amplification (iTPA) system

In the ICA method, which relies on the strand displacement activity of DNA polymerase and the RNA-degrading activity of RNase H, two displacement events occur in the presence of four specially designed primers that lead to high specificity for the target sequence. In the CPT method, a DNA-RNA-DNA chimeric probe is hybridized with the target DNA, and the RNA region of the duplex is specifically cleaved by RNase H. The cleaved probe fragment is disassociated from the target DNA and another intact probe is again hybridized and then cleaved. In this cycling event, a single target DNA molecule results in a large number of cleaved probe fragments, which can be designed to generate fluorescence signals (Kim *et al.* 2011).

## 2. Various PCR methods approaches for the detection of *Salmonella* spp.

### 2.1 Rapid and simultaneous detection of five pathogenic bacteria by a novel multiplex PCR assay: *Salmonella* spp., *Escherichia coli* O157:H7, *Listeria monocytogenes*, *Staphylococcus aureus* and *Vibrio parahaemolyticus*

According to Centers for Disease Control (CDC), about 5 millions food mediated diseases are killing 4,000 people every year. *Salmonella* was the most frequently found pathogenic bacteria in food poisoning : 1 ~ 4 millions of people were infected, 2,000 (0.1%) of them were dead. *Salmonella* is an important pathogen associated with bacterial foodborne outbreaks in the United states, accounting for 24% of all food outbreaks and 18% of produce-related outbreaks between 1990 and 2009 (Center for Science in the Public Interest, 2009). An outbreak in 2009 associated with *Salmonella*-contaminated peanut butter and peanut containing products caused nine deaths in 46 states as of 17 March 2009. This outbreak led to the largest recall of food items in the United States resulting in over 2100 products being voluntarily recalled by more than 200 companies (FDA, 2009). Recently, more than 500 million eggs were recalled after dangerous levels of *Salmonella* were detected in the eggs from two Iowa producers, who distributed the eggs in 14 US states. Nearly 2000 illnesses were reported between May and July 2010 (CDC, 2010). Food poisoning by E. coli O157:H7 broke out in 10000 people, 300 of them were dead. As for Listeria monocytogenes, 1500 people were infected and 400 were dead. This shows that stock farm products which were contaminated by these four bacteria (*E. coli* O157:H7, *Salmonella* spp., *Listeria monocytogene* and *Staphylococcus aureus*) is seriously threatening consumer's health. In korea, 50% of food poisoning are caused by meat or processed meat products, and *Salmonella* strains (50%), *S. aureus* (20%) are two major sources. Different molecular targets have been used to characterize the presence of food-borne pathogenic bacteria. In this study, genes encoding the virulence determinants and their expression regulator have been used to characterize numerous bacteria. A molecular test based on the detection of shiga-like toxin (verotoxin type II), femA (cytoplasmic protein), toxR (trans-membrane DNA binding protein), iap (invasive associative protein), and invA (invasion protein A) genes has been applied for identification of *E. coli* O157:H7 (Jinneman *et al.*, 2003; Kaneko *et al.*, 2001; Karpman *et al.*, 1998; Schmidt *et al.*, 1995; Wang *et al.*, 2002), *Staphylococcus aureus* (Mehrotra *et al.*, 2000), *Vibrio parahaemolyticus* (Karpman *et al.*, 1998; Cabrera-Garcia *et al.*, 2004), *Listeria monocytogenes* (Bubert *et al.*, 1992; Bubert *et al.*, 1999; Volokhov *et al.*, 2002), and *Salmonella spp.* (Chiu *et al.*, 1996).

To our knowledge, there is not a single acceptable method which is available to detect these five food-borne pathogenic bacteria simultaneously in food samples. The objective of the present work, therefore, was to establish a multiplex PCR assay method to detect the specific bacterial genus simultaneously and to analyze their distribution in contaminated foods. Our results indicate, that this method is rapid and specific for the simultaneous detection of *E. coli* O157:H7, *Staphylococcus aureus, Vibrio parahaemolyticus, Listeria monocytogenes* and *Salmonella* spp.

#### 2.1.1 Materials & methods [bacterial strains]

Bacterial strains were obtained from the American Type Culture Collection (ATCC; Manassas, Va.), the Korean Collection for Type Culture (KCTC; Daejeon, South Korea), and the Korean Culture Center of Microorganisms (KCCM; Seoul, South Korea), Also the strains isolated from various food samples were used in this study (Table 1).

All bacterial strains were grown on Luria-Bertani broth (LB; Bactopeptone 10 g, Yeast extract 5 g, and NaCl 10 g, each per Liter) at 37°C. All *Vibrio* species were grown in LB broth with supplementary 2% sodium chloride. Cultures were grown in LB, and a population of visible microorganisms was obtained by plating 10-fold serial dilutions of broth cultures on to plate count agar (Difco, Sparks, USA) and incubating the plates at 37°C for 16 hours. At each sampling dilution ratio, all bacterial cultures were mixed, and 100 μl (approximately $10^7$ CFU) of the suspension was used as DNA templates for PCR.

| Strain | Source [a] | Cultural medium |
|---|---|---|
| *Vibrio* spp. | | |
| *V. algosus* | KCCM41677 | Trypticase Soy Broth with 2.5% NaCl |
| *V. carchariae* | KCCM40865 | Marine Broth |
| *V. cholerae* | KCCM41626 | Nutrient Broth |
| *V. cincinnatiensis* | KCCM41683 | Marine Broth |
| *V. diazotrophicus* | KCCM41666 | Trypticase Soy Broth with 1% NaCl |
| *V. fischeri* | KCCM41685 | Marine Broth |
| *V. fluvialis* | KCCM40827 | Marine Broth |
| *V. furnissii* | KCCM41679 | Trypticase Soy Broth with 1% NaCl |
| *V. hollisae* | KCCM41680 | Marine Broth |
| *V. marinagilis* | KCCM41673 | Marine Broth |
| *V. marinofulvus* | KCCM41674 | Marine Broth |
| *V. marinovulgaris* | KCCM41675 | Marine Broth |
| *V. mediterranei* | KCCM40867 | Marine Broth |
| *V. metschnikovii* | KCCM41681 | Trypticase Soy Broth with 1% NaCl |
| *V. natriegens* | KCCM40868 | Nutrient Broth with 1.5% NaCl |
| *V. navarrensis* | KCCM41682 | Marine Broth |
| *V. penaeicida* | KCCM40869 | Marine Broth |
| *V. proteolyticus* | KCCM11992 | Nutrient Broth with 3% NaCl |
| *V. salmonicida* | KCCM41663 | Trypticase Soy Broth with 1% NaCl |
| *V. vulnificus* | KCCM41665 | Trypticase Soy Broth with 1% NaCl |
| *V. parahaemolyticus* | KCCM11965 | LB Broth with 1% Nacl |
| *V. parahaemolyticus* | KCCM41664 | LB Broth with 1% Nacl |
| *V. parahaemolyticus* | Inha university | LB Broth with 1% Nacl |
| Other bacteria | | |
| *Staphylococcus xylosus* | KCCM41465 | LB Broth |
| *Bacillus licheniformis* | KCTC1831 | LB Broth |
| *Yersinia enterocolitica* | KCCM41657 | LB Broth |
| *Staphylococcus aureus* | KCCM11764 | LB Broth |
| *Staphylococcus cohnii* | KCTC3574 | LB Broth |
| *Bacillus subtilis* | KCTC2213 | LB Broth |

| Strain | Source [a] | Cultural medium |
|---|---|---|
| *Bacillus cereus* | KCTC1661 | LB Broth |
| *Bacillus cereus* | KCTC 3624 | LB Broth |
| *Salmonella typhimurium* | KCTC 2421 | LB Broth |
| *Bacillus subtilis* | KCTC 3013 | LB Broth |
| *Staphylococcus arlettae* | KCTC 3588 | LB Broth |
| *Citrobacter freundii* | KCCM 11931 | LB Broth |
| *Bacillus licheniformis* | KCTC 3006 | LB Broth |
| *Salmonella choleraesuis* | KCCM 41575 | LB Broth |
| *Shigella sonnei* | KCTC 2009 | LB Broth |
| *Stphylococcus aureus* | KCTC 1916 | LB Broth |
| *Salmonella typhimurium* | KCTC 2515 | LB Broth |
| *Shigella bongori* | KCCM 41758 | LB Broth |
| *Staphylococcus caprae* | KCTC 3583 | LB Broth |
| *Salmonella typhimurium* | ATCC 14028 | LB Broth |
| *Staphylococcus warneri* | KCTC 3340 | LB Broth |
| *Salmonella enterica* | KCTC 2929 | LB Broth |
| *Staphylococcus aureus* | KCTC 1927 | LB Broth |
| *Listeria grayi* | ATCC 700545 | LB Broth |
| *Listeria ivanovii* | ATCC 49953 | LB Broth |
| *Listeria grayi* | ATCC 25400 | LB Broth |
| *Listeria innocuia* | ATCC 33091 | LB Broth |
| *Listeria murroy* | ATCC 25403 | LB Broth |
| *Listeria ivanovii* | ATCC 49954 | LB Broth |
| *Escherichia coli* O157:H7 | NVRQ | LB Broth |
| *Listeria innocuia* | ATCC 33090 | LB Broth |
| *Staphylococcus aureus* | KCTC 1928 | LB Broth |

[a] KCCM, Korean Culture Center of Microorganisms
KCTC, Korean Collection for Type Culture
ATCC, American Type Culture Collection
NVRQS, National Veterinary Research and Quarantine Service
KACC, Korean Agricultural Culture Collection

Table 1. Bacterial strains used in this study

**[Enrichment procedures for detection of food-borne microorganisms]**

All food-borne pathogens were grown for 16 hours in LB broth at 37°C in a shaking water bath. Cells were diluted from 1:10 to 1:$10^8$ in 10 ml of Luria-Bertani broth and manipulated as described above to make approximate cell count from 10 to $10^8$ CFU / ml. In each dilution ratio, single enrichment broth samples (1 ml) were collected into 1.5 ml micro-centrifuge tubes and used for DNA extraction (Fig. 1).

**[Extraction and preparation of DNA templates for PCR assay]**

Individual samples (1 ml) were centrifuged at 10,000 X g for 3 min. The cell pellets were resuspended in RNase free water (100 μl) and placed in a 100°C heating block for 20 min. The samples were cooled for 2 min at room temperature and centrifuged at 16,000 X g for 5 min. The supernatant fluids (5 μl) were used to make 25 μl of a multiplex PCR reaction mixture, which included 5 μl of 5 X reaction buffer (2.5 mM $MgCl_2$ and 0.8 mM concentration of each dNTP), 4 μl of the primer mixtures of the five food-borne bacteria, 1 μl of Super Taq plus polymerase (Rexgene Biotech., Cheongwon, South Korea), and 10 μl of DNase free water in a single tube. The multiplex PCR was run for 35 cycles on a Tpersonal cycler (Whatman Biometra, Goettingen, Germany) under the following conditions : denaturation at 94°C for 30 sec, primer annealing at 60°C for 30 sec, and extension at 72°C for 30 sec. The final cycle included an additional 5 min of extension time at 72°C. A 5 μl aliquot of the reaction mixture was then electrophoresis on a 2% agarose gel electrophoresis in 0.5 X Tris-borate buffer at 100 V for 25 min. The amplification products were stained with ethidium bromide and visualized by UV trans-illumination.

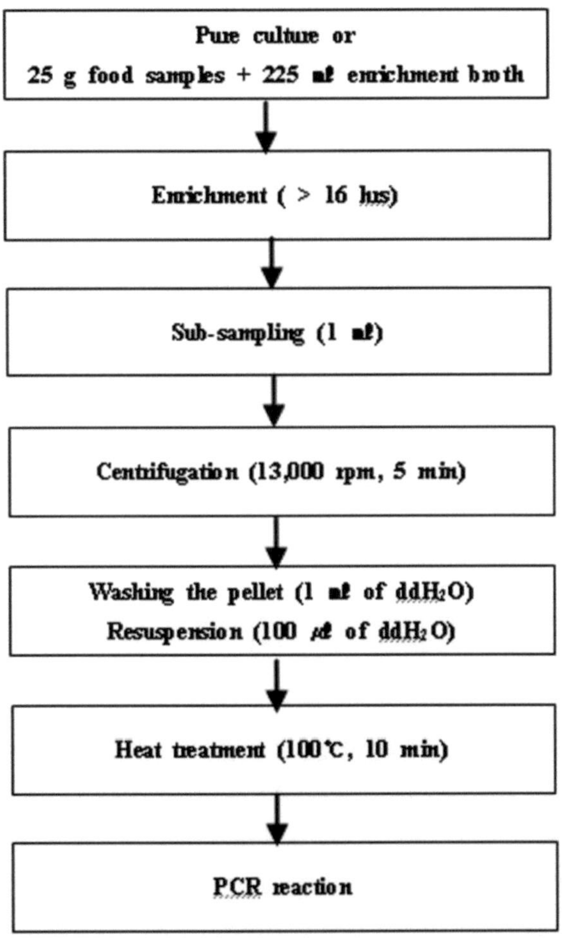


Fig. 4. Flow diagram of experimental protocols for PCR template preparation

**[Oligonucleotides]**

The oligonucleotide primers designed with Primer 3.0 software (Whitehead Institute, Cambridge, Mass.) were based on sequences obtained from Genbank and were used to amplify chromosomal DNA for the five food-borne pathogens (Table 2). The oligonucleotides and all reagents for PCRs were synthesized and purchased from Incorporation Bioneer (Daejeon, South Korea) and KoGene BioTech. (Seoul, South Korea).

| Strains | Primer name | Primer direction | Sequences (5`→3`) | Target gene | PCR product (bp) |
|---|---|---|---|---|---|
| *Vibrio parahaemolyticus* | VP | Forward<br>Reverse | CTCATTTGTACTGTTGAAC GCCTAAATAGA<br>AGGCAACCAGTTGTTGAT | *toxR* | 219 bp |
| *Salmonella* spp. | SAL | Forward<br>Reverse | GAATCCTCAGTTTTTCAAC GTTTC<br>TAGCCGTAACAACCAATAC AAATG | *invA* | 678 bp |
| *Staphylococcus aureus* | SA | Forward<br>Reverse | AATTTAACAGCTAAAGAGT TTGGT<br>TTCATTAAAGAAAAAGTGT ACGAG | *femA* | 264 bp |
| *E. coli* O157:H7 | EC | Forward<br>Reverse | GATAGACTTTTCGACCCAA CAAAG<br>TTGCTCAATAATCAGACGA AGATG | shiga-like toxin | 208 bp |
| *Listeria monocytogenes* | LM | Forward<br>Reverse | CTGGCACAAAATTACTTAC AACGA<br>AACTACTGGAGCTGCTTGT TTTTC | p60 protein | 454 bp |

Table 2. Oligonucleotide primers used in this study

**[Specificity of the primer pairs and the multiplex PCR]**

To evaluate the specificity of each oligonucleotide primer pair for its target gene, a PCR assay was carried out by testing all the reference strains reported in Table 2.1. The multiplex PCR was developed specifically and efficiently using amplified reactions and the same PCR program. The reaction was performed in a total volume of 25 μl that contained 5 to 15 μl (50 ng) of template.

**[Food sample processing and multiplex PCR assay]**

A sample of ham (CJ, Seoul, South Korea) from the Korea Food & Drug Administration was used for all tests. Equal concentration of the bacteria were used for inoculation of the ham. *E. coli* O157:H7, *Staphylococcus aureus, Listeria monocytogenes, V. parahaemolyticus* and *Salmonella typhimurium* were inoculated either single or as two or three species simultaneously. Media bottles (500 ml) containing 25 g of crushed ham were inoculated with bacteria at 100 CFU of each species alone or with 2 X $10^3$ CFU for inoculation of the three species together. inoculated ham was vigorously mixed by shaking for about 30sec to distribute the bacteria. After inoculation, 225 ml of freshly made LB broth was added to each bottle containing ham. To suspend the bacteria, the bottles were shaken for 10 min at 200 rpm and then incubated at 37°C for 16 hours (Kim *et al.*, 2006). Raw pork was also processed as described method above.

The five bacterial species were inoculated simultaneously in raw pork. Water and milk were directly inoculated with five strains; 1 ml of medium containing each strain was added to 9 ml of water and milk and diluted 10 times from 1:10 to 1:$10^8$.

### 2.1.2 Results and discussion

**[Multiplex PCR assay]**

Five PCR products of different sizes were amplified simultaneously from five food-borne pathogenic bacteria with the multiplex PCR assay used in this study (Fig. 2). For all of the bacteria tested, the optical density (absorbance value) at 600 nm was 0.010 and 0.080. The different sizes of the amplification products allowed rapid and specific discrimination of *Vibrio parahaemolyticus*, *Salmonella* spp., *Staphylococcus aureus*, *E. coli* O157:H7 and *L. monocytogenes*. The annealing temperature, extension time, and primer concentrations used in this multiplex PCR assay were optimized. The PCR products were separated by agarose gel electrophoresis, and the negative controls used with the multiplex PCR produced negative results. Using the multiplex primers, another single amplification was conducted to confirm the chromosomal DNA from samples contaminated with single specific pathogenic bacteria. In the multiplex PCR with mixed DNA samples, five different bands of specific sizes corresponding to the target genes (Table 2) were detected simultaneously after amplification of the contents of a single tube (Fig. 2).

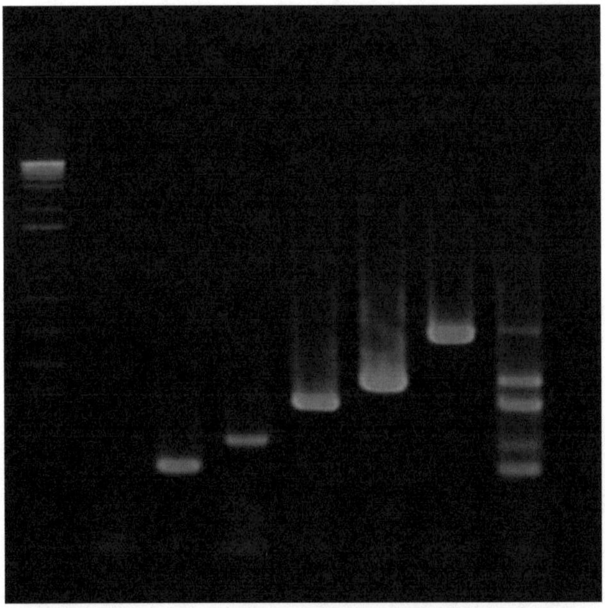


Fig. 5. Agarose gel electrophoresis showing the result of multiplex PCR amplification of five target gene segments from purified DNA of the five microbial pathogens

M, 100 bp size marker; lane 1, negative control (no template); lane 2, *E. coli* O157:H7 NVRQS; lane 3, *Staphylococcus aureus* KCTC1927; lane 4, *Vibrio parahaemolyticus* KCCM41654; lane 5, *Listeria monocytogenes* ATCC15313; lane 6, *Salmonella enteritidis* ATCC10376; lane 7, Multiplex PCR amplification of all five target genes.

**[Specificity and sensitivity for selected primer sets]**

The sensitivity and specificity of the PCR assay were evaluated with 67 food-borne pathogenic bacteria (Table 1). Fig. 3 shows the result of amplification from a representative sample of *Salmonella* spp. The multiplex primer is highly specific for the five pathogenic bacteria target sequence; all *Salmonella* serovars tested produced amplicons of the expected size (678 bp) without spurious priming and without cross-reactivity with non-*Salmonella* species. Results for the other four bacterial species also highly specific (data not shown). Fig. 4 illustrates the detection sensitivities of the multiplex PCR assay, which were evaluated using whole cell cultures of *S. choleraesuis* KCCM41035 and *S. bongori* KCCM41758, cell cultures diluted 10-fold from 1:10 to 1:$10^8$ were tested. Based on these results, the multiplex PCR assay detection limits were approximately $10^5$ CFU / ml. Detection results for the other four bacteria with this assay were similar (data not shown).

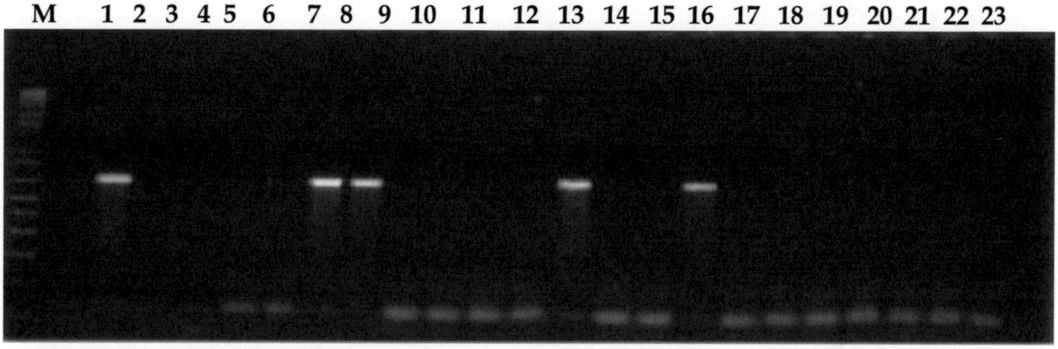


Fig. 6. Specificity for five food pathogenic bacteria using the multiplex primer sets for the detection of *Salmonella* spp.

M,100 bp size marker; lane 1, Negative control(no template); lane 2, *S. bongori* KCCM41757; lane 3, *B. subtilis* KCTC2213; lane 4, B. cereus KCTC1526; lane 5, Listeria monocytogenes ATCC15313; lane 6, *L. innocula* ATCC3091; lane 7, *S. enteritidis* ATCC13076; lane 8, *S. typhimurium* KCTC2421; lane 9, *Shigella boydii* ATCC12034; lane 10, *Shigella flexneri* ATCC12022; lane 11, *Shigella flexneri* KCTC2517; lane 12, *Shigella sonnei* KCTC2009; lane 13, *S. enteritidis* KCCM12021; lane 14, *Shigella sonnei* KCTC2518; lane 15, *Shigella sonnei* KCCM41282; lane 16, *S. choleraesuis* KCCM41035; lane 17, *Shigella sonnei* KCCM41282; lane 18, *Y. enterocolitica* KCCM41657; lane 19, *B. cereus* KCTC1661; lane 20, *B. lichniformis* KCTC3006; lane 21, *B. thuringiensis* KCTC1510; lane 22, *Citrobacter fruendii* KCCM11931; lane 23, *Listeria murray* ATCC25402.

The non-autoclaved ham samples were representative of samples that would be collected from a commercial food processing environment. The detection limit for the five pathogens inoculated individually onto non-autoclaved ham was 2 CFU / ml after enrichment. For non-autoclaved ham incubated with two or three organisms together, the sensitivity was the same as that achieved when the pathogens were evaluated singly (Fig. 5). Without enrichment of the bacterial culture, the detection limits after inoculation of non-autoclaved ham with *E. coli* O157:H7, *S. aureus* and *L. monocytogenes* together were 20,000 cells, respectively (data not shown).

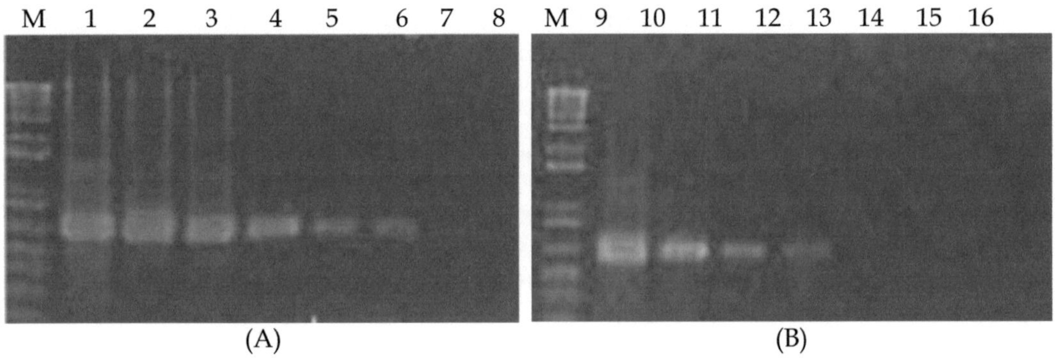


Fig. 7. Sensitivity of the multiplex PCR assay for *Salmonella choleraesuis* KCCM41035 (A) and *Salmonella bongori* KCCM41757 (B)

M, 100 bp size marker; lane 1, 1.2 X $10^8$ CFU / ml; lane 2, 1.2 X $10^7$ CFU / ml; lane 3, 1.2 X $10^6$ CFU / ml; lane 4, 1.2 X $10^5$ CFU / ml; lane 5, 1.2 X $10^4$ CFU / ml; lane 6, 1.2 X $10^3$ CFU / ml; lane 7, 1.2 X $10^2$ CFU / ml; lane 8, 1.2 X 10 CFU / ml; lane 9, 1.2 X $10^8$ CFU / ml; lane 10, 1.2 X $10^7$ CFU / ml; lane 11, 1.2 X $10^6$ CFU / ml; lane 12, 1.2 X $10^5$ CFU / ml; lane 13, 1.2 X $10^4$ CFU / ml; lane 14, 1.2 X $10^3$ CFU / ml; lane 15, 1.2 X $10^2$ CFU / ml; lane 16, 1.2 X 10 CFU / ml

**[Validity of the multiplex PCR assay for food samples]**

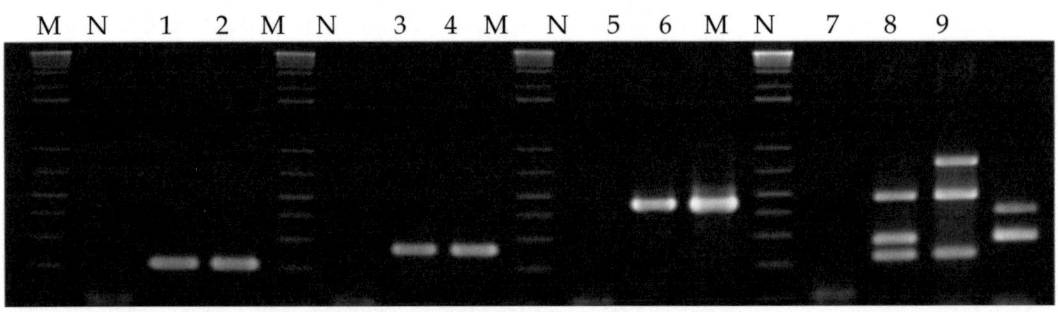


Fig. 8. Amplification products obtained with the multiplex PCR assay

M, 100 bp size marker; N, negative control; lane 1, PCR with *E. coli* O157:H7; lane 2, PCR with *E. coli* O157:H7 DNA (100 pg); lane 3, PCR with *S. aureus*; lane 4, PCR with *S. aureus* DNA (100 pg); lane 5, PCR with *L. monocytogenes*; lane 6, PCR with *L. monocytogenes* DNA (100 pg); lane 7, PCR with 100 pg DNA each from *E. coli* O157:H7, *S. aureus* and *L. monocytogenes*; lane 8, PCR with 100 pg DNA each from *E. coli* O157:H7, *L. monocytogenes* and *Salmonella typhimurium*; lane 9, PCR with 100 pg DNA each from *S. aureus* and *V. parahaemolyticus*

This multiplex PCR assay offers the advantages of significantly short processing time and saving cost. Only one composite DNA sample is required rather than separate samples for each target gene to be analyzed (Kim *et al.*, 2006). To test the efficacy of this PCR assay for detecting pathogenic bacteria in food, *Salmonella typhimurium* ATCC19585 (10 CFU / g of food) was inoculated into samples of selected foods (milk, raw pork and raw chicken) that had been previously screened for detectable pathogenic microbial contamination. The inoculated samples were then incubated aerobically at 37°C for 8 hours (enrichment culture step). The PCR assay detected bacterial cells in all inoculated samples. However, when a 5 hours instead of 8 hours enrichment culture step was used, no bacteria were detected (data not shown).

Thus, our PCR assay requires at least 8 hours of enrichment to detect the added pathogenic bacteria in these foods with a detection sensitivity ranging from 10 to 100 CFU / g. Therefore, the enrichment step is required in this PCR protocol for detection of food-borne pathogenic bacteria. The five specific primer sets tested for *Vibrio parahaemolyticus, Salmonella* spp., *Staphylococcus aureus, E. coli* O157:H7 and *L. monocytogenes* can be used specifically and simultaneously. These five food pathogens were clearly detected from both culture medium artificially inoculated water, milk and raw pork. Thus, the protocol developed in this study could have important application for the rapid and simultaneous detection and identification of up to five food-borne pathogenic bacteria in many foods. This simple method is expected to enable rapid risk assessment of pathogen contamination of foods at a low cost. The cost of detection could be reduced from the $ 50 (approximately $ 10 per pathogen) for the traditional method to less than $ 1 for this multiplex PCR method.

## 3. The development of rapid real-time PCR detection system for *Salmonella* spp.

Previously, we developed multiplex conventional PCR assay from the conventional PCR methods (Kim *et al.*, 2007). Conventional PCR methods for the detection of food-borne bacterial pathogens are time consuming and insensitive that it can not provide adequate screening of samples for the presence of potential pathogens. With the advent of automated real-time PCR suspected food-borne contaminants can be detected in less than an hour. This technique, using TaqMan PCR, has been successfully adapted for the detection of pathogenic bacteria, including *Salmonella enterica, Listeria monocytogenes, Escherichia coli* O157:H7, and *Yersinia pestis* (Bassler *et al*, 1995; Bellin *et al*, 2001; Higgins *et al*, 1998; Hoorfar *et al*, 2000; Jothikumar *et al*, 2002; Knutsson *et al*, 2002; Oberst *et al*, 1998; Sharma *et al*, 1999).

Can there be a better method which has the same sensitivity with nested PCR and can be performed with one PCR reaction? It will be more effective if there is more sensitive optical instrument and staining dye which can detect very small amount of product than naked eyes and EtBr. Micro PCR, which was developed for this purpose, uses real-time PCR machine as a detector and SYBR Green reagent as a staining dye. Real-Time PCR is currently used for the diagnosis of *Escherichia coli* strain O157:H7 (Ibekwe *et a*l, 2002) and *Plesimonas shigelloides* (Loh *et al*, 2001) in stool specimens. To develop micro PCR, following factors were studied. First, selection of specific primers; primer size (17~25 mer), hybridization ability, secondary structure within primer, GC content (40~60%), melting temperature (Tm) (55~65°C). Second, factors affecting Tm; product size, GC contents of product. Third, effect of commercial SYBR Green reagent; Takara, A&B, Qiagen and in house reagent. Forth, product size; 60, 100, 200, 300, 400, 500, 600 and 700bp Fifth, condition of PCR. To enable simultaneous detection, each PCR products were designed to have different melting temperature, at least 2°C apart from each other (Fig. 1).

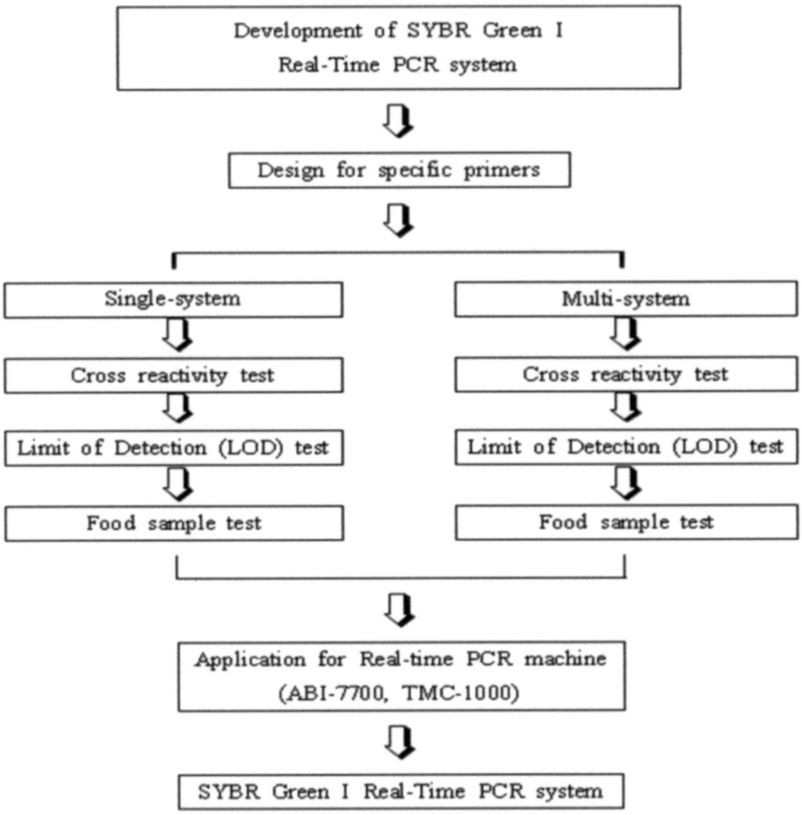


Fig. 9. Strategy for the development of SYBR Green I real-time PCR detection system.

### 3.1 Materials & methods

**[Oligonucleotides ]**

The oligonucleotide primers were designed by Primer version 3.0 software (Whitehead Institute), referring to Genbank in order to amplify a chromosomal DNA of *Salmonella* spp. (Table 1). The oligonucleotides and all reagents for PCR used in this study were synthesized and purchased from Bioneer (Daejeon, Korea) and Kogene Biotech Inc. (Seoul, Korea).

50 ng of template DNA was used in a 20 µl reaction mixture that included 2X SYBR Green I premix Ex Taq (Takara, Japan), 1X ROX Dye (Takara, Japan), 20 pmol of forward and reverse specific primer (Bioneer, Korea). Cycling conditions began with an initial hold at 94°C for 5 min, followed by 35 cycles consisting of 94°C for 30 s, 60°C for 30 s and 72°C for 30 s. and final extension time carry out 72°C for 5 min. Following amplification, melting curves were acquired on the SYBR channel using a ramping rate of 1°C / 30 s for 60 ~ 94°C. The differentiated data were analysed by 7500 software V1.3.0. with the digital filter set as none.

| Strains | Direction (5' → 3') | Primer sequence | Size (bp) |
|---|---|---|---|
| | Forward | GAA TCC TCA GTT TTT CAA CGT TTC | |
| *Salmonella* spp. | Reverse | CCA GAC GAA AGA GCG TGG TAA | 60 |
| | | GAA GCC CGA ACG TGG CGA | 137 |
| | | GTA TGC CCG GTA AAC AGA TGA GT | 284 |
| | | AAA GGA ACC GTA AAG CTG GCT | 330 |
| | | GGG TCA TCC CCA CCG AAA TAC | 424 |

Table 3. Oligonucleotide primers for *Salmonella* spp. used in this study

**[SYBR Green I PCR assay using ABI 7500]**

**[Detection studies with diversity food samples]**

Before inoculating into food, five bacterial strains were incubated in 5 ml LB broth for overnight. 100 μl of each culture broth was inoculated in 25 g of each food material. These food samples were then mixed with 225 ml of LB broth and incubated for overnight. Food segments in sample solution must be removed before assay because PCR can be inhibited by them. Among the 10 samples, water contaminated with *Salmonella* spp. were analyzed without any pre-treatment, other samples were filtered through gauze before assay. 1 ml of each prepared sample solution was transferred to 1.5 ml e-tube and centrifuged at 12,000 rpm for 10 min. The supernatant was removed and the pellet was re-suspended in 500 ml deionized water. Centrifugation and re-suspension in deionized water was performed one more time for exact assay. 150 μl of Deionized water and 50 μl of 10% chelex resin was added to the pellet and mixed throughly. The solution was heated at 100°C for 10 min, and centrifuged at 12,000 rpm for 10 min. 5 μl aliquot of this solution was taken for SYBR Green I assay. PCR using ABI 7500 (Perkin-elmer, USA) was cycled 35 times as follows: 30 sec denaturation at 94°C, 30 seconds annealing at 60°C, and 30 seconds polymerization at 72°C. The products of real-time PCR were run on 2% agarose gel electrophoresis and melting curves were acquired on the SYBR channel using a ramping rate of 1°C / 30 seconds for 60 ~ 94°C.

### 3.2 Results and discussion

**[Primers design and specificity]**

Fig. 2 is the result of PCR reaction performed with various primer sets which are designed for *Salmonella* spp. Specific PCR reaction was observed with primer sets of which product sizes are 60 bp, 284 bp and 678 bp, respectively. However, primer sets of 137 bp, 330 bp and 551 bp showed non-specific products in the place of negative control, meaning that these primers are not available. As for the primers of 424 bp, bacterial DNA was not amplified. Therefore, primer sets of 60 bp, 284 bp, and 678 bp were selected.

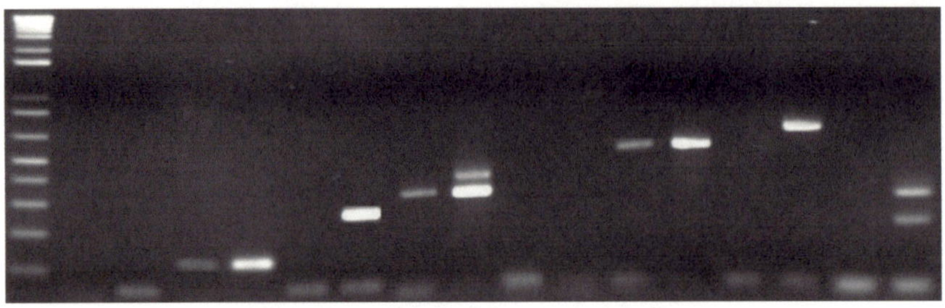


Fig. 10. PCR amplification of *Salmonella* spp. using each primer set

M, 100 bp DNA ladder; lane 1, 2, 60 bp primer; lane 3, 4, 137 bp primer; lane 5, 6, 284 bp primer; lane 7, 8, 330 bp primer; lane 9, 10, 424 bp primer; lane 11, 12, 551 bp primer; lane 13, 14, 678 bp primer; lane 15, 16, 787 bp primer; odd lane number, negative control; even lane number, positive control.

**[Real-time PCR system]**

It will be more effective if there is more sensitive optical instrument and staining dye which can detect very small amount of product than naked eyes and EtBr. Micro PCR, which was developed for this purpose, uses real-time ABI 7500 PCR machine as a detector and SYBR Green I reagent as a staining dye. First, selection of specific primers; primer size (17~25 mer), hybridization ability, secondary structure within primer, GC contents (40~60%), melting temperature (Tm) (55~65°C). Second, factors affecting Tm; product size, GC content of product. Third, effect of commercial SYBR green reagent; Takara, A&B, Qiagen and in house reagent. Fourth, products size; approximately 60, 100, 200, 300, 400, 500, 600 and 700 bp. Fifth, running conditions of real-time PCR. to enable simultaneous detection, each PCR products were designed to have different melting temperature, at least 2°C apart from each other.

As shown in Fig. 3 primer of 60 bp showed two peaks of positive and negative control at the same position. Primer of 284 bp did not showed non-specific products at all but it was also unavailable because the peak of positive control was too weak. The Tm value was 86.8°C. Only the primer of 678 bp was proved to be available. Although a weak undesired peak was appeared beneath 75°C, it is ignorable because its temperature is sufficiently low. The Tm value was measured as 86.7°C. Therefore, the primer of 678 bp is finally selected for SYBR Green I system.

A. 60 bp

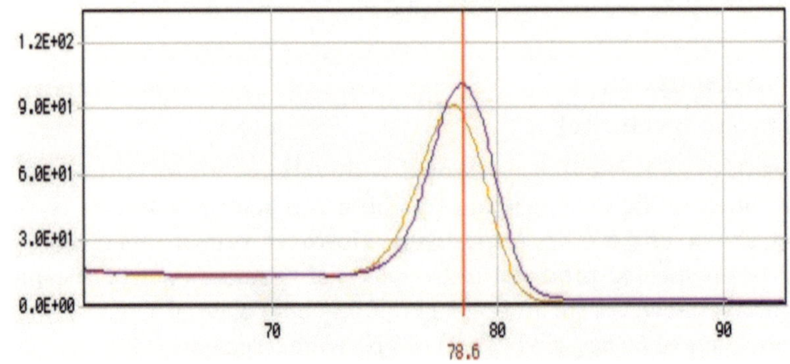

B. 284 bp

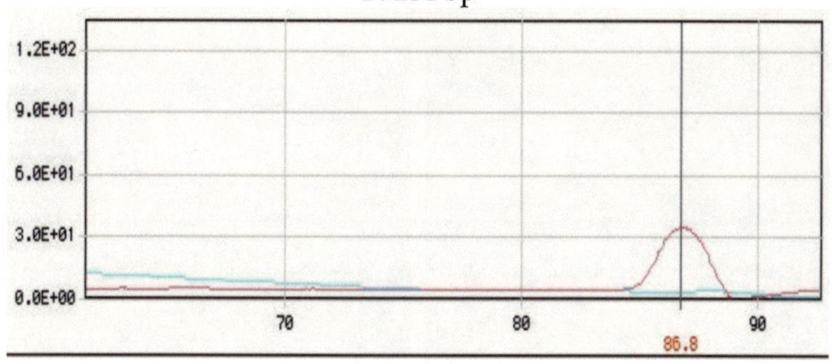


C. 678 bp

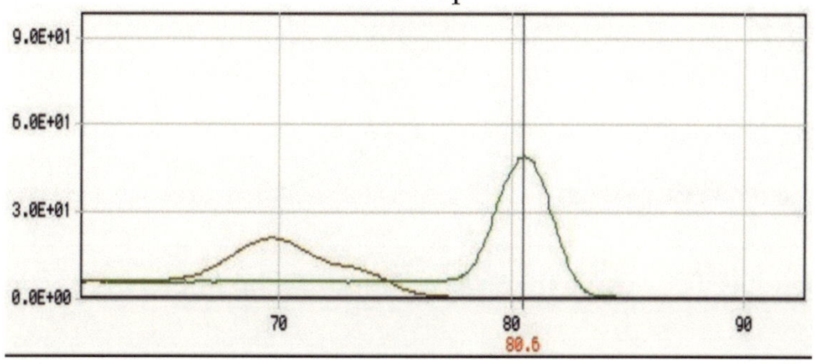


Fig. 11. Melting curve analysis for *Salmonella* spp. A ~ C : melting curve of 60, 284, 678 bp primer sets

**[Application of Real-time SYBR Green I PCR system to food]**

To apply real-time SYBR Green I system to food, various food samples were artificially contaminated by the Salmonella and incubated for enrichment. After overnight enrichment, *Salmonella* spp. gave positive PCR reaction. No signals were observed in negative (un-inoculated) controls. As shown in this result, no other strains but the inoculated *Salmonella enteritidis* was detected (Fig. 4). In conclusion, the SYBR Green I PCR assay combined with DNA extraction using boiling method offers rapid and non-sequence-specific detection of amplicons.

M, 100 bp ladder; N, negative control; lane 1, hamburger patty contaminated with *Escherichia coli* O157:H7; lane 2, ground poultry with *Escherichia coli* O157:H7; lane 3 , soondae (a sausage made of bean curd and green-bean sprouts stuffed in pig intestine) with *Staphylococcus aureus*; lane 4, kimbob (rice rolled in dried laver) with *Staphylococcus aureus*; lane 5, sea water with *Vibrio parahaemolyticus*; lane 6, shrimp with *Vibrio parahaemolyticus*; lane 7, salad with *Listeria monocytogenes*; lane 8, ice-cream with *Listeria monocytogenes*; lane 9, frozen chicken with *Salmonella enteritidis*.; lane 10, salad with *Salmonella enteritidis*.; lane 11, Soybean paste with *B. cereus*; lane 12, korean red pepper paste with *B. cereus*; lane 13, bottled water with *Yersinia enterocolitica*; lane 14, milk with *Yersinia entercolitica*; lane 15, spring water with *Shigella* spp.; lane 16, oyster with *Shigella* spp.; P, Positive control (100 pg)

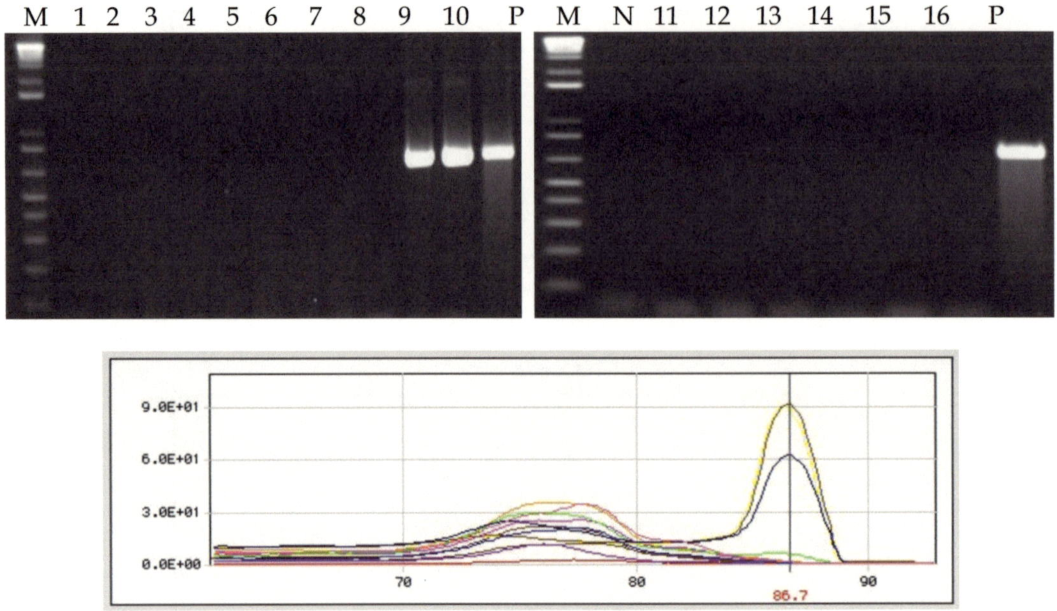


Fig. 12. Detection specificity using the *Salmonella* spp. 674 bp primer in contaminated variety food samples

The minimum detection limit was 10 cells / ml with pure culture, which is far more sensitive than conventional PCR which has detection limit of 10,000 cells / ml. In conclusion, we developed a highly sensitive and specific real-time PCR assay for detection of the five food-borne pathogenic bacteria in food samples. This newly developed assay was successfully used to monitor the dynamics of this novel bacterium in food (Abu *et al*, 2005).

## 4. Rapid and simple detection of *invA* gene in *Salmonella* spp. by isothermal target probe amplification (iTPA)

Nucleic acid amplification methods are widely used for detection of food-borne pathogens and the PCR is the most popular and useful method, requires a high precision thermal cycling instrument, which often prevents PCR from being used in routine food pathogen detection by the food industry. Recently, Jung *et al.* (Jung et al. 2010) developed a new highly sensitive and specific isothermal amplification and detection system called isothermal target and probe amplification (iTPA) by employing DNA-RNA-DNA chimeric primers and a FRET probe. The iTPA reaction is done under isothermal conditions between 55 and 65°C using a simple incubator such as a water bath or block heater which is sufficient for amplification. The detection of the fluorescence signal is acquired directly from the amplification reaction tube without any post-amplification handling that reduces the risk of any amplicon-carryover cross-contamination. The iTPA assay is highly specific for the target sequence because the primers and probe recognize five distinct regions on the targeted DNA. The iTPA method is based on a combination of novel ICA (isothermal chain amplification) and FRET cycling probe technology (CPT). In the ICA method, which relies on the strand displacement activity of DNA polymerase and the RNA degrading activity of

RNase H, two displacement events occur in the presence of four specially designed primers that lead to powerful amplification of target DNA. Since the amplification is initiated only after hybridization of the four primers, the ICA method leads to high specificity for the target sequence. In the CPT method, a DNA-RNA-DNA chimeric probe is hybridized with the target DNA, and the RNA region of the duplex is specifically cleaved by RNase H. The cleaved probe fragments are disassociated from the target DNA and another intact probe is again hybridized and then cleaved. In the cycling events, a single target DNA molecule results in a large number of cleaved probe fragments, which can be designed to generate fluorescent signals (Fig. 1). In the present study, a sensitive and specific iTPA assay for detecting *Salmonella* spp. in experimentally inoculated food samples was developed.

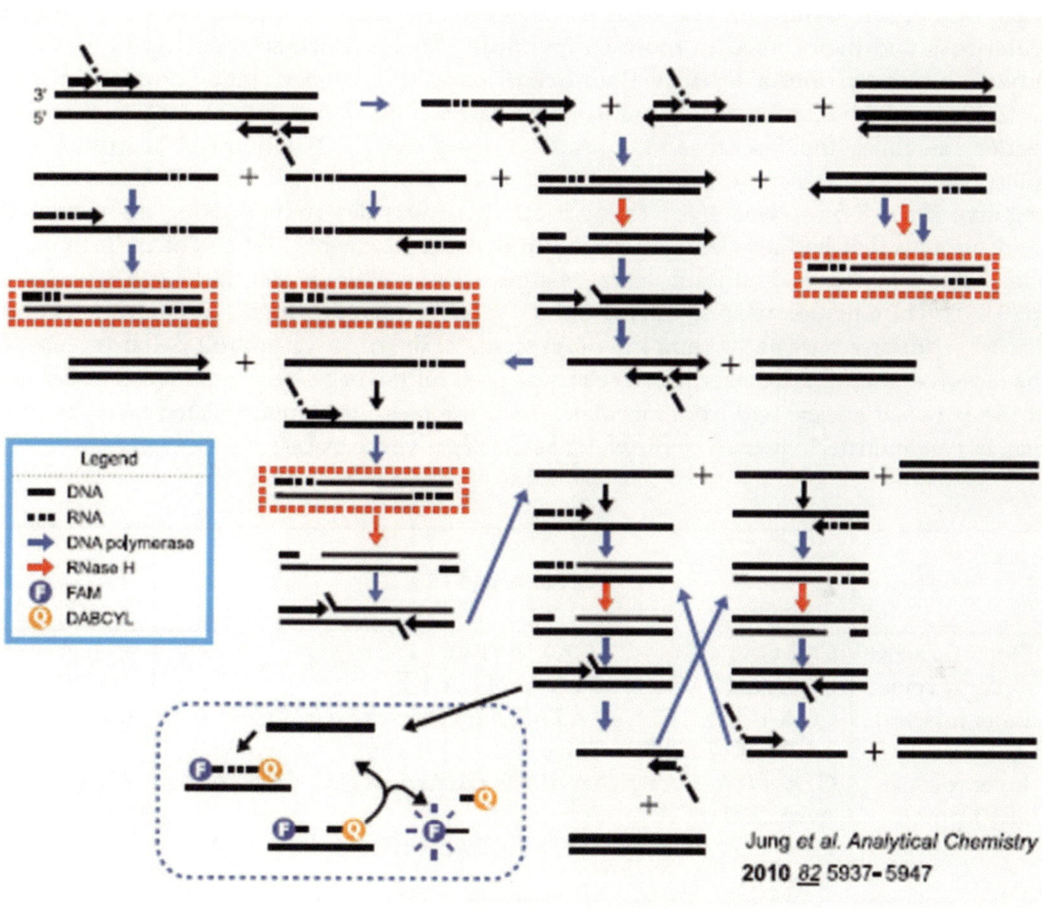


Fig. 13. The process for the Isothermal target & Probe amplification

### 4.1 Materials & methods

**[iTPA primers, FRET probe, and reaction conditions]**

The *Salmonella invA* gene (GenBank: EU348369) was used as the target for iTPA primer and probe design. Four primers, two outer and two inner, and one FRET probe which recognized five distinct regions of the target sequence were designed using the DNASTAR software (Maison, WI). Oligonucleotide sequences and locations of the primers and the probe are shown in Table 1. The DNA primers were synthesized by Genotech (Daejeon, South Korea). The chimeric primers and a FRET probe were synthesized by IDT (San Diego, CA). The iTPA reaction mix in a 20 *µl* volume consisted of the following: 10 mmol / L of Tris-HCl (pH 8.5), 22 mmol / L of $MgSO_4$, 10 mmol / L of KCl, 10 mmol / L of $(NH_4)_2SO_4$, 0.05 mg ml / L of acetylated BSA, 3 mmol / L of DTT, 0.4 mmol / L of deoxynucleotide triphosphate (dNTP), 0.22 mol / L of each outer primers, 2.2 mol / L of each inner primers, 100 nmol / L of the FRET probe, 5 units of *bst* polymerase (NEB, Ipswich, MA), 5 units of RNase H (Epicentre, Madison, WI), 6 units of RNase inhibitor (Solgent, South Korea), and 2 µl l of DNA template (2 µl of sterilized water was used for a negative control). The iTPA reaction mix was incubated at 58°C for 60 min in a water-bath and then cooled to room temperature. After a quick spin-down, the reaction tube was inserted into a RF-1000 fluorescent reader (Raplegene, Inc., Sungnam, South Korea) to read the relative RFU (fluorescence relative unit) signal. The RF-1000 fluorescent reader calculates the F-score and it is display on the LCD window. The result was interpreted as a *Salmonella* spp. positive if the F-score was ≥35 or a *Salmonella* spp. negative if the F-score was < 35. This cut-off value was determined using uninoculated food samples that had also undergone cultural pre-enrichment. F-scores of uninoculated egg yolk samples and chicken meat samples were 20±9.5 and 20±7.2 respectively ($p \leq 0.001$). The equation used to calculate the F-score is the following:

F-score = [(fluorescence of the sample - fluorescence of the negative control) / fluorescence of the negative control] x 100. Sterilized water was used for the negative control reaction instead of the extracted nucleic acid from inoculated food samples. Since uninoculated food samples may be contaminated, we used sterile water as the negative control.

| Name | Sequence (5′-3′) | Position# |
|---|---|---|
| Outer forward | CCT GAT CGC ACT GAA TAT C | 99-117 |
| Outer reverse | CGA AAG AGC GTG GTA ATT AAC | 195-215 |
| Inner forward | CGA TGA CTG ACT ATA CAA GrUrA rCrGC TGG CGA TAT TGG TGT TTA TG | 121-131 |
| Inner reverse | CTA GTA CAT GAA GCT rArArA rGAC CGC AGG AAA CGT TGA A | 174-191 |
| FRET probe | FAM-CGT TCT ACA TTrG rArCrA rGrAA TCC TCA G-DABCYL | 146-170 |

Table 4. iTPA primers and FRET probe used in this study to detect Salmonella spp.

**[iTPA specificity and detection limits]**

Fifty bacterial strains were used to determine the iTPA specificity. DNA templates were prepared from bacterial cultures and aliquots were subjected to the iTPA assay. For *Salmonella* strains, the genomic DNA was isolated from the overnight culture grown in LB medium and then quantified. One picogram of genomic DNA was used as the template. For non-*Salmonella* strains, the genomic DNA was isolated from the overnight culture grown in LB medium and then 2 L of the DNA extraction TE buffer solution was used. Specificity tests were repeated 10 times. To determine iTPA detection limits, serial 10-fold dilutions of a mid-log phase *S. typhimurium* KCTC2515 culture (*ca.* $10^8$ CFU) grown in LB broth were prepared in PBS and quantified using the standard plating method. The detection limit tests were repeated 10 times and the lower limits of detection (CFU per assay) were reported.

**[iTPA testing in experimentally inoculated food samples]**

Three kinds of foods were used for the study: peanut butters, egg yolk and chicken breasts. Food samples were processed as described in a previous study (Kim *et al.* 2007) with slight modifications. Briefly, A 500 ml Erlenmeyer flask (LB broth 225 ml) containing 25 g of chicken breast was incubated at 37°C overnight and then 9 ml of this solution was transferred into a 10 ml conical tube followed by adding 1 ml of inoculated buffered peptone water of *Salmonella* spp.(1.0 x $10^9$ CFU / ml) to prepare a stock solution. Plastic food bags containing 25 g of chicken breast were inoculated with 1 ml of serial dilutions (1:10 to 1:$10^8$) of the stock solution and vigorously mixed using a homogenizer (Pro-media SH-001, ELMEX Ltd., Tokyo, Japan) for about 30 sec to distribute the bacteria followed by adding 225 ml of freshly made LB broth to prepare pre-enriched solutions. The sample preparations for peanut butters and other food samples were the same except that for peanut butters which required an additional washing with a washing solution (0.05% NaOH, 0.5% Tween 20 in PBS buffer solution) due to the high viscosity. 100 L of the pre-enriched solution was mixed with the washing solution and centrifuged at 10,770 x g for 5 min followed by discarding the supernatant. The pellet was washed with 100% ethanol and then with TE buffer solution twice. The washed pellet was suspended in 200 L of TE buffer solution and heated at 100°C for 10 min in a dry heating block. The crude cell lysate was centrifuged at 10,770 x g for 5 min and an aliquot (2 L) of the supernatant was used for the iTPA assay. For negative samples, the same amount of aliquot (2 L) of uninoculated food samples that had also undergone cultural pre-enrichment was used. The inoculated food sample tests were repeated 10 times and the lower limits of detection (CFU per assay) were reported.

### 4.2 Results and discussion

**[Inclusivity and exclusivity of the iTPA assay]**

The *Salmonella* spp. *invA*-based iTPA assay, which required only a water bath and the RF-1000 fluorescent reader successfully detected 10 *Salmonella* spp. strains while showing negative results for 40 non-*Salmonella* spp. strains (Table 1), indicating that the *invA*-based iTPA assay was specific for *Salmonella* spp.. The PCR assay using iTPA outer primers yielded amplicons of the expected size (117 bp) for all 10 Salmonella spp. strains. (data not shown) Two sample t-tests were performed for negatives and positives in pure culture. The mean F-score of the negatives was 3.97±0.44 and the mean F-score of the positives was 82.9±6.1 ($p \leq 0.001$, data not shown). For a rigorous exclusivity comparison, the positive strains were used at a low concentration of the genomic DNA (1pg, ca. $10^2$ CFU) as the template while the negative strains were used at very high concentration of the genomic DNA (ca. $10^5$ CFU). Neither false positive nor false negative results for the 50 bacterial strains were observed by the iTPA assay using two primer sets and a FRET probe, indicating good specificity. (Table 1)

**[Detection limits of the iTPA assay]**

The detection limits of the iTPA assay using serial in *S.* Typhimurium strain were determined. KCTC2515 were determined and the lowest number of cells detected was 4 x $10^1$ CFU per iTPA reaction (Table 2).

| | Dilution | No. of Bacteria (CFU) | iTPA reaction (F-score#) |
|---|---|---|---|
| *S. Typhimurium* KCTC2515 | $10^{-4}$ | 4 x $10^4$ | 142±9 |
| | $10^{-5}$ | 4 x $10^3$ | 96±30 |
| | $10^{-6}$ | 4 x $10^2$ | 82±35 |
| | $10^{-7}$ | 4 x $10^1$ | 69±18 |
| | $10^{-8}$ | 4 | 0 |

# F-score = [(fluorescence of the sample - fluorescence of the negative control) / fluorescence of the negative control] x 100

Table 5. Sensitivity of the iTPA assays

**[Detection of *Salmonella* spp. cells in inoculated food samples]**

The detection limits of *Salmonella* spp. inoculated in three food samples are shown in Table 3. In inoculation experiments, the *invA*-based iTPA assay using the serial dilution platforms consistently detected at an initial inoculums level of less than 10 CFU in the pre-enriched food samples (egg yolk, chicken breast, and peanut butter). In Table 4 the results of the F-score measurement for the iTPA reaction for 60 min at 58°C in the artificially contaminated samples are shown. For statistics, one-way analysis of variance (ANOVA) test was performed (Clarke and Cooke 1998). The mean F-scores for uninoculated peanut butter, egg yolk and chicken breast were 14±4.7, 20±10, and 20±7.2, respectively. The mean F-scores for inoculated peanut butter, egg yolk and chicken breast were 87.34±30.24, 59.09±36.16 and 68.24±26.33($p \leq 0.001$), respectively. The lowest detection limit achieved in this study was a less than 10 CFU per 25 g of food samples.

In this study, we designed a set of DNA-RNA-DNA chimeric primers and a FRET probe to specifically target the *Salmonella* spp. *invA* gene. So, a novel and rapid DNA detection system has been developed which we have termed isothermal target and probe amplification (iTPA). By simultaneously utilizing the dual amplification powers of the target DNA and FRET probe, we have demonstrated that iTPA can be used to rapidly detect less than 10 CFU of *Salmonella* spp. in food samples after pre-enrichment. The four chimeric primers and one FRET probe were designed from five regions of the *Salmonella* spp. *invA* gene coding sequence that are highly specific for *Salmonella* spp. (Table 1). In conclusion, we have developed a DNA detection system which is conveniently performed by requiring only a water bath and a fluorometer and has great potential in applications for hand-held or point-of-care-testing (POCT) diagnostics. The *invA*-based iTPA assay developed in this study is a specific, sensitive, and rapid method for the detection of *Salmonella* spp. in food samples. This simple method is expected to enable a rapid risk assessment of pathogen contamination of foods at a low cost. (Kim *et al.* 2011)

| Food samples | Dilution | No. of Bacteria#(CFU) | F-score |
|---|---|---|---|
| Peanut butter | $10^{-5}$ | $1.7 \pm 0.4 \times 10^{3}$ | 87±5.7 |
| | $10^{-6}$ | $1.7 \pm 0.4 \times 10^{2}$ | 86±6.6 |
| | $10^{-7}$ | $1.7 \pm 0.4 \times 10^{1}$ | 82±12 |
| | $10^{-8}$ | $1.7 \pm 0.4 \times 10^{0}$ | 82±13 |
| | $10^{-9}$ | $1.7 \pm 0.4 \times 10^{-1}$ | 39±40 |
| | | un-inoculated | 14±4.7 |
| Egg yolk | $10^{-5}$ | $1.7 \pm 0.4 \times 10^{3}$ | 72±4.0 |
| | $10^{-6}$ | $1.7 \pm 0.4 \times 10^{2}$ | 73±4.0 |
| | $10^{-7}$ | $1.7 \pm 0.4 \times 10^{1}$ | 69±7.3 |
| | $10^{-8}$ | $1.7 \pm 0.4 \times 10^{0}$ | 44±3.4 |
| | $10^{-9}$ | $1.7 \pm 0.4 \times 10^{-1}$ | 11±26 |
| | | un-inoculated | 20±10 |
| Chicken meat | $10^{-5}$ | $1.7 \pm 0.4 \times 10^{3}$ | 72±3.6 |
| | $10^{-6}$ | $1.7 \pm 0.4 \times 10^{2}$ | 72±2.3 |
| | $10^{-7}$ | $1.7 \pm 0.4 \times 10^{1}$ | 71±4.8 |
| | $10^{-8}$ | $1.7 \pm 0.4 \times 10^{0}$ | 56±19 |
| | $10^{-9}$ | $1.7 \pm 0.4 \times 10^{-1}$ | 34±29 |
| | | un-inoculated | 20±7.2 |

# Seven *Salmonella* spp. strains were tested: *S. typhimurium* (KCTC 2515, KCTC 2412, ATCC 14028), *S. choleraesuis* (KCTC 2929, KCCM 41575), *S. enetritidis* (KCCM 12021), *S. bongori* (KCCM 41758)

Table 6. Detection limits for inoculated food samples by iTPA assay

## 5. References


Abu, S. M, Piyaunch, B., Teruo, S., Apinya, A., Masaru, W., and Atsushi Y. (2005) Development and assessment of a real-time PCR assay for rapid and sensitive detection of a novel termotolerant bacterium, Lactobacillus thermotolerans, in chicken feces. Amer. micro 71: 4214-4219.

Bassler, H. A., S. J. Flood, K. J. Livak, J. Marmaro, R. Knorr, and C. A. Batt. (1995) Use of a fluorogenic probe in a PCR-based assay for the detection of Listeria monocytogenes. Appl. Environ. Microbiol 61, 3724-3728.

Bellin, T., M. Pulz, A. Matussek, H. G. Hempen, and F. Gunzer. (2001) Rapid detection of enetrohemorrhagic Escherichia coli by real-time PCR with fluorescent hybridization probes. J. Clin. Microbiol 39, 370-374.

Bubert, A., I. Hein, M. Rauch, A. Lehner, B. S. Yoon, W. Goebel, and M. Wagner (1999) Detection and Differentiation of Listeria spp. by a Single Reaction based on Multiplex PCR. Appl. Envir. Microbiol 65: 4688-4692.

Bubert, A., S. Kohler, and W. Goebel (1992) The homologous and heterologous regions within the iap gene allow genus- and species-specific identification of Listeria spp. by polymerase chain reaction. Appl. Envir. Microbiol 58: 2625-2632.

Cabrera-García, M. E., C. Vázquez-Salinas, and E. I. Quiones-Ramrez (2004) Serologic and Molecular Characterization of Vibrio parahaemolyticus Strains Isolated from Seawater and Fish Products of the Gulf of Mexico. Appl. Envir. Microbiol 70: 6401-6406.

Centers for Disease Control and prevention (2010) Investigation update: multistate outbreak of human Salmonella enteritidis infections associated with shell eggs. Available at: http://www.cdc.gov/salmonella/enteritidis/index.html (accessed 2 December 2010)

Centers for Science in the public Interest (2009) Outbreak alert 2007. Available at: http://www.cspinet.org/foodsafety/outbreak_alert.pdf (accessed 3 February 2009)

Chiu, C. H., and J. T. Ou (1996) Rapid identification of Salmonella serovars in feces by specific detection of virulence genes, invA and spvC, by an enrichment broth culture-multiplex PCR combination assay. J. Clin. Microbiol 34: 2619-2622.

Heid, C. A., J. Steven, K. J. Livak, and P.M. Williams (1996) Real time PCR. Genome Res. 6: 986-994

Higgins, J. A., J. Ezzell, B. J. Hinnebusch, M. Shipley, E. A. Henchal, and M. S. Ibrahim. (1998) 5' nuclease PCR assay to detect Yersinia pestis. J. Clin. Microbiol 36, 2284-2288.

Higuchi, R., C. Fockler, G. Dollinger, and R. Watson (1993) Kinetic PCR analysis: Real-time PCR monitoring of DNA amplification reactions. Biotechnol 11: 1026-1030

Holland, M. T., R. D. Abramson, R. Watson, and D. H. Gelfand (1991) Detection of specific polymerase chain reaction product by utilizing the 5′-3′ exonuclease activity of Thermus aquaticus DNA polymerase. Proc. Natl. Acad. Sci. USA 88: 7276-7280

Hoofar, J., P. Ahrens, and P. Radstrom. (2000) Automated 5' nuclease PCR assay for identification of Salmonella enterica. J. clin. Microbiol 38, 3429-3435.

Ibekwe, A. M., P. M. Watt, C. M. Grieve, V. K. Sharma, and S. R. Lyons. (2002) Multiplex fluorogenic real-time PCR for detection and quantification of Escherichia coli O157:H7 in dairy wastewater wetlands. Appl. Environ. Microbiol 68, 4853-4862.

Jinneman, K. C., K. J. Yoshitomi, and S. D. Weagant (2003) Multiplex Real-Time PCR Method To Identify Shiga Toxin Genes stx1 and stx2 and Escherichia coli O157:H7/H-Serotype. Appl. Envir. Microbiol 69: 6327-633.

John Maurer (2006) PCR methods in foods. Springer Inc. Food microbiology and food safety series

Jothikumar, N., and M. W. Griffiths. (2002) Rapid detection of Escherichia coli O157;H7 with multiplex real-time PCR assays. Appl. Environ. Microbiol 68, 3169-3171.

Jung, C. H., Chung, J. W., Kim, U. O., Kim, M. H. and Park, H. G. (2010) An Isothermal target and probe amplification (iTPA) method, based on a combination of an isothermal chain amplification (ICA) technique and a FRET cycling probe technology (CPT). Anal Chem 82, 5937-5943

Kaneko, K., N. Kiyokawa, Y. Ohtomo, R. Nagaoka, Y. Yamashiro, T. Taguchi, T. Mori, J. Fujimoto, and T. Takeda (2001) Apoptosis of renal tubular cells in Shiga-toxin-mediated hemolytic uremic syndrome. Nephron 32: 182-185.

Karpman, D., A. Hakansson, M.T.R. Perez, C. Isaksson, E. Carlemalm, A. Caprioli, and C. Svanborg (1998) Apoptosis of renal cortical cells in the hemolytic-uremic syndrome: In vivo and in vitro studies. Infect. Immun 66: 636-644.

Kim J.S., Jahng M.S., Lee G.G., Lee K.J., Chae H.K., Lee J.H., and Lim M.H (2011) Rapid and simple detection of the invA gene in Salmonella spp. By isothermal target and probe amplification (iTPA). Letters in Applied Microbiology Vol 52. No 4.: 399-405

Kim, J. S., Lee, G. G., Park, J. S., Jung, Y. H., Kwak, H. S., Kim, S. B., Nam, Y. S., and Kwon, S. T. (2007) A novel multiplex PCR assay for rapid and simultaneous detection of five pathogenic bacteria: Escherichia coli O157:H7, Salmonella, Staphylococcus aureus, Listeria monocytogenes, and Vibrio parahaemolyticus. J Food Prot 70, 1656-1662

Kim, J., T. Demeke, R. M. Clear, and S. K. Patrick (2006) Simultaneous detection by PCR of Escherichia coli, Listeria monocytogenes and Salmonella typhimurium in artificially inoculated wheat grain. J. Food Micro Articleinpress.

Kim, J.S., Jahng, M.S., Lee, G.G., Lee, K.J., Chae, H.K., Lee, J.H., Lee, J.H., and Kim, M.H. (2011) Rapid and simple detection of the invA gene in Salmonella spp. by isothermal target and probe amplification (iTPA). Letters in Applied Microbiology 52, 399-405

Kim, J.S., Lee. G.G., Park, J.S., Jung, Y.H., Kwak, H.S., Kim, S.B., Nam, Y.S. and Kwon, S.-T. (2007) A novel multiplex PCR assay for rapid and simultaneous detection of five pathogenic bacteria: Escherichia coli O157:H7, Salmonella, Staphylococcus aureus, Listeria monocytogenes, and Vibrio parahaemolyticus. J. Food Prot 70, 1656-1662.

Knutsson, R., C. Lofstrom, H. Grage, J. Hoorfar, and P. Radstrom. (2002) Modeling of 5' nuclease real-time responses for optimization of a high -throughput enrichment PCR procedure for Salmonella enetricolitica. J. clin. Microbiol 40, 52-60.

Loh, J. P., and E. P. H. Yap. (2001) Rapid and specific detection of Plesiomonas shigelloides directly from stool by LightCycler PCR, p.161-169. In U. Reischl, C. Wittwer, and E. R. Cockerill (ed.), Rapid cycle real-time PCR, methods and applications, microbiology and food analysis. Springer-Verlag, Berlin, Germany.

Mullah, B., K. Livak, A. Andrus, and P. Kenney (1998) Efficient synthesis of double dye-labeled oligodeoxyribonucleotide probes and their application in a real tome PCR assay. Nucleic Acids Res. 26: 1026-1031

Narayanan, J., Xiaowen, W., and Masel W. G. (2003) Real-Time Multiplex SYBR Green I-Based PCR Assay for Simultaneous Detection of Salmonella Serovars and Listeria monocytogenes. J. Food Prot 66, 2141-2145.

Oberst, R. D., M. P. Hays, L. K. Bohra, et al. (1998) PCR-based DNA amplification and presumptive detection of Escherichia coli O157;H7 with an internal fluorogenic probe and the 5' nuclease (TaqMan) assay. Appl. Environ. Microbiol 64, 3389-3396.

Panicker, G., D. R. Call, M. J. Krug, and A. K. Bej (2004) Detection of pathogenic Vibrio spp. In shellfish by using multiplex PCR and DNA microarrays. Appl. Environ. Microbiol 70: 7436-7444

Schmidt, H., C. Knop, S. Franke, S. Aleksic, J. Heesemann, and H .Karch (1995) Development of PCR for screening of enteroaggregative Escherichia coli. J. Clin. Microbiol 33: 701-705.

Sharma, V. K., E. A. Dean-Nystrom, and T. A. Casey. (1999) Semi-automated fluorogenic PCR assays (TaqMan) for rapid detection of E. coli O157:H7 and other shiga toxigenic E. coli. Mol. Cell. Probes 13, 291-302.

Volokhov, D., A. Rasooly, K. Chumakov, and V. Chizhikov (2002) Identification of Listeria Species by Microarray - Based Assay. J. Clin. Microbiol 40: 4720-4728.

Wang, G., C. G. Clark, and F. G. Rodgers (2002) Detection in Escherichia coli of the Genes Encoding the Major Virulence Factors, the Genes Defining the O157:H7 Serotype, and Components of the Type 2 Shiga Toxin Family by Multiplex PCR. J. Clin. Microbiol 40: 3613-3619.